Clinical Anesthesia Procedures of the Massachusetts General Hospital

Clinical Anesthesia Procedures of the Massachusetts General Hospital

Fourth Edition

Department of Anesthesia
Massachusetts General Hospital
Harvard Medical School

Edited by
J. Kenneth Davison, M.D.
William F. Eckhardt III, M.D.
Deniz A. Perese, M.D.

Little, Brown and Company
Boston/Toronto/London

Fifth Printing

Previous editions copyright © 1978, 1982 by Little, Brown and Company
(Inc.); 1988 by Department of Anesthesia, Massachusetts General
Hospital

Library of Congress Cataloging-in-Publication Data

Clinical anesthesia procedures of the Massachusetts General Hospital /
    Department of Anesthesia, Massachusetts General Hospital [and]
    Harvard Medical School. — 4th ed. / edited by J. Kenneth Davison,
    William F. Eckhardt III, Deniz A. Perese.
        p.   cm.
    Includes bibliographical references and index.
    ISBN 0-316-17714-8 (pbk.)
    1. Anesthesiology—Handbooks, manuals, etc.   I. Davison, J.
    Kenneth.   II. Eckhardt, William F.   III. Perese, Deniz A.
    IV. Massachusetts General Hospital.   Dept. of Anesthesia.
    V. Harvard Medical School.
    [DNLM: 1. Anesthesiology.   WO 200 C6413 1993]
    RD82.2.C54   1993
    617.9′6—dc20
    DNLM/DLC
    for Library of Congress   92-48517
                                                                    CIP

Printed in the United States of America

MART

Sponsoring Editor: Elizabeth A. Thompson
Development Editor: Laurie Anello
Production Editor: Karen Feeney
Copyeditor: Debra Corman
Indexer: Julia Figures
Production Supervisor: Louis C. Bruno, Jr.
Cover Designer: Louis C. Bruno, Jr.

To
RICHARD J. KITZ, M.D.

**Henry Isaiah Dorr Professor and Chairman,
Department of Anesthesia,
Massachusetts General Hospital**

The fourth edition coincides with Dr. Kitz's final years as Chairman, and we dedicate this book to his primary goal of attracting and educating outstanding residents and fellows from around the world. His enthusiastic support in initiating and updating this book is appreciated by all who have contributed to it.

Contents

Preface

The fourth edition of *Clinical Anesthesia Procedures of the Massachusetts General Hospital* was undertaken by the residents and clinical fellows of the Department of Anesthesia to reflect the most current practices at Massachusetts General Hospital, Massachusetts Eye and Ear Infirmary, Shriners Burns Institute, Brigham and Women's Hospital, The Children's Hospital, New England Deaconess Hospital, The Cambridge Hospital, Beth Israel Hospital, and Mount Auburn Hospital. The emphasis is still on the clinical fundamentals involved in the safe administration of anesthesia.

This handbook is designed to complement readings in textbooks and journals and thus assumes some prior knowledge of anesthesia or critical care. It is designed to be an accessible and accurate source of information for the practicing anesthesiologist, anesthesia resident, nurse anesthetist, medical student, medical or surgical resident, nurse, and respiratory therapist involved in ICU or perioperative care. Each chapter contains a complete Suggested Reading list for those who desire more in-depth information.

As with previous editions, this book has been expanded to maintain state-of-the-art coverage of an increasingly complex field. Although five new chapters have been added and every chapter has been revised and updated, the basic format is similar to that of the third edition. The section dealing with preanesthetic evaluation has been expanded to include discussion of anesthesia for the patient with an AICD or pacemaker, the cardiac transplant patient, the patient status post repair of a congenital heart defect, and anesthetic implications of carcinoid syndrome, as well as current reviews of hepatitis, acquired immunodeficiency syndrome, and tuberculosis. The editors gratefully acknowledge the contributions of Drs. Leslie Shaff, John Allyn, Kenneth Haspel, Michael Bailin, and Charles Jeffrey. The section on administration of anesthesia has been extensively edited and five new chapters have been added: Airway Evaluation and Management; Monitoring; Intravenous and Inhalation Anesthetics; Spinal, Epidural, and Caudal Anesthesia; and Regional Anesthesia. This emphasis reflects the many changes and improvements in anesthetic care. New topics include use of the laryngeal mask airway; fiberoptic laryngoscopy; management of the difficult airway; monitoring techniques such as pulmonary artery catheters, ICP bolts, and transesophageal echocardiography; new IV and inhalation anesthetic agents; new muscle relaxants; expanded coverage of intraanesthetic problems; anesthesia for lung transplantation; and a comprehensive review of regional anesthesia of the brachial plexus and nerves of the upper extremity, as well as lumbosacral plexus and nerves of the leg. The following faculty members provided valuable critical discussion: Drs. Jeffrey Cooper, Mark Dershwitz, Robert Peterfreund, Mavis Shure, Dolly Hansen, Martin Acquadro, Susan Vassallo, John M. R. Bruner, Salvatore Basta, Andrew Jeon, William Latta, Neelakanthan Sunder, Paul Alfille, Charles Vacanti, William Kimball, Lee Kearse, Laurie Shapiro, Michael Long, and Sanjay Datta.

ix

The final section, Patient Care in Other Settings, contains completely revised chapters on pain and adult, pediatric, and newborn resuscitation. The appendix has been updated and reformatted to provide accurate and useful information regarding the vast spectrum of medications used in the perioperative and intensive care setting, including new coverage of common antibiotics. These chapters owe much to the contributions of Drs. Daniel Carr, Carl Rosow, Jesse D. Roberts, Michael D'Ambra, James T. Roberts, Alberto DeArmendi, William Hurford, Frederic deBros, Marlene Meyer, Nick Goudsouzian, and William Denman.

We have continually strived to make this book accurate and clinically useful for the practitioner. Our illustrations and tables have been chosen with this in mind. Again, we have chosen to reproduce an algorithm for the treatment of malignant hyperthermia on the inside front cover.

Finally, we thank Ms. Donna Cutillo for providing us with a quiet sanctuary; and Ms. Susan Pioli and her colleagues at Little, Brown and Company for their guidance and encouragement.

J.K.D.
W.F.E.
D.A.P.

Clinical Anesthesia Procedures of the Massachusetts General Hospital

Notice
The indications and dosages of all drugs in this book have been recommended in the medical literature and conform to the practices of the general medical community. The medications described do not necessarily have specific approval by the Food and Drug Administration for use in the diseases and dosages for which they are recommended. The package insert for each drug should be consulted for use and dosage as approved by the FDA. Because standards for usage change, it is advisable to keep abreast of revised recommendations, particularly those concerning new drugs.

Evaluating the Patient Before Anesthesia

General Preanesthetic Evaluation

Thomas J. Long

I. **Overview.** The preanesthetic evaluation has specific objectives, which include becoming familiar with the present surgical illness and coexisting medical conditions, establishing a doctor-patient relationship, developing a management strategy for perioperative anesthetic care, and obtaining informed consent for the anesthetic plan. The consultation is detailed in the patient's record and concludes with the anesthetic options and their attendant risks and benefits. The **overall goal** of the preoperative visit is to reduce perioperative morbidity and mortality.

II. **History.** Knowledge of the patient's general state of well-being is extremely helpful. Patients' daily activity level, ability to care for themselves, eating habits, weight loss, and understanding of their medical condition all provide an insight into how well they may cope during the perioperative period. Relevant information regarding the present surgical illness and coexisting medical conditions is obtained by a chart review followed by the patient interview. A knowledge of the patient's history when beginning the interview is reassuring to the anxious patient. When old records or recent surgical/medical admission notes are not available, the history obtained from the patient may be supplemented by direct discussion with the medical and surgical staff.

A. The **present surgical illness** should note initial symptoms, diagnostic studies performed, presumptive diagnosis, treatment, and responses. For inpatients, the vital sign trends and fluid balance should be ascertained.

B. **Coexisting medical illnesses** may complicate the surgical and anesthetic course. They should be evaluated in a systematic "organ systems" approach with an emphasis on recent changes in symptoms and treatment. Specific preanesthetic considerations with coexisting cardiac, pulmonary, renal, hepatic, endocrine, or infectious diseases are found in Chaps. 2–7. In certain circumstances, specialty consultation may be advisable preoperatively. Such consults are most valuable when answering specific questions regarding the interpretation of unusual laboratory tests, unfamiliar drug therapies, or changes from the patient's baseline status. These consultants are not asked for a general "clearance" for anesthesia, as this is the specific responsibility of the anesthesiologist.

C. **Medications** may be used to treat present or coexisting illnesses; the doses and schedules must be ascertained. Of special importance are antihypertensive, antianginal, antiarrhythmic, anticoagulant, anticonvulsant, and specific endocrine medication. The decision to continue these medications during the preanesthetic period depends on the severity of the underlying illness, the potential consequences of discontinuing treatment, the medication's half-life, and the likelihood of deleterious interactions with proposed anesthetic agents. However, as a general rule, medications can be continued up to the time of surgery. Specific medications used to treat diabetes mellitus, hypertension, angina pectoris, and other common diseases are discussed in Chaps. 2–7.

D. **Allergies and drug reactions.** Unusual, unexpected, or unpleasant reactions to perianesthetic medications are not uncommon. Unfortunately the task of determining the exact nature of the "reaction" may be difficult. **True allergic reactions** are much less common than nonallergic responses such as adverse reactions, side effects, and drug-drug interactions. However patients frequently label all of these as "allergic" phenomena.

1. **True allergic reactions.** Any agent that (by direct observation, chart documentation, or description by the patient) when administered leads to skin manifestations (pruritus with hives or flushing), facial or oral swelling, shortness of breath, choking, wheezing, or vascular collapse should be considered to have elicited a true allergic reaction until proved otherwise.

   a. **Antibiotics** are the most common precipitants, especially sulfa, penicillin, and cephalosporin derivatives.

   b. **Allergy to the induction agents** thiopental sodium and propofol is uncommon. With thiopental, patients may remember postoperative nausea, vomiting, and "grogginess" and consider this an allergy. Propofol contains soybean oil and egg yolk components, so allergy to these foods may preclude its safe use.

   c. **Known allergy to shellfish and seafood** is important to document, since allergic cross reactions with intravenous (IV) contrast dye and the heparin-reversing agent protamine may occur when the agents are administered intraoperatively.

   d. A history of "allergy" to **halothane or succinylcholine** (in either the patient or any close relative) warrants special attention, since this may actually represent the occurrence of malignant hyperthermia.

   e. True allergy to the **amide-type local anesthetics** is exceedingly rare, although a syncopal episode in the dentist's chair or prior to starting an IV with injection of local anesthetic may be falsely labeled as allergic. However, **ester-type local anesthetics** can produce anaphylaxis (see Chap. 15).

2. **Adverse reactions and side effects.** Many of the medications the anesthesiologist uses in a conscious patient produce memorable, unpleasant effects (e.g., nausea, vomiting, and pruritus after narcotic administration). Inquiring as to what patients usually take for headache and pain and how they respond to such medications may provide insight regarding abnormal drug sensitivities and altered requirements.

3. **Certain rare but important drug interactions** must be anticipated because of their life-threatening nature. For example, thiopental may precipitate a

fatal episode of acute intermittent porphyria, and meperidine may produce a hypertensive crisis when administered to patients treated with monoamine oxidase inhibitors.

E. Anesthetic history
1. **Old anesthesia records** should be reviewed for the following information:
   a. Response to sedative/analgesic premedications and anesthetic agents.
   b. Ease of mask ventilation, direct laryngoscopy, and the size/type of laryngoscope blade and endotracheal tube used.
   c. Difficulty with and types of vascular access and invasive monitoring.
   d. Perianesthetic complications such as adverse drug reactions, cardiorespiratory instability, postoperative myocardial infarction or congestive heart failure, unexpected admission to an intensive care unit, and prolonged wake-up or intubation.
2. Patients should be asked about **prior anesthetics,** including
   a. Common complaints such as postoperative nausea and hoarseness.
   b. Warnings from previous anesthetists describing prior anesthetic problems.

F. Family history. A history of adverse anesthesia outcomes in family members should be evaluated. This history is perhaps best obtained with open-ended questions, such as "Has anyone in your family experienced unusual or serious reactions to anesthesia?" Patients should be specifically asked about a family history of malignant hyperthermia.

G. Social history
1. **Smoking.** A history of exercise intolerance or the presence of a productive cough or hemoptysis may indicate a need for further pulmonary evaluation or treatment. Eliminating cigarette use for 2–4 weeks prior to elective surgery may reduce airway hyperreactivity and perioperative pulmonary complications.
2. **Drugs and alcohol.** Although self-reporting of the use of drugs and alcohol typically **underestimates actual use,** it is still helpful to define the types of drugs used, routes of administration, frequency of use, and most recent use. Stimulant abuse may lead to palpitations, true angina, weight loss, and lowered thresholds for the precipitation of serious arrhythmias and convulsions. Acute alcohol intoxication will lower anesthetic requirements and predispose to hypothermia and hypoglycemia, while withdrawal from ethanol may precipitate severe hypertension, tremors, delirium, and seizures and may markedly increase anesthetic requirements. The routine use of narcotics and benzodiazepines (whether prescribed or illegal) may significantly increase the doses needed to induce and maintain anesthesia or to provide adequate postoperative analgesia.

H. **Review of systems.** Acute or chronic lung disease, ischemic heart disease, hypertension, and gastroesophageal reflux are examples of commonly encountered coexisting conditions that increase the risk of perianesthetic morbidity and mortality. Hence, a minimum review of systems survey should seek to elicit any history of the following:

1. **Asthma.** Acute, severe bronchospasm may follow the induction of anesthesia and endotracheal intubation. Asthma may also be accompanied by airway mucous plugging, pneumothorax, and an increased susceptibility to postoperative pneumonia.

2. **A recent history of an upper respiratory infection**, especially in children, predisposes patients to pulmonary complications including bronchospasm and laryngospasm during the induction of and emergence from general anesthesia.

3. **Untreated hypertension** is frequently associated with blood pressure lability during anesthesia. If associated with left ventricular hypertrophy, hypertension leads to a higher incidence of postoperative complications (stroke, myocardial infarction). Diuretic therapy often leads to hypovolemia and electrolyte imbalances, especially in the elderly.

4. The patient with preexisting **unstable angina** may experience worsening myocardial ischemia, ventricular dysfunction, or frank myocardial infarction with the stress of surgery and anesthesia.

5. **Hiatal hernia with esophageal reflux symptoms** increases the risk of pulmonary aspiration and may alter the anesthetic plan (e.g., a "rapid sequence" style of induction may be chosen).

6. **Pregnancy.** All women of childbearing age should be questioned regarding last menses and the likelihood of current pregnancy, since premedications and anesthetic agents may adversely influence uteroplacental blood flow or act as teratogens.

III. **Physical examination**

A. The physical examination should be thorough but focused. Special attention is directed toward evaluation of the airway, heart, lungs, and neurologic examination. When regional anesthetic techniques are to be applied, detailed assessment of the extremities and back is necessary.

B. **As a minimum**, the physical examination should consist of the following:

1. **Vital signs**

a. **Height and weight** are useful in estimating therapeutic drug dosages and in determining volume requirements and the adequacy of perioperative urine output.

b. **Blood pressure** should be recorded in both arms and any disparity between upper extremities noted (significant differences may imply disease of the thoracic aorta or its major branches).

c. **Resting pulse** is noted for rhythm, perfusion (fullness), and rate. Pulses may be slow in the beta-blocked patient or rapid and bounding in the patient with fever, aortic regurgitation, or sepsis. Anxious and dehydrated patients frequently have rapid, "thready" (weak) pulses.

   d. Respirations are observed for rate, depth, and "pattern" while at rest. Rapid, deep breathing may be seen with acidosis and central nervous system disease. A shallow, slow pattern with uncoordinated-appearing chest wall and abdominal movements may herald narcotic overdose or impending apnea.

2. **Head and neck.** The details of a thorough head and neck examination are outlined in Chap. 13. During the preoperative examination, one should
   a. Note the size of the oral opening and tongue.
   b. Document loose or chipped teeth, "caps," dentures, and other orthodontic appliances.
   c. Note the range of cervical spine motion in flexion, extension, and rotation.
   d. Document tracheal deviation, cervical masses, and carotid bruits.
3. **Precordium.** Auscultation of the heart may reveal murmurs, gallop rhythms, or a pericardial rub.
4. **Lungs.** Auscultation may reveal wheezing, rhonchi, or rales, which should be correlated with observation of the ease of breathing and use of accessory muscles of respiration.
5. **Abdomen.** Any evidence of distention, masses, or ascites should be noted, as these might predispose to regurgitation or compromise ventilation.
6. **Extremities.** Muscle wasting and weakness must be documented, as well as general distal perfusion, clubbing, cyanosis, and cutaneous infection (especially over sites of planned vascular cannulation or regional nerve block).
7. **Back.** Any deformity, bruising, or infection is noted.
8. **Neurologic.** At a minimum, document mental status, cranial nerve function, cognition, and peripheral sensorimotor function.

IV. **Laboratory studies**
   A. Routine laboratory screening tests rarely uncover abnormalities not already apparent from the history and physical examination. However, certain tests are currently considered necessary to meet presurgical "standard of care" requirements for healthy patients.
   1. **Recent hematocrit/hemoglobin.** There is **no universally accepted minimum hematocrit prior to anesthesia.** Hematocrits in the 25–30% range are usually well tolerated by otherwise healthy people but may result in ischemia in patients with coronary artery disease. Each case must be evaluated individually for the etiology and duration of anemia. If there is no obvious explanation for anemia, a delay of surgery may be indicated.
   2. **Serum chemistries** and **coagulation screens** are ordered only when specifically indicated by the history and physical examination.

      a. Hypokalemia is not uncommon in patients on diuretics and is usually readily corrected by preoperative oral potassium supplementation. Efforts to correct hypokalemia rapidly with IV infusion may lead to arrhythmias and even cardiac arrest. In the face of demonstrated hypokalemia with arrhythmia, a delay in surgery to allow cautious IV correction is reasonable.

      b. The **bleeding time** may be useful in assessing platelet function in those patients who have recently been on nonsteroidal antiinflammatory drugs (NSAIDs) or aspirin, although the most important information is a detailed history regarding easy bruising or excessive bleeding with minor cuts.

      c. Generally, **coagulation studies** are ordered only when clinically indicated (history of a bleeding diathesis or serious systemic illness).

   3. Electrocardiogram (ECG) is advisable for all patients over the age of 40. ECG abnormalities of significance to the anesthetist include new Q waves, ST-segment depression or elevation, T-wave inversions, and rhythm disturbances (premature ventricular contractions, atrial fibrillation or flutter, left bundle branch block, and second- or third-degree atrioventricular block). These findings on a preoperative ECG mandate correlation with history, physical examination, and prior ECGs and may require further workup and consultation with a cardiologist prior to surgery.

   4. Chest x-ray is obtained only when clinically indicated (e.g., heavy smokers, the elderly, and patients with major organ system disease).

V. The anesthesiologist-patient relationship

  A. The perioperative period is emotionally stressful for many patients with fears about **surgery** (cancer, physical disfigurement, postoperative pain, and even death) and **anesthesia** (loss of control, fear of not waking up, postoperative nausea, confusion, pain, paralysis, and headache). The anesthesiologist can alleviate many of these fears and foster trust by

    1. Conducting an unhurried, organized **interview** where you convey to the patient that you are interested and understand his or her fears and concerns.

    2. Reassuring the patient that you will see the patient in the operating room. If there is going to be another person administering the anesthetic, the patient should be so advised and reassured that his or her concerns and needs will be competently addressed.

    3. Informing the patient of the events of the perioperative period, including

      a. The time after which the patient must have nothing to eat or drink (NPO).

      b. The estimated time of surgery.

      c. The need for sedative premedications (see sec. **VI.B**) and which daily medications should be continued as usual.

      d. Induction area tasks to occur on the day of surgery

(e.g., placement of IV or arterial catheters, routine monitoring devices, epidural catheters) with reassurance that supplemental IV sedation and analgesia will be provided as necessary during this period.

  e. Postoperative recovery either in the postanesthesia care unit (PACU) or intensive care unit (ICU) for close observation.

  Note that the above discussion should be restricted to those endeavors specific to anesthesia; opinions regarding the medical diagnosis, prognosis, and issues of surgical technique should be conveyed by the surgeon.

B. **Informed consent** involves discussing the anesthesia management plan, alternatives, and potential complications in terms understandable to the layperson.

  1. Certain aspects of anesthetic management are outside the realm of common experience and, therefore, must be explicitly defined and discussed beforehand. Examples include intubation and mechanical ventilation, complex hemodynamic monitoring, regional anesthesia techniques, blood product transfusion, and postoperative ICU care.

  2. **Alternatives** to the suggested management plan should be presented, as they may become necessary if the planned procedure fails or if there is a change in clinical circumstances (e.g., the patient's ability to cooperate).

  3. It is the anesthesiologist's duty to **disclose the risks** associated with anesthesia-related procedures in a way that a reasonable person (in the patient's position) would find helpful in making a decision. In general, disclosure applies to complications that occur with a relatively **high frequency**, not to all remotely possible risks. However, the anesthesiologist should be familiar with the most frequent and severe complications of commonly employed procedures, including (but not limited to) the following:

    a. **Regional anesthesia.** Headache, infection, local bleeding, nerve injury, and drug reactions. In patients for whom a regional technique is planned, a discussion of general anesthesia and its attendant risks is suggested, since general anesthesia "backup" may be necessary.

    b. **General anesthesia.** Sore throat, hoarseness, nausea and vomiting, dental injury, allergic drug reactions, cardiac dysfunction, and aspiration pneumonia.

    c. **Blood transfusion.** Fever, infectious hepatitis, HIV infection, and hemolytic reactions.

    d. **Vascular cannulations.** Peripheral nerve, tendon, or blood vessel injury; hemo- or pneumothorax; and infection.

  Note: Further detail may be found in the reference by Ross and Tinker in **Suggested Reading.** In cases where risk has not been objectively defined, the patient should be so informed.

   4. Extenuating circumstances. Anesthesia procedures may proceed without informed consent (e.g., in dire emergency) or with limited consent (e.g., the Jehovah's Witness patient who agrees to anesthesia with the understanding that transfusion will be withheld).

VI. The anesthesia consultant's note. The preoperative anesthesia note is a medicolegal document in the permanent hospital record. As such, it should contain:

A. A concise, legible statement of the date and time of the interview, the planned procedure, and a description of any extraordinary circumstances regarding the anesthesia (e.g., locations outside the operating room).

B. Relevant positive and negative findings from the history, physical examination, and laboratory studies.

C. A problem list that delineates all disease processes, their treatments, and current functional limitations; medications and allergies are included.

D. An overall impression of the complexity of the patient's medical condition, with assignment to one of the **American Society of Anesthesiologists (ASA) Physical Status Classes.**

  1. Class 1. A healthy patient.

  2. Class 2. A patient with mild systemic disease.

  3. Class 3. A patient with severe systemic disease that limits activity but is not incapacitating.

  4. Class 4. A patient with an incapacitating systemic disease that is a constant threat to life.

  5. Class 5. A moribund patient not expected to survive 24 hours with or without operation.

  Note: If the procedure is performed as an emergency, an *E* is added to the previously defined ASA Physical Status.

E. The anesthesia plan in the hospital record is used to convey a general management strategy (e.g., suggestions for further preoperative evaluation, premedications, intraoperative monitoring, and postoperative care). If the author of the plan is not scheduled to actually administer care on the day of surgery, this person should avoid defining precise details of the anesthetic agents or techniques to be employed, as these will be determined by the anesthesia team providing care. In the healthy, uncomplicated (i.e., same-day admission) patient, completion of a preanesthesia form is adequate, but when the history needs to be detailed (i.e., the patient with cardiovascular disease), it should be in a formal, legible style in the progress note. It is also imperative in the complicated patient to convey this information to the anesthesia team responsible **in advance** of the surgery.

VII. Premedication

A. The **goals** of administering sedatives and analgesics prior to surgery are to allay the patient's anxiety; prevent pain during vascular cannulation, regional anesthesia procedures, or positioning; and facilitate a smooth induction of anesthesia. It has been shown that the requirement for these drugs is reduced after a thorough preoperative visit by an anesthesiologist.

1. In elderly, debilitated, or acutely intoxicated patients, as well as in those with upper airway obstruction or trauma, central apnea, neurologic deterioration, or severe pulmonary or valvular heart disease, doses of sedatives and analgesics should be reduced or held.

2. Patients addicted to narcotics and barbiturates should be premedicated sufficiently to prevent withdrawal during or shortly after anesthesia.

3. Premedication schemes for patients with selected illnesses are found in Chaps. 2–7.

B. **Sedatives** are given to calm the anxious patient and help provide a restful night of sleep before surgery.

   1. **Benzodiazepines**

      a. **Diazepam** (Valium) is an effective tranquilizer that rarely produces significant cardiovascular or respiratory depression at recommended doses. A dose of 5–10 mg PO 1–2 hours before surgery usually suffices. Diazepam should not be given IM because injection is painful and absorption unpredictable.

      b. **Lorazepam** (Ativan) may also be used (1–4 mg IM or PO) but may cause more intense amnesia and prolonged postoperative sedation.

      c. **Midazolam** (Versed), 1–5 mg IV or IM, is most frequently used in the induction area as a supplemental premedicant and provides excellent amnesia and sedation with low risk of respiratory depression.

   2. **Barbiturates** are rarely used for preoperative sedation, although they are occasionally used by nonanesthetists for sedation for diagnostic procedures (endoscopy, magnetic resonance imaging, and computed tomography scans). Examples include **pentobarbital** (Nembutal) and **secobarbital** (Seconal), intermediate-acting drugs that are sedating and hypnotic but not analgesic. At doses of 1–4 mg/kg IM, their onset of action is 30 minutes, with a peak at 60 minutes and a duration of 2–3 hours.

   3. **Droperidol** (Inapsine) is a butyrophenone that produces long-acting sedation in doses of 0.03–0.14 mg/kg IM. It is most frequently used in combination with fentanyl and midazolam to ease the stress of elective awake intubation. It is also a useful antiemetic at low dose (1.25–2.5 mg IV) when given intra- or postoperatively. Side effects include systemic vasodilation leading to hypotension due to alpha-adrenergic blockade, flushing, and extrapyramidal symptoms from its antidopaminergic qualities. Particularly when used alone, droperidol may also cause an unpleasant dissociative reaction, which is sometimes reversible with physostigmine (Antilirium), 1–2 mg IV, a centrally active cholinesterase inhibitor.

   4. The phenothiazine **promethazine** (Phenergan) and the piperazine **hydroxyzine** (Vistaril), in doses of 25–75 mg IM, are mild tranquilizers, antiemetics, and H_1 blockers; they also potentiate the sedating and

analgesic properties of narcotics. Lower doses (25 mg IM) are selected when given in combination with narcotics.

C. **Narcotics** are most frequently given in the preoperative setting to relieve pain (e.g., patient with a painful hip fracture) and occasionally when the placement of extensive invasive monitoring devices is planned. **Morphine** is the primary narcotic employed, as it has both analgesic and sedative properties. Usual doses are 5–10 mg IM, 60–90 minutes prior to coming to the operating room.

D. **Anticholinergics** are seldom used preoperatively. However, specific agents still occasionally used include the following:

1. **Glycopyrrolate** is given IV during ketamine induction and during oral/dental surgery as an antisialagogue. The dosage is 0.2–0.4 mg IV for adults and 10–20 μg/kg for pediatric patients.

2. **Scopolamine,** given in combination with morphine IM before cardiac surgery, provides additional amnesia and sedation. The adult dose is 0.3–0.4 mg IM with morphine.

E. **Prophylaxis for pulmonary aspiration** may be beneficial for patients at high risk for aspiration pneumonitis, including the parturient and those with a hiatal hernia and reflux symptoms, difficult airway, ileus, obesity, or central nervous system depression.

1. **Histamine H_2 antagonists** produce a dose-related decrease in basal, nocturnal, and stimulated gastric acid production. Cimetidine (Tagamet), 200–400 mg PO, IM, or IV, and ranitidine (Zantac), 150–300 mg PO or 50–100 mg IV or IM, significantly reduce both the volume of gastric juice secreted and its hydrogen ion concentration. Multidose regimens (i.e., the night before and morning of surgery) are the most effective, although parenteral administration may be used to achieve a rapid (<1 hour) onset. Cimetidine has been shown to prolong the elimination of theophylline, diazepam, propranolol, and lidocaine, potentially leading to toxicity of these agents. Ranitidine has not been associated with such side effects and is just as effective and longer acting than cimetidine.

2. **Nonparticulate antacids.** Colloidal antacid suspensions are the most effective neutralizers of stomach acid but can produce serious pneumonitis if aspirated. Nonsuspension antacids, such as citric acid solutions (30–60 ml, 30 minutes prior to induction), may be somewhat less effective in raising gastric pH, but their aspiration is less harmful.

3. **Metoclopramide** (Reglan) is a dopamine antagonist that enhances gastric emptying by increasing lower esophageal sphincter tone while simultaneously relaxing the pylorus. A dose of 10 mg should be given 1 hour prior to anesthesia or IV in the induction area as soon as the IV is inserted. When administered IV, it should be given slowly so as not to precipitate abdominal cramping. Metoclopramide also has an antiemetic effect.

SUGGESTED READING

Barash, P. G. Preoperative cardiac evaluation for noncardiac surgery: A functional approach. *Anesth. Analg.* 74:586, 1992.

Egbert, L. D., et al. The value of the preoperative visit by an anesthetist. *J.A.M.A.* 185:553, 1963.

Olsson, G. L., et al. Aspiration during anesthesia: A computer-aided study of 185,358 anesthetics. *Acta Anaesthesiol. Scand.* 30:84, 1986.

Ross, A. F., and Tinker, J. H. Anesthesia Risk. In R. D. Miller (ed.), *Anesthesia* (3rd ed.). New York: Churchill Livingstone, 1990. Pp. 715–742.

Shorten, G. D., and Roberts, J. T. The prediction of difficult intubation. *Anesthesiol. Clin. North Am.* 9:63, 1991.

Vandam, L. D. *To Make the Patient Ready for Anesthesia: Medical Care of the Surgical Patient.* Menlo Park, CA: Addison-Wesley, 1980.

Velanovich, V. The value of routine preoperative laboratory testing in predicting postoperative complications: A multivariate analysis. *Surgery* 109:236, 1991.

White, P. F. Pharmacologic and clinical aspects of preoperative medication. *Anesth. Analg.* 65:963, 1986.

2

Specific Considerations with Cardiac Disease

Steve Rotter

I. **Ischemic heart disease.** More than one million people with heart disease undergo anesthesia every year, and cardiovascular complications are a leading cause of postoperative morbidity and mortality. Understanding the pathophysiology and treatment of heart disease is of major importance to the anesthesiologist.

A. **Physiology**

1. **Oxygen supply-demand balance.** Myocardial ischemia occurs when cardiac metabolic demands exceed supply.

a. **Supply.** The heart relies on oxygenated blood provided by the coronary arteries. The **left coronary artery** branches into the **left anterior descending (LAD)** and **circumflex** arteries to supply the left ventricle (LV). The **right coronary artery (RCA)** supplies the right ventricle (RV). The **dominant** vessel supplies the posterior diaphragmatic portion of the interventricular septum, the atrioventricular node, and the inferoposterior portion of the LV. The RCA is dominant in 85% of patients, and the sinus node is supplied by the RCA in 60% of patients. Various rhythm and conduction abnormalities may result from diminished perfusion to these areas.

(1) **Coronary blood flow** is determined by perfusion pressure divided by coronary resistance. Coronary perfusion pressure is determined by the difference between aortic diastolic pressure and central venous pressure (CVP). The majority of antegrade flow in the coronary arteries occurs during diastole. With exercise or stress, coronary flow may increase four- or fivefold to compensate for the increase in oxygen consumption ($M\dot{V}O_2$).

(2) **Heart rate.** As heart rate increases, diastolic filling time and coronary blood flow decrease. Patients with coronary artery disease (CAD) often become ischemic at higher heart rates.

(3) **Oxygen content.** Arterial blood enters the heart approximately 95–100% saturated with oxygen, and venous blood is returned via the coronary sinus at approximately 30% saturation. Oxygen content (CaO_2) is determined by hemoglobin concentration, arterial oxygen saturation (SaO_2), and dissolved oxygen (PaO_2) (see Chap. 35). It is of critical importance for patients with CAD to have well-oxygenated blood and adequate hemoglobin concentration to avoid ischemia. Since oxygen is nearly maximally extracted at rest, increased demand can only be met by an increase in coronary blood flow, oth-

erwise a shift to anaerobic metabolism will occur.

b. Demand or myocardial oxygen consumption ($M\dot{V}O_2$) is difficult to quantify but is affected by a number of factors:

   (1) Systolic work of the heart is a function of heart rate, blood pressure, and stroke volume.

   (2) Inotropic state or contractility is independent of the load on the heart and varies directly with sympathetic stimulation. Positive inotropic agents like digitalis or beta-adrenergic agonists increase $M\dot{V}O_2$, while beta-adrenergic antagonists, calcium channel blockers, and inhalation agents decrease $M\dot{V}O_2$.

   (3) Ventricular wall tension. Since Laplace's law states that the tension in the wall of a sphere is directly related to the radius of the sphere, cardiac enlargement leads to greater wall tension and an increase in $M\dot{V}O_2$.

c. Supply and demand balance

   (1) Etiology. Although atherosclerosis is the most common etiology for supply-demand imbalances, other conditions may cause myocardial ischemia. Marked ventricular hypertrophy, prolonged systole, and high intraventricular pressure may lead to an increase in $M\dot{V}O_2$ that exceeds supply, even in the setting of normal coronary anatomy. Examples include aortic stenosis, systemic hypertension, or hypertrophic cardiomyopathy.

   (2) Treatment that may improve the supply-demand balance includes the following:

      (a) Increase supply

         i. Increase perfusion pressure with fluid administration or drugs such as alpha agonists to increase aortic diastolic pressure.

         ii. Increase oxygen content by increasing hemoglobin concentration or oxygen saturation.

      (b) Decrease demand

         i. Decrease heart rate with beta antagonists or narcotics to increase diastolic filling time and improve coronary perfusion.

         ii. Decrease ventricular size

            i **IV nitroglycerin** may treat coronary ischemia and decrease end-diastolic volume.

            ii **Inotropes** may improve contractility.

         iii. Intraaortic balloon counterpulsation

            i This augments aortic diastolic pressure and improves coronary artery perfusion.

            ii Afterload, or resistance to ventricular ejection, is decreased.

B. **Preoperative predictors of cardiac morbidity.** There
    are many risk factors associated with cardiac disease.
    Primary risk factors directly influence onset, duration,
    intensity of heart disease, and risk of cardiac morbidity,
    while secondary risk factors are associated with and
    influenced by the primary risk factors.
    1. **Primary risk factors**
       a. **Congestive heart failure (CHF)** is one of the most
          important predictors of cardiac mortality, carrying
          a 5-year survival rate of less than 50%. There is a
          fourfold increased risk of perioperative complica-
          tions in these patients. An ejection fraction less
          than 0.40 has been found to be predictive of periop-
          erative myocardial infarction (MI), reinfarction, and
          perioperative ventricular dysfunction.
       b. **Angina** can be classified as stable or unstable.
          Stable angina is exercise- or stress-induced, re-
          solves with rest, and can be controlled with medica-
          tion. **Unstable angina** occurs at rest or when a
          stable pattern exhibits increasing severity or fre-
          quency of attacks. New-onset angina is also consid-
          ered unstable. Unstable angina is poorly controlled
          with medication and carries with it a significantly
          higher risk. Myocardial ischemia may occur without
          pain and may be manifest by fatigue, arrhythmias,
          or pulmonary edema. The electrocardiogram (ECG)
          may demonstrate ischemic changes, but approxi-
          mately 50% of patients with chronic stable angina
          experience daily episodes of silent ischemia demon-
          strated by continuous ECG monitoring. Thirty per-
          cent of MIs are silent, and 50% of all perioperative
          MIs are asymptomatic.
       c. **Previous MI.** The nature of a prior MI (e.g., date,
          anatomic location, symptoms, and sequelae) will
          contribute to the relative risk for a future cardiac
          event. The risk of reinfarction with anesthesia is
          significant in the immediate postinfarction period
          and decreases over the ensuing 6 months.
       d. **Hypertension** is a risk factor for ischemic heart
          disease, CHF, and stroke but is not a predictor of
          cardiac risk as an isolated factor.
       e. **Arrhythmias.** A documented ventricular arrhyth-
          mia or nonsinus rhythm increases the risk of peri-
          operative cardiac complications. The ventricular
          rate, duration of arrhythmia, and hemodynamic
          effect determine the overall consequence.
       f. **Prior cardiac surgery**, whether coronary artery
          bypass grafting (CABG) or valve replacement, may
          imply an increased cardiac risk for a future proce-
          dure. Old records should be obtained, if possible, to
          determine the nature and adequacy of the repair
          (saphenous vein graft or left internal mammary ar-
          tery [LIMA]), postoperative complications, and the
          nature of current cardiac symptomatology. The in-
          cidence of postoperative MI in patients undergoing
          noncardiac surgery is reduced after CABG surgery,

though the overall mortality rate is unchanged. It is important to determine the type of valvular prosthesis, the anticoagulation regimen, and whether there are symptoms to suggest valve failure or endocarditis. There are no data on the effect of coronary angioplasty or valvuloplasty in patients undergoing subsequent noncardiac surgical procedures.

2. **Secondary risk factors**

   a. **Diabetes mellitus** is a risk factor for CAD. The incidence of silent ischemia or infarction is greater in patients with diabetes mellitus. Cardiac morbidity is greater and survival rate is lower in diabetic patients who have an MI.

   b. **Cigarette smoking and hypercholesterolemia** are the major modifiable risk factors for heart disease. Many studies have demonstrated that smokers have approximately twice the risk of CAD as nonsmokers. Both smoking and hypercholesterolemia are independent risk factors that may act synergistically with other risk factors.

   c. **Obesity,** defined as an increase of 20% above ideal body weight, adversely affects both health and longevity and has a direct relationship with most of the other risk factors.

   d. **Age** does not appear to affect resting ejection fraction, end-diastolic volume, or regional wall motion. Increasing age does impair the heart's response to stress, exercise, or drugs and may influence the severity of other risk factors.

   e. **Genetics** can influence risk factors. A family history of significant cardiac morbidity and mortality is a strong but indirect risk factor.

   f. **Vascular disease** such as peripheral vascular and cerebrovascular disease is commonly associated with CAD. Patients who undergo a vascular procedure have an increased risk of cardiac morbidity.

C. **Preoperative evaluation**

   1. **History.** Exercise limitations, daily activities, and life-style are important questions in assessing cardiac disease.

      a. **Angina,** if present, should be characterized as to symptoms, duration, and precipitating and palliative factors. Anginal equivalents (e.g., nausea, shortness of breath, or diaphoresis) should be sought. Current medication regimen and recent changes should be noted.

      b. **Congestive heart failure.** Shortness of breath, orthopnea, paroxysmal nocturnal dyspnea, pedal edema, dyspnea on exertion, and fatigue should be elicited. Digitalis and diuretic therapy requirements must be determined.

      c. **Arrhythmias.** Palpitations, syncope, and light-headedness are common symptoms. A Holter monitor evaluation may provide useful information.

      d. **Hypertension.** Duration, medication compliance, and current therapy should be noted.

      e. Hospitalizations. Visits to the emergency room and intensive care unit admissions for angina or CHF should be elicited.

      f. Infarction. History of "heart attack" or ECG evidence of old infarction should be noted.

      g. Murmurs. The presence of a murmur and history of congenital heart disease (CHD) or rheumatic fever should be noted. The extent of the workup and need for antibiotic therapy should be reviewed.

      h. Medications. Current regimen, recent changes, side effects, or adverse reactions should be determined.

      i. Previous studies. ECG, stress test, Holter monitor, and coronary angiogram must be reviewed.

2. Physical examination is discussed in Chap. 1.

      a. In the patient with cardiac disease, evidence of **jugular venous distention** and **carotid bruits** should be sought.

      b. The **chest examination** should document rales, rhonchi, wheezing, and evidence of pleural effusion.

      c. The **cardiac examination** should document the presence of heaves, thrills, murmurs, rubs, and gallops.

      d. The **abdominal examination** may reveal evidence of an aortic aneurysm (pulsatile mass, bruits) or cardiac dysfunction (pulsatile liver, hepatomegaly, or hepatojugular reflux).

      e. Extremities. Peripheral pulses should be evaluated and blood pressure measured in each arm. Cyanosis, edema, and clubbing of the extremities are noted.

3. Laboratory studies

      a. Routine laboratory tests should include a hematocrit. Other studies (electrolytes, blood urea nitrogen, and creatinine) are ordered as needed.

      b. Twelve-lead ECG should always be obtained to document rate, rhythm, conduction disturbances, and evidence of ischemia or infarction.

      c. Chest radiographs may demonstrate cardiomegaly, pulmonary edema, and pleural effusions.

4. Noninvasive testing

      a. Exercise stress testing is a noninvasive method to evaluate patients with known CAD or atypical chest pain. Exercise stress testing provides information concerning ischemia, ventricular dysfunction, and arrhythmias. Various protocols increase the workload of the heart and quantitate the hemodynamic and ECG response. Exercise stress tests are highly predictive of cardiac morbidity when ST changes are characteristic, greater than 2 mm, immediate (within 1–4 minutes), sustained into recovery, or associated with hypotension. The relationship of ischemia to clinical symptoms is determined. The results can be used to decide further evaluation, to aid in perioperative care, and to serve as a prognostic indicator.

b. **Continuous ECG monitoring** (Holter) is useful for detecting episodes of ischemia or arrhythmias and correlating them with symptoms. Episodes of asymptomatic ST-segment depression are common and probably represent myocardial perfusion abnormalities. The presence of a significant degree of ischemia serves as a predictor of unfavorable outcome and is more sensitive than the standard 12-lead ECG.

c. **Echocardiography** is an important noninvasive test to evaluate global ventricular function, wall motion abnormalities, and valvular function. An echocardiogram performed during exercise may give a more dynamic measure of cardiac function. Patients with an ejection fraction less than 0.30 have a 1-year mortality rate of 30%.

d. **Transesophageal echocardiography (TEE)** is used to evaluate valvular function, to characterize mural or atrial thrombi, to assess dissecting aortic aneurysms and intracardiac shunts, and to evaluate regional and global ventricular function. TEE is used as an intraoperative monitor to evaluate valve function (e.g., after mitral valve reconstruction) and ischemia.

e. **Radionuclide imaging** is a safe and effective method to assess myocardial perfusion, infarction, and function.

   (1) **Thallium 201** is a radioactive tracer that is injected intravenously, has minimal lung uptake, is cleared from the blood rapidly, and is avidly extracted by cardiac muscle as a potassium analogue. Myocardial distribution of thallium is closely related to regional myocardial blood flow. In a thallium study, initial images are taken soon after thallium is injected. Regions of decreased tracer activity due to diminished or absent perfusion will demonstrate little thallium uptake (i.e., a cold spot). There is an ongoing equilibrium between myocardium and blood, and initial defects (areas not perfused with thallium) may appear to "fill in" or "redistribute" to normal zones when studied 3–4 hours later. This is due to continued uptake in regions that are underperfused but still viable. They are called **areas of redistribution.** These areas are considered to represent **myocardium at risk.** A significantly positive scan identifies redistribution in the area perfused by the left main coronary artery or an extensive area representing three-vessel disease. If there is no increased thallium activity on the delayed image, the area is felt to represent scar tissue (an old MI) and is called a **fixed defect.** Lack of homogeneity in the myocardial images may be due to factors other than diminished flow such as attenuation artifacts, regions of asymmetry or

hypertrophy, or overlap of activity in the RV, lung, or splanchnic vessels. Normally, the lung retains about 5–10% of the injected thallium dose, while the myocardium retains up to 85%. However, with slower transit of thallium through the lung or with pulmonary edema, lung extraction can increase to 25%. Increased lung uptake indicates LV dysfunction, possible severe CAD, and a worse prognosis. These tests may be performed with stress (exercise or dipyridamole) to unmask regional differences in coronary perfusion not evident at rest. Only stenoses of 90% or greater produce flow abnormalities at rest, while stenoses of 50% or greater may be detected with stress. Patients unable to exercise adequately are given dipyridamole (Persantine), which dilates coronary arteries via the mediator adenosine. The sensitivity and specificity of dypyridamole thallium are comparable to exercise thallium studies. The effect is negated or reversed with aminophylline, and dipyridamole cannot be used in patients taking aminophylline. A relative contraindication to dipyridamole is a history of asthma or bronchospasm.

(2) **Technetium 99m** is a radionuclide that is injected into a vein, and using a technique called infarct-avid myocardial scintigraphy ("hot-spot imaging"), newly infarcted myocardium can be visualized. First-pass radionuclear angiography using technetium provides information about ventricular function, both RV and LV ejection fraction, intracardiac shunts, and LV end-diastolic volume. The gated blood pool scan measures regional wall motion and ejection fraction. These radionuclide studies can be performed both at rest and with exercise (or with dipyridamole) and provide a sensitive noninvasive method of evaluating the heart.

5. **Cardiac catheterization** is considered the "gold standard" for evaluating cardiac disease. Information obtained includes anatomy, hemodynamics, and function of the heart (see Chap. 23).

6. **Cardiac consultation** may be helpful in identifying patients at risk. The consultant should provide guidance in deciding which tests are helpful and may expedite and interpret the results. The consultant also helps to maximize perioperative medical therapy and provides follow-up after automatic internal cardioverter-defibrillator (AICD) or pacemaker insertion.

D. **Anesthetic considerations**

1. Patients with ischemic heart disease are often very apprehensive and need **reassurance** during the perioperative period.

2. **Cardiac medications** are usually continued on the day of surgery. Possible exceptions include long-acting beta antagonists, diuretics for hypertension, or digoxin,

unless needed for heart rate control. Patients on oral or sublingual nitrates may bring them to the operating room. Sedatives are discussed in Chap. 1.

3. **Supplemental oxygen** should be provided to patients with significant ischemic or valvular heart disease. It should be written as part of the preanesthetic orders (i.e., O_2 via nasal cannula at 2–3 L/min).

4. **Monitors.** A detailed discussion of monitoring is found in Chap. 10.

5. **Perioperative issues**
   a. **General versus regional anesthesia.** There have been no convincing outcome data regarding the benefits of a well-conducted general anesthetic versus a well-conducted regional anesthetic in patients with cardiac disease. Individual evaluation should be made for the type of surgery.
   b. **Site of surgery** can be a predictor of perioperative cardiac morbidity. Patients undergoing thoracic or upper abdominal surgery have a two- to threefold higher risk for myocardial ischemia and infarction. Patients with CAD undergoing major vascular surgery have an increased risk for perioperative cardiac complications.

II. Valvular heart disease

A. **Subacute bacterial endocarditis prophylaxis.** Transient bacteremia following surgical and dental procedures may cause endocarditis in select individuals. Blood-borne bacteria may lodge on damaged or abnormal valves or on congenital anatomic defects. Endocarditis prophylaxis is currently recommended for patients with prosthetic cardiac valves, previous endocarditis, most congenital malformations, rheumatic valvular disease, hypertrophic cardiomyopathy, and mitral valve prolapse *with* valvular regurgitation. Endocarditis prophylaxis is *not* recommended for patients with mitral valve prolapse *without* regurgitation, cardiac pacemakers, and implanted defibrillators. Tables 2-1 and 2-2 indicate appropriate antibiotic coverage for surgical procedures.

B. **Aortic stenosis**
   1. **Etiology** is usually progressive senile calcification and narrowing of a normal or bicuspid valve. This results in increased obstruction to LV ejection, increased wall tension, and ventricular hypertrophy.
   2. **Symptoms** appear late in the disease process. Life expectancy is usually 5 years after the onset of angina, 3 years after syncope, and 2 years after CHF.
   3. The **ventricle** becomes hypertrophied and stiff, and atrial contraction is often critical to provide adequate ventricular filling and stroke volume. The ventricle is also susceptible to ischemia even in the absence of CAD, due to increased intraventricular pressure, increased muscle mass, and decreased aortic diastolic pressure.
   4. **Anesthetic considerations**
      a. It is important to maintain **sinus rhythm and adequate preload.** Hypotension should be aggressively treated to maintain adequate coronary perfu-

Table 2-1. Antibiotics for dental, oral, or upper respiratory tract procedures

Drug	Dosage regimen
PO Regimen	
Amoxicillin	3 gm PO 1 hr before procedure, then 1.5 gm PO 6 hr after initial dose
For penicillin-allergic patients	
Erythromycin	1 gm PO 2 hr before procedure, then 500 mg PO 6 hr after initial dose
Clindamycin	300 mg PO 1 hr before procedure, then 150 mg PO 6 hr after dose (alternate regimen)
IV Regimen	
Ampicillin	2 gm IV 30 min before procedure, then 1 gm IV 6 hr after initial dose
For penicillin-allergic patients	
Clindamycin	300 mg IV 30 min before procedure and 150 mg 6 hr after initial dose
For high-risk patients	
Ampicillin, gentamicin, and amoxicillin	Ampicillin, 2 gm IV, plus gentamicin, 1.5 gm/kg, 30 min before procedure; followed by amoxicillin, 1.5 gm PO 6 hr after initial dose, or ampicillin, 2 gm IV, and gentamicin, 1.5 mg/kg, 8 hr after initial dose
For penicillin-allergic patients	
Vancomycin	1 gm IV 1 hr before the procedure

sion pressure. Tachycardia (causing increased $M\dot{V}O_2$ and decreased diastolic filling) or bradycardia (causing decreased cardiac output) is poorly tolerated in patients with severe aortic stenosis.

   b. **Patients with severe aortic stenosis** (aortic valve area $< 0.6\,cm^2$) may benefit from a pulmonary artery catheter, but it is important to realize that measurement of pulmonary capillary wedge pressure (PCWP) will underestimate left ventricular end-diastolic pressure (LVEDP), and higher "filling pressures" may be needed for optimal cardiac output.

   c. **The treatment of ischemia** is directed at increasing oxygen delivery or decreasing $M\dot{V}O_2$. Nitrates should be used with extreme caution, as small reductions in ventricular volume may lead to marked reduction in cardiac output.

C. **Idiopathic hypertrophic subaortic stenosis (IHSS)**
   1. **Etiology.** IHSS results from asymmetric hypertrophy

Table 2-2. Antibiotics for genitourinary or gastrointestinal procedures

Drug	Dosage regimen
Ampicillin, gentamicin, and amoxicillin	Ampicillin, 2.0 gm IV, and gentamicin, 1.5 mg/kg IV, 30 min before procedure, followed by amoxicillin, 1.5 gm PO, 6 hr after initial dose
For penicillin-allergic patients Vancomycin and gentamicin	Vancomycin, 1 gm IV, and gentamicin, 1.5 mg/kg IV, before procedure; followed by same 8 hr after initial dose

of the interventricular septum leading to outflow obstruction during systole. The anterior leaflet of the mitral valve opposes the septum and increases the amount of outflow obstruction.

2. Factors that **worsen outflow obstruction** include decreased arterial pressure, decreased intraventricular volume, and increased contractility.

3. **The clinical implications** are similar to those for aortic stenosis.

4. **Anesthetic considerations**

   a. Sinus rhythm should be maintained, and cardioversion should be considered for supraventricular tachycardia.

   b. Beta-adrenergic antagonists or calcium channel blockers should be continued until surgery.

   c. Preload should be maintained, and hypotension should be corrected with volume and alpha-adrenergic agonists (phenylephrine).

   d. Inotropes must be used cautiously, as they may exacerbate outflow obstruction.

D. **Aortic regurgitation**

   1. **Etiologies** include rheumatic heart disease, endocarditis, trauma, collagen vascular diseases, and any process that dilates the aortic root (aneurysm, Marfan's disease, or syphilis).

   2. **Pathophysiology.** A distinction is made between acute and chronic aortic regurgitation.

      a. **Acute aortic regurgitation** may cause sudden volume overload on the LV with increased PCWP and LVEDP. Manifestations include tachycardia, vasoconstriction, decreased cardiac output, and acute CHF.

      b. **Chronic aortic regurgitation** causes eccentric ventricular hypertrophy with increased LV volume and slightly increased LV pressure. Symptoms may be minimal until late-onset CHF occurs.

   3. **Anesthetic considerations**

      a. Optimal hemodynamics include maintaining a normal or slightly increased heart rate to minimize regurgitation and maintain aortic diastolic and coronary artery perfusion pressure.

   b. Adequate preload should be maintained.
   c. Vasodilators can improve forward flow and decrease LVEDP and myocardial wall tension.

E. **Mitral stenosis**
   1. **Etiology** is almost always rheumatic heart disease.
   2. **Pathophysiology**
      a. Increased left atrial pressure and volume overload increase left atrial size (hypertrophy) and often lead to atrial fibrillation.
      b. Pulmonary venous pressure and increased pulmonary artery pressure lead to vascular engorgement and chronic pulmonary hypertension.
      c. Increased pulmonary artery pressure leads to RV failure, a decrease in cardiac output, and tricuspid regurgitation.
      d. Tachycardia is poorly tolerated because it diminishes diastolic filling time and will decrease LV preload and cardiac output. Pulmonary edema may occur, and lung compliance is decreased, predisposing to ventilation-perfusion ($\dot{V}/\dot{Q}$) mismatch.
   3. **Anesthetic considerations**
      a. **Avoid tachycardia.** If the patient is in atrial fibrillation, control the ventricular response with digoxin or beta antagonists. Continue preoperative digoxin or beta antagonists on the day of surgery.
      b. **Avoid pulmonary hypertension** by maintaining normocarbia, adequate oxygenation, and preventing acidosis (Table 2-3).
      c. **Hypotension is rarely directly caused by hypovolema.** If RV failure is present, consider dopamine, dobutamine, nitroprusside, or prostaglandin E_1 (PGE_1).
      d. A **pulmonary artery catheter** is useful, but placement may be difficult if tricuspid regurgitation or RV hypertrophy is present.
         (1) There may be an increased risk of pulmonary artery rupture with balloon inflation.
         (2) Pulmonary artery diastolic pressure is not an accurate estimate of left atrial pressure or LVEDP.
      e. **Premedication** should be adequate to prevent anxiety and tachycardia but should be used judi-

Table 2-3. Factors altering pulmonary vascular resistance (PVR)

Increase PVR	Decrease PVR
Hypoxia	Oxygen
Hypercarbia	Hypocarbia
Acidosis	Alkalosis
Atelectasis	
Sympathomimetics	

ciously in patients with hypotension or low cardiac output.

F. **Mitral regurgitation**
  1. **Etiologies** include mitral valve prolapse, ischemic heart disease, endocarditis, and papillary muscle rupture from infarction.
  2. Mitral regurgitation allows blood to be ejected into the left atrium during systole. The amount of regurgitant flow depends on the ventricular-atrial pressure gradient, the size of the mitral orifice, and the duration of ejection.
  3. **Pathophysiology**
    a. **Acute mitral regurgitation** usually occurs in the setting of MI. Acute volume overload of the left atrium and ventricle leads to symptoms of LV dysfunction. Ventricular filling pressures increase, and cardiac output is reduced.
    b. **Chronic mitral regurgitation.** Gradual left atrial and ventricular dilatation and hypertrophy compensate for volume overload.
    c. **Measurement of ejection fraction** does not quantify forward versus backward flow, as the incompetent valve permits immediate ejection of blood with the onset of ventricular systole. Patients with mitral regurgitation and depressed ejection fraction are at high risk for perioperative cardiac complications.
  4. **Anesthetic considerations**
    a. A faster heart rate is desirable, as it decreases ventricular volume. Bradycardia is associated with increased LV volume and regurgitation.
    b. Afterload reduction is beneficial, and use of an intraaortic balloon pump may be lifesaving. Avoid increased systemic vascular resistance, as this will increase regurgitant flow.
    c. Maintain preload. Titrate potential myocardial depressants carefully.

G. **Mitral valve prolapse**
  1. Mitral valve prolapse has a prevalence of 5–10%.
  2. **Clinical features.** Symptoms may include atypical chest pain, palpitations, anxiety, and shortness of breath. Associated findings include conduction defects, supraventricular and bradyarrhythmias, nonspecific ECG changes, mitral regurgitation, endocarditis, and a midsystolic click.
  3. **Diagnosis** is confirmed by echocardiography.
  4. **Subacute bacterial endocarditis prophylaxis** is recommended for patients with regurgitation (see sec. II.A).
  5. **Anesthetic considerations** are those appropriate for coexisting disease.

III. **Congenital heart disease (CHD).** Patients with CHD are either unrepaired or have had surgery and may be considered "cured," "corrected," or "palliated," depending on the nature of the lesion and type of procedure. Preoperative information must be obtained from the pediatrician, internist, or cardiologist managing the patient, and review of old records is valuable. Noninvasive studies of cardiac function and anatomy should be performed. Many of the patients will present for noncardiac surgery where surgeons unfamiliar with the physiologic restrictions of CHD will perform stressful procedures, and cardiopulmonary bypass is not available for circulatory support.

A. **General considerations.** When patients present for noncardiac surgery after surgical correction of congenital heart lesions, certain basic maneuvers must be performed.

1. **Systemic air emboli** are a constant danger, particularly due to the dynamic nature of shunting. IV lines must be purged of air bubbles, and air filters should be used.

2. **Cyanotic patients** are often polycythemic and at risk for strokes or other thrombotic problems. IV hydration is important, and erythrophoresis may be required if preoperative hematocrits are greater than 60–70%.

3. **Prevention of bacterial endocarditis** is mandatory in this patient population with few exceptions (see Tables 2-1 and 2-2).

B. **Unrepaired** congenital heart defects may lead to more severe hemodynamic derangements in adulthood than in childhood. **Atrial septal defect** is the most common congenital lesion that is diagnosed in adults.

1. **Left-to-right shunting** of blood leads to RV overload, increased pulmonary blood flow, and pulmonary hypertension.

2. Patients often present with a flow murmur, arrhythmia, atrial fibrillation, or CHF. Although these findings usually resolve after surgery, **Eisenmenger's physiology** (irreversibly elevated pulmonary vascular resistance) may persist postoperatively. Other problems following repair include conduction defects and supraventricular and ventricular arrhythmias.

C. **Repaired** congenital lesions may be truly corrected, "corrected," or "palliated." True corrections include the following:

1. **Patent ductus arteriosus**, once ligated, rarely has any long-term sequelae. Percutaneous closure is now a successful and minimal risk procedure.

2. **Atrial septal defect.** Repair of a secundum-type atrial septal defect early in life results in normal physiology and function. Repair of a primum-type atrial septal defect with mitral valve cleft or sinus venosus defect with partial anomalous pulmonary venous drainage may lead to residual mitral regurgitation.

D. **"Corrected" lesions** result in markedly prolonged life expectancy but with some degree of cardiovascular impairment.

1. **Coarctation of the aorta.** Even after successful repair, labile blood pressure may occur.

   a. Residual coarctation occurs in 10% of patients.

   b. If a subclavian flap is used to repair the coarctation,

blood pressures obtained from the left arm may not be equal to those from the right.

   c. Hypertension is a late-developing complication in 65% of patients after repair.
   d. Occult aortic valve disease should be considered in any patient requiring anesthesia after repair of coarctation.

2. **Transposition of the great arteries** (TGA)
   a. TGA has been corrected by means of an **intraatrial baffle** that reroutes blood return to the appropriate great vessel (e.g., Mustard or Senning procedure). Long-term postoperative problems include residual atrial septal defect, RV dysfunction, conduction disturbances, supraventricular tachyarrhythmias, caval or pulmonary venous obstruction, and tricuspid regurgitation. Cardiovascular function at rest may be relatively normal in patients after atrial repair of TGA. However, physiologic response to moderate and maximal exercise is grossly abnormal from RV dysfunction when it functions as the systemic ventricle. There is a 10% incidence of late sudden death of unclear etiology occurring 10 years after TGA repair.
   b. Currently an **arterial switch procedure** (Jatene repair) is employed; postoperative sequelae include LV dysfunction, biventricular outflow tract obstruction, aortic regurgitation, and coronary insufficiency, but with much lower incidence than for the Mustard or Senning procedure.

3. **Ventricular septal defects**, even after repair, may leave **residual RV and pulmonary artery hypertension** and **CHF.**
   a. Residual ventricular septal defects, tricuspid regurgitation, elevated pulmonary vascular resistance, and respiratory insufficiency may all occur in the early postoperative period.
   b. His' bundle injury can lead to complete heart block, especially in patients with right bundle branch block.
   c. Percutaneous transcatheter umbrella closure of ventricular septal defects is a new therapeutic option.

4. **Tetralogy of Fallot**, after correction, usually shows normalization of the RV/PA systolic gradient.
   a. Most patients have **residual RV dysfunction and right bundle branch block** but can still respond to exercise with an increase in cardiac output. Some show **residual RV outflow obstruction or peripheral pulmonic stenosis**, which can lead to RV failure and ventricular arrhythmias.
   b. **Persistent pulmonary vascular hyperreactivity** can result in an increased PCWP with exercise. Shunting can occur, which usually is mild and does not alter the oxygen saturation.
   c. **Pulmonic regurgitation** is common but usually does not affect cardiac output.

       d. A few patients have **residual ventricular septal defects** or LV dysfunction.

       e. There is an increased incidence of ventricular tachy-arrhythmias and **sudden death.**

E. Palliative procedures result in prolonged life expectancy but with markedly abnormal cardiovascular function. Palliative procedures include the following:

1. **Cardiac transplantation for hypoplastic left heart syndrome** (HLHS).

2. **Pulmonary atresia.** Systemic-to-pulmonary shunts (e.g., Blalock-Taussig, Potts, Waterston shunt) were performed in the past. Currently, synthetic grafts are used to shunt between either the ascending aorta to the main pulmonary artery or subclavian artery to the right or left pulmonary artery. The purpose of these is to increase pulmonary blood flow and to unload the RV. Late complications may include CHF and progressive pulmonary hypertension.

3. The **Fontan procedure** is a commonly performed procedure used to treat aortic atresia, mitral or tricuspid atresia, and all types of "single functioning ventricle" (e.g., HLHS). Since the pulmonary and systemic circulations are separate, the goal is to provide all systemic venous return directly to the pulmonary artery. This is accomplished by atrial septal defect closure and anastomosis of the right atrium to the right or main pulmonary artery. **Late complications** include

    a. Persistent pericardial and pleural effusions.

    b. Limited cardiac reserve with exercise or stress (e.g., anesthesia and surgery).

    c. Hemodynamic instability when hypovolemia, arrhythmias (e.g., atrial fibrillation), or increased intrathoracic pressure occurs.

F. The postcardiac transplant patient

1. As the frequency of cardiac transplantation increases, more of these patients will present for noncardiac surgery. Recent statistics reveal that more than 2500 cardiac transplants, including 225 pediatric transplants, are performed annually with a 90% 1-year survival rate and a more than 70% 5-year survival rate.

2. Postcardiac transplant patients typically require surgery related either to their underlying vascular disease or to a complication of chronic steroid therapy or immunosuppression (infection).

3. **Physiology of the postcardiac transplant heart**

    a. There is no histologic evidence of cardiac reinnervation, and patients do not experience anginal pain. Since transplanted hearts demonstrate accelerated graft atherosclerosis, these patients are at risk for silent myocardial ischemia.

    b. Hemodynamics in the transplanted heart

       (1) Cardiac impulse formation and conduction are normal, though resting heart rate is elevated.

       (2) The Frank-Starling effect is intact, and these hearts respond normally to circulating catecholamines.

        (3) Metabolic control of coronary blood flow is intact.

        (4) During stress or exercise when cardiac output is increased, the postcardiac transplant heart will meet these demands by increasing stroke volume via the Frank-Starling effect, followed by a delayed increase in heart rate due to circulating catecholamines.

  c. Drug effects

        (1) Drugs that act only via the autonomic nervous system (e.g., atropine) are ineffective in these patients.

        (2) Direct-acting vasoactive agents are effective in the postcardiac transplant patient. Commonly used agents include isoproterenol to increase heart rate and norepinephrine or phenylephrine to increase blood pressure.

        (3) Beta-adrenergic receptors are intact and may have increased density.

4. Anesthetic considerations

  a. The patient's activity level and exercise capacity must be determined. A cardiology consultant can provide recent data concerning function and anatomy as measured by echocardiography and catheterization.

  b. Underlying CAD is usually asymptomatic, so evidence of ischemia may include a history of dyspnea, signs of reduced cardiac function, and arrhythmias.

  c. A baseline 12-lead ECG must be obtained. This may demonstrate multiple P waves (from both the donor and recipient sinus nodes) and right bundle branch block.

  d. A chest radiograph is useful.

  e. Baseline laboratory studies should include complete blood count, electrolytes, blood urea nitrogen, creatinine, glucose, and liver function tests, particularly as such patients require lifelong immunosuppression.

  f. Strict aseptic technique is required for all interventions (e.g., IV access, intubation).

  g. Monitoring. Invasive monitoring is used when dictated by the patient's cardiopulmonary status and the proposed surgical procedure. If central access is required, the right internal jugular vein should be spared, as this is the access site for endomyocardial biopsy.

  h. Anesthesia

        (1) All types of anesthesia have been administered to postcardiac transplant patients, including general, regional, and spinal anesthesia.

        (2) **Hemodynamic goals**

            (a) Maintain preload.

            (b) Avoid sudden vasodilation, as compensatory changes are dependent on the Frank-Starling effect and *not* an increase in heart rate.

            (c) If sudden hypotension occurs, administer volume and a direct-acting vasopressor such as phenylephrine or norepinephrine.

IV. Pacemakers
A. Definitions
1. **Unipolar pacing** is accomplished by placing a negative stimulating electrode within the atrium or ventricle and a positive ground electrode distant from the heart.
2. **Bipolar pacing** places both positive and negative electrodes in the chamber paced or sensed.
3. An **asynchronous generator** is a simple generator that only forms electrical impulses. It has no sensing function.
4. **Synchronous generators** have circuits for impulse formation and for sensing functions.
5. **Nomenclature.** A five-letter code describes the pacemaker. The first position designates the **chamber paced.** The second position describes the **chamber sensed.** The third position defines the **pacemaker's response** to sensed events. The fourth position details programmability, and the fifth signifies antitachycardia response. The letter O denotes none, and D is both. For example, a VVI pacemaker will pace the ventricle. If an R wave is detected, the pacemaker will inhibit and not fire. A DDD pacemaker is known as a universal, as it can sense and pace both chambers.

B. Indications
1. **Permanent.** Generally accepted indications for permanent pacemakers (PPM) include
   a. **Sinus node dysfunction**
      (1) Symptomatic bradycardia refractory to drug therapy.
      (2) Sick sinus syndrome.
   b. **Atrioventricular block (AV block)**
      (1) Complete heart block.
      (2) Type 2 second-degree AV block.
   c. **Fascicular block**
      (1) Symptomatic bifascicular block.
      (2) Trifascicular block.
2. **Temporary.** The indications are similar to those for PPM. Additional indications might include
   a. Bifascicular block and/or second-degree AV block following MI.
   b. Patients with malfunctioning PPM.
   c. Patients with severe aortic stenosis or aortic insufficiency undergoing major surgery.

C. Physiology
1. **Atrial versus ventricular pacing.** Advantages of atrial or AV pacing include
   a. Maintenance of atrial contraction, especially in patients with decreased LV compliance.
   b. Improved mitral and tricuspid valve function.
   c. Normal sequence of electrical and mechanical activation.
   d. Suppression of atrial and ventricular ectopy.
2. **Rate responsive pacemakers** have recently been developed to alter pacing rate to meet the demands of increased cardiac output. Pacemakers adjust rate

based on increased physical activity, increased minute ventilation, or other variables.

D. Preoperative evaluation of patients with PPM

1. Define symptoms requiring PPM.

2. Type of PPM (e.g., date of insertion, baseline pacing rate).

3. Current symptoms and cardiac status.

4. Pacemaker dependence—is the majority of beats paced or spontaneous?

5. Pacemaker function—it is important to evaluate an ECG or Holter monitor to determine the pacemaker's ability to sense and pace properly.

6. If central access (CVP, pulmonary artery line) is required, consideration should be made for fluoroscopy if a pacemaker has been placed within 6 weeks to avoid dislodging a lead.

E. Intraoperative management

1. The **dispersal electrode ("grounding pad")** for the electrocautery should be placed as far away from the pulse generator as possible.

2. **Monitor blood flow** during electrocautery by a precordial or esophageal stethoscope, pulse oximeter, arterial line, or a finger on the pulse.

3. A **magnet** will convert a demand (VVI) pacemaker into an asynchronous (VOO) pacemaker by placing it over the pulse generator. This is rarely necessary, as most PPM will spontaneously convert to an asynchronous mode during prolonged periods of electromagnetic interference (electrocautery).

4. **Postoperative evaluation of PPM** is indicated if significant electrocautery use occurred.

F. Perioperative pacing options

1. **Transcutaneous.** External pacing can be performed via large pads placed on the anterior and posterior thorax. This is an easy and inexpensive method of ventricular pacing.

2. **Transvenous**
   a. A temporary pacing electrode is easily inserted via a central vein into the RV.
   b. Various pulmonary artery catheters exist that have pacing options (see Chap. 10).

3. **Transesophageal.** The left atrium is easily paced through the esophagus with a pacing esophageal stethoscope.

V. The automatic internal cardioverter-defibrillator (AICD) has dramatically changed the treatment of patients at high risk for sudden death. Electrical countershock is the only reliable treatment for ventricular fibrillation. The AICD is essentially a box implanted in the abdomen connected to two defibrillating electrodes (patches), one on the right atrium or ventricle and one on the cardiac apex. A separate electrode is used for pacing and sensing. AICDs can sense ventricular tachycardia or fibrillation and deliver a countershock of 20–30 joules during up to four consecutive attempts. AICD failure during anesthesia may occur, as defibrillation thresholds may change. An external defibrillator should be available, and some advocate the placement of external defibrillation pads preoperatively. The anesthetic technique does not need to be altered, and monitoring should be guided by the underlying disease and surgical procedure. Electromagnetic interference (electrocautery) may cause inappropriate inhibition or discharge of the AICD. The pulse generator should be deactivated if electrocautery is planned. A magnet can easily deactivate the AICD and reactivate it at the conclusion of surgery. Patients with AICD devices should not enter a room with an MRI, and the devices should be deactivated prior to lithotripsy. One must be aware of potential pacemaker-AICD interaction in the presence of a tachyarrhythmia.

SUGGESTED READING

Bailey, P. L., and Stanley, T. H. Anesthesia for patients with prior cardiac transplant. *J. Cardiothorac. Anesth.* 4(Suppl. 1):38, 1990.

Barash, P. G., Cullen, B. F., and Stoelting, R. K. *Clinical Anesthesia.* Philadelphia: Lippincott, 1989.

Boucher, C. A., et al. Determination of cardiac risk by dipyridamole-thallium imaging before peripheral vascular surgery *N. Engl. J. Med.* 312:389, 1985.

Bridges, N. D., et al. Preoperative transcatheter closure of congenital muscular ventricular septal defects. *N. Engl. J. Med.* 324:1312, 1991.

Dajani, A. S., et al. Prevention of bacterial endocarditis: Recommendations by the American Heart Association. *J.A.M.A.* 264:2919, 1990.

Deutsch, N., et al. Perioperative management of the patient undergoing automatic internal cardioverter-defibrillator implantation. *J. Cardiothorac. Anesth.* 4:236, 1990.

Eagle, K. A., et al. *The Practice of Cardiology* (2nd ed.). Boston: Little, Brown, 1980.

Eagle, K. A., et al. Combining clinical and thallium data optimizes preoperative assessment of cardiac risk before major vascular surgery. *Ann. Intern. Med.* 110:859, 1989.

Goldman, L., et al. Multifactorial index of cardiac risk in noncardiac surgical procedures. *N. Engl. J. Med.* 297:845, 1977.

Hickey, P. R. Anesthesia for the Reconstructed Heart. In R. K. Stoelting (ed.), *Advances in Anesthesia.* Chicago: Year Book, 1991. Vol VII, pp. 91–113.

Kaplan, J. A. *Cardiac Anesthesia* (2nd ed). New York: Grune & Stratton, 1987.

Mangano, D. T. Perioperative cardiac morbidity. *Anesthesiology* 72:153, 1990.

Miller, R. D. *Anesthesia* (2nd ed.). New York: Churchill Livingstone, 1986.

Zaidan, J. R. Pacemakers. *Anesthesiology* 60:319, 1984.

3

Specific Considerations with Pulmonary Disease

Paul L. Epstein

I. **General considerations.** The incidence of postoperative pulmonary complications is second only to cardiovascular complications as a cause of perioperative mortality.
   A. Patients with significant chronic pulmonary disease are at greater risk for postoperative respiratory failure than the general population, since anesthesia and surgery more easily produce hypoventilation, hypoxemia, and retention of secretions in patients with limited respiratory reserve.
   B. Patients with moderate to severe chronic lung disease and those having thoracic and upper abdominal operations have a higher morbidity and mortality rate.
   C. Postoperative morbidity and mortality can be reduced by identifying patients at risk for perioperative respiratory complications, optimizing their medical therapy, and instituting a program of chest physiotherapy prior to surgery.

II. **Classification of pulmonary disease**
   A. **Obstructive airway disease** is characterized by an increase in airway resistance.
      1. **Obstructive disease states**
         a. **Emphysema** involves the destruction of alveoli and support structures, leading to loss of the normal elastic recoil of the lung with subsequent premature airway closure (collapse) at higher than normal lung volumes during exhalation. These patients often maintain normal arterial blood gases by compensatory increased minute ventilation (**"pink puffers"**). Carbon dioxide retention and hypoxemia may occur as late signs.
         b. **Chronic bronchitis** is characterized by excessive production of mucus, with subsequent narrowing of small and large airways. The most common precipitant is cigarette smoking. Blood gases in these **"blue bloaters"** may show evidence of hypercarbia and hypoxemia, with late cor pulmonale, characterized by pulmonary artery hypertension and right ventricular dysfunction.
         c. **Bronchial asthma** is characterized by reversible airway constriction resulting from a combination of airway hyperreactivity, mucous secretion, and airway edema. Known precipitants of airway hyperreactivity include cold temperature, exercise, infection, medications, and occupational exposure.
         d. **Cystic fibrosis** leads to the secretion of highly viscous mucus and abnormal sweat. This results in airway obstruction, fibrosis, and predisposition to pulmonary infection. Late changes include bron-

chiectasis with hypoxemia, carbon dioxide retention, and respiratory failure.

2. The **mechanism of hypoxemia in obstructive disease** is primarily through regional mismatching of ventilation and perfusion ($\dot{V}/\dot{Q}$ mismatch). Dyspnea, secondary to increased work of breathing, is caused by the elevated airway resistance.

B. **Restrictive pulmonary disease** is characterized by a decrease in lung compliance and may be intrinsic or extrinsic. Airway resistance is usually normal, while lung volumes are reduced.

1. **Intrinsic**

a. **Adult respiratory distress syndrome.** Pulmonary capillary membranes leak protein-rich fluid into the interstitium and alveoli. This is often associated with sepsis and hemorrhage.

b. **Aspiration pneumonitis** occurs following damage to both alveoli and capillary endothelium, classically inflicted by regurgitation of gastric contents.

c. **Pulmonary edema** occurs when fluid accumulates in the parenchymal interstitium or alveoli leading to hypoxemia. Common etiologies include cardiogenic and neurogenic pulmonary edema.

d. **Pulmonary interstitial disease** causes loss of lung elasticity and fibrosis of interstitium, alveoli, or vascular beds. The latter may lead to pulmonary hypertension and cor pulmonale. Examples include sarcoidosis, chronic hypersensitivity pneumonitis, and radiation fibrosis.

2. **Extrinsic**

a. **Pleural disease**, either fibrosis or effusion.

b. **Chest wall deformity** such as kyphoscoliosis, pectus excavatum, or burns.

c. **Diaphragmatic compression** by obesity, ascites, or pregnancy or from retraction during abdominal surgery.

3. As in obstructive disease, the primary cause of **hypoxemia** in restrictive states is $\dot{V}/\dot{Q}$ mismatch (sec. **II.A.2**). Often patients have multiple reasons for pulmonary dysfunction, as well as both mixed obstructive and restrictive defects. Proper diagnosis requires a careful history and physical examination. Pulmonary function testing may be required to differentiate obstructive from restrictive defects and can be used to assess a patient's response to therapy.

III. **Identification of the patient at risk**

A. **History**

1. The history should detail preexisting lung disease including risk factors such as: occupational exposure, wheezing, productive cough, prior hospitalizations, and medications.

2. **Chronic cough** may suggest bronchitis. If productive, sputum should be examined for evidence of acute infection and, if appropriate, sent for Gram's stain, culture, or cytology.

3. **Smoking** history should be quantitated in pack years

(number of packs smoked per day multiplied by the number of years smoked). A smoking history is directly proportional to increased risk of malignancy, chronic obstructive pulmonary disease (COPD), and postoperative pulmonary complications.

4. **Dyspnea** is the subjective sensation that ventilation is inadequate to meet demands and may be due to decreased reserve (functional residual capacity [FRC]) or increased work of breathing. The activity level should be defined; severe exertional dyspnea (occurring at minimal activity or rest) may be a predictor of both poor ventilatory reserve and the need for postoperative ventilatory support.

B. **Physical findings**

1. **Body habitus and general appearance**

   a. **Obesity, pregnancy, and kyphoscoliosis** result in reduction in lung volumes (FRC, total lung capacity) and pulmonary compliance with a predisposition toward atelectasis and hypoxemia.

   b. **Cachectic**, malnourished patients have blunted respiratory drive and decreased muscle strength and are predisposed to pneumonia.

   c. **Cyanosis** requires a minimum reduced hemoglobin concentration of 5 gm/dl. The appearance of cyanosis depends on many factors, including arterial oxygen uptake, tissue blood flow, blood volume, oxygen uptake of the tissue, and hemoglobin concentration.

2. **Respiratory signs.** Respiratory rate, pattern, diaphragmatic coordination, and the use of accessory muscles should be assessed.

   a. **Tachypnea**, a respiratory rate greater than 25 breaths/min, is usually the earliest sign of respiratory distress.

   b. **Respiratory pattern**

      (1) **Pursed-lip breathing** and **visible expiratory effort** may indicate airway obstruction.

      (2) **Accessory muscle use** increases with fatigue of the diaphragm and intercostal muscles. Important accessory muscles include the scalene and sternocleidomastoid muscles.

      (3) **Asymmetry of chest wall expansion** may result from pneumothorax, pleural effusion, lung consolidation, or unilateral phrenic nerve injury (causing an elevated hemidiaphragm).

      (4) **Tracheal deviation** may suggest mediastinal disease with tracheal compression. This may cause difficulty during intubation or airway obstruction during induction of general anesthesia.

      (5) **Inspiratory paradox.** Normally the abdominal wall should move outward with the chest wall during inspiration. Inspiratory paradox occurs when the abdomen collapses as the chest wall expands during inspiration and suggests paralysis or severe fatigue of the diaphragm.

   c. **Auscultation**

        (1) **Diminished breath sounds** may indicate local consolidation or pleural effusion.

        (2) **Rales**, usually in dependent portions, may indicate atelectasis or congestive heart failure (CHF).

        (3) **Wheezing** may indicate obstructive airway disease.

        (4) **Stridor** may indicate upper airway obstruction.

3. Cardiovascular signs

  a. Pulsus paradoxus is defined as a fall in blood pressure of greater than 10 mm Hg during inspiration. A paradoxical pulse reflects increased afterloading of the left ventricle and may be seen in COPD and pericardial tamponade.

  b. Pulmonary hypertension occurs in COPD as a result of elevated pulmonary vascular resistance. Pulmonary hypertension may lead to right atrial and right ventricular hypertrophy and eventual failure (cor pulmonale).

    (1) **Physical signs** include splitting of the second heart sound with an accentuated pulmonic component, jugular venous distention, hepatomegaly, hepatojugular reflux, and peripheral edema.

    (2) **Factors that may increase pulmonary vascular resistance** include hypoxia, hypercarbia, acidosis, sepsis, and application of positive end-expiratory pressure (PEEP).

C. Laboratory Studies

1. Chest x-ray

  a. It may show hyperinflation and increased vascular markings, characteristic of COPD.

  b. Air space disease including CHF, consolidation, atelectasis, lobar collapse (bronchial obstruction), or pneumothorax is an important predictor of $\dot{V}/\dot{Q}$ mismatch and hypoxemia.

  c. Pleural effusion, pulmonary fibrosis, and skeletal abnormalities (kyphoscoliosis, rib fractures) may predict restrictive disease states.

  d. Specific lesions including pneumothorax, emphysematous blebs, and cysts may preclude the use of nitrous oxide.

  e. Tracheal narrowing or deviation from mediastinal compression. Further workup with computed tomography (CT) scan and tomograms may be of value in detailing the precise location and degree of obstruction of tracheal/bronchial lesions.

2. Electrocardiogram. Electrocardiographic signs of significant pulmonary dysfunction include

  a. Low voltage and poor R-wave progression due to hyperinflation.

  b. Signs of pulmonary hypertension and cor pulmonale, such as

    (1) Right-axis deviation.

    (2) P pulmonale (P waves greater than 2.5 mm in height).

(3) Right ventricular hypertrophy.

(4) Right bundle branch block.

3. Arterial blood gases

a. Partial pressure of oxygen (PaO$_2$). Hypoxemia is considered severe when PAO$_2$ is less than 60 mm Hg on room air. Patients with severe hypoxemia have significant pulmonary dysfunction and are at increased risk for postoperative pulmonary complications.

b. Partial pressure of carbon dioxide (PaCO$_2$). Hypercarbia occurs when PaCO$_2$ is greater than 45 mm Hg. Patients who are **carbon dioxide retainers** have end-stage lung disease with little or no reserve and are at increased risk for postoperative pulmonary complications.

c. pH in conjunction with PaCO$_2$ allows determination of acid-base disturbances.

4. Pulmonary function tests measure pulmonary mechanics and functional reserve and provide an objective assessment of lung function. They may help to

a. Predict the risk of postoperative pulmonary complications.

b. Predict the need for postoperative ventilatory support.

c. Evaluate the clinical response to therapy such as preoperative bronchodilators.

d. Estimate residual lung function following pulmonary resection, as measured by split-function studies (which quantitate dysfunction in both the right and left lung).

e. Define the nature of pulmonary disease as being either obstructive, restrictive, or mixed.

IV. Effects of anesthesia and surgery on pulmonary function. General anesthesia decreases lung volumes and promotes mismatching of pulmonary ventilation and perfusion. Many anesthetic drugs blunt the ventilatory response to hypercarbia and hypoxia. Postoperatively, atelectasis and hypoxemia commonly result, especially in patients with preexisting pulmonary disease. Pulmonary function is further compromised by postoperative pain, which can limit coughing and lung expansion.

A. Respiratory mechanics and gas exchange

1. General anesthesia and the supine position decrease FRC. Atelectasis occurs when lung volumes during tidal breathing fall below the volume at which airway closure occurs (closing capacity). Positive-pressure ventilation with large tidal volumes and PEEP can minimize this effect.

2. Positive-pressure ventilation compared to spontaneous breathing leads to $\dot{V}/\dot{Q}$ mismatching. During positive-pressure ventilation, nondependent portions of the lung receive a greater proportion of ventilation than do dependent portions. The distribution of pulmonary blood flow is determined by gravity, as blood flow tends to be increased in dependent portions of the lung. The end result is a variable increase in both physiologic dead space and shunt compared to spontaneous ventilation.

3. **Diaphragmatic dysfunction.** In the supine position, the diaphragm is displaced cephalad by abdominal contents. The addition of general anesthesia, muscle paralysis, and positive-pressure ventilation alters diaphragmatic motion, causing nondependent portions of the diaphragm to move more than dependent portions (the opposite of the case during spontaneous ventilation). These changes may further alter the distribution of ventilation and perfusion within the lungs.

B. **Regulation of breathing**

1. The ventilatory response to **hypercarbia** is reduced by inhalation anesthetics, barbiturates, and opioids. Carbon dioxide tension ($PaCO_2$) is elevated with spontaneous ventilation during general anesthesia, as is the apneic threshold (the $PaCO_2$ at which patients hyperventilated to apnea resume spontaneous ventilation).

2. The ventilatory response to **hypoxia** may also be blunted by inhalation anesthetics, barbiturates, and opioids. This effect may be particularly important in patients with severe chronic lung disease who normally retain carbon dioxide and depend on a hypoxic drive for ventilation.

C. **Effect of surgery.** Postoperative pulmonary function is affected by the site of surgery. The ability to cough is reduced after abdominal operations compared with peripheral procedures and appears related to the pain produced by coughing. Vital capacity is reduced by 75% after upper abdominal procedures and by approximately 50% after lower abdominal or thoracic operations. Recovery of normal pulmonary function may take several weeks. Peripheral procedures have little impact on vital capacity or the ability to clear secretions.

D. **Effect on ciliary function.** The upper respiratory tract normally warms and humidifies inspired air, providing an ideal environment for normal function of respiratory tract cilia and mucus. General anesthesia, often conducted with unhumidified gases at high flow rates, dries secretions and can easily damage respiratory epithelium. Endotracheal intubation exacerbates this problem by bypassing the nasopharynx. Secretions become thickened, ciliary function is reduced, and the patient's resistance to pulmonary infections is decreased. These problems may be partially prevented by lowering fresh gas flows and including a heated humidifier in the anesthesia circuit.

V. **Preoperative treatment in pulmonary disease.** The goals of preoperative treatment are to improve those aspects of disease that may be reversible.

A. **Cessation of smoking** for 24–48 hours prior to surgery may reduce carboxyhemoglobin levels, promoting better tissue oxygen transport via shift of the oxyhemoglobin dissociation curve to the right. Cessation of smoking for greater than 4 weeks may reduce the risk of postoperative pulmonary complications by improving ciliary function and reducing airway secretions and irritability.

B. Acute infection should be treated prior to elective surgery. Therapy is guided by sputum Gram's stain and culture.

C. Hydration and humidification of inspired gases will aid clearance of bronchial secretions.

D. Chest physiotherapy (voluntary deep breathing, coughing, incentive spirometry, and chest percussion and vibration combined with postural drainage) will improve mobilization of secretions and increase lung volumes, reducing the incidence of postoperative pulmonary complications.

E. Medical treatment

1. **Sympathomimetics**, or beta-agonist drugs, cause bronchodilation via cyclic adenosine monophosphate (cAMP)–mediated relaxation of bronchial smooth muscle.

   a. **Drugs with mixed beta-1 and beta-2 effects** include epinephrine (Adrenalin), isoproterenol (Isuprel), and isoetharine (Bronkosol). The tachycardia and arrhythmogenic potential of these drugs, notably epinephrine and isoproterenol, is of concern in patients with cardiac disease.

   b. **Drugs with beta-2 selectivity include** albuterol (Ventolin), terbutaline (Brethine), and metaproterenol (Alupent) and are less prone to beta-1-mediated cardiac effects. These agents are most commonly administered by inhalation.

2. **Phosphodiesterase inhibitors** (e.g., theophylline).

   a. These cause bronchodilation by increasing the intracellular concentration of cAMP through inhibition of the enzyme phosphodiesterase.

   b. Many patients with bronchial **asthma or COPD** receive chronic therapy with oral theophylline, usually with doses of 300–1500 mg/day. Serum theophylline levels should be checked and dosage adjusted to keep levels to 10–20 µg/dl. These medications should be continued to the morning of surgery.

   c. Patients who experience an **acute exacerbation** or who will **remain NPO for an extended period** should receive IV aminophylline (a soluble ethylene diamine salt containing 85% theophylline by weight). For patients already on theophylline, an infusion rate may be estimated based on the patient's total daily requirement, divided by 24 (divided again by 0.85, since theophylline = 0.85 × aminophylline). For patients not currently taking theophylline, a loading dose of 5–6 mg/kg IV may be given over 20 minutes followed by infusion rates of 0.5–0.9 mg/kg/hr. Smokers and adolescents may require higher doses, reflecting rapid metabolism. Patients who are elderly, have CHF or liver disease, or are taking cimetidine, propranolol, or erythromycin should receive reduced doses, reflecting slower aminophylline metabolism.

 d. Signs of toxicity occur frequently when drug levels exceed 20 µg/ml and include nausea, vomiting, headache, anxiety, tachycardia, arrhythmias, and seizures.

3. Corticosteroids are often used in patients not responding to theophylline and beta-adrenergic agonists. Their therapeutic effect may take up to 12 hours, and their mechanism of action is believed to be a reduction of mucosal edema and membrane stabilization of mast cells with reduction of histamine release.

 a. Commonly used drugs include **hydrocortisone** (Solu-Cortef), 100 mg IV q8h, and **methylprednisolone** (Solu-Medrol), 40–50 mg IV q4–6h. Regimens are usually tapered in dose, frequency, and route of administration as dictated by clinical response.

 b. Steroids may also be administered by inhalation (e.g., beclomethasone) with decreased systemic effects.

4. Cromolyn sodium is an inhaled medication used as prophylactic therapy for asthma. Its mechanism of action is mast cell membrane stabilization, inhibiting the IgE-mediated release of histamine and leukotrienes (which are both bronchoconstrictors). It is of no utility in the acute treatment of bronchospasm.

5. Parasympatholytics. Anticholinergics such as atropine and glycopyrrolate may have a direct bronchodilating effect by blocking formation of cyclic guanine monophosphate (cGMP) and may improve forced expiratory volume (FEV_1) in patients with COPD when administered by inhalation. Specific agents include

 a. Atropine sulfate, which has considerable systemic absorption, causing tachycardia and thus limiting usefulness.

 b. Glycopyrrolate (0.4–0.8 mg by nebulizer).

 c. Ipratropium bromide (Atrovent, 2 puffs q6h, metered dose inhaler).

6. Mucolytics

 a. Acetylcysteine (Mucomyst), administered by nebulizer, decreases the viscosity of mucus by breaking the disulfide bonds in mucoproteins. Acetylcysteine is an airway irritant and should be preceded by a bronchodilator (beta-adrenergic agonist) to minimize bronchospasm.

 b. Hypertonic saline has also been used to decrease mucus viscosity. When given by nebulizer, an osmotic shift of water to mucus enhances mucus volume and promotes clearance. Hypertonic saline, like acetylcysteine, may increase airway resistance.

VI. Premedication. The goals of premedication are to allay anxiety and to facilitate smooth induction of anesthesia.

A. Oxygen therapy, if required preoperatively, should be continued during transport to the operating room and clearly written as a preoperative "order." Consider starting oxygen (i.e., 2 L/min by nasal cannula) if the patient has marginal reserve.

B. If the patient is taking **inhaled beta sympathomimetics or corticosteroids**, these should accompany the patient to the operation room.

C. **Anticholinergics are rarely indicated.** Parenteral administration will not cause bronchodilation but will cause drying of secretions, increasing viscosity of mucus.

D. **H_2 antagonists (cimetidine, ranitidine)** may exacerbate bronchospasm in patients with asthma, as blockage of H_2 receptors may result in unopposed H_1-mediated bronchoconstriction.

E. **Benzodiazepines** are effective anxiolytics but may cause excessive sedation and respiratory depression in compromised patients.

F. **Narcotics** provide analgesia as well as sedation but must be carefully titrated to avoid respiratory depression. In patients with severe pulmonary dysfunction, narcotics are best avoided.

VII. **Anesthetic technique**

A. **Regional anesthesia**, including peripheral nerve blockade or local anesthesia, may be the best choice of anesthetic for patients with pulmonary disease when the site of operation is peripheral, such as eye or extremity procedures.

B. **Spinal or epidural anesthesia** is a reasonable choice for lower extremity surgery. Patients with severe COPD depend on accessory muscle use, including intercostals for inspiration and abdominal muscles for forced exhalation. Spinal anesthesia may be deleterious if motor blockade decreases FRC, reduces a patient's ability to cough and clear secretions, or precipitates respiratory insufficiency or failure. Combined epidural and general anesthetic techniques ensure airway control, provide adequate ventilation, and prevent hypoxemia and atelectasis. Prolonged peripheral procedures are probably best performed with a general anesthetic.

C. **General anesthesia** is indicated for upper abdominal and thoracic procedures, although combined general and epidural anesthesia is often provided. Inhalation agents provide bronchodilation as well as an adequate depth of anesthesia to decrease the hyperreactivity of sensitive airways.

VIII. **Postoperative care.** All patients who are identified as high risk should be admitted to a monitored postoperative unit where chest physiotherapy and suctioning can be performed. The possibility of ventilatory support should be anticipated and discussed with the patient. Postoperative pain management is critical to decreasing respiratory complications.

SUGGESTED READING

Bowe, E. A., and Llein, E. F., Jr. Acid Base, Blood Gas, Electrolytes. In P. G. Barash, B. Cullen, and R. K. Stoelting (eds.), *Clinical Anesthesia.* Philadelphia: Lippincott, 1989. Pp. 669–685.

Eisenkraft, J. B., Cohen, E., and Kaplan, J. A. Anesthesia for Thoracic Surgery. In P. G. Barash, B. Cullen, and R. K. Stoelting (eds.), *Clinical Anesthesia*. Philadelphia: Lippincott, 1989. Pp. 905–942.

Harrison, R. A. Respiratory Function and Anesthesia. In P. G. Barash, B. Cullen, and R. K. Stoelting (eds.), *Clinical Anesthesia*. Philadelphia: Lippincott, 1989. Pp. 877–902.

Stoelting, R. K., Dierdorf, S. F., and McCammon, R. L. Obstructive Airways Disease. In R. K. Stoelting, S. F. Dierdorf, and R. L. McCammon (eds.), *Anesthesia and Co-existing Disease*. New York: Churchill Livingstone, 1988. Pp. 195–223.

Stoelting, R. K., Dierdorf, S. F., and McCammon, R. L. Restrictive Pulmonary Disease. In R. K. Stoelting, S. F. Dierdorf, and R. L. McCammon (eds.), *Anesthesia and Co-existing Disease*. New York: Churchill Livingstone, 1988. Pp. 227–233.

West, J. B. *Respiratory Physiology—The Essential*. Baltimore: Williams & Wilkins, 1990.

4

Specific Considerations with Renal Disease

Peter G. Kovatsis

I. **Normal renal physiology**
   A. **The primary role of the kidney** is to maintain the volume, composition, and distribution of body fluids and excrete toxic materials. This is accomplished by the following:
      1. **Renin-angiotensin-aldosterone (RAA) system.** The kidney secretes renin in response to renal hypoperfusion, volume depletion (i.e., decreased Na^+), and increased sympathetic activity. Renin cleaves angiotensinogen to form **angiotensin I**, which is then converted to **angiotensin II** in the lung by angiotensin converting enzyme.
         a. **Angiotensin II** produces arteriolar vasoconstriction and stimulates aldosterone release.
         b. **Aldosterone** is a mineralocorticoid released by the adrenal cortex in response to angiotensin II, increased K^+ levels, decreased Na^+ content, and adrenocorticotropic hormone. Aldosterone acts on the distal tubule to increase the resorption of Na^+ in exchange for K^+ and H^+.
      2. **Antidiuretic hormone (ADH)** is released by the posterior pituitary gland in response to increased osmolality, decreased extracellular volume, positive-pressure ventilation, or surgical stimuli. ADH acts to increase the permeability of the collecting duct to water. Thus, ADH conserves water and concentrates the urine.
      3. **Atrial natriuretic factor (ANF)** is released by specialized atrial cells in response to atrial distention (i.e., increased intravascular volume). ANF causes a diuresis and acts to counter the RAA system.
      4. **Prostaglandins** (PGE_2, PGI_2) and **kinins** are stimulated by renin release and stress. They cause renal vasodilation and decreased Na^+ absorption.
   B. **Secondary roles of the kidney** include extrarenal regulatory and metabolic functions.
      1. **Erythropoietin** is produced to stimulate red blood cell production.
      2. **Vitamin D** is converted to its most active form.
      3. **Parathyroid hormone** acts on the kidney to conserve Ca^{2+}, inhibit PO_4^{2-} resorption, and increase conversion of vitamin D by the kidney.
      4. **Peptides** and **protein hormones** such as insulin are metabolized, accounting for the generally decreased insulin requirements as renal failure progresses.
   C. **Renal blood flow** represents 20–25% of cardiac output and is autoregulated over a wide range of mean arterial blood pressure (70–180 mm Hg).

II. **Fluids and electrolytes**

A. Fluid compartments
   1. Total body water (TBW) equals 60% of body weight.
      a. Two-thirds of TBW is intracellular fluid.
      b. One-third of TBW is extracellular fluid. Approximately two-thirds of extracellular fluid is interstitial, and one-third is intravascular.
   2. TBW is proportional to lean body mass.
B. Normal fluid balance
   1. Daily water intake is approximately 2600 ml: 1400 ml in liquids, 800 ml in solid food, and 400 ml from metabolism.
   2. Daily water loss is normally the same: 1500 ml in urine, 400 ml from respiration, 500 ml from skin evaporation, and 200 ml in stool.
   3. Losses will be increased by fever (about 500 ml/°C/day), sweating, low humidity, solute diuresis as with hyperglycemia and contrast dyes, drug therapy, bowel preparations, and adrenal disease.
C. Electrolyte disorders
   1. **Hyponatremia** (increased TBW relative to Na^+).
      a. TBW may be low, high, or normal.
      b. Hyponatremia often results in **reduced plasma osmolality.** This is calculated by the following formula:

$$Osmolality\ (mOsm) = 2[Na^+\ (mEq/L)] + K^+\ (mEq/L)]$$
$$+ \frac{urea\ (mg\%)}{2.8} + \frac{glucose\ (mg\%)}{18}$$

If larger concentrations of osmotically active substances (glucose, urea, mannitol, methyl alcohol) are present, measured osmolality will be high despite low serum Na^+.
      c. Clinical features. Symptoms not only reflect underlying volume status but also include malaise, headache, and lethargy progressing to seizures and coma. Hyponatremia causes decreased cell excitability, decreased cardiac function, and arrhythmias, and symptoms are more likely if Na^+ is less than 120 mEq/L or there is a rapid decrease in concentration.
      d. Treatment relies on determining the volume status of the patient.
         (1) Hypovolemic patients (e.g., secondary to diuretics, vomiting, or bowel preparations) should have their intravascular volume repleted with isotonic crystalloid solutions.
         (2) Hypervolemic patients (e.g., secondary to renal failure, congestive heart failure, cirrhosis, nephrotic syndrome) should have their free water intake restricted and undergo gentle diuresis.
         (3) Normovolemic patients (e.g., secondary to syndrome of inappropriate ADH secretion, hypothyroidism, drugs that impair renal water excre-

tion, water intoxication) should have their free water intake restricted and undergo diuresis with replacement of urinary Na^+ and K^+ losses. Hypertonic saline (3% NaCl) or mannitol should be reserved for emergency management of severe central nervous system (CNS) or cardiac symptoms. Both must be used cautiously to prevent circulatory overload.

(4) Acute normalization of the serum Na^+ is not necessary, since most symptoms are relieved by raising the concentration to 125 mEq/L.

2. **Hypernatremia** (decreased TBW relative to Na^+).

   a. **TBW** may be low, high, or normal.

   b. **Clinical features** include tremulousness, weakness, irritability, and mental confusion progressing to seizures and coma.

   c. **Treatment** relies on determining the volume status of the patient.

   (1) **Hypovolemic patients,** secondary to water loss exceeding Na^+ loss (diarrhea, vomiting, osmotic diuresis) or inadequate water intake (impaired thirst mechanism, altered mental status).

   (a) If hemodynamic instability or evidence of hypoperfusion is present, initial volume therapy should consist of 0.45% or even 0.9% NaCl.

   (b) After volume replenishment, the remaining free water deficit should be replaced with 5% dextrose until the Na^+ concentration decreases, and 0.45% saline may then be administered.

   (2) **Hypervolemic patients,** secondary to Na^+ overload from mineralocorticoid excess, dialysis with hypertonic solutions, and treatment with hypertonic saline or sodium bicarbonate ($NaHCO_3$).

   (a) The excess total body Na^+ (i.e., volume) may be removed by dialysis or with diuretic therapy and the water deficit replaced with 5% dextrose in water (5% D/W) as estimated by the following formula:

   $$Normal\ TBW\ (L) = 0.6 \times body\ weight\ (kg)$$

   $$\frac{Normal\ serum\ Na^+}{Current\ serum\ Na^+} \times TBW = current\ TBW$$

   $$H_2O\ deficit = normal\ TBW - current\ TBW$$

   (b) The deficit should be replaced slowly, especially in chronic cases, to avoid cerebral edema and seizures. Normally, half of this deficit is replaced in the first 24 hours and the remaining deficit in the next 24–48 hours. As treatment progresses, it should be guided by serial determinations of Na^+.

   (3) **Normovolemic patients,** secondary to diabetes

insipidus. Therapy consists of treating the underlying etiology, correction of free water deficit with 5% D/W, and the use of exogenous vasopressin in neurogenic diabetes insipidus (see Chap. 6).

3. Hypokalemia

   a. Etiologies

     (1) Total body K^+ deficit.

     (2) Shifts in the distribution of K^+ (extracellular to intracellular).

   b. Serum K^+ is a poor index of total body potassium stores, as 98% of body potassium is located intracellularly. Thus, large K^+ deficits must be present prior to seeing a decrease in serum K^+. In a 70-kg man with normal pH, a fall in serum K^+ from 4 to 3 mEq/L reflects a deficit of 100–200 mEq. Below 3 mEq/L, each fall of 1 mEq/L reflects an additional deficit of 200–400 mEq.

   c. Sources of K^+ loss include:

     (1) Gastrointestinal tract (vomiting, diarrhea, or obstructed ileal loops).

     (2) Kidney (diuretics, mineralocorticoid and glucocorticoid excess, renal tubular acidosis).

   d. Changes in K^+ distribution occur with alkalosis, as H^+ shifts to the extracellular fluid and K^+ moves intracellularly. Thus, rapid correction of acidosis, as by artificial ventilation or $NaHCO_3$ administration, may produce fatal hypokalemia.

   e. Clinical features rarely appear until K^+ is less than 3 mEq/L or the rate of fall is rapid.

     (1) **Signs** include weakness, augmentation of neuromuscular block, ileus, and disturbances of cardiac contractility.

     (2) **Electrocardiographic (ECG) changes** include flattened T waves, U waves, increased P–R and Q–T intervals, ST-segment depression, and atrial and ventricular dysrhythmias. Ventricular ectopy is more likely with concomitant digitalis therapy.

     (3) Serum K^+ less than 2.0 mEq/L is associated with vasoconstriction and rhabdomyolysis.

   f. Treatment consists of managing the underlying etiology and K^+ supplementation (0.2 mEq/kg/hr IV). There is no need to correct chronic hypokalemia ($K^+ \geq 2.5$ mEq/L) prior to induction of anesthesia. Rapid replacement of K^+ may cause more problems than hypokalemia itself. Intraoperatively, avoidance of hyperventilation would be prudent. Hypokalemic-induced conduction disturbances or diminished contractility are treated with K^+ (0.5–1.0 mEq IV q3–5 min) until resolution. Serum K^+ must be closely followed.

4. Hyperkalemia

   a. Etiologies

     (1) Decreased excretion (renal failure, hypoaldosteronism).

(2) **Extracellular shift** (acidosis, ischemia, rhabdomyolysis, and drugs such as succinylcholine).

(3) Administration of blood, potassium penicillins, and salt substitutes to renal failure patients.

(4) Artifactual elevation is seen with hemolysis.

b. **Clinical features** are more likely with acute changes than with chronic elevation.

(1) **Signs and symptoms** include muscle weakness, paresthesias, and cardiac conduction abnormalities, which become dangerous as K^+ levels approach 7 mEq/L. Bradycardia, ventricular fibrillation, and cardiac arrest may result.

(2) **ECG findings** include high peaked T waves, ST-segment depression, prolonged P–R interval, loss of the P wave, diminished R-wave amplitude, QRS widening, and prolonged Q–T interval.

c. **Treatment** depends on the nature of ECG changes and serum levels.

(1) ECG changes are treated with slow IV administration of 0.5–1.0 gm of calcium chloride ($CaCl_2$). The dose may be repeated in 5 minutes if changes persist.

(2) $NaHCO_3$ shifts K^+ intracellularly, and 50 mEq may be given IV over 5 minutes, with a repeated dose in 10–15 minutes. Hyperventilation will cause an intracellular shift of K^+.

(3) Glucose and insulin also shift K^+ intracellularly. Regular insulin (10 units) is given IV simultaneously with 25 gm of glucose (1 ampule of a 50% solution) over 5 minutes.

(4) The above therapies are short-term measures to decrease K^+ via cellular shifts. Cation exchange resins (sodium polystyrene sulfonate [Kayexalate], 50 gm with sorbitol) will slowly remove K^+ from the body and should be employed as soon as possible. Serum K^+ can also be lowered by dialysis.

III. Renal failure

A. **Acute renal failure (ARF)** is a sudden decrease in renal function characterized by anuric, oliguric (< 20 ml/hr), or nonoliguric states. Mortality in ARF is significant, being greater than 50% in surgical and trauma patients.

1. **Etiologies**

a. **Prerenal** (e.g., volume contraction, low cardiac output). Early correction of the underlying cause usually results in rapid reversal of renal dysfunction, but continued renal hypoperfusion may result in intrinsic renal damage.

b. **Intrarenal** (e.g., acute tubular necrosis) secondary to prerenal causes or drugs, renovascular disease, acute glomerulonephritis, or acute interstitial nephritis.

c. **Postrenal** (e.g., obstructive uropathy) due to renal calculi, thrombi, or prostatic disease (Table 4-1).

2. **Clinical features**

a. **Hypervolemia** due to impaired ability to excrete

Table 4-1. Urine and serum diagnostic indexes

	Prerenal	Renal	Postrenal
Urine (Na)	<10 mEq/L	>20 mEq/L	> 20 mEq/L
Urine (CL)	<10 mEq/L	>20 mEq/L	
FEna	<1%	>2%	>2%
Urine osmolarity	>500	<350	<350
Urine/serum (creatinine)	>40	<20	<20
Renal failure index (RFI)	<1%	>2%	>2%
Urine/serum (urea)	>8	<3	<3
Serum (BUN) /creatinine	>20	=10	=10

FEna = (Una/Pna) ÷ (Ucr/Pcr) × 100.
RFI = Una ÷ (Ucr/Pcr).
FEna = fractional excretion of sodium.
RFI = renal failure index.
Una = urine concentration of sodium.
Pna = plasma concentration of sodium.
Ucr = urine concentration of creatinine.
Pcr = plasma concentration of creatinine.

water and Na^+ with resultant hypertension and peripheral edema.
   - **b.** Potential **hypovolemia** due to lack of urine concentrating ability.
   - **c.** K^+ **retention.**
   - **d.** **Impaired excretion** of drugs and toxins.
   - **e.** **Potential progression** to chronic renal failure.
- **B. Chronic renal failure (CRF)** is characterized by a permanent decrease in glomerular filtration rate (GFR) with a rise in serum creatinine and azotemia. Patients may be well compensated until late in the course of CRF.
   1. **Etiologies.** Common causes are hypertension, diabetes mellitus, chronic glomerulonephritis, tubulointerstitial disease, renovascular disease, and polycystic kidney disease.
   2. **Clinical features**
      - **a.** **Hypervolemia** and **hypertension,** ultimately resulting in CHF and edema.
      - **b.** **Accelerated atherosclerosis,** which may increase the risk of coronary artery disease.
      - **c.** **Uremic pericarditis** and **pericardial** effusions.
      - **d.** **Hyperkalemia, hypermagnesemia,** and **hyponatremia** may also occur.
      - **e.** **Hypocalcemia** and **hyperphosphatemia** due to elevated parathyroid hormone, resulting in renal osteodystrophy.
      - **f.** **Metabolic acidosis** due to the inability to excrete endogenously produced acid.
      - **g.** **Chronic anemia** secondary to decreased erythropoietin production and decreased red blood cell survival, which is relatively well tolerated since it parallels the slow decline in renal function.

h. **Prolonged bleeding time** due to decreased platelet adhesiveness.

i. **Increased gastric volume, acid production,** and **delayed gastric emptying** and an increased incidence of nausea, vomiting, and peptic ulceration.

j. **Increased susceptibility to infection** even in the absence of immunosuppressive therapy.

k. **CNS changes** varying from mild changes in mentation to severe encephalopathy and coma. Peripheral and autonomic neuropathies are common.

l. **Glucose intolerance,** type IV hyperlipidemia, and abnormal thyroid function tests.

m. **Altered pharmacodynamics** of most drugs due to changes in compartment volumes, electrolytes, pH, total protein, and rates of excretion.

C. **Dialysis** is indicated in ARF and CRF for hyperkalemia, acidosis, volume overload, uremic complications (pericarditis, tamponade, encephalopathy), and severe azotemia.

1. **Hemodialysis** uses an artificial semipermeable membrane that separates the patient's blood from dialysate and allows for the exchange of solutes by diffusion. It requires vascular access via either a central venous Quinton catheter or via a surgically created arteriovenous (AV) fistula in the arm or leg and systemic or regional anticoagulation. Hemodialysis is typically performed 2 or 3 times a week, and serum electrolyte and volume abnormalities are corrected by adjusting the dialysis bath fluid. Blood samples taken immediately after dialysis will be inaccurate, as redistribution of fluid and electrolytes takes about 6 hours. Complications include AV fistula infection or thrombosis, dialysis disequilibrium or dementia, hypotension, pericarditis, and hypoxemia.

2. **Ultrafiltration** and **hemofiltration** allow for the removal of volume with minimal removal of waste products. These techniques are useful in volume-overloaded patients. As with standard hemodialysis, anticoagulation is required.

a. **Ultrafiltration** utilizes hemodialysis equipment to employ a hydrostatic driving force across the membrane without a dialysate on the opposing side. Thus, an ultrafiltrate of serum is removed. If large volumes of fluid are removed rapidly, hypotension may ensue.

b. **Hemofiltration** (continuous arteriovenous hemofiltration) uses a highly permeable membrane and the patient's own systemic arterial pressure to remove an ultrafiltrate. Fluid is removed more slowly than with ultrafiltration and is useful for patients unable to tolerate rapid volume shifts.

3. **Peritoneal dialysis** uses the capillaries of the peritoneum as a semipermeable exchange membrane with the dialysate infused into the peritoneal cavity via an indwelling peritoneal catheter. Peritoneal dialysis may be used acutely in ARF or chronically. Advantages

over hemodialysis include less hypotension or disequilibrium and no need for heparinization. However,
peritoneal dialysis is less efficient and limited in catabolic states when compared to hemodialysis. Complications include infection, hyperglycemia from the dextran in the dialysate, and increased protein loss into
the dialysate.

D. **Specific causes of renal failure.** An understanding of
the pathophysiology and other systemic manifestations of
renal failure is important to achieve optimal patient
management.

   1. **Acute glomerulonephritis** is caused by inflammation
   of the glomerulus, usually due to deposition of antigen-
   antibody complexes. It usually presents as acute nephrotic syndrome, characterized by hematuria, proteinuria, hypertension, and edema. Serious complications
   include hypertension, encephalopathy, heart failure,
   and progression to renal failure. Etiologies are varied,
   including postinfection and collagen vascular disease.

   2. **Nephrotic syndrome** is defined as massive proteinuria (> 3.5 gm/day), hypoalbuminemia, hyperlipidemia, and edema. Anesthetic issues include intravascular volume depletion with decreased oncotic
   pressure, increased risk of infection, increased risk of
   atherosclerosis, and a potentially hypercoagulable
   state. Therapy with diuretics and corticosteroids is
   common. There are multiple etiologies for this syndrome, including diabetes mellitus, systemic lupus
   erythematosus (SLE), and toxemia of pregnancy.

   3. **Diabetes mellitus** commonly involves the kidney, particularly in type I diabetes of greater than 10 years'
   duration. Renal disease usually presents with proteinuria that becomes progressively worse, culminating
   in nephrotic syndrome. CRF usually follows the onset of
   proteinuria within 5 years. Renal disease may also manifest as type IV renal tubular acidosis (hyporeninemic
   hypoaldosteronism). There is a strong correlation between renal dysfunction and diabetic neuropathy.

   4. **Connective tissue diseases** such as SLE, rheumatoid
   arthritis, and periarteritis nodosa can involve the
   kidney and progress to renal failure.

   5. **Tubulointerstitial diseases** primarily affect the renal
   tubules and interstitium, resulting in interstitial inflammation. Secondary glomerular changes may also
   be seen. Involvement of the proximal convoluted tubule
   may result in HCO_3^- wasting and acidosis, or wasting
   of organic acids, PO_4, amino acids, and glucose, as in
   Fanconi's syndrome. Involvement of the loop of Henle
   and medulla will affect concentrating ability. Involvement of the distal convolutional tubule and collecting
   duct will cause loss of acid secretion, acidemia, salt
   wasting, and decreased ability to excrete K^+ with
   resultant hyperkalemia. Thus, tubulointerstitial diseases may present with alterations in osmotic balance,
   acid-base balance, volume homeostasis, and metabolic
   and mineral homeostasis. There are many possible

etiologies (radiation, heavy metals, nephrocalcinosis, multiple myeloma, immune disorders, and hyperuricemia). The more common causes are pyelonephritis, hypersensitivity nephritis (interstitial nephritis), and polycystic kidney disease.

    a. Pyelonephritis is an acute or chronic infection of the kidney that is due to retrograde infection of the urinary tract by gram-negative bacteria.

        (1) The acute form is characterized by flank pain, fever, dysuria, and symptoms of cystitis. Presentation may mimic an acute abdomen. Renal impairment is often not present acutely, but medullary dysfunction may occur as well as prerenal ARF from dehydration and volume depletion. Complications include papillary necrosis, pyelonephrosis, and perinephric abscess.

        (2) The chronic form can be confused with renal ischemia, chronic interstitial nephritis, radiation injury, and obstruction. There is early impairment of urinary concentrating ability with K^+ wasting.

        (3) Deranged fluid balance and hypovolemia are seen in both forms.

    b. Hypersensitivity nephritis is an allergic reaction to drugs, which affects the renal interstitium. A classic example is methicillin-induced interstitial nephritis. Common causes include penicillins, cephalosporins, sulfonamides, and diuretics. Clinical manifestations include fever, urine and peripheral eosinophilia, and rash. Proteinuria, concentrating defects, and hypertension are common findings. Treatment includes corticosteroids.

    c. Adult polycystic kidney disease is inherited as an autosomal dominant disease. Approximately 25% of patients by age 50 and 50% by age 75 will have end-stage renal disease. Early manifestations include concentration deficits, hematuria, proteinuria, and mild hypertension. These diseases normally do not present until 20–25 years of age. Cysts may be found in the liver or CNS (intracranial aneurysm).

IV. Pharmacology and the kidney

    A. Diuretics are used to increase urine output (Table 4-2), treat hypertension, and manage electrolyte, fluid, and acid-base disturbances.

    B. Dopamine. At a dosage of 1–4 µg/kg/min, dopamine will increase renal blood flow, GFR, and Na^+ excretion. These effects are mediated by dopaminergic receptors that preferentially reduce regional arterial resistance of the kidney (mesenteric dilation also occurs). Dopamine is used widely as an adjunct to maintain or improve renal function or treat ARF. In the clinical setting, the renal effects of dopamine may be overridden by other physiologic processes such as the RAA system, therefore limiting dopamine's clinical benefit. Additional physiologic effects include inotropy, chronotropy (at dosages of 4–10 µg/kg/min), and vasoconstriction (> 10 µg/kg/min).

Table 4-2. Diuretics

	Primary site of action	Primary effect	Side effects	Comments
Nonosmotic				
Loop (Lasix, edecrin, bumex)	Thick ascending loop of Henle, active Na^+Cl^- pump	Moderate to severe naturesis, chloruresis	Hypokalemia, alkalosis, volume contraction	Interferes with both urinary concentration and dilution
Thiazides (Diuril, dyazide, metolazone)	Distal tubules (Na^+-H^+, Na^+-K^+ exchange)	Mild to moderate naturesis	Hyponatremia, hypokalemia, alkalosis, volume contraction	Interferes with urinary dilution, tends to be ineffective in renal failure and CHF
Carbonic anhydrase inhibitors, acetazolamide (Diamox)	Proximal tubule Na^+-H^+ exchange	Mild naturesis	Hyperchloremia, hypokalemia	Used primarily for ophthalmology; self limiting renal effect
Potassium sparing (aldactone, triamterene, amiloride)	Collecting duct, Na^+-K^+, Na^+-H^+ exchange	Mild to moderate naturesis	Hyperkalemia	Used in conjunction with K^+ losing diuretics or in hyperaldosterone states
Osmotic				
Mannitol	Intratubular osmotic load	Moderate to severe diuresis	Early: vasodilation, volume expansion Late: Hyperosmolality, volume contraction	Draws intracellular fluid into intravascular space

C. **Anesthetic effects on the kidney.** Patients with normal kidneys experience transient postanesthetic alterations in renal function. These alterations may occur despite insignificant changes in blood pressure and cardiac output, suggesting that changes in intrarenal distribution of blood flow are responsible.

1. **Indirect effects.** Halothane, enflurane, isoflurane, and thiopental may cause myocardial depression, hypotension, and a mild to moderate increase in renal vascular resistance, leading to a decrease of renal blood flow and GFR. Compensatory catecholamine secretion causes redistribution of renal cortical blood flow. ADH levels do not change during halothane or morphine anesthesia but increase with the onset of surgical stimulation. Hydration before the induction of anesthesia attenuates the rise in ADH produced by painful stimuli. Spinal and epidural anesthesia produce decreases in renal blood flow, GFR, and urine output.

2. **Direct effects.** The direct toxicity of fluorinated agents is of concern, since fluoride (F^-) inhibits metabolic processes, affects urine concentrating ability, and can cause proximal tubular swelling and necrosis. The magnitude of serum F^- elevation is concentration and duration dependent. Levels above 50 $\mu M/L$ are associated with detectable renal dysfunction.

   a. **Methoxyflurane** is no longer in use because of its fluoride-induced nephrotoxicity.

   b. Only 2% of absorbed **enflurane** is metabolized to fluoride ion, thus producing low levels of F^- (typically < 15 $\mu M/L$). There is a theoretic concern that use of enflurane in patients with renal dysfunction may lead to F^- accumulation and additional nephrotoxicity.

   c. **Isoflurane** is not associated with significant release of F^-.

   d. **Halothane** has a different structure and metabolism and results in the lowest F^- level.

3. With brief anesthesia, changes in renal function are reversible (renal blood flow and GFR return to normal within a few hours). With extensive surgery and prolonged anesthesia, impaired ability to excrete a water load or concentrate urine is seen and may last for several days.

V. **Pharmacology and renal failure**

A. **Alterations in drug action** seen in renal failure may be due to the following:

1. Changes in volume of distribution.

2. Decreased serum protein concentration results in increased bioavailability of protein-bound drugs.

3. Acidemia results in a higher percentage of nonionized drug.

4. Electrolyte abnormalities.

5. Impaired biotransformation.

6. Decreased renal elimination.

7. Uremia may be associated with CNS depression, reducing the requirement for sedation by up to 50%.

B. **Lipid-soluble drugs,** in general, are poorly ionized and metabolized by the liver to water-soluble forms before elimination by the kidney. With few exceptions, the metabolites have little biologic activity.

   1. **Atropine** and **glycopyrrolate** are eliminated by the kidney, and reduced dosages must be used in severe renal failure.

   2. **Benzodiazepines, phenothiazines,** and **butyrophenones** are metabolized in the liver to both active and inactive compounds, which are then eliminated by the kidney. Benzodiazepines are 90–95% protein-bound. Lorazepam, in particular, is not recommended for patients with severe renal failure due to its potential for accumulation. Great care must be used with diazepam because of its long half-life and its active metabolites. Benzodiazepines are not appreciably removed by dialysis. The alpha-adrenergic blockade of phenothiazine derivatives may accentuate cardiovascular instability, particularly in recently dialyzed patients.

   3. **Barbiturates, etomidate,** and **propofol** are highly protein-bound, and in hypoalbuminemic patients, a much greater proportion will be available to reach receptor sites. Acidosis and changes in the blood-brain barrier will further reduce the requirements. Lower initial doses are recommended in renal failure.

   4. **Narcotics** are metabolized in the liver but may have a more intense and prolonged effect in patients with renal failure, particularly in hypoalbuminemic patients, in whom protein binding will be reduced.

C. **Ionized drugs.** Drugs that are highly ionized at physiologic pH tend to be eliminated unchanged by the kidney, and their duration of action may be prolonged by renal dysfunction.

   1. **Muscle relaxants** (see Chap. 12).

   2. **Cholinesterase inhibitors** (see Chap. 12). With impaired renal function, the elimination of the reversal drugs is decreased and their half-lives prolonged. Prolongation is similar or greater than the duration of blockade from pancuronium or d-tubocurarine, so that the return of muscle relaxation after adequate reversal (recurarization) is rarely seen.

   3. **Vasoactive agents**
      a. **Catecholamines with alpha-adrenergic effects** (norepinephrine, epinephrine, phenylephrine, ephedrine) constrict the renal vasculature and reduce renal blood flow.
      b. **Isoproterenol** also reduces renal blood flow but to a lesser extent.
      c. **Dopamine** (see sec. **IV.B**).
      d. **Sodium nitroprusside** contains cyanide and is metabolized to renally excreted thiocyanate. Toxicity, primarily neurologic from excessive accumulation of thiocyanate, is thus more likely in renal failure patients.

4. Digoxin is excreted in the urine, and blood levels should be determined prior to surgery.

VI. **General principles of management in renal failure patients**

A. **Preoperative assessment.** The etiology of renal failure should be elucidated (e.g., diabetes mellitus, glomerulonephritis, polycystic kidney disease). Elective surgery should be postponed pending resolution of the acute disease process. The degree of residual renal function is the most important consideration for anesthetic management.

1. **History**

   a. **Signs and symptoms.** Polyuria, polydipsia, dysuria, edema, and dyspnea should be sought.

   b. **Relevant medications** should be detailed. Diuretics, antihypertensives, K^+ supplements, digitalis, and nephrotoxic agents (aminoglycosides, exposure to heavy metals, and recent radiographic dye).

   c. **Dialyzed patients.** Dialysis schedule, wet and dry weights, and any problems during dialysis should be determined.

2. **Physical examination**

   a. Patients should be thoroughly examined for stigmata of renal failure as described in sec. **III.B.2.**

   b. **AV fistulae** should be evaluated for patency and infection. IV access and blood pressure determination should be performed in the opposite limb.

3. **Laboratory studies**

   a. **Urinalysis** provides a qualitative assessment of general renal function.

      (1) Positive findings include abnormal pH, proteinuria, pyuria, and casts.

      (2) The kidney's ability to concentrate urine is often lost before other changes become apparent. A specific gravity of 1.018 or greater following an overnight fast suggests that concentrating ability is intact. However, radiographic dye and osmotic agents will elevate specific gravity and invalidate this test.

   b. **Urine electrolytes, osmolality,** and **urine creatinine** will help in determining volume status and concentration ability and are used to help differentiate between prerenal and intrarenal disease (see Table 4-1).

   c. **Blood urea nitrogen (BUN)** is an insensitive measure of GFR, as it is influenced by volume status, cardiac output, diet, and body habitus. The ratio of BUN to creatinine is normally 10 to 20 : 1; disproportionate elevation of the BUN may reflect hypovolemia, low cardiac output, or gastrointestinal bleeding.

   d. **Serum creatinine (Cr)** normally is 0.6–1.2 mg/dl but is affected by the patient's skeletal muscle mass and activity level. Cr is inversely proportional to GFR such that a doubling of the Cr generally corresponds to a 50% reduction in GFR.

e. **Creatinine clearance** (C_{Cr}, normally 80–120 ml/min) provides the best estimate of renal reserve. C_{Cr} can be estimated as follows:

$$C_{Cr} = \frac{(140 - \text{age}) \times \text{weight (kg)}}{72 \times Cr}$$

Multiply by 0.85 for women. This formula is invalid in the presence of gross renal insufficiency or changing renal function. Mild dysfunction occurs with values between 50 and 80 ml/min.

f. **Serum Na^+, K^+, Cl^-, and HCO_3^-** will usually be normal until renal failure is advanced. Careful consideration of the risk and benefit of proceeding with elective surgery should be made if Na^+ is less than 131 or greater than 150 mEq/L or K^+ is less than 2.5 or greater than 5.9 mEq/L, because these abnormalities may exacerbate dysrhythmias and compromise cardiac function.

g. **Serum Ca^{2+}, PO_4^-, and Mg^+** are altered as outlined in sec. **III.B.2.d** and **e.**

h. **Hematologic studies** verify anemia, platelet dysfunction, and coagulation abnormalities.

i. **Total protein** may be decreased in renal disease secondary to proteinuria or inadequate nutrition.

j. **Arterial blood gases** can delineate the extent of acid-base abnormalities.

k. **ECG** may reveal myocardial ischemia or infarction, pericarditis, and the effects of electrolyte abnormalities (see sec. **II.C.3.e** and **4.b**).

l. **Chest radiographs** may reveal evidence of fluid overload, pericardial effusion, infection, uremic pneumonitis, and cardiomegaly.

B. **Identification of patients at high risk for perioperative ARF**

1. Elderly patients, as renal reserve and GFR decrease with advancing age.

2. Patients with preexisting renal disease

   a. Patients with greater than 50% normal creatinine clearance (i.e., $C_{Cr} > 50$ ml/min) may be managed as usual.

   b. If C_{Cr} is 25–50 ml/min, early evidence of renal failure will be evident. Special attention should be made to optimize the patient's medical status prior to surgery and maintain renal blood flow perioperatively.

   c. Patients with C_{Cr} less than 20 ml/min will manifest more severe symptoms of uremia and renal failure and are usually on dialysis.

3. Patients with cardiac dysfunction or those requiring cardiac surgery.

4. Patients undergoing angiographic procedures or requiring vascular surgery.

5. Patients with major trauma and burns.

6. Patients with inadequate intravascular volume (e.g., shock, sepsis, nephrotic syndrome, cirrhosis).

7. Patients with malignant hyperthermia.

C. **Dialysis patients** should be dialyzed prior to surgery, allowing time between dialysis and surgery to permit equilibration of fluid and electrolytes. Patients are usually dialyzed in the morning and undergo surgery in the afternoon. Since renal failure patients respond to anesthesia as if hypovolemic, preoperative dialysis should attempt to minimize fluid reduction unless the patients are symptomatically volume overloaded.

D. **Premedication** should be administered carefully, as renal failure patients have increased sensitivity to CNS depressants. A combination of antacids, H_2 blockers, and antiemetics should be considered.

E. **Anesthetic technique.** Either general or regional anesthesia is acceptable. Prior to proceeding with regional anesthesia, the current coagulation status should be determined, and the presence of uremic neuropathy documented.

F. **Intraoperative management**
   1. **Routine monitoring** as described in Chap. 10 should be used. The need for invasive hemodynamic monitoring should be based on concomitant disease, clinical status, and anticipated volume shifts during surgery.
   2. **Positioning** should be done carefully, as these patients are prone to fractures because of their renal osteodystrophy.
   3. **Induction.** The dose of induction agents may need to be reduced and their rate of administration slowed to avoid hypotension. Phenylephrine may be required, although it can decrease renal perfusion.
      a. **The airway should be protected with a cuffed endotracheal tube because of the increased risk of aspiration in these patients** (see sec. **III.B.2.i).** The need for a rapid sequence induction must be evaluated on an individual basis.
   4. **Anesthesia** is typically maintained with nitrous oxide, oxygen, and isoflurane. Narcotics are carefully administered, and muscle relaxants (atracurium, vecuronium) are administered if needed.
   5. **Fluid administration** should proceed cautiously.
      a. For brief, noninvasive procedures, insensible losses should be replaced with 0.9% normal saline.
      b. For more extensive procedures, a central venous pressure or pulmonary artery catheter may help guide fluid management.
   6. **Hypertension** is a common postoperative problem aggravated by fluid overload. For those not on dialysis, diuretics and short-acting antihypertensives are effective. For those on dialysis, postoperative dialysis may be required.

SUGGESTED READING

Barash, P. G., Cullen, B. F., and Stoelting, R. K. (eds.). *Clinical Anesthesia.* Philadelphia: Lippincott, 1989.

Blitt, C. D. (ed.). *Monitoring in Anesthesia and Critical Care Medicine* (2nd ed.). New York: Churchill Livingstone, 1990.

Cousins, M. J., Skowronski, G., and Plummer, J. L. Anaesthesia and the kidney. *Anaesth. Intensive Care* 11:292, 1983.

Cronnelly, R., et al. Renal function and the pharmacokinetics of neostigmine in anesthetized man. *Anesthesiology* 51:222, 1979.

Dunajaa, W. C., and Ridner, M. L. (eds.). *Manual of Medical Therapeutics* (26th ed.). Boston: Little, Brown, 1989.

Gilbert, P. C., and Stein, R. Preoperative evaluation of patients with chronic renal disease. *Mt. Sinai J. Med.* 58:69, 1991.

Klein, L. A. Evaluation of function in the preoperative kidney. *Urol. Clin. North Am.* 3:293, 1976.

Laragh, J. H. Atrial natriuretic hormone. *N. Engl. J. Med.* 313:1330, 1985.

Levinsky, N. G. Pathophysiology of acute renal failure. *N. Engl. J. Med.* 296:1453, 1977.

Maddern, P. J. Anaesthesia for the patient with impaired renal function. *Anaesth. Intensive Care* 11:321, 1983.

Mazze, R. I., and Cousins, M. J. Renal Diseases. In J. Katz, J. Benumof, and L. B. Kadis (eds.), *Anesthesia and Uncommon Diseases* (2nd ed.). Philadelphia: Saunders, 1981.

Mazze, R. I., Sievenpiper, T. S., and Stephenson, J. Renal effects of enflurane and halothane in patients with abnormal renal function. *Anesthesiology* 60:161, 1984.

Miller, R. D. (ed.). *Anesthesia* (3rd ed.). New York: Churchill Livingstone, 1990.

Myers, B. D., and Moran, S. M. Hemodynamically mediated acute renal failure. *N. Engl. J. Med.* 314:97, 1986.

Nancarrow, C., and Mather, L. E. Pharmacokinetics in renal failure. *Anaesth. Intensive Care* 11:350, 1983.

Narin, R. G., et al. Diagnostic strategies in disorders of fluid, electrolytes and acid-base homeostasis. *Am. J. Med.* 72:496, 1982.

Rose, B. D. *Clinical Physiology of Acid-Base and Electrolyte Disorders* (2nd ed.). New York: McGraw-Hill, 1984.

Schrier, R. W. *Renal and Electrolyte Disorders* (3rd ed.). Boston: Little, Brown, 1986.

Sladen, R. N. Effect of anesthesia and surgery on renal function. *Crit. Care Clin.* 3:373, 1987.

Stoelting, R. K. *Pharmacology and Physiology in Anesthetic Practice* (2nd ed.). Philadelphia: Lippincott, 1991.

Stoelting, R. K., Dierdorf, S. F., and McCammon, R. L. *Anesthesia and Co-Existing Disease* (2nd ed.). New York: Churchill Livingstone, 1988.

Textor, S. C., et al. Critical perfusion pressure for patients with bilateral atherosclerotic renovascular disease. *Ann. Intern. Med.* 102:308, 1985.

Tinley, N. L., and Lazarus, S. M. Acute renal failure in surgical patients: Causes, clinical patterns, and care. *Surg. Clin. North Am.* 63:357, 1983.

Vitez, T. S., et al. Chronic hypokalemia and intraoperation dysrhythmias. *Anesthesiology* 63:130, 1985.

Weil, P. H., and Chung, F. F. Anesthesia for patients with chronic renal disease. *Can. Anesth. Soc. J.* 31:468, 1984.

Wilkes, B. M., and Mailoux, L. U. Acute renal failure: Pathogenesis and Prevention. *Am. J. Med.* 80:1129, 1986.

Zaologa, G. P., and Hughes, S. S. Oliguria in patients with normal renal function. *Anesthesiology* 72:598, 1990.

5

Specific Considerations with Liver Disease

D. Jay Iaconetti

I. **Hepatic blood supply.** The hepatic artery and portal vein supply the liver with approximately 25% of the total cardiac output.
   A. The **hepatic artery** carries arterialized oxygen-rich blood and supplies approximately **one-third of the total hepatic blood flow** while providing about one-half of the total oxygen delivered to the liver.
   B. The **portal vein** carries a venous effluent from the abdominal viscera that is lower in oxygen content but rich in nutrients (carbohydrates, lipids, amino acids), hormones (e.g., insulin, glucagon, gastrin, vasoactive intestinal peptide, cholecystokinin), drugs, and toxins.
   C. The dual blood supply generally protects the liver from ischemia secondary to interruption of one or the other blood supply, although some degree of liver dysfunction may become evident with time. In the face of preexisting liver disease and reduced hepatic reserve, however, a reduction in hepatic blood flow from either source may lead to ischemia.

II. **Functions of the liver**
   A. **Synthetic functions**
      1. **Protein synthesis**
         a. **Albumin** is a high-molecular-weight protein manufactured exclusively by the liver. It maintains plasma oncotic pressure and is a carrier protein for bilirubin, certain hormones, and many lipophilic and acidic drugs. Liver disease that results in **hypoalbuminemia** can therefore cause intravascular volume depletion and extravascular volume expansion (in the form of ascites and edema) and increase the volume of distribution for water-soluble drugs. This will reduce their effective concentration but increase their half-life. Hypoalbuminemia also results in diminished protein binding, increasing the "effective" free fraction of lipophilic drugs like barbiturates, benzodiazepines, and lipophilic narcotics. This will increase their physiologic effects, especially with bolus administration, and increase their rate of clearance, thereby shortening their half-life.
         b. **Alpha-1 acid glycoprotein** is an "acute-phase reactant" secreted by the liver and increased during states of inflammation and stress. It binds basic drugs like muscle relaxants, local anesthetics, beta antagonists, and some narcotics. The clinical effects of these drugs may be prolonged in the face of trauma, surgery, burns, malignancy, and myocardial infarction because of an increase in their protein binding.
         c. **Clotting factors.** Most of the clotting factors, in-

cluding fibrinogen and prothrombin, are manufactured by the liver. The notable exception is factor VIII, which is manufactured and secreted by the vascular endothelium. Generally, a clinical coagulopathy will only become manifest with severe liver disease when factor levels are reduced below 30–50% of normal values. In addition, the vitamin K–dependent factors II, VII, IX, and X rely on the liver's ability to synthesize bile in order to absorb vitamin K (a coenzyme necessary for their activation) from the gut. Since vitamin K is produced by colonic flora, a vitamin K deficiency that results in a clinical coagulopathy generally results from decreased absorption of vitamin K from the gut. This may be due to hepatic dysfunction with resultant decreased bile production, biliary obstruction with decreased bile flow, or antibiotic therapies that reduce colonic flora (second- and third-generation cephalosporins).

  d. **Plasma cholinesterase, pseudocholinesterase,** or **nonspecific cholinesterase** is a 320,000–molecular weight protein manufactured by the liver. It is responsible for the degradation of succinylcholine, mivacurium, and ester-type local anesthetics. It is manufactured in quantities far in excess of those normally required. It is only in the presence of severe liver disease or genetic enzyme deficiency when levels are reduced by approximately 75% that there is clinically significant prolongation of succinylcholine and mivacurium activity or an increased potential for ester-type local anesthetic toxicity.

2. **Bile production.** Bile contains both primary bile salts (manufactured by the liver) and secondary bile salts (synthesized from primary bile salts by normal colonic flora). In addition to these major constituents, bile contains cholesterol, fatty acids, proteins, carbohydrates, electrolytes, and bililrubin and serves as a carrier for metabolic waste products and drug metabolites released by the liver. Bile also acts as a fat emulsifier, facilitating fat absorption by the small intestine. Therefore failure either to manufacture or release bile causes an inability to absorb fat, resulting in jaundice, steatorrhea, and fat-soluble vitamin deficiencies (vitamins A, D, E, and K).

3. **Gluconeogenesis.** The normal liver is able to store enough glycogen to provide a source of glucose for the body during a fast of approximately 12 hours. After this time, glucose is derived from gluconeogenesis. Most elective surgery patients are required to fast for approximately 8–10 hours prior to their surgical procedure. This makes them dependent on gluconeogenesis for their energy needs intraoperatively. The stress hormones normally released prior to and during surgery (e.g., epinephrine, norepinephrine, cortisol, glucagon) promote gluconeogenesis and often result in hyperglycemia. Patients with liver disease, however,

have decreased hepatic glycogen stores, decreased end-organ receptor sensitivity to hormones, and decreased capacity to generate glucose. They are therefore at significant risk for developing perioperative hypoglycemia.

B. Metabolism and detoxification

1. Bilirubin

  a. Bilirubin is the final metabolite of heme-containing substances (primarily hemoglobin, but also myoglobin and the cytochromes). Bilirubin is very lipophilic and requires binding to albumin for its transport to the liver. There it is taken up by hepatocytes and "conjugated" with glucuronic acid to form water-soluble, conjugated bilirubin and then excreted into the bile.

  b. **Hyperbilirubinemia** is an important marker for hepatobiliary disease. Unconjugated hyperbilirubinemia is commonly due to excess bilirubin production (e.g., massive transfusion, absorption of large hematomas, or hemolysis) or faulty uptake of unconjugated bilirubin by the hepatocyte (i.e., Gilbert's syndrome). Conjugated hyperbilirubinemia generally occurs with hepatocellular disease (e.g., alcoholic or viral hepatitis, cirrhosis), disease of the small bile ducts (e.g., primary biliary cirrhosis, Dubin-Johnson syndrome), or obstruction of the extrahepatic bile ducts (e.g., pancreatic carcinoma, cholangiocarcinoma, gallstones).

2. Ammonia.
Amino acids in excess of those needed for the synthesis of proteins and other biomolecules are "deaminated" to produce ammonia, which is then converted to urea by the liver. Thus, in severe liver disease the blood urea nitrogen (BUN) levels are often low, while serum ammonia levels are high. Serum ammonia levels are often used to assess the degree of hepatic dysfunction, but they do not directly correlate with the development of hepatic encephalopathy. Other factors have been implicated in its development, including the formation of amines that act as false neurotransmitters and an increase in the neurotransmitter gamma-aminobutyric acid.

3. Steroid hormones.
Because the liver is the major site of steroid hormone degradation, hepatic failure results in steroid excess. Elevations of serum aldosterone and cortisol result in enhanced resorption of sodium and water (contributing to edema and ascites) and loss of potassium in the urine. Decreased metabolism of estrogens and impaired conversion to androgens cause the clinical stigmata of liver disease, that is, spider angiomata, gynecomastia, palmar erythema, and testicular atrophy.

4. Drugs

  a. **Mechanisms.** Most compounds are initially metabolized by a family of mixed-function oxidases (cytochrome P-450) in a first-phase oxidative reaction. The products of this reaction are then conjugated to glycine, glucuronic acid, or sulfate in a second-phase conjugative reaction to enhance their water solubility for excretion in bile and urine. Some metabolites are more active (prednisolone > prednisone) or have longer half-lives (desmethyldiazepam > diazepam) than the original drug. Severe liver disease can therefore impact on the pharmacologic effect and duration of drug action by altering the degree to which a drug is metabolized and eliminated.

b. **Induction of enzymes.** Certain drugs (i.e., barbiturates, benzodiazepines, corticosteroids, antihistamines, ethanol, phenytoin, and chloral hydrate), when administered in increasing concentrations, can induce the enzymes that metabolize them to increase their number and activity. This predisposes to **dispositional tolerance** where increasing doses of drug are needed to attain a given pharmacologic effect, since more drug is being metabolized at a faster rate. Enzyme induction is nonspecific, and cross-tolerance between drugs does occur.

c. **Halogenated inhalation agents** are metabolized by the liver to varying degrees to produce inorganic fluoride ion (F^-), which is nephrotoxic at high levels (see Chap. 4).

   (1) **Isoflurane.** Only 0.2% of absorbed isoflurane undergoes hepatic metabolism, generating insufficient amounts of F^- to cause nephrotoxicity.

   (2) **Enflurane.** Only 2% of absorbed enflurane is metabolized by the liver to produce F^-. It is thus unlikely to generate a sufficient amount of F^- to cause nephrotoxicity. The coadministration of enflurane and isoniazid (which is known to induce cytochrome P-450) does have the potential to create nephrotoxic levels of F^-.

   (3) **Halothane.** About 20% of absorbed halothane is metabolized. The majority undergoes oxidative metabolism with the subsequent release of **trifluoroacetic acid, chloride, bromide,** and only **trace amounts of fluoride.** Reductive metabolism of halothane by the cytochrome P-450 system may also occur in the presence of hypoxia. This generates free radicals that have been postulated to cause direct hepatocellular damage (see sec. **VII.C** for a discussion of halothane-associated hepatitis).

d. **Barbiturates.** Long- and intermediate-acting barbiturates (phenobarbital, pentobarbital, secobarbital), whose durations of action are determined by metabolism, will have prolonged effects in liver failure. The short-acting barbiturates (thiopental, thiamylal, and methohexital), whose duration of action are determined by redistribution, must still be used cautiously in liver disease not only because of decreased metabolism but also because preexisting hypoalbuminemia will reduce the degree of protein binding and increase the active free fraction.

e. **Neuromuscular blocking agents** are generally very polar compounds and are predominantly excreted in the urine unchanged. (Note that ordinarily a small proportion of curare and pancuronium is excreted in the bile.) Exceptions are vecuronium and doxacurium, which are excreted in the bile, and atracurium, which is degraded via Hofman elimination and by plasma esterases. The duration of action of most muscle relaxants is prolonged in liver failure but results from different mechanisms. Those that are predominantly excreted by the kidney are prolonged secondary to an increase in their volume of distribution, while vecuronium and doxacurium are prolonged because of decreased biliary excretion. Although atracurium partially depends on esterases manufactured in the liver for its degradation, only severe liver disease will reduce these enzymes to a level prolonging atracurium's clinical effect.

f. **Vasoactive amines and cardiovascular drugs**

(1) The **catecholamines,** including norepinephrine, epinephrine, isoproterenol, dopamine, and dobutamine, are rapidly inactivated in the body. The liver is rich in both of the enzymes that are responsible for their degradation, catechol-O-methyltransferase and monoamine oxidase. The liver's role is important but not essential in this process. Thus, endogenous levels of the natural-occurring catecholamines are not affected by liver disease because these enzymes are widely distributed throughout the body. On the other hand, when pharmacologic doses of these drugs are administered to patients with severe liver disease, there is a potential for increased sensitivity secondary to decreased metabolism.

(2) The **noncatecholamines,** including amphetamines, ephedrine, phenylephrine, metaproterenol, and terbutaline, are all capable of being absorbed from the gastrointestinal tract in addition to being administered parenterally. As such they are subject to a first-pass effect. Although only a portion of their metabolism and excretion may be dependent on hepatic metabolism, one should expect an increase in their duration of action and pharmacologic effect in severe hepatocellular disease and portosystemic shunting.

(3) **Beta antagonists** (propranolol, esmolol, atenolol, and metoprolol) and **calcium channel blockers** (diltiazem, nifedipine, and verapamil) are also metabolized extensively by the liver. When given orally, they too undergo first-pass metabolism and are capable of reaching toxic levels if dosages are not reduced in liver failure. Intravenous doses must also be reduced accordingly.

(4) **Narcotics, benzodiazepines,** and **amide local anesthetics** are metabolized primarily in the liver and have significantly prolonged half-lives with liver failure.

III. Specific hepatic disorders

A. **Hepatitis.** Acute hepatitis may be caused by viruses (hepatitis A, B, C; Epstein-Barr, cytomegalovirus, herpes simplex, Coxsackie virus, ECHO virus, and yellow fever), drugs (methyldopa, acetaminophen, phenytoin, isoniazid, alcohol, propylthiouracil, estrogens, and tetracycline), or toxins. Serum transaminases (aspartate aminotransferase [AST], alanine aminotransferase [ALT]) will generally be elevated out of proportion to the alkaline phosphatase and bilirubin.

1. **Hepatitis A** is spread predominantly by fecal-oral contact. In general, it is a mild disorder with many subclinical cases and recovery usually within 2 months. The reported mortality is less than 1/1000. If anesthesia and surgery are performed during incubation or the prodromal period, however, the mortality is increased significantly, reaching as high as 100% in patients with fulminant hepatitis. Therefore elective surgery should be postponed until recovery has occurred.

2. **Hepatitis B and C** are primarily transmitted by transfer of body fluids and have higher intrinsic mortality rates than hepatitis A—approximately 5% for hepatitis B and 1–3% for hepatitis C. Both can induce a chronic carrier state, chronic persistent hepatitis, chronic active hepatitis leading to cirrhosis and hepatocellular carcinoma, or fulminant hepatic necrosis. There are a number of other manifestations associated with acute hepatitis B infections, including nausea, vomiting, rash, diarrhea, arthralgias, pancreatitis, bradycardia, pleural effusion, and pancytopenia. The mortality associated with anesthesia and surgery performed on a patient with active hepatitis is exceedingly high, warranting postponement of elective surgery. Patients with biopsy-proven **mild** chronic active hepatitis and chronic persistent hepatitis appear to be at no increased risk when undergoing anesthesia and surgery. The anesthetic should be tailored to avoid the use of potentially hepatotoxic drugs.

B. **Cholestatic liver disease** results in an elevation of alkaline phosphatase out of proportion to serum transminases. Cholestasis without an anatomic obstruction can occur in infancy, during pregnancy, after anesthesia, during sepsis, in viral hepatitis, and with certain drugs (e.g., alcohol, oral contraceptives, oral hypoglycemics, phenothiazines, thiazide diuretics, sulfonamides, and erythromycin estolate).

C. **Chronic liver disease and cirrhosis** may result from chronic active hepatitis, alcoholism, hemochromatosis, primary biliary cirrhosis, or congenital metabolic disorders such as Wilson's disease, alpha$_1$-antitrypsin deficiency, glycogen storage disease, or hereditary tyrosinemia. The end result of chronic liver disease is **cirrhosis,** exemplified by a scarred, shrunken liver that causes significant resistance to portal blood flow. This in turn elevates portal venous pressure, resulting in portal hypertension and esophageal varices. The combination of portal hypertension and decreased production of albumin and coagulation factors sets the stage for the development of ascites, coagulopathy, gastrointestinal bleeding, and encephalopathy. As a result, many of these patients will present for procedures aimed at reducing these manifestations (portacaval, mesocaval, and LeVeen shunts) as well as orthotopic liver transplantation.

IV. **Preoperative evaluation of the patient with liver disease**

   A. A **history** of jaundice, hepatitis, alcohol abuse, intravenous drug abuse and propensity for bleeding, acholic stools, and weight loss should be sought.

   B. **Physical findings** might include hepatosplenomegaly, ascites, peripheral edema, spider angiomata, testicular atrophy, caput medusae, hemorrhoids, asterixis, gynecomastia, and temporal wasting.

   C. **Laboratory data** indicative of hepatic dysfunction should be obtained, including direct and indirect bilirubin, serum transaminases, and alkaline phosphatase. It should be noted that skeletal and cardiac muscle release transaminases as well. In addition, alkaline phosphatase elevations can be seen in bone disease. Further differentiation can be obtained with 5'-nucleotidase or gamma-glutamyl transferase, specific to the liver. Hepatic synthetic function may be assessed by the serum albumin or prothrombin time (PT).

   D. **The gastrointestinal consultant.** When there is doubt concerning the significance of a patient's history of liver disease or abnormal liver function tests, it is often prudent to involve a hepatologist.

   E. **Operative risk assessment**

      1. The Child's classification system evaluates the operative risk for **cirrhotic** patients. A low-risk patient (**class A**) has a bilirubin less than 2.0 mg/dl, albumin greater than 3.5 gm/dl, and no ascites or encephalopathy. The highest risk patient (**class C**) has bilirubin greater than 3.0 mg/dl, albumin less than 3.0 gm/dl, and advanced ascites and/or encephalopathy.

      2. Poor nutritional status, dementia, and encephalopathy indicate very poor risk.

      3. Active gastrointestinal bleeding or a history of variceal bleeding increase the operative risk.

      4. Associated medical problems increase risk significantly.

      5. Albumin, bilirubin, and PT abnormalities are markers of increased risk.

      6. Uncontrolled ascites puts the patient at greater risk than if preoperative correction or control of ascites is performed.

      7. Preoperative correction of as many preexisting medical problems as possible is beneficial.

      8. Avoid anesthetizing patients with possible viral hepatitis because of high postoperative mortality rates.

V. **Anesthetic considerations in end-stage liver disease.**
Regardless of the cause, end-stage liver disease will affect
most other organ systems. Meticulous attention to intravascular volume, acid-base status, and vital organ perfusion is
needed to prevent multiple organ failure.

A. **Central nervous system.** The severity of hepatic encephalopathy ranges from mild confusion to deep coma.
Encephalopathic patients may become deeply depressed
by sedatives, due to both pharmacodynamic and pharmacokinetic factors. Aspiration, especially in the presence of
ascites, is more likely. Premedication is avoided or used
sparingly in these patients.

B. **Cardiovascular system**
1. **Alcoholic cardiomyopathy** may be present. Diuretics given to reduce total body fluid overload may cause
intravascular volume depletion. They may also cause
hypokalemia (furosemide) or hyperkalemia (spironolactone). Significant arteriovenous shunting may reduce peripheral resistance. Cardiac output is generally
increased to maintain blood pressure in the face of this
reduced peripheral resistance. Invasive monitoring
(central venous pressure, pulmonary artery catheter)
may be required to guide fluid management.
2. **Portal hypertension and coagulopathy** combine to
produce an increased incidence of bleeding from varices, diffuse gastritis, and peptic ulcers.

C. **Respiratory system**
1. **Airway protection** is often vital, for reasons mentioned in sec. **A** and because the stomach may be filled
with blood. Awake or rapid sequence inductions should
be considered.
2. **Gas exchange** is often abnormal. Encephalopathy
seems to cause an inappropriate central hyperventilation, resulting in hypocarbia and respiratory alkalosis.
Hypoxemia may be present secondary to basilar atelectasis from abdominal distention, as well as intrapulmonary arteriovenous shunting.

D. **Renal system**
1. Intravascular volume depletion from hypoalbuminemia and diuretic therapy may result in **prerenal
azotemia.** BUN may be deceptively low because of the
liver's inability to synthesize urea from ammonia.
2. Renal failure may result from **hepatorenal syndrome,** the etiology of which is unknown but may be
related to circulating factors that alter intrarenal
hemodynamics. Since the renal parenchyma is not
reversibly damaged, normal renal function may return
if liver failure resolves.

E. **Coagulopathy** occurs from clotting factor deficiency and
thrombocytopenia often secondary to hypersplenism. Portosystemic shunting in the abdominal wall, esophagus,
rectal veins, and retroperitoneum makes surgery in these
areas prone to hemorrhage. Clotting studies should be
checked prior to proceeding with regional techniques, and
appropriate blood products ordered in advance of surgery
(e.g., fresh-frozen plasma, platelets).

F. **Carbohydrate support.** Because diminished reserves of glycogen will tend to decrease blood glucose levels, patients with hepatic failure should be given continuous infusions of glucose-containing solutions, and their blood glucose levels should be intermittently checked.

VI. **Effects of anesthesia on the liver**

A. **Hepatic blood flow.** Anesthesia and surgery generally decrease hepatic blood flow. The decrease in hepatic blood flow is usually proportional to the decrease in systemic blood pressure. Although total blood flow decreases, hepatic artery blood flow tends to increase as portal blood flow decreases. This holds true whether the cause of relative hypotension is secondary to general or regional anesthesia. There is some evidence, however, that halothane may increase the resistance of the hepatic artery when portal blood flow diminishes, thus exacerbating the reduction in total hepatic blood flow. In addition to the type of anesthesia used, there are a number of factors that tend to reduce hepatic blood flow further and should be avoided or minimized, including hypovolemia, compromised patient position, hypocapnia, positive-pressure ventilation, beta antagonists, sympathomimetics, vasodilators, and surgical packs. Hepatic blood flow is generally compromised in severe hepatic disease. Further reduction can only exacerbate hepatic dysfunction.

B. **Histamine (H_2) receptor antagonists** are common premedications, especially in patients with liver disease because of the increased risk of pulmonary aspiration. Cimetidine is known to inhibit the cytochrome P-450 system, which in turn can prolong the duration of many hepatically cleared drugs including warfarin-type anticoagulants, phenytoin, propranolol, diazepam, lidocaine, theophylline, and metronidazole. Ranitidine has a much lower affinity for the P-450 system and therefore has less of an effect on drug metabolism. Both drugs are capable of lowering hepatic blood flow, presumably by decreasing gastric metabolic activity via reduction in gastric acid production.

VII. **Postoperative hepatic dysfunction.** Liver dysfunction after surgery and anesthesia is not an uncommon occurrence. It can range from mild enzyme elevations to fulminant hepatic failure. Etiologies for postoperative hepatic dysfunction include the following:

A. **Surgical interventions** that impair hepatic blood flow or obstruct the biliary system. Postoperative serum elevations in hepatocellular enzymes or bilirubin can also be caused by increased bilirubin loads after massive transfusion, resorption of hematoma, or hemolysis caused by prosthetic valves, sepsis, or glucose 6-phosphate dehydrogenase deficiency. A picture of "benign postoperative intrahepatic cholestasis" is usually a marker of a systemic process (e.g., sepsis) rather than intrinsic hepatic dysfunction. Overt hepatic failure can occur after or during shock of any etiology, especially if there has been a history of prolonged pressor use that has resulted in long-standing hepatic ischemia.

B. **Nonsurgical causes.** Hepatic dysfunction from common entities like viral hepatitis, alcoholism, and cholelithiasis can exist preoperatively (but may not be detected) or can occur postoperatively as mere coincidence. The stresses of surgery can convert a nonicteric illness into one of frank jaundice. Drug therapy in the postoperative period must also be evaluated as a cause of jaundice.

C. **Halothane-associated hepatitis.** Following the administration of halothane, hepatic dysfunction may develop that is clinically indistinguishable from viral hepatitis. The presentation covers a broad spectrum; it may occur as an asymptomatic elevation in serum transaminases, fever of unknown origin, clinical jaundice, or, very rarely, massive hepatic necrosis and death. Theoretic predisposing factors include previous halothane exposure (especially when associated with previous mild hepatic dysfunction or fever of unknown origin), other drug allergies, obesity, advanced age, and the female gender. The problem is virtually unknown in pediatric patients. Currently, the diagnosis is one of exclusion. There appears to be no distinctive hepatic pathology.

1. **The United States National Halothane Study** found that otherwise unexplained massive hepatic necrosis following halothane exposure was an exceedingly rare complication and occurred in only 1/35,000 exposures. Risks were highest in the adult population who received multiple halothane exposures and in those who underwent procedures that carried a higher intrinsic mortality rate. Seven cases of unexplained massive hepatic necrosis occurred in 250,000 exposures to halothane; four of the seven had received an earlier halothane anesthetic in the previous 6 weeks.

2. **Possible mechanisms.** It is now recognized that two types of halothane-induced hepatic dysfunction exist. They include a mild subclinical form that is manifested by abnormal liver function tests and may occur in up to 20% of patients who are exposed to halothane. This could be due to either genetic predisposition or reductive metabolic processes in a hypoxic environment causing the development of hepatotoxic metabolites. The rarer, more fulminant form is probably an immunologic phenomenon whereby oxidative metabolites of halothane, trifluoroacetyl molecules, bind to hepatocytes, creating an antigenic structure to which antibodies may be generated with resulting hepatocellular damage.

3. **Recommendations concerning the use of halothane.** Halothane possesses special attributes that, in certain circumstances, may make it more useful than other potent inhalation anesthetics. The Massachusetts General Hospital has established suggested guidelines for the use of halothane in adults. There are no restrictions on the use of halothane in pediatric patients. Halothane use in adults should be restricted to patients with severe airway compromise or bronchospasm. A specific informed consent should include the

indications for halothane use and the possible risks. A staff anesthesiologist confirms the informed consent and the indications for its use and includes an evaluation of the patient's hepatic function and outcome of prior exposures to halothane. Multiple, frequent exposures to halothane should be minimized, and unexplained deterioration of liver function following previous exposure should be determined. Halothane should not be routinely stored in any vaporizer, and at the conclusion of the anesthetic, halothane remaining in the vaporizer should be drained and discarded.

SUGGESTED READING

Brown, R. (ed.). *Anesthesia and Hepatic and Biliary Disease*. Philadelphia: Davis, 1988.

Bunker, J. P. (ed.). *The National Halothane Study*. Bethesda: NIGMS, National Institutes of Health, 1965.

Dykes, M. H. M., et al. Halothane and the liver: A review of the epidemiological, immunologic and metabolic aspects of the relationship. *Can. J. Surg.* 15:4, 1972.

Mazze, R. I. Metabolism of the inhaled anesthetics: Implications of enzyme induction. *Br. J. Anaesth.* 56:27s, 1984.

Strunin, L., and Davies, J. M. The liver and anaesthesia. *Can. Anaesth. Soc. J.* 30:2, 1983.

6

Specific Considerations with Endocrine Disease

William Dylewsky

I. Diabetes mellitus

A. Diabetes is a chronic **systemic** disease due to the absolute or relative lack of insulin. It occurs frequently and increases perioperative mortality fivefold.

B. **Physiology.** Insulin is manufactured in the pancreas and stored in granules in its beta cells. It facilitates glucose and potassium transport across cell membranes, increases glycogen synthesis, and inhibits lipolysis. Its release is stimulated by sugars, growth hormone, and acetylcholine. Catecholamines inhibit the release of insulin through their action at the alpha receptor. The production of insulin continues during fasting periods to prevent catabolism and ketoacidosis. There is a peripheral resistance to the effects of insulin during times of stress, including surgery and cardiopulmonary bypass. Insulin is metabolized by the liver and kidney and may have a prolonged action in the presence of renal insufficiency.

C. **Type I diabetes** is also referred to as **juvenile** or **insulin-dependent** (IDDM) diabetes. These patients generally present at a younger age, are not obese, and are prone to ketosis.

D. **Type II diabetes** is also referred to as **noninsulin-dependent diabetes mellitus** (NIDDM) or **adult-onset diabetes mellitus** (AODM). These patients generally have a functioning pancreas but are peripherally resistant to the effects of insulin. They represent 90% of all diabetics and generally are older, obese, and ketosis-resistant, but prone to hyperosmolar complications. They are usually managed with diet alone or in combination with oral hypoglycemic agents. These agents act by increasing both pancreatic insulin release and peripheral insulin responsiveness. They can induce hypoglycemia up to 50 hours after administration in the fasting patient. These medications increase the effectiveness of thiazide diuretics, barbiturates, and anticoagulants.

E. **Other causes of insulin insufficiency.** Pancreatic hyposecretion is seen in cystic fibrosis, pancreatic surgery/resection, chronic pancreatitis, and hemochromatosis. The effects of insulin may be overwhelmed in patients with glucagonomas, pheochromocytomas, acromegaly, or glucocorticoid excess.

F. **Acute complications of diabetes**

1. **Ketoacidosis.** Stress (e.g., infection, surgery, and trauma) may lead to an increased resistance to insulin and ketoacidosis. This occurs more commonly in type I diabetics.

   a. Ketoacidosis is associated with depressed myocardial contractility and peripheral tone, hyperglycemia (and concurrent hyperosmolarity), intracellular dehydration, and an osmotic diuresis leading to profound hypovolemia.

b. Electrolyte abnormalities include hyperglycemia (although glucose is usually less than 500 mg/dl), hyperkalemia, and hyponatremia. The total body K^+ is actually depressed (3–10 mEq/kg body weight) but appears elevated because there is insufficient insulin to drive it into cells. Sodium concentration is artificially lowered 1.6 mEq/L for every 100 mg/dl that the glucose is elevated.

c. Treatment. Regular insulin should be given initially as a bolus (10 units IV) and then as a continuous infusion, intravascular volume replaced with normal saline, and K^+ replaced as indicated. Phosphorus and magnesium may need to be replaced and bicarbonate may be given if pH is less than 7.1 and hemodynamic instability is present.

G. Hyperosmolar state

1. It is often triggered by infection or dehydration and may occur in diabetic (type II) and nondiabetic patients. Characteristics include glucose greater than 600 mg/dl, hypovolemia with an osmotic diuresis, electrolyte abnormalities, hemoconcentration, and central nervous system (CNS) dysfunction (such as seizure or coma). There is no evidence of ketosis.

2. **Treatment** includes normal saline replacement and insulin administration. These patients may be sensitive to insulin, and smaller doses should be used. When glucose falls below 300 mg/dl, treatment should progress slowly to avoid cerebral edema. Electrolyte abnormalities must be corrected.

H. Chronic complications of diabetes

1. **Atherosclerosis.** Middle-aged and elderly diabetics have diffuse vascular disease. Significant coronary artery disease, cerebrovascular disease, microangiopathic renal dysfunction, and retinal degeneration are common.

2. **Neuropathy.** Autonomic neuropathy may result in silent ischemia, postural hypotension, gastroparesis, and bladder atony. There is an increased risk of perioperative sudden cardiac death due to autonomic cardiac dysfunction and a diminished central ventilatory response to hypoxia and drugs that depress the CNS. Peripheral neuropathies may cause pain and/or numbness.

3. **Other manifestations.** Infection and poor wound healing are major postoperative complications.

I. Agents. See Table 6-1.

J. Anesthetic considerations

1. Ketoacidosis or hyperosmolar coma must be corrected before elective surgery.

2. Surgical procedures should be planned as the first case in the morning.

3. **Glucose and insulin management**

a. Ketoacidosis or hyperosmolar coma must be prevented without inducing hypoglycemia. Optimal serum glucose intraoperatively is 120–200 mg/dl.

Table 6-1. Hypoglycemic agents

Agent	Typical time to onset (hours)	Typical duration of action (hours)
Insulins (SQ administration)		
Regular	1	8
Semilente	1	14
NPH	2	24
Lente	2	24
Protamine zinc	4	36
Ultralente	4	36
Sulfonylureas		
Tolbutamide (Orinase or Oramide)	1	8–12
Glipizide (Glucotrol)	1	8–24
Acetohexamide (Dymelor)	1	12–24
Tolazamide (Tolinase)	4–6	12–16
Glyburide (Micronase or Diabeta)	1–4	18–24
Chlorpropramide (Diabinese)	1–4	24–72

  b. Patients on oral hypoglycemic agents should not receive them within 24 hours of surgery. If they have been taken, IV glucose supplementation is necessary during the fasting period. For IDDM patients having minor procedures of short duration (e.g., in the ambulatory care setting), the morning insulin can be held until the patient is alert postoperatively and able to eat. Glucose may be checked by finger stick immediately before and after the procedure.

  c. For more substantial procedures, patients should receive one-half of their total normal morning dose of insulin in the form of an intermediate- or long-acting subcutaneous (SQ) dose. A glucose-containing infusion should be started simultaneously at 100 ml/hr. Increased rates of infusion or supplemental doses of regular insulin may be indicated by frequent (every 2–4 hours intraoperatively) monitoring of blood sugar. Doses should be decreased in renal failure. Patients on split-dose insulin regimens preoperatively should receive reduced doses of any long- or intermediate-acting insulin the night before surgery. Intravenous dosing is preferable when there is hemodynamic instability or the patient is on vasoconstrictors because of unreliable SQ absorption.

4. Patients with evidence of **severe heart disease** or **autonomic dysfunction** should be considered for perioperative invasive monitoring.

5. Patients with **peripheral neuropathy** are vulnerable to positioning injury and should have neuropathies documented prior to initiating regional anesthesia.

6. Patients with **autonomic neuropathy** have delayed gastric emptying and may be less able to compensate for positional changes or the sympathectomy of re-

gional anesthesia. They should receive aspiration prophylaxis and a rapid sequence induction if a general anesthetic is planned.

7. **Protamine** to reverse heparin must be administered very cautiously in the diabetic chronically receiving NPH insulin.

K. **Hypoglycemia**

1. **Etiologies.** Hypoglycemia is an uncommon entity and may be due to pancreatic adenoma or carcinoma, cirrhosis, hypopituitarism, adrenal insufficiency, hepatoma, sarcoma, or ethanol ingestion.

2. Patients may exhibit **symptoms** of adrenergic excess including tachycardia, diaphoresis, palpitations, and tremulousness or **neuroglycopenia** including headache, confusion, stupor, seizure, and coma.

3. **Anesthetic considerations** include providing a continuous glucose infusion and periodically checking serum glucose.

II. **Thyroid disease**

A. **Physiology.** Thyroid hormone is one of the major regulators of cellular metabolic activity. It alters the speed of reactions and the total oxygen consumption and heat production of the body. Under the control of thyroid-stimulating hormone (TSH) from the anterior pituitary, iodine is taken up into the thyroid gland and incorporated into tyrosine residues, and the hormones **triiodothyronine** (T_3) and **thyroxine** (T_4) are formed and stored. Peripheral tissues convert T_4 to T_3, which is 3 times more potent than T_4 and has a shorter half-life. Both forms of thyroid hormone are partially bound to the plasma protein thyroid binding globulin (TBG), although only the free (unbound) concentration is pharmacologically active. TBG can increase with acute liver disease, pregnancy, acute intermittent porphyria, and medications (e.g., oral hypoglycemics, exogenous estrogens, clofibrate, and opioids) and can decrease with chronic liver disease, nephrotic syndrome, anabolic steroids, and acromegaly. TBG plays no direct role in cell metabolism, but its concentration can alter diagnostic test results when checking for thyroid disease.

B. **Laboratory studies.** Total T_4 is a useful screening test for thyroid dysfunction. Since TBG concentration may alter the measured T_4, a resin T_3 uptake (RT_3) can be ordered. This will distinguish between protein binding abnormalities and true metabolic changes associated with hypo- or hyperthyroidism. The most sensitive measure of hypothyroidism remains TSH, although it may be artificially lowered by starvation, steroids, stress, or fever (Table 6-2).

C. **Hyperthyroidism**

1. **Etiologies.** An increase in thyroid function resulting from an excess supply of thyroid hormones is associated with Graves' disease, TSH overproduction, and pregnancy. In subacute thyroiditis, excess thyroid hormone leaks out of the gland due to inflammation. Extrathyroid gland hormone may be produced by ovarian

Table 6-2. Screening tests for thyroid function in diseased states

Disease	T_4	RT_3	TSH
Hyperthyroidism	Inc	Inc	Dec or NL
Primary hypothyroidism	Dec	Dec	Inc
Secondary hypothyroidism	Dec	Dec	Dec
Pregnancy	Inc	Dec	NL

T_4 = thyroxine; RT_3 = triiodothyronine resin uptake; TSH = thyroid-stimulating hormone; Inc = increased; Dec = decreased; NL = normal.

tumors or metastatic thyroid carcinoma. Exogenous consumption of thyroid hormone can also lead to hyperthyroidism.

2. **Clinical features**

   a. Patients present with nervousness, heat intolerance, muscle weakness, and tremors. Cardiovascular signs include dysrhythmias (e.g., sinus tachycardia, atrial fibrillation), systolic murmurs, and congestive heart failure.

   b. **Thyroid storm** may be precipitated by surgical stress but is usually seen 6–18 hours postoperatively. Its manifestations include diarrhea, vomiting, and hyperpyrexia leading to hypovolemia, irritability, delirium, or coma. Thyroid storm may mimic malignant hyperthermia, sepsis, hemorrhage, or transfusion/drug reaction.

3. **Treatment.** Chronic thyroid hormone excess is treated by gland ablation with surgery, radioactive iodine, or specific antithyroid drugs (e.g., **propylthiouracil** [PTU] and **methimazole**). Side effects of PTU include leukopenia, thrombocytopenia, and hypothrombinemia. Thyroid storm therapy includes active cooling, hydration, beta-adrenergic blockade, steroids if there is any indication of adrenal insufficiency, and institution of long-term therapy with PTU or iodine. Six weeks is required to become euthyroid.

4. **Anesthetic considerations.** Only emergency surgery should be performed in thyrotoxic patients. Premedication including beta blockers should be generous. Sympathetic stimulation (pain, ketamine, pancuronium) should be avoided. The eyes of patients with Graves' disease should be well protected. Clinically, drug metabolism and anesthetic requirements appear to be increased. Myasthenia gravis may be seen in some hyperthyroid patients so relaxants should be titrated carefully. Hypotension should be treated with direct-acting agents such as phenylephrine. Regional anesthesia may be beneficial in thyrotoxic patients, since it blocks sympathetic response. Local anesthetics with epinephrine may lead to further arrhythmias.

D. **Hypothyroidism**

1. **Etiologies.** Insufficient synthesis of thyroid hormone may be congenital, postablative, or postradiation therapy. Goitrous conditions (e.g., iodine deficiency), drug

therapy (lithium or phenylbutazone), or Hashimoto's thyroiditis also may be causative. Hashimoto's thyroiditis is the most common cause of hypothyroidism in adults and can be associated with other autoimmune processes including myasthenia gravis, primary adrenal insufficiency, pernicious anemia, or Sjögren's syndrome.

2. **Clinical features**
   a. Patients can experience lethargy, constipation, cold intolerance, facial edema with an enlarged tongue, a reversible cardiomyopathy, pericardial effusion, ascites, anemia, and an adynamic ileus with delayed gastric emptying. There may be adrenal atrophy with decreased cortisol production, dilutional hyponatremia, and decreased water excretion. There is a decreased cardiac output, bradycardia, hypovolemia, and diminished baroreceptor reflexes. The electrocardiogram demonstrates diminished QRS amplitude.
   b. **Myxedema coma** (profound hypothyroidism) may be triggered by trauma, infection, and CNS depressants, leading to respiratory depression, congestive heart failure, and depressed consciousness.

3. **Treatment.** Chronic treatment involves the exogenous supplementation of thyroid hormone. T_4 requires 10 days to have an effect. T_3 begins to have an effect in 6 hours.

4. **Anesthetic considerations.** Elective surgery must be postponed in any patient who is clinically hypothyroid. In hypothyroid patients who must undergo emergency procedures, the following should be considered:
   a. **Preoperative sedation should be avoided** because of the profound CNS and respiratory sensitivity to depressants. Cortisol supplementation should be considered, intravascular volume optimized, and anemia corrected.
   b. **Anesthetic techniques** must take into consideration airway problems associated with a large tongue, poor gastric emptying, and increased sensitivity to all depressant medications.
   c. **Postoperative observation** should be arranged.

III. **Calcium metabolism and parathyroid disease**
   A. The parathyroid glands are responsible for the maintenance of extracellular calcium concentration. **Parathyroid hormone** (PTH) acts on the kidney to decrease renal clearance of calcium, on the intestine to increase calcium absorption, and on the skeletal system to increase bone resorption. Antagonizing the effects of PTH is **calcitonin,** a hormone produced in the thyroid gland that lowers both calcium and phosphorous concentrations. Alterations in PTH function are reflected in the relative availability of calcium.
   B. **Calcium** is essential for coagulation, muscle contraction, neurotransmitter release, and endocrine secretion. It is the free ionic calcium form that is physiologically important, and this can be measured directly.

1. **Hypercalcemia**
   a. **Etiologies** include hyperparathyroidism, malignancy, sarcoidosis, vitamin D intoxication, thyrotoxicosis, and adrenal insufficiency.
   b. **Clinical features** include anorexia, nausea/vomiting, constipation, peptic ulcer disease, depression, lethargy, nephrolithiasis, polyuria, and ECG changes (e.g., prolonged P–R interval with a short Q–T interval).
   c. **Treatment.** Hypercalcemia is considered an emergency when values are greater than 15 mg/dl. Treatment includes limiting PO intake, administration of large quantities of IV normal saline (6–10 L/day) and diuresis with furosemide or ethacrynic acid. Administration of phosphate will limit intestinal absorption and increase skeletal reuptake of calcium. Mithramycin and calcitonin decrease bone resorption. Steroids increase urinary calcium excretion (especially for patients with hematologic and breast cancers).
2. **Hypocalcemia**
   a. **Clinical features.** Acute hypocalcemia (e.g., after removal of the parathyroid glands) can result in stridor, laryngospasm, apnea, and focal or grand mal seizures unresponsive to conventional therapy. Bedside demonstration of facial nerve irritability to percussion (**Chvostek's sign**) or carpal spasm with tourniquet ischemia (**Trousseau's sign**) indicates the need for supplementation. Chronic signs and symptoms include peripheral and perioral paresthesias, mental status changes, bronchospasm, hypotension with relative insensitivity to beta agonists, and a prolonged Q–T interval leading to 2 : 1 heart block.
   b. **Treatment.** Calcium should be repleted (acutely, as 1–4 gm of calcium chloride or gluconate IV; chronically, as 1–8 gm/day of calcium carbonate, often with vitamin D supplementation) until the ionized calcium reaches normal levels and symptoms resolve. Phosphorus and magnesium should also be evaluated and corrected if low.
C. **Hyperparathyroidism**
   1. **Etiologies.** Hyperparathyroidism is characterized by hypercalcemia and hypophosphatemia caused by a secretory lesion such as carcinoma or adenoma, with only 10% being due to hyperplasia. It may also be caused by the **multiple endocrine neoplasia complex.** Treatment involves removal of the parathyroid gland or glands. Pseudohyperparathyroidism is due to secretion of a PTH-like molecule from tumors of the lung, breast, gut, urinary tract, or lymphoproliferative system.
   2. **Anesthetic considerations.** Hypercalcemia should be corrected as discussed in sec. **B.1.c.** Intravascular volume and other electrolyte abnormalities should be normalized. Hypercalcemia has an unpredictable effect

on neuromuscular blockade so relaxants should be carefully titrated. Careful positioning is required, since these patients can be osteopenic. Postoperatively, patients may suffer from transient or complete hypocalcemia requiring supplementation.

D. **Hypoparathyroidism**

1. **Etiologies.** Hypoparathyroidism is due to underproduction of PTH or resistance to its effects by end-organ tissues. This may occur after neck surgery where the parathyroid glands have been damaged or excised. Symptoms are usually seen weeks to months later, but occasionally acute hypocalcemia has been observed in the immediate postoperative period. Other causes include postradiation therapy, granulomatous disease, hemosiderosis, infiltrative processes like malignancy or amyloidosis, and severe hypomagnesemia. Extensive burns and pancreatitis cause sequestration of calcium and suppression of PTH function.

2. **Anesthetic considerations.** Calcium and other electrolyte abnormalities should be corrected. Hypocalcemia can be worsened by respiratory or metabolic alkalosis, rapid infusions of blood products, hypothermia, and renal dysfunction. Coagulation factors must be followed carefully.

IV. **Adrenal cortical disease**

A. **Physiology.** Three types of hormones are produced in the adrenal cortex: glucocorticoids, mineralocorticoids, and androgens.

1. **Glucocorticoids.** Cortisol is the principal hormone of this class produced in response to adrenocorticotropic hormone (ACTH) from the anterior pituitary. About 20 mg of cortisol is produced daily. It has multiple effects on carbohydrate, protein, and fatty acid metabolism. It decreases cellular uptake of glucose and promotes gluconeogenesis and hepatic glycogen synthesis. It is crucial to the conversion of norepinephrine to epinephrine in the adrenal medulla. It acts as an antiinflammatory by stabilizing microsomes and promoting capillary stability. Cortisol is metabolized by the liver and filtered and excreted unchanged by the kidney.

2. **Mineralocorticoids.** Aldosterone is a major regulator of extracellular fluid volume and potassium homeostasis. Its production is principally regulated by the renin-angiotensin system and the potassium concentration (see Chap. 4).

3. **Androgens.** Abnormal secretion of these sex hormones may indicate abnormalities in biosynthesis of multiple steroids, including cortisol.

B. **Pharmacology.** A variety of synthetic steroids are available with varying potencies and ratios of glucocorticoid to mineralocorticoid effects (Table 6-3).

C. **Hyperfunction**

1. **Etiologies.** Most cases are due to adrenal hyperplasia secondary to excess secretion of ACTH (either from a pituitary tumor or ectopic production by carcinoids or

Table 6-3. Adrenal cortical hormones

	Relative potency		
Steroid	Glucocor-ticoid	Mineralocor-ticoid	Equivalent dose (mg)
Short-acting (8–12 hours' duration)			
Cortisol	1.0	1.0	20
Cortisone	0.8	0.8	25
Aldosterone	0.3	3000	—
Intermediate (12–36 hours' duration)			
Prednisone	4.0	0.8	5
Prednisolone	4.0	0.8	5
Methylprednisolone	5.0	0.5	4
Fludrocortisone	10.0	125	—
Long-acting (> 48 hours' duration)			
Dexamethasone	25–40	0	0.5

tumors of the kidney, pancreas, thymus, or lung). Other causes include adrenal tumors or exogenous steroid administration.

2. **Clinical features.** Patients can present with truncal obesity, hypertension, hypernatremia, excess intravascular volume, hyperglycemia, hypokalemia, muscle weakness, osteopenia, hypercoagulability with thromboembolism, and infection.

3. **Anesthetic considerations.** There is no specific anesthetic technique required for adrenalectomy. Excess intravascular volume can be reduced with diuretics, but potassium must be replaced. Serum glucose must also be monitored intraoperatively. Osteopenia makes careful positioning necessary. Steroid replacement should begin postoperatively, either in unilateral or bilateral adrenalectomy. Both glucocorticoid and mineralocorticoid replacement is necessary. In unilateral resection, the remaining adrenal gland should resume normal steroid output eventually.

D. **Hypofunction**
   1. **Loss of adrenal gland function**
      a. **Etiologies** include idiopathic autoimmune atrophy, surgical removal, radiation therapy, metastatic invasion, infection (e.g., fungus, tuberculosis, HIV), or loss of ACTH stimulation from a pituitary tumor. Exogenous steroid administration can cause suppression of the pituitary-adrenal axis that can persist for up to 12 months.
      b. **Primary adrenal insufficiency** (Addison's disease) is associated with weight loss, anorexia, nausea/vomiting, abdominal pain, diarrhea or constipation, and hyperpigmentation. Lack of catecholamines may result in hypotension and be difficult to distin-

guish from an acute surgical abdomen. Mineralocorticoid deficiency will lead to decreasing urinary sodium conservation, decreased response to circulating catecholamines, and hyperkalemia.

2. **Anesthetic considerations**
   a. **Acute adrenal insufficiency** (addisonian crisis) is a medical emergency, and treatment includes fluids, steroid replacement, inotropes as necessary, and electrolyte correction. If surgery is required, drugs must be titrated carefully, as these patients are exquisitely sensitive to drug-induced myocardial depression. Perioperative steroid replacement should be tailored to the patient's requirements. **Primary adrenal insufficiency** requires both glucocorticoid and mineralocorticoid replacement.
   b. Any patient who has received **more than a 5-day treatment with steroids in the past year** should receive glucocorticoid supplementation (i.e., **"stress steroid coverage"**). Hydrocortisone IV, 25 mg preoperatively, 100 mg intraoperatively, and then 50 mg q8h for the first 24 hours and 25 mg q8h for the second 24 hours, is recommended for major elective surgery.
   c. Patients chronically receiving **high-dose steroid therapy** are at increased risk for glucose intolerance, fluid retention with hypertension, aseptic osteonecrosis, pancreatitis, benign intracranial hypertension, peptic ulceration, glaucoma, mental status changes, infection, and poor wound healing.
   d. **Etomidate** should be avoided due to adrenal suppression (see Chap. 11).

V. **Adrenal medullary disease**
   A. **Physiology.** Preganglionic fibers of the sympathetic nervous system end in the adrenal medulla and stimulate release of norepinephrine (20%) and epinephrine (80%). Peripheral effects of these catecholamines include chronotropic and inotropic stimulation of the heart, vasomotor changes, enhanced hepatic glycogenolysis, and inhibition of insulin release. They are biotransformed in the kidney and liver primarily to **metanephrine** and **vanillylmandelic acid** (VMA).
   B. **Pheochromocytoma**
      1. Pheochromocytoma is a tumor of the adrenal medulla, although it may occur in a variety of other locations including spleen, ovary, bladder, and right atrium. The majority is solitary, but 10% are bilateral and 10% are metastatic in the adult. This tumor can occur as part of multiple endocrine neoplasia syndrome types IIa and IIb and can be associated with von Recklinghausen's disease. The majority of tumors secretes both epinephrine and norepinephrine, and their release is independent of neurogenic control.
      2. **Clinical features.** The majority of signs and symptoms is due to excess catecholamine release. The classic triad includes palpitations, headache, and diaphoresis in a hypertensive patient. Other symptoms include

flushing, mental status changes, hyperglycemia, and hypovolemia-induced orthostatic hypotension, polycythemia, and weight loss. Chronic exposure to high catecholamine concentrations may produce a cardiomyopathy. Twenty-four hour urine collection for catecholamines and their metabolites is the routine screening procedure. Sometimes multiple samples are necessary to make the diagnosis. Once diagnosed, the tumor is then surgically removed.

3. **Perioperative considerations**
   a. **Preoperative preparation.** With adequate preparation, perioperative mortality falls from 45 to 0.3%. Alpha-receptor blockade is usually started with oral phenoxybenzamine, a long-acting alpha-1 and alpha-2 blocker (starting with 20–30 mg/day and increasing to 60–250 mg/day until blood pressure is controlled). This may require 10–14 days for adequate alpha-receptor blockade as evidenced by postural hypotension, nasal stuffiness, and decreased sweating. Alternatively, prazosin, a shorter-acting alpha-1 blocker, may be used. Adequate volume repletion should be provided as reflected by a fall in the hematocrit. Beta blockade is instituted after the onset of adequate alpha blockade if tachycardia persists.
   b. **Anesthetic considerations.** The overall goal is to avoid sympathetic outflow that commonly occurs with induction and surgical stimulation. The need for invasive monitors (central venous pressure, pulmonary artery catheter) depends on the patient's underlying medical condition and response to preoperative preparation. Their placement should be done with generous sedation or deferred until after induction of anesthesia. A combined technique using a spinal or epidural catheter is effective in ablating sympathetic responses while providing profound muscle relaxation. Arrhythmias and severe hypertension may occur with tumor manipulation, requiring treatment with sodium nitroprusside and beta blockers. When the tumor is isolated and its veins ligated, a sudden drop in blood pressure may be seen (especially with a spinal- or epidural-induced sympathectomy), requiring fluid administration and, if necessary, a direct short-acting vasopressor such as phenylephrine. Endogenous catecholamine levels should return to normal within a few days after successful removal of the tumor.

VI. **Pituitary disease**
   A. **Anterior**
      1. **Physiology.** The anterior pituitary secretes a variety of hormones including luteinizing hormone, follicle-stimulating hormone, TSH, ACTH, growth hormone, and prolactin. The control over their production comes from hypothalamic releasing factors. Adenomas may lead to excess secretion (i.e., prolactin).
      2. **Acromegaly**

        a. Clinical features. Excess growth hormone secretion in the adult will lead to prognathism, soft-tissue overgrowth of the lips, tongue, epiglottis, and vocal cords, and subglottic narrowing of the trachea. Connective tissue overgrowth can cause recurrent laryngeal nerve paralysis and carpal tunnel syndrome. These patients often develop peripheral neuropathies, glucose intolerance, and an increased incidence of coronary artery disease, congestive heart failure, and arrhythmias.

        b. Anesthetic considerations. Mask airways are often difficult to achieve, and intubation can be a challenge. Awake intubation with or without a fiberoptic scope is often chosen using smaller endotracheal tubes (see Chap. 13). Serum glucose levels should be carefully maintained and muscle relaxants titrated using a peripheral nerve stimulator in patients with a history of skeletal muscle weakness.

    3. Hyposecretion (panhypopituitarism)

        a. Sheehan's syndrome (postpartum patients) is seen where hemorrhagic shock has caused vasospasm and subsequent pituitary necrosis. Other causes of pituitary failure include trauma, radiation therapy, and surgical hypophysectomy. Deliberate surgical-removal of the pituitary is carried out for tumor resection, for treatment of diabetic retinopathy or exophthalmos, and to encourage the regression of hormone-dependent tumors elsewhere. Chemical hypophysectomy with alcohol is sometimes accomplished to reduce the pain associated with metastatic carcinoma.

        b. Anesthetic considerations. Hypoadrenocorticism does not ensue in these patients until 4–14 days after destruction or removal of the pituitary. Glucocorticoid, not mineralocorticoid, replacement is required. Hypothyroidism does not occur until 4 weeks after pituitary removal.

B. Posterior

    1. Physiology. Antidiuretic hormone (ADH), also known as vasopressin, and oxytocin are stored in the posterior pituitary. ADH regulates plasma osmolarity and maintenance of extracellular fluid volume. When released it facilitates the resorption of water in the kidney by the renal tubules and therefore causes urinary osmolarity to rise. ADH is stimulated by decreases in intravascular volume, painful stimulation secondary to trauma or surgery, positive airway pressure, and positive end-expiratory pressure.

    2. Diabetes insipidus (DI)

        a. Etiologies. DI represents the loss of ADH secretion by the posterior pituitary (**central DI**) or failure of the renal tubules to respond to ADH (**nephrogenic DI**). Central DI can be caused by intracranial trauma, hypophysectomy, neoplastic invasion, or sarcoidosis. Renal DI can be caused by hypokalemia, hypercalcemia, sickle cell anemia, obstructive uropathy, chronic renal insufficiency, or lithium.

b. **Clinical features** include polydipsia and polyuria with poorly concentrated urine despite a high serum osmolarity.

c. **Anesthetic considerations.** Treatment includes careful monitoring of urine output, plasma volume, and plasma osmolarity. Isotonic fluids may be administered until osmolarity is greater than 290; then hypotonic fluids are necessary. Central DI may be treated with desmopressin (DDAVP) at 0.3 µg/kg. Side effects of desmopressin include hypotension and coronary artery vasospasm.

3. **Syndrome of inappropriate ADH secretion.** (SIADH) can be caused by nicotine, narcotics, chlorpropamide, clofibrate, vincristine, vinblastine, cyclophosphamide, pulmonary infections (especially *Legionella*), hypothyroidism, hypoadrenocorticism, intracranial tumors, porphyria, and ectopically by carcinoma of the lung (especially undifferentiated small-cell carcinoma). The diagnosis is made by examining serum and urine sodium and osmolarity values: Urine osmolarity is high (higher than serum value), urine sodium is greater than 20 mEq/L, and serum sodium is less than 130 mEq/L. If serum sodium falls below 110 mEq/L, cerebral edema and seizures may result. Fluid restriction using sodium-containing solutions and slow correction of hyponatremia (no faster than 0.5 mEq/L/hr, as overly aggressive replacement can result in central pontine myelinolysis) are required.

VII. Carcinoid

A. The majority of carcinoid tumors is found in the gastrointestinal tract, most commonly in the appendix. Other sites include breast, head/neck, lung, gonads, genitourinary system, and thymus. Ten percent of carcinoid tumors secrete humoral mediators or vasoactive substances, producing the **carcinoid syndrome.**

B. **Physiology.** While many mediators can be secreted by these tumors, including serotonin, bradykinin, histamine, prostaglandins, and kallikrein, the biochemical hallmark of carcinoid syndrome is the overproduction of **serotonin** and elevation of its degradation product, **5-hydroxyindoleacetic acid,** in the urine. Stimuli for the release of mediators include catecholamines, histamine, and tumor manipulation.

C. **Clinical features** of the carcinoid syndrome depend on the tumor's location and extent of metastasis to the liver. Compounds released by the tumor are typically metabolized during the first bypass through the liver, and symptoms are only seen when there are extensive hepatic metastases or with a tumor not located in the portal system. Symptoms include flushing, diarrhea, bronchoconstriction, mild hyperglycemia, and supraventricular tachycardias. Cardiac valve cusp distortions from metastases can cause tricuspid regurgitation and pulmonary stenosis. Peripheral vasodilation can produce profound hypotension.

D. Anesthetic considerations
  1. Perioperative care of the **symptomatic carcinoid patient** can be difficult. Pretreatment with the somatostatin analogue **sandostatin** (Octreotide), which may block the peripheral actions of serotonin and kinins and prevent the release of other mediators, followed by its administration intraoperatively, should be considered.
  2. If a **carcinoid crisis,** notable for refractory hypotension and bronchoconstriction, does occur, then treatment should be initiated with sandostatin (50–100 μg IV), fluid resuscitation, and a direct-acting vasopressor (e.g., phenylephrine).

VIII. Porphyria

A. Etiology. Porphyria results from the abnormal accumulation of porphyrins, the metabolic intermediates formed during the creation of heme. There are a variety of forms, depending on where the exact biochemical aberration occurs.

B. Acute intermittent porphyria
  1. **Etiology.** This autosomal dominant disease is the most common and one of the more serious forms of porphyria. It is caused by the accumulation of porphobilinogen.
  2. **Clinical features** include abdominal pain and central nervous system degeneration caused by neuron demyelination. This can lead to motor weakness, depressed reflexes, autonomic dysfunction, cranial nerve palsies, and mental status changes. The typical patient is a young to middle-aged female, and pregnancy can worsen its course.
  3. **Attacks can be stimulated** by certain stresses including starvation, dehydration, and sepsis. Drugs that may provoke an attack include barbiturates, ketamine, ethanol, phenytoin, etomidate, benzodiazepines, meprobamate, and pentazocine.
  4. **Drugs considered safe for anesthesia** include inhalation agents, narcotics (except pentazocine), droperidol, chlorpromazine, anticholinergics, anticholinesterases, and depolarizing and nondepolarizing muscle relaxants.

SUGGESTED READING

Foster, W. W., and McGarry, J. D. The metabolic derangements and treatment of diabetic ketoacidosis. *N. Engl. J. Med.* 309:159, 1983.

Litt, L., and Rosen, F. Anesthetic and surgical risk in hypothyroidism. *Arch. Intern. Med.* 144:657, 1984.

Meulemen, J., and Katz, P. The immunologic effects, kinetics, and use of glucocorticosteroids. *Med. Clin. North Am.* 69:805, 1985.

Napolitano, L. M., and Chernow, B. Guidelines for corticosteroid use in anesthetic and surgical stress. *Int. Anesthesiol. Clin.* 26:226, 1988.

Wilson, J. D., and Foster, D. W. *Textbook of Endocrinology* (7th ed.). Philadelphia: Saunders, 1985.

7

Specific Considerations with Infectious Diseases and Immunosuppression

Gary D. Thal

I. **Operating environment.** The operating room environment and the administration of anesthesia provide numerous means for the transmission of infectious diseases. Careful consideration must be given to the risks of transmission from patient to patient (via the environment and anesthesia equipment), patient to anesthesiologist, and anesthesiologist to patient. Surgical patients may enter the operating room with their immune defenses already compromised by injury, illness, or immunosuppressive agents. Basic defenses such as intact skin and mucous membranes are violated by the routine insertion of IV and arterial catheters. Endotracheal intubation eliminates the protective function of pharyngeal reflexes and filtration by the nasal passages. Inhalation agents may impair mucociliary function, and general anesthesia affects leukocyte function. The appropriate disinfection or disposal of all potentially contaminated equipment is, therefore, essential.

A. **Work area.** Work surfaces should be kept organized and clean. Spills of blood or other body fluids must be cleaned up as quickly as possible. Contaminated gloves should be changed immediately to prevent potential spread of fluids to other surfaces and equipment (including the anesthesia record, syringes, and IV bags and tubing). Surfaces of the anesthesia machine and cart should be wiped clean between each case using 70% isopropyl alcohol. The operating room floor and the operating table must also be cleaned between each case. Washing one's hands before and after contact with a patient and changing contaminated clothing are basic yet important steps.

B. **Anesthesia machine.** The exterior of the anesthesia machine, including monitors, should be cleaned at least daily and whenever visible contamination occurs. The interior of the machine, due to significant variations in humidity and temperature, relatively high oxygen concentration, and metal surfaces, provides a hostile environment for bacteria, and the anesthesia machine itself has not been implicated as a significant source of cross contamination. Nevertheless, routine periodic cleaning and disinfection of the machine are recommended.

C. **Airway and breathing circuit equipment.** All nondisposable equipment having direct contact with mucosal surfaces or body fluids should be appropriately sterilized between uses. This includes laryngoscopes, oral and nasal airways, face masks, Magill forceps, and nondisposable laryngeal mask airways and endotracheal tubes (when used). Likewise, the breathing circuit and reservoir bag may become contaminated with respiratory and oral secretions, particularly during coughing and emergence, and must be sterilized if not disposable. The efficacy of bacterial filters in the breathing circuit (e.g., the Pall HME filter) to reduce postoperative respiratory infections has not been clearly demonstrated. Humidifiers are potential reservoirs for organisms and should be changed and sterilized between cases. Soda lime containers should be cleaned each time the soda lime is changed.

D. Equipment that comes in contact only with intact, noninfected skin, such as blood pressure cuffs, pulse oximeter probes, and head straps, should be wiped clean after each use.

E. A basin or bag on the anesthesia machine or cart to hold used, nondisposable equipment not only will keep the work surface clean but also will facilitate removing this equipment for proper cleaning before reuse.

II. Routine procedures

A. Endotracheal intubation. The use of sterilized airway equipment has been discussed (see sec. **I.C**). Special care must be taken to prevent contamination of other equipment. Used laryngoscopes, airways, and masks should be kept apart from other materials on the work surface. Intubation is usually followed by other activities, and it is important to keep in mind that one's gloves may be exposed to saliva, blood, respiratory secretions, and vomitus during intubation. One way to avoid cross contamination is to wear two pairs of gloves during intubation, removing the outer, contaminated pair while still being protected by the second pair from subsequent contact with the patient's body fluids.

B. Intravenous catheters. The placement and use of IVs are routine procedures, but one must always use aseptic technique. Insertion should include skin preparation with an antimicrobial agent, avoiding contact with the catheter during placement, and appropriately securing the catheter with an occlusive dressing to avoid contamination of the entry site. IV tubing should be connected sterilely, and injections made via stopcocks or by use of clean needles into injection ports that have been swabbed with alcohol before use. Patients who are immunosuppressed, have valvular heart disease, or have indwelling prostheses should be treated aseptically, and sterile gloves should be used.

C. Invasive monitoring. The placement of central venous lines, pulmonary artery catheters, and arterial catheters must be done with strict aseptic technique. Sterile gloves, gown, and mask are worn during placement of pulmonary artery catheters. As with IVs, all connections, tubing, and fluids must be sterile.

D. Regional anesthesia and peripheral nerve blockade should also be performed with sterile technique, including prepping and draping the site. Sites that are themselves infected or in close proximity to an infected area should be avoided. Indwelling catheters (e.g., epidural) should be properly secured, the site checked at appropriate intervals postoperatively, the injection port covered with an occlusive cap, and each new connection or injection performed with sterile technique.

III. Anesthesia for patients with infections

A. General considerations. The anesthesiologist should be aware of any special precautions required for a patient and take appropriate steps to continue these measures (e.g., respiratory precautions for a patient with pulmonary tuberculosis or varicella infection). "Reverse isolation" is used in some settings for immunocompromised patients.

B. Associated conditions. Patients who are febrile may have higher anesthetic requirements to achieve a given depth of anesthesia. Oxygen and fluid requirements are also increased by fever. Malnutrition, hypoalbuminemia, and anemia may be encountered in a chronically infected patient, and venous access may be difficult to perform in patients receiving chronic IV antibiotics.

C. A patient's **antibiotic** regimen should always be reviewed and continued. Alterations may be indicated by the nature and location of the procedure. Many antibiotics have multiorgan effects and drug interactions that must be considered (e.g., aminoglycoside antibiotics enhance neuromuscular blocking drugs).

IV. The immunocompromised patient.
A variety of immune defects with numerous etiologies predispose patients to a broad spectrum of infections. Careful attention to aseptic technique must be maintained to prevent potentially life-threatening iatrogenic infections.

A. Specific defects in host defenses

1. **Skin and mucous membranes.** Burns, extensive trauma, diabetic and decubitus ulcers, IV catheters, and urinary catheters create a route for secondary infection from organisms via the skin. Respiratory mucosal damage from burns, inhalation of toxic substances, and viral infections predispose to respiratory infection. Tracheal intubation alters the ability to clear secretions and pathogens.

2. **Humoral immunity.** Immunoglobulin deficiency may be caused by lymphoma, multiple myeloma, agammaglobulinemia, and immunosuppressive drug therapy, predisposing such patients to infection by encapsulated organisms.

3. **Neutropenia** results in defects in the phagocytic system and is associated with an increased incidence of fever. Aplastic anemia and immunosuppressive chemotherapy may result in neutropenia. Abnormal neutrophil function due to hyperglycemia, uremia, and immune complexes can be seen in patients with diabetes, renal failure, and diseases such as rheumatoid arthritis and systemic lupus erythematosus, respectively.

4. **Cell-mediated immunity** is abnormal in human immunodeficiency virus (HIV) infection (see sec. **VI.B**), Hodgkin's disease, sarcoidosis, and other conditions due to defective lymphocyte-monocyte function. Predisposition to tuberculosis, candidiasis, and disseminated viral infections is seen.

   5. Splenectomy is known to predispose patients to severe bacterial infection, especially pneumococcal infection.
 B. **Drug-induced immune defects**
   1. **Antibiotics.** Broad-spectrum or multiple-drug regimens predispose patients to superinfection, often by resistant organisms.
   2. **Glucocorticoids** alter host immune defenses by decreasing mobilization of neutrophils and interfering with cell-mediated immunity. Dermal changes such as thinning of the skin may impair host defenses and create technical difficulties with placement of IVs or other invasive lines.
   3. **Immunosuppressive agents.** A host of drugs (e.g., steroids and some cytotoxic agents) are prescribed for a variety of disorders, including malignancies, rheumatologic disease (rheumatoid arthritis, systemic lupus erythematosus), vasculitides, and glomerulopathies and to suppress transplant rejection.
V. **Chemotherapy.** Chemotherapeutic drugs inhibit or destroy malignant cells. However, normal host cells are also affected. Tissues with high proliferative capacities (e.g., bone marrow, gastrointestinal mucosa, skin, and hair follicles) are particularly susceptible, but major organ toxicity (e.g., heart, lungs, kidneys, liver, and central nervous system) occurs as well (Table 7-1). Preoperative assessment of patients who have received chemotherapy should include complete blood count, platelet count, serum electrolytes (sodium, potassium, calcium, magnesium), blood urea nitrogen, creatinine, liver function tests, bilirubin, amylase, fasting blood sugar, urinalysis, electrocardiogram, and chest x-ray. Where appropriate, coagulation profile, pulmonary function tests, and arterial blood gases should be obtained. A thorough neurologic examination, particularly in patients with known neurologic symptoms or deficits, should be documented preoperatively.
 A. **Myelosuppression and decreased cell life span** are caused by all chemotherapeutic agents and lead to anemia, leukopenia, and thrombocytopenia. These generally resolve within 1–6 weeks after cessation of chemotherapy.
 B. **Immunosuppression** results from the use of most agents, particularly the alkylating agents.
 C. **Pulmonary toxicity** is seen most frequently with bleomycin (causing interstitial pneumonitis and fibrosis) but may occur with other agents (Table 7-1). The effect of bleomycin is similar to that of radiation, and the two may have synergistic toxicities. Initial manifestations include cough, dyspnea, and bibasilar rales, which may progress to severe hypoxia with radiographic abnormalities. Symptomatic patients should have arterial blood gases monitored. An increased incidence of adult respiratory distress syndrome is seen postoperatively. The incidence of severe pulmonary complications may be reduced by avoiding high inspired oxygen concentrations perioperatively and use of colloid rather than crystalloid for fluid replacement.
 D. **Cardiac toxicity.** Doxorubicin and daunorubicin are associated with a 10% incidence of electrocardiographic

Table 7-1. Side effects of chemotherapeutic agents

Agents	Anemia	Thrombocytopenia	Leukopenia	Hemolytic anemia	Coagulation defects	Immunosuppression	Pumonary toxicity	Hepatic toxicity	Renal toxicity	Anticholinesterase effect
Alkylating agents										
Mechlorethamine	+++	+++	+++	++		+	+			+
Busulfan	++	+++	+++	++	+	+	++		++	+
Chlorambucil	+	++	+	++		+	+			++
Cyclophosphamide	++	+++	+	++		+++	+++	+	+	++
Melphalan	++	+++	++	++		+++	+			+
Thiotepa	+++	+++	++	++		+++	+			+
Antimetabolites										
Methotrexate	+++	++	+++			++++		++	++	
Mercaptopurine	+++	+++	++			++++		+++	++	
Fluorouracil	+++	+++	+++			++++				
Cytarabine (ara-C)	+++	+++	+++			+++		+		
Plant alkaloids										
Vinblastine	+	+	+++			++	+			
Vincristine	+	+	++			++				
VP-16		+	+							
Antibiotics										
Doxorubicin	++	++	+++					+		
Daunorubicin	++	++	++							
Bleomycin	+	+	+				+++			
Mithramycin	+++	+++	++		++			+	+	
Mitomycin-C	+++	+++	+++		+		+++	+	+	
Nitrosoureas										
Carmustine (BCNU)	++	+++	++				+			
Lomustine (CCNU)	++	+++	+++				+			
Enzymes										
L-Asparaginase	+	+	+		+	+		+++	+	
Random synthetics										
Cisplatin	++	++	++			+++			++++	
Hydroxyurea	++	+++	+++			+				
Procarbazine	++	+	+++	+		+++				

abnormalities (shortened QRS interval, supraventricular arrhythmias, and left axis deviation). Sudden death has also been reported. These effects are not dose-related but occur during administration of the drugs and generally resolve after cessation of treatment. A severe dose-dependent, usually irreversible, cardiomyopathy can occur up to 6 months after discontinuation of therapy. The incidence is approximately 2% but may be as high as 25% with cumulative doses over 550 mg/m^2. Evaluation of ventricular function should be considered preoperatively. Anesthetic agents associated with significant myocardial depression should be avoided.

E. **Hepato- or nephrotoxicity** occurs following the use of a number of chemotherapeutic agents (Table 7-1). Anesthetic considerations are discussed in Chaps. 4 and 5.

F. **Anticholinesterase effects.** Alkylating agents may significantly prolong the effect of succinylcholine, and dosage should be adjusted accordingly.

VI. **Infectious risks to anesthesiologists**

A. **Viral hepatitis**

1. **Hepatitis A** usually causes an acute, self-limited infection without a chronic or carrier state. It is transmitted by the fecal-oral route and rarely, if ever, by blood transfusion. It generally poses minimal risk to the anesthesiologist, but there is a risk of exposure from a patient who is incubating the virus at the time of surgery. A single dose of gamma globulin within 2 weeks of exposure to hepatitis A is recommended.

2. **Hepatitis B** produces an acute infection, a chronic active hepatitis that may lead to cirrhosis or hepatocellular carcinoma, and also an asymptomatic carrier state. Transmission occurs through contact of the recipient's blood, mucosal surfaces, or nonintact skin with infected blood, blood products, and body fluids, including urine and saliva, or through sexual contact. It is estimated that 0.1–1.0% of healthy adults in the United States are potentially infectious with the hepatitis B virus (HBV).

   a. **Serologic evidence** of HBV surface antigen (HB_sAg) diagnoses infection in the acute, chronic, or carrier state. Presence of IgM antibody to the viral core antigen (IgM anti-HB_c) indicates that the infection is acute, and presence of HBV e antigen (HB_eAg) is a marker of increased infectivity. Anti-HB_s indicates prior exposure and immunity. Acute HBV infection is followed by full recovery in approximately 90% of patients, with 5–10% leading to a carrier state, and less than 1% resulting in fulminant disease. There is a 60% mortality rate in this latter group.

   b. **Vaccination.** Given the risk of exposure to HBV in training and in practice, vaccination for all anesthesiologists is strongly recommended unless anti-HB_s seropositive from a previous exposure. Two forms of vaccine exist (made from purified plasma of carriers or by recombinant techniques). Both offer safe and effective protection against HBV with minimal side effects, and induction of protective antibody titers occurs in 95% of immunocompetent adults. Strict adherence to universal precaution guidelines will reduce the risk of exposure (see sec. **VIII**).

    c. **Treatment** following exposure to HB_sAg-positive patients should include both hepatitis B immunoglobulin (HBIG) and the hepatitis B vaccine, ideally within 24–48 hours of exposure.

3. **Non-A, non-B hepatitis** is the cause of approximately 90% of posttransfusion hepatitis. The etiology of most cases is **hepatitis C** (HCV), a virus identified by an assay for anti-HCV. HCV is also responsible for 20–50% of cases of sporadic viral hepatitis in the United States, and anti-HCV has been found in up to 67% of IV drug abusers and 10–30% of patients on chronic hemodialysis.

    a. Hepatitis C is characterized by a striking propensity to progress to chronic disease. Chronic fluctuating elevations in transaminase levels are seen in 50% of cases, and cirrhosis occurs in up to 20% of chronic carriers.

    b. The routes of transmission of hepatitis C are similar to hepatitis B, and the same safety precautions should be taken to prevent exposure. There is currently no vaccine available for HCV.

B. **Acquired immunodeficiency syndrome (AIDS)**

1. **AIDS** is caused by the retrovirus, human immunodeficiency virus (HIV). The virus attacks and eventually kills CD4 (T4) lymphocytes (often called T helper cells) and can also attack macrophages and cells within the central nervous system. Immune function is further compromised by functional abnormalities of B cells, natural killer cells, and monocytes/macrophages. The presence of antibodies to HIV confirms infection, although seroconversion does not connote active disease.

2. **A nonspecific viral syndrome** may follow HIV infection within several days, with fever, malaise, rash, arthralgias, and lymphadenopathy. These symptoms, which appear in only a minority of cases, resolve and are generally followed by a prolonged asymptomatic period. Seroconversion occurs up to 6 months after infection, and months or years may pass before any clinical evidence is apparent. Manifestations of full-blown AIDS vary widely and may include weight loss, fatigue, anemia, leukopenia, chronic diarrhea, and progressive dementia. Initial presentation may be with a secondary malignancy, commonly Kaposi's sarcoma or non-Hodgkin's lymphoma. The hallmark of AIDS, however, is a susceptibility to opportunistic infections such as *Pneumocystis carinii* pneumonia, toxoplasmosis, cryptosporidiosis, candidiasis, cryptococcosis, histoplasmosis, cytomegalovirus, herpes simplex virus, progressive multifocal leukoencephalopathy, and atypical mycobacteria.

3. **AIDS is transmitted** through blood and body fluids,

including semen and vaginal secretions. Although HIV has been isolated from saliva, tears, and urine, transmission via these fluids has not been documented. Those at greatest risk of HIV infection include intravenous drug users, homosexual men, recipients of blood products, the sexual partners of any person in a high-risk group, and children born to infected mothers.

   a. Needlestick or other sharp puncture injuries are the anesthesiologist's greatest risk of exposure to HIV. Exposed mucous membranes, conjunctiva, and nonintact skin also pose a risk. Percutaneous exposure (e.g., needlestick) carries an approximate risk of 1 in 1000 (0.1%) of seroconversion, compared with hepatitis B, with a risk of 1 in 10 (10%).

   b. Because HIV infection may have an extended asymptomatic period, all patients could potentially be HIV seropositive. Since routine preoperative screening for HIV is neither practical nor recommended at this time, universal precautions should be used at all times (see sec. **VIII**).

C. Herpes simplex virus (HSV)

   1. HSV type I usually presents with oral or conjunctival infections (e.g., cold sores) and **type II** with genital lesions (although both viruses can infect either area).

   2. Herpetic whitlow is an HSV infection of the fingers, occurring after exposure of nonintact skin to oral secretions. Since this may occur with trivial skin trauma, gloves are protective against infection. The presence of oral lesions is not necessary for viral shedding to occur. HSV can be spread from herpetic vesicles, and personnel with active herpetic whitlow should not be involved in direct patient care until all lesions have dried and crusted. It is important to differentiate the herpetic lesions from cellulitis or abscess (paronychia or felon), since incision and drainage may significantly worsen the course of whitlow infection.

D. Varicella zoster virus, another herpesvirus, is more contagious than HSV. It is transmitted by direct contact, as well as by airborne and droplet spread. Nonimmune anesthesiologists are at risk when exposed to patients with active shingles, chickenpox, and varicella pneumonia. If contact cannot be avoided altogether, gowns, gloves, and masks should be worn. Varicella-zoster immune globin (VZIG) is available for those with known exposure.

E. Active pulmonary tuberculosis infection, whose incidence has recently increased, presents a threat to the anesthesiologist. After decades of declining incidence prior to 1980, the incidence of pulmonary tuberculosis has increased by 3–6% annually. More than 25,000 cases were reported to the Centers for Disease Control in 1990. Proper respiratory precautions should be followed. A PPD should be checked regularly and followed up with a chest x-ray and appropriate medical therapy if conversion occurs.

VII. **Blood products.** The greatest infectious risks associated with the administration of blood and blood products are the transmission of HIV and viral hepatitis. Routine screening of donated blood for antibodies to HIV, HBV, and HCV has significantly reduced the incidence of transfusion-related infection. There is a "window period" of seronegativity following infection with HIV, and blood products containing the virus may test negative for this reason. Indications for administration of blood products are discussed in Chap. 33.

VIII. **Universal precautions for transmission control** have been recommended by the Centers for Disease Control (CDC) and mandated by the Occupational Safety and Health Administration (OSHA). Blood and body fluids of **all** patients should be considered potentially infectious and the following safety precautions adopted.

A. Appropriate **barrier precautions** should be used to prevent skin and mucous membrane exposure whenever contact with blood or body fluids is anticipated (this may include gloves, masks, protective eye wear or face shields, gowns, or aprons).

B. **Immediate washing of hands or other skin surfaces** if exposed to blood or body fluids. Hands should be washed after gloves are removed.

C. **Special care should be employed when using, cleaning, or disposing of needles, scalpels, and other sharp instruments.** Needles should not be recapped, bent, broken, or removed from disposable syringes. Used "sharps" should be placed in puncture-resistant containers located in close proximity to areas of use (e.g., operating room, intensive care unit).

D. **Appropriate ventilation equipment should be available** to eliminate the need to perform emergency mouth-to-mouth resuscitation. Stopcocks inserted in the IV tubing allow for drug administration while reducing the risk of needlestick exposure.

E. **Other special devices** that may reduce the risk of percutaneous exposure include needleless injection ports on IV tubing and stands that hold uncapped needles or enable safe reinsertion of needles into caps.

F. **Following exposure to known or suspected HIV-infected blood or body fluids** through percutaneous or mucous membrane exposure, our institutional policy recommends the following:

1. Immediately report to the employee health service, the infection control unit, or the emergency department (after hours).

2. File an incident report to document the circumstances of the exposure.

3. A baseline blood sample from the exposed worker should be drawn and sent. HIV testing should be repeated at 5 weeks, 3 months, and 1 year after exposure.

4. If the worker is not HBV immune, test the patient for HBV.

5. The worker has the option of beginning therapy with zidovudine (azidothymidine, AZT) immediately after

exposure, with supplies available 24 hours a day through employee health, the operating room pharmacy, and the emergency room. There are reports that if initiated within several hours of exposure to HIV, AZT therapy reduces the infectivity of the virus on lymphocytes. Current dosing is 100 mg PO q6h for 3 days, followed by 100 mg 5 times a day for 4 weeks. Definitive evidence of the efficacy of AZT treatment is lacking, and therapy is not without significant side effects. Each health worker exposed to known or suspected HIV-positive blood or body fluid must determine individually if AZT therapy is to be instituted.

SUGGESTED READING

Bernardo, J. Tuberculosis: A disease of the 1990s. *Hosp. Pract.* 26(10):195, 1991.

Berry, A. J. Infection control in anesthesia. *Anesthesiol. Clin. North Am.* 7(4):967, 1989.

Berry, A. J., et al. A multicenter study of the epidemiology of hepatitis B in anesthesia residents. *Anesth. Analg.* 64(7):672, 1985.

Browne, R. A., and Chernesky, M. A. Infectious diseases and the anaesthetist. *Can. J. Anaesth.* 35(6):655, 1988.

Centers for Disease Control. Recommendations for prevention of HIV transmission in health-care settings. *M.M.W.R.* 36(29):39, 1987.

Ciresi, S. A. The anesthetic implications of chemotherapy. *J. Am. Assoc. Nurse Anesth.* 51(1):26, 1983.

Ergun, G. A., and Miskovitz, P. F. Viral hepatitis: The new ABC's. *Postgrad. Med.* 88(5):69, 1990.

Masur, H., and Fauci, A. S. Infections in the Compromised Host. In J. D. Wilson et al. (eds.), *Harrison's Principles of Internal Medicine* (12th ed.). New York: McGraw-Hill, 1991. Pp. 464–468.

Rosenquist, R. W., and Stock, M. C. Decontaminating anesthesia and respiratory therapy equipment. *Anesthesiol. Clin. North Am.* 7(4):951, 1989.

Schlech, W. F. The risk of infection in anaesthetic practice. *Can. J. Anaesth.* 35(3):S46, 1988.

Selvin, B. L. Cancer chemotherapy: Implications for the anesthesiologist. *Anesth Analg.* 60(6):425, 1981.

Trepanier, C. A. Transmission of hepatitis and AIDS: Risks for the anaesthetist and the patient. *Can. J. Anaesth.* 38(4):R102, 1991.

II

Administration of
Anesthesia

8

Safety in Anesthesia

Jeffrey B. Cooper

I. **The risk of anesthesia**
   A. There is no accurate measure of the overall risk of anesthesia nor can the risk to an individual patient be predicted. It was estimated in the 1950s that aspects of anesthesia care contributed to three deaths in 10,000 surgical procedures. Experience with muscle relaxants, controlled ventilation, improved resuscitation practice, and the introduction of newer drugs have significantly decreased this incidence. Mortality rates for healthy patients presenting for elective surgery are now considered to be in the range of 1/50,000 to 1/150,000. The rate of serious morbidity (e.g., permanent neurologic injury) is also unknown but may add an additional 30% above the rate of anesthesia-contributory mortality. Unexpected, undesirable events requiring intervention by the anesthesiologist, such as hypotension, hypovolemia, airway obstruction, and bronchospasm, occur frequently. The anesthesiologist must promptly correct potentially harmful disturbances in homeostasis and be prepared to intervene quickly to prevent minor problems from evolving into an adverse outcome.
   B. Serious mishaps are typically the result of a combination of errors, lapses in vigilance, environmental influences, and human-factor deficiencies, all of which can combine to obscure the prompt detection or correction of a problem.
   C. Some of the factors frequently associated with critical anesthesia incidents and mishaps include
      1. Failure to prepare adequately for anesthesia, including a complete patient history and thorough inspection of equipment and apparatus.
      2. Inadequate familiarity with instrumentation or equipment, the surgical procedure, or the anesthetic technique.
      3. Poor communication with the surgical team.
      4. Haste and carelessness.
      5. Obstruction of the visual field.
      6. Inattention and fatigue.
II. **General safety strategies.** The anesthesiologist must adopt a strategy for preventing adverse outcomes. Some tactics are as follows:
   A. **Preoperative preparation.** Construct a sound anesthesia plan, prepare the patient, prepare the workspace (including backup equipment), and label all medications.
   B. **Optimize perception.** Arrange equipment and monitors in a way that facilitates scanning; avoid blocking access to the airway when possible.
   C. Employ appropriate intraoperative **monitoring** (see sec. III.A).
   D. **Crisis preparation.** Be prepared for critical events; call for help early.

III. Standards and procedures

A. Standards for basic intraoperative monitoring. The American Society of Anesthesiologists has standards for preanesthesia care, intraoperative monitoring, and postanesthesia care, all with the objective of enhancing patient safety. The standards for basic intraoperative monitoring apply to all anesthesia care, although in emergency circumstances appropriate life-support measures take precedence. These standards may be exceeded at any time based on the judgment of the responsible anesthesiologist. They are intended to encourage high-quality patient care, but observing them cannot guarantee any specific patient outcome. This set of standards addresses only the issue of basic intraoperative monitoring, which is one component of anesthesia care. In certain rare or unusual circumstances, some of these methods of monitoring may be clinically impractical, and appropriate use of the described monitoring methods may fail to detect untoward clinical developments. Brief interruptions of continual monitoring may be unavoidable.

1. **Standard I.** Qualified anesthesia personnel shall be present in the operating room throughout the conduct of all general anesthetics, regional anesthetics, and monitored anesthesia care.

2. **Standard II.** During all anesthetics, the patient's oxygenation, ventilation, circulation, and temperature shall be continually evaluated.

   a. Oxygenation

   (1) **Inspired gas.** During every administration of general anesthesia using an anesthesia machine, the concentration of oxygen in the patient breathing system shall be measured by an **oxygen analyzer** with a low oxygen concentration limit alarm in use.

   (2) **Blood oxygenation.** During all anesthetics, adequate illumination and exposure of the patient are necessary to assess the patient's skin color. While this and other qualitative clinical signs may be adequate, there are quantitative methods, such as **pulse oximetry,** that are encouraged.

   b. Ventilation

   (1) Every patient receiving general anesthesia shall have the adequacy of ventilation continually evaluated. While qualitative clinical signs such as chest excursion, observation of the reservoir breathing bag, and auscultation of breath sounds may be adequate, quantitative monitoring of the carbon dioxide content and/or volume of expired gas is encouraged.

   (2) When an endotracheal tube is inserted, its correct positioning in the trachea must be verified. Clinical assessment is essential, and **end-tidal carbon dioxide analysis**, in use from the time of endotracheal tube placement, is encouraged.

   (3) When ventilation is controlled by a mechanical

ventilator, there shall be in continuous use a device that is capable of detecting disconnection of components of the breathing system. The device must give an audible signal when its alarm threshold is exceeded.

(4) During regional anesthesia and monitored anesthesia care, the adequacy of ventilation shall be evaluated, at least, by continual observation of qualitative clinical signs.

c. **Circulation.** To ensure the adequacy of the patient's circulatory function during all anesthetics:

(1) Every patient receiving anesthesia shall have the **electrocardiogram** continuously displayed from the beginning of anesthesia until preparing to leave the anesthetizing location.

(2) Every patient receiving anesthesia shall have arterial blood pressure and heart rate determined and evaluated at least every 5 minutes.

(3) Every patient receiving general anesthesia shall have, in addition to the above, circulatory function continually evaluated by at least one of the following: palpation of a pulse, auscultation of heart sounds, monitoring of a tracing of intraarterial pressure, ultrasound peripheral pulse monitoring, or pulse plethysmography or oximetry.

d. **Body temperature.** To aid in the maintenance of appropriate body temperature in all anesthetics, there shall be readily available a means to measure the patient's temperature continuously. When changes in body temperature are intended, anticipated, or suspected, the temperature shall be measured.

B. **Guideline for action following an adverse anesthesia event.** The Department of Anaesthesia of Harvard Medical School has adopted other standards and guidelines for patient safety including standards for preoperative anesthesia machine inspection (see Chap. 9), standards for non-operating-room anesthetizing locations (see Chap. 31), and the following guideline for action after an adverse anesthesia event, which should be used when a patient has died or has been injured from causes suspected to be related to anesthesia management:

1. The **objectives** are to limit patient injury from a specific adverse event associated with anesthesia and to ensure that the causes of the event are identified so that a recurrence can be prevented. The activities aim at ensuring care of the patient, preventing loss or alteration of equipment or supplies related to the event, documenting information, informing appropriate personnel, and providing necessary guidance and support to caregivers.

2. The guidelines indicate **responsibilities** for the primary anesthesiologist, the incident supervisor (preferably someone other than the primary anesthesiologist[s] involved in the event), the equipment manager, and a follow-up supervisor.

3. The **anesthesiologist** involved in an adverse event should
   a. Concentrate on continuing care.
   b. Notify the anesthesia operating room administrator (or, if a resident or certified registered nurse anesthetist, the attending staff) as soon as possible.
   c. Not discard supplies or tamper with equipment.
   d. Document events in the patient record.
   e. Not alter the record.
   f. Stay involved with follow-up care.
   g. Contact consultants as needed.
   h. Submit a follow-up report.
   i. Document continuing care in the patient's record.
C. **Relief protocol**
   1. It is the policy at the Massachusetts General Hospital to provide periodic breaks for the primary individual providing anesthesia. No firm rule is enforced; rather, the decision is based on the individual's needs. However, current practice is to afford a 20-minute break approximately every 2–3 hours.
   2. Relief should be avoided in short cases and should be used with caution in cases characterized by complexity, that is, where the primary anesthesiologist's intuitive sense of anesthetic management cannot be satisfactorily transferred to another person.
   3. When an anesthesiologist is relieved, the record should indicate the time of the change.
   4. During a relief changeover, the following information should be exchanged and actions taken before the original anesthesiologist exits:
      a. **The situation**
         (1) Presentation of the patient's diagnosis, operation, past medical history, allergies, abnormal laboratory values, chest x-ray, and electrocardiogram.
         (2) Description of the anesthetic technique and reasoning behind it.
      b. **Surgical course**
         (1) Determination of anesthetic course and the status of the surgical procedure.
         (2) Assessment of blood loss and adequacy of fluid replacement.
         (3) Inspection of IV catheters and monitoring lines.
         (4) Present level of anesthesia (lightening or deepening); time at which the patient will need additional medications.
         (5) Inspection of drug administration syringes and containers for drug names and concentrations.
         (6) Determination of current settings of gas flows and anesthetic concentration, readings on the oxygen analyzer, and the cylinder and pipeline supply pressures.
         (7) Measurement of current clinical vital signs.
      c. **Anticipated course**
         (1) The availability of blood products.

(2) The anesthetic plan, including fluid and drug therapies.

(3) The plan for postoperative respiratory and drug support.

IV. **Quality assurance.** A quality assurance program includes a spectrum of activities aimed at maintaining and improving the quality of care and minimizing the risk of injury from anesthesia. It involves the following:

A. An **incident report** must be completed for any unusual occurrence, especially if follow-up action may be required to prevent recurrence. The report should document only the **relevant facts** in the incident, avoiding judgmental statements. Incidents should be reviewed by the departmental quality assurance committee, which receives additional information from those involved in the event and may suggest remedial steps as systematic factors are identified. Cases with special educational value should be presented at **departmental case conferences,** which provide a forum for discussion of important and controversial clinical issues.

B. A **postoperative visit** by the anesthesiologist is a key component of quality care and is required by the Joint Commission on Accreditation of Hospitals. Adverse outcomes may be discovered by this route and discussed at departmental case conferences.

SUGGESTED READING

Cheney, F. W., et al. Standard of care and anesthesia liability. *J.A.M.A.* 261:1599, 1989.

Cooper, J. B., and Gaba, D. M. A strategy for preventing anesthesia accidents. *Internatl. Anesthesiol. Clin. North Am.* 27:148, 1989.

Derrington, M. C., and Smith, G. A review of studies of anaesthetic risk, morbidity and mortality. *Br. J. Anaesth.* 59:815, 1987.

Eichhorn, J. H., et al. Anesthesia practice standards at Harvard: A review. *J. Clin. Anesth.* 1:55, 1988.

Forrest, J. B., et al. Multicenter study of general anesthesia: III. Predictors of severe perioperative adverse outcomes. *Anesthesiology* 76:3, 1992.

Gaba, D. M. Anesthetic mishaps: Breaking the chain of accident evolution. *Anesthesiology* 66:670, 1987.

Keats, A. S. Anesthesia mortality in perspective. *Anesth. Analg.* 71:113, 1990.

9

Equipment

Kenneth Giuffre and Jeffrey B. Cooper

I. **Overview.** Anesthesia equipment is used to deliver oxygen and inhalation anesthetics, to control ventilation, and to monitor the function of that equipment. The **anesthesia machine** provides a controlled flow of oxygen, nitrous oxide, air, and inhalation anesthetic vapors. These are delivered to a breathing system, which provides a means to deliver positive-pressure ventilation and to control alveolar carbon dioxide (PCO_2) by minimizing rebreathing or by absorbing carbon dioxide. A **ventilator** is connected to the breathing system, freeing up the anesthesiologist's hands for other tasks. Several types of **monitors** are used to observe the function of the system, to detect equipment failures, and to provide information about the patient. There are different types of each component of the anesthesia system; the common features are described here. The components described above must be available regardless of the anesthetic technique in preparation for the possibility of a need for general anesthesia. A source of oxygen and a backup means of positive-pressure ventilation (self-inflating bag [e.g., Ambu]) should be available for any anesthetic procedure.

II. **Anesthesia machine** (Fig. 9-1)

   A. **Gas supplies**

   1. **Wall outlets** are available for a supply of oxygen and nitrous oxide at a pressure of 50–55 pounds/inch^2 (psi). These outlets and the supply hoses to the machine are **diameter indexed** and **color coded** (oxygen—green, nitrous oxide—blue) to prevent misconnection.

   2. **Cylinder supplies** (E size)

   a. Oxygen cylinders containing 660 liters (at atmospheric pressure and room temperature) at 2000–2200 psi are mounted on the machine. The oxygen cylinder pressure gauge decreases in proportion to the amount of oxygen in the cylinder.

   b. Nitrous oxide cylinders contain 1500 liters at 750 psi when full. The nitrous oxide gauge does not decrease until the liquid content is exhausted, at which time one-quarter remains.

   c. Air cylinders (yellow) contain 630 liters at 1800 psi and are present on some machines.

   B. **Pressure regulators** reduce the high pressure from oxygen and nitrous oxide sources to about 45 psi in the machine. When pressure in the line falls below about 25 psi, the supply of other gases is automatically shut off. This oxygen-pressure **"fail-safe" system** reacts only to the oxygen supply pressure and does not prevent a hypoxic gas mixture from being delivered.

   C. **Flowmeters** (rotameters) are supplied with gas from the regulator. Each flowmeter is a calibrated, tapered glass tube in which a bobbin or ball floats to indicate the flow of gas. Newer machines have safety systems to prevent a

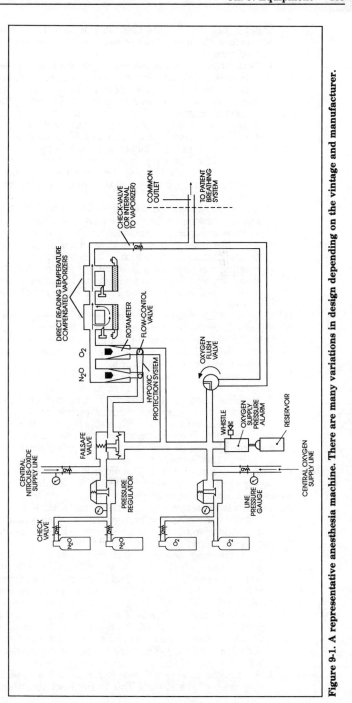

Figure 9-1. A representative anesthesia machine. There are many variations in design depending on the vintage and manufacturer.

hypoxic gas mixture less than 25% oxygen from being delivered to the breathing system.

D. **Vaporizers**

1. **Temperature-compensated vaporizers,** calibrated to deliver a specific volume percent of anesthetic, are located downstream from the flowmeters. A small portion of the total gas flow is directed through the vaporizing chamber, where it is saturated with anesthetic vapor and then mixed with the bypassed flow. The concentration is proportional to the amount of gas passing through the chamber and is varied by a dial on the vaporizer. These vaporizers compensate for temperature, are calibrated for a specific anesthetic, and have pin-indexed filling adapters to prevent inadvertent mixing of anesthetics.

2. A **copper kettle** vaporizer receives oxygen from a separate flowmeter. This oxygen flow is saturated with anesthetic vapor and is added to the flow from the other flowmeters. This type of vaporizer is useful for the rare situation in which a high concentration of anesthetic is required (e.g., during inductions for tracheal surgery). These vaporizers are temperature dependent and nonanesthetic specific and are not pin-indexed.

E. **Oxygen flush value,** 100% oxygen at 45 psi, comes directly from the pressure regulator to the common gas outlet. Flushing permits rapid filling of the breathing system but will dilute the contained anesthetic gases. Oxygen flow can be 40–60 L/min.

F. The **common gas outlet** is the port where gases exit the machine to be connected to the breathing system.

G. A separate **oxygen flowmeter is mounted on most anesthesia machines for administering oxygen** by nasal cannula or face mask. When this is not available, a No. 5 tracheal tube connector can be inserted into the common gas outlet and the oxygen tubing connected directly to this connector.

III. **Breathing system** (Fig. 9-2). The circle system is the most commonly used system for adults, while the Mapleson configuration is used in pediatrics.

A. The **circle system** prevents rebreathing of exhaled carbon dioxide, allowing low fresh gas flows, which conserve use of expensive inhalation anesthetics while maintaining higher humidity.

1. Two **one-way valves** (inspiratory and expiratory) ensure that exhaled gas is not rebreathed without passing through a carbon dioxide absorber. **Sodalyme** ($CaOH_2$ + NaOH + KOH + silica) or **Baralyme** ($BA[OH]_2$ + $Ca[OH]_2$) contained in the absorber combine with carbon dioxide, forming $CaCO_3$, liberating heat and moisture (H_2O). A pH-sensitive dye changes to a blue-violet color, indicating exhaustion of the absorbing capacity. The canister should be changed when 25–50% of the contents has changed color.

2. An **oxygen analyzer** sensor is placed in the inspiratory limb of the circuit. This is the most important

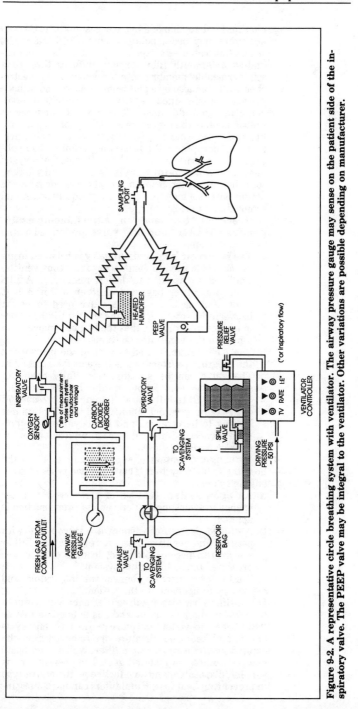

Figure 9-2. A representative circle breathing system with ventilator. The airway pressure gauge may sense on the patient side of the inspiratory valve. The PEEP valve may be integral to the ventilator. Other variations are possible depending on manufacturer.

monitor for detection of a hypoxic gas mixture. Oxygen analyzers may use a polarographic (Clark electrode) sensor fabricated as a replacement cartridge (approximately a 9-month life). Oxygen diffuses through a semipermeable membrane, after which it is electrochemically reduced by a platinum cathode. The cathode voltage is maintained negative with respect to a silver/silver chloride anode. The current produced is proportional to the concentration of oxygen. A galvanic fuel cell is more commonly used. It functions similarly to a polarographic cell but does not require the application of external voltage. For all types of oxygen analyzers, a **warm-up time** is usually required. Sensors should be placed in an upright position to avoid accumulation of moisture. They may require occasional removal and drying.

3. A **reservoir bag** and an **adjustable-pressure-limiting (APL)** or **"pop-off" valve** are located on the expiratory limb.

   a. The **reservoir bag** accumulates gas between inspirations. It is used to visualize spontaneous ventilation and to assist ventilation manually. Adults require a 3-liter bag, and children a 2-liter bag. Most new machines have a valve used to switch between the reservoir bag and the ventilator. Older machines may require that the bag be removed and a hose to the ventilator be connected.

   b. The **APL valve** is used to control the pressure in the breathing system and is the exit for excess gas. The valve can be adjusted from fully open (for spontaneous ventilation, minimal peak pressure $1–3$ cm H_2O) to fully closed (maximum pressure 75 cm H_2O or greater). Dangerously high pressures leading to barotrauma and hemodynamic compromise may occur if the valve is left unattended in the fully or partially closed position.

4. A **scavenging system** channels waste gases to the hospital vacuum system. There are two types of scavenging systems:

   a. An **open system** consists of a reservoir canister opened to atmosphere at one end to which suction is applied.

   b. A **closed system** consists of a reservoir bag with positive and negative pressure relief valves. Either system can become occluded, leading to excessive pressures in the breathing system.

5. A **Y adapter** is used to connect the inspiratory and expiratory components to the patient.

6. **Humidifiers** are either **active** (i.e., energy is required to warm a water reservoir and gas is bubbled into or flows over the water) or **passive** (i.e., no energy is added, and heat and moisture are removed from the expired gas by a hygroscopic filter, which then heats and humidifies the inspired gas). The passive type is simpler, disposable, and as effective as the active type in preventing heat loss. Humidifiers can harbor organ-

isms if not disinfected periodically. Heated humidifiers without a servomechanism may overheat, leading to potentially harmful airway temperatures and must be observed carefully. Some active warmers contain one-way valves that can impede airflow if placed into the breathing system in the wrong orientation.

7. A **positive end-expiratory pressure (PEEP) valve** can be connected to the absorber on the expiratory limb of the system. Newer machines have built-in PEEP capability.

B. **Mapleson breathing circuits.** There are several types of Mapleson breathing circuits, all of which contain no valves or carbon dioxide absorber. Inspired carbon dioxide concentration is controlled by the fresh gas flow and/or minute ventilation (Fig. 9-3).

1. **The Mapleson D circuit** is commonly used with children. The fresh gas flow washes out expired gas and must be high enough to prevent substantial rebreathing (at least 2–3 times normal minute ventilation). Capnography is used to verify sufficient wash-out.

2. **The Bain circuit** is the Mapleson D circuit modified so that the fresh gas flow travels coaxially within a longer tube for warming and simplicity.

3. **The Jackson-Rees/Ayres T-piece** modification of the Mapleson D has no APL valve. A hole at the distal end of the reservoir bag can be occluded for manual ventilation.

IV. The **anesthesia ventilator** consists of a bellows within a chamber (and an electronic control system). The bellows is compressed by oxygen or air directed into the chamber. **Ventilator controls** vary between makes and models. Some ventilators require setting of minute ventilation, rate, and inspiratory-expiratory (I/E) ratio to produce a desired tidal volume; other ventilators allow direct adjustment of tidal volume, with I/E ratio being dependent on the inspiratory flow rate, which is set independently. A portion of the fresh gas flow delivered by the machine adds to the set tidal volume during the **inhalation** phase. For example, an increase in total fresh gas flow from 3 L/min to 6 L/min will increase delivered minute ventilation by an additional 1 L/min at an I/E ratio of 1 : 2 or by 1.5 L/min at an I/E ratio of 1 : 1 (more inspiratory time in the latter).

A. A **low-pressure alarm** is triggered by a 30-second period of no pressure in the system (Omehda 7810 series) or when pressure drops below 6 cm H_2O over 3 breaths (in the Frasier Harlake 2000 series). This usually indicates a disconnection or large leak in the system.

B. A **high-pressure alarm** may have a variable or preset (65 cm H_2O) limit. A high-pressure alarm may indicate obstruction in the tubing or endotracheal tube or a change in pulmonary compliance (e.g., from broncho-spasm or pneumothorax).

V. **Pulse oximetry**

A. **Blood oxygen content (CaO_2)** is the volume of oxygen contained in 100 ml of blood. Since oxygen is both

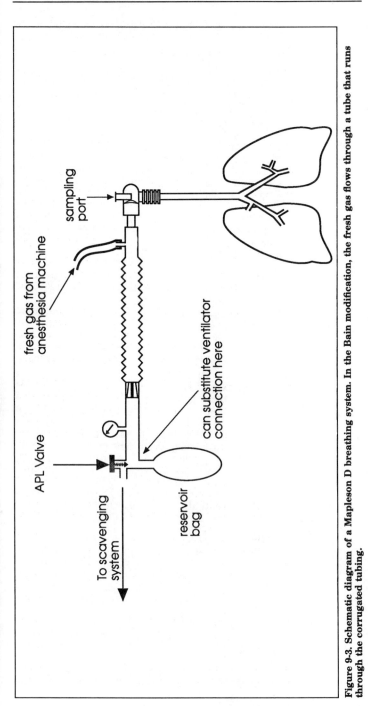

Figure 9-3. Schematic diagram of a Mapleson D breathing system. In the Bain modification, the fresh gas flows through a tube that runs through the corrugated tubing.

dissolved in the plasma and bound to hemoglobin, the calculation of the CaO_2 content has two terms:

$$CaO_2 = [(1.37) (Hgb) (SaO_2)] + [(0.003) (PaO_2)]$$

where 1.37 = the milliliters of oxygen bound to 1 gm of fully saturated hemoglobin, Hgb = the hemoglobin concentration in gm/dl, SaO_2 = the oxygen saturation, 0.003 = the solubility K of oxygen in plasma in ml oxygen/dl blood/mg Hg oxygen, and PaO_2 = the arterial oxygen tension.

B. Pulse oximetry uses **spectrophotometry** to measure changes in light absorption in blood. Two different wavelengths of light are used, one an infrared frequency and the other a visible red frequency. At each frequency, oxyhemoglobin and reduced hemoglobin absorb light differently. The light comes from light-emitting diodes (LED), which are housed in a sensor placed around a vascular bed (usually the finger). The amount of light reaching the detector (a light-sensitive resistor) on the other side of the sensor changes for two reasons:

1. Each arterial pulse causes a proportional increase in the amount of light absorbed at both wavelengths due to the increased blood volume between the LED and the detector.

2. A change in the concentration of either hemoglobin or oxyhemoglobin relative to the other (i.e., changes in saturation) causes a change in the amount of each wavelength absorbed relative to the other. This ratio of absorbed red light to absorbed infrared light is proportional to oxygen saturation.

C. **Light absorption measurements** are made only during the pulsatile component of the cycle, thereby subtracting the absorption from the nonpulsatile components, such as venous blood, tissue, and pigment. This feature of pulse detection allows pulse oximeters to select arterial blood, but it is also responsible for measurement problems, for example, loss of reading due to a loss of pulse and erroneous readings because sensor movement mimics a "pulsatile" signal. Due to inaccuracies caused by the scattering of light as it passes through tissues, all pulse oximeters are calibrated empirically, mostly from healthy volunteers, hence their decreasing accuracy at saturations less than 70%.

D. The light source and detector must be aligned properly. A sufficient peripheral pulse is required. Different probes for other locations are available (nasal, ear, foot, neonatal/pediatric size) for special situations. Disposable probes can be used for convenience, but reusable probes are recommended because they are considerably cheaper and sufficiently reliable.

VI. Gas analysis. Several methods are used to monitor concentrations of carbon dioxide (capnography) and other inhalation anesthetic gases (nitrous oxide, halothane, ethrane, forane, nitrogen) in the breathing system.

A. Infrared analysis uses spectrophotometry and Beer's law to measure the concentration of an agent in a gas mixture. Typically, some gas is withdrawn from the breathing system at a steady rate (50–300 ml/min) and passed into a small measurement chamber in the instrument. Pulses of infrared energy at a wavelength that is absorbed only by the gas of interest are beamed through the gas and the difference in energy absorbed is used to determine the gas concentration.

In some capnographs, a miniaturized measurement chamber and sensor are placed in the breathing system. In most infrared instruments, only one preselected volatile anesthetic can be measured at a time. Infrared analyzers can also measure nitrous oxide, but not nitrogen or water vapor, and may include a paramagnetic oxygen analyzer.

B. Mass spectrometry. A sample of gas is withdrawn through a side port in the breathing system near the Y piece and carried through a nylon catheter to a central mass spectrometer. The sample is ionized in an electron beam. The resulting fragments are accelerated through a high-voltage field and then subjected to a deflecting magnetic field. The specific fragments are detected on collectors, and the relative concentration of each agent is determined. Calibration is performed automatically at the central system. The instrument measures the concentration of oxygen, carbon dioxide, nitrogen, nitrous oxide, and the common potent inhalation anesthetics. By a switching system, the mass spectrometer samples from as many as 32 locations. The time between measurements in each room may be one or several minutes depending on the number of rooms "on line." A "stat" sample may be requested. One system also provides a breath-to-breath carbon dioxide analysis in real time. This mode of monitoring provides excellent tracking of the process of inhalation anesthetic uptake and distribution.

C. Raman spectroscopy uses a laser light source and the Raman effect, which involves the scattering and wavelength change of light that interacts with the gas molecules. Raman-based instruments measure the volatile anesthetics, oxygen, nitrogen, nitrous oxide, and carbon dioxide.

VII. Anesthesia equipment checkout recommendations. This checkout, or a reasonable equivalent, should be conducted before administration of anesthesia. These recommendations are only valid for an anesthesia system that conforms to current and relevant standards, including an ascending bellows ventilator and at least the following monitors: capnograph, pulse oximeter, oxygen analyzer, respiratory volume monitor (spirometer), and breathing system pressure monitor with high- and low-pressure alarms. This is a guideline that users are encouraged to modify to accommodate differences in equipment design and variations in local clinical practice. Such local modifications should have appropriate peer review. Users should refer to the operator's manual for specific procedures and precautions.

A. Emergency ventilation equipment. Verify that backup ventilation equipment is available and functioning (e.g., self-inflating bag, Ambu).

B. **High-pressure system**
  1. Check **oxygen cylinder** supply.
     a. Open oxygen cylinder, and verify that it is at least half full (about 1000 psi).
     b. Close cylinder.
  2. Check **central pipeline** supplies. Check that hoses are connected and pipeline gauges read 45–55 psi.

C. **Low-pressure system**
  1. Check **initial status** of low-pressure system.
     a. Close flow control valves, and turn vaporizers off.
     b. Check fill level, and tighten vaporizer filler caps.
     c. Remove oxygen analyzer sensor from circuit.
  2. Perform **leak check** for machine low-pressure system.
     a. Verify that the machine master switch and flow control valves are **off.**
     b. Attach "suction bulb" to common (fresh) gas outlet.
     c. Squeeze bulb repeatedly until fully collapsed.
     d. Verify that bulb stays **fully** collapsed for at least 10 seconds.
     e. Open one vaporizer at a time and repeat c and d as above.
     f. Remove suction bulb, and reconnect fresh gas hose.
  3. Turn on **machine master switch** and all other necessary electrical equipment.
  4. Test **flowmeters.**
     a. Adjust flow of all gases through their full range, checking for smooth operation of floats and undamaged flow tubes.
     b. Attempt to create a hypoxic oxygen–nitrous oxide mixture, and verify correct changes in flow and/or alarm.

D. **Breathing system**
  1. Calibrate **oxygen** analyzer.
     a. Calibrate to read 21% in room air.
     b. Reinstall sensor in circuit, and flush breathing system with 100% oxygen.
     c. Verify that monitor now reads greater than 90%.
  2. Check **initial status** of breathing system.
     a. Set selector switch to "Bag" mode.
     b. Check that breathing circuit is complete, undamaged, and unobstructed.
     c. Verify that carbon dioxide absorbent is adequate.
  3. Install **breathing circuit accessory equipment** to be used during the case.
  4. Perform **leak check** of the breathing system.
     a. Set all gas flows to zero (or minimum).
     b. Close APL valve, and occlude Y piece.
     c. Pressurize breathing system to 30 cm H_2O with oxygen flush.
     d. Ensure that pressure remains at 30 cm H_2O for at least 10 seconds.

E. **Scavenging system.** Check **APL valve** and **scavenging system.**
  1. Pressurize breathing system to 50 cm H_2O, and ensure its integrity.
  2. Open APL valve, and ensure that pressure decreases.

    3. Ensure proper scavenging connections and waste gas vacuum.
    4. Fully open APL valve, and occlude Y piece.
    5. Ensure absorber pressure gauge reads zero when
        a. Minimum oxygen is flowing.
        b. Oxygen flush is activated.
F. **Manual and automatic ventilation systems.** Test **ventilation systems** and **unidirectional valves.**
    1. Place a second breathing bag (simulated lungs) on Y-piece.
    2. Set appropriate ventilator parameters for next patient.
    3. Set oxygen flow to 250 ml/min, other gas flows to zero.
    4. Switch to automatic ventilation (Ventilator) mode.
    5. Turn ventilator **on,** and fill bellows and breathing bag with oxygen flush.
    6. Verify that
        a. During inhalation, ventilator bellows compresses to correct tidal volume and breathing bag appropriately distends.
        b. During exhalation, breathing bag contracts and ventilator bellows inflates completely.
        c. Volume monitor reading is consistent with ventilator parameters.
        d. Bellows moves freely during cycle.
    7. **Check for proper action of unidirectional valves.**
    8. Test breathing circuit accessories to ensure proper function.
    9. Turn ventilator **off,** and switch to manual ventilation (Bag/APL) mode.
    10. Ventilate manually, and ensure inflation and deflation of artificial lungs and appropriate feel of system resistance and compliance.
    11. Remove second breathing bag from Y piece.
G. **Monitors.** Check, calibrate, and/or set **alarm limits** of all monitors: capnometer, pulse oximeter, oxygen analyzer, respiratory volume monitor (spirometer), and pressure monitor with high- and low-pressure alarms.
H. **Final position.** Check final status of machine.
    1. Vaporizers off.
    2. APL valve open.
    3. Selector switch to "Bag."
    4. All flowmeters to zero (or minimum).
    5. Patient suction level adequate.
    6. Breathing system ready to use.
I. **Periodic inspection.** All anesthesia apparatus should be inspected systematically at 6-month intervals and inspection and service records maintained.
J. An **identifying number** affixed on the front surface of each anesthesia machine should be noted on the anesthesia record so that, in the event of an actual or suspected problem, the equipment used can be identified.

VIII. **Airway accessories**
   A. **Oral airway(s)** (size 3–5 for adults).
   B. **Nasal airway(s)** (sizes 28–30 for women and 32–34 for men).
   C. **Endotracheal tubes** (cuffed 7.0–8.0 mm internal diam-

eter [ID] for women and 8.0–9.0 mm ID for men; for small children, uncuffed tubes roughly [age + 16]/4 mm ID).
D. An endotracheal tube **stylette.**
E. An airtight-fitting **anesthesia mask(s)** (small to medium for women, and medium to large for men).
F. A **head strap** to help maintain an airtight mask fit.
G. **Laryngoscope** with blades(s) of appropriate size (a Macintosh No. 3 is the most commonly used blade in adults, but other sizes and different blades should be available if a difficult intubation is anticipated).
H. A **working suction** with both rigid tonsil-tip and flexible appliances available.

IX. **Standard drug setup tray**
A. Prior to every induction, this tray should include
  1. A **hypnotic** (i.e., thiopental, propofol, etomidate, or ketamine).
  2. **Narcotics** (i.e., morphine, fentanyl, sufentanil, meperidine, or Alfentanil).
  3. **Muscle relaxants.** Succinylcholine and an appropriate nondepolarizing relaxant.
  4. **Atropine.**
  5. **Ephedrine** (5–10 mg/cc).
  6. **Phenylephrine** when a regional anesthetic technique is employed.
B. **Labeling.** All syringes should be clearly identified with a label that includes the name and concentration of the medication. Medications should never be administered from a syringe unless labeled as described.

X. **Other drugs that should be available in the operating room** include
A. **Antiarrhythmics** (e.g., lidocaine, procainamide, bretylium, verapamil, esmolol, and adenosine).
B. **Antihypertensives** (e.g., propranolol, labetalol, esmolol, hydralazine, nitroprusside, nitroglycerin, trimethaphan, or calcium channel blockers).
C. **Anticholinesterase agents** (e.g., neostigmine).
D. **Anticholinergics** (e.g., atropine, glycopyrrolate).
E. **Miscellaneous drugs** (e.g., antibiotics, steroids, mannitol, furosemide, diphenhydramine, and naloxone). These should be available, possibly in a separate cart or drawer(s).

XI. **Fluid warmers** should be prepared if substantial blood loss is anticipated. General types include coil and countercurrent heat exchangers.
A. **Coil-type warmers** consist of either a heated fluid reservoir in which a plastic tubing coil is submerged or a warmed metal interface opposed to a disposable plastic grid through which fluid travels. These produce significant resistance to flow and vary in their efficiency.
B. **Countercurrent heat exchange columns** (e.g., "Level-One") provide a minimum of resistance to fluid and are very efficient warmers. Air entrapment devices eliminate air produced when fluid is warmed, but their efficiency may decrease after blood has been infused. An air-detecting safety shutoff device has been placed in-line to prevent accidental air infusion. Very high flows are

achieved during trauma and larger blood loss cases. This safety feature should not be bypassed.

XII. A **flashlight** should be available for use.

SUGGESTED READING

Andrews, J. L. The Anatomy of Modern Anesthesia Machines. In P. G. Barash, S. Deutsch, and J. Tinker (eds.), *American Society of Anesthesiology Refresher Courses in Anesthesiology*. Philadelphia: Lippincott, 1990. Vol. 18, pp. 1–6.

Dorsch, J. A., and Dorsch, S. E. (eds.). *Understanding Anesthesia Equipment: Construction, Care, and Complications* (2nd ed.). Baltimore: Williams & Wilkins, 1984.

Eisencraft, J. A. Anatomy and Physiology of the Anesthesia Machine. *Lecture Notes of the 38th Annual Anesthesiology Review Course*. Danemiller Memorial Education Foundation, San Antonio, 1991.

Petty, C. *The Anesthesia Machine*. New York: Churchill Livingstone, 1987.

Severinghaus, J. W. and Kelleher, J. F. Recent developments in pulse oximetry. *Anesthesiology* 76(6): 1018, 1992.

10

Monitoring

Stephen Small

I. **Standard monitoring.** The proliferation of perioperative monitoring devices has given rise to a certain level of standard of care in anesthesiology.
   A. Standard monitoring for a **general anesthetic** includes electrocardiogram, blood pressure, respiratory rate, oxygen saturation, end-tidal carbon dioxide, and inspired oxygen concentration (FIO_2).
   B. Standard monitoring for a **regional anesthetic** includes electrocardiogram, blood pressure, respiratory rate, and oxygen saturation.

II. **Cardiovascular monitoring**
   A. **Electrocardiogram (ECG)**
      1. **Purpose.** The ECG is monitored in all patients undergoing surgery. It is used for the detection of arrhythmias, myocardial ischemia, electrolyte imbalance, and pacemaker function.
      2. **Electrode placement.** ECG monitoring requires the proper placement of two sensing electrodes and a third reference (ground) electrode. Four electrodes may be used to allow any of the limb lead configuration selections. Since the ECG is a small electrical signal (about 1 mV), its measurement is very susceptible to electrical interference from other sources, especially power cords, electrosurgical instruments, and motion. Improper application of electrodes is an important source of electrical noise. Electrodes should have adequate gel and be applied to a clean, dry skin area. Wires should be securely fastened into the cable.
      3. **Lead II** is most commonly monitored because the P wave is easily seen, allowing detection of arrhythmias. Inferior ischemia may also be detected.
      4. **Lead V5** is monitored for the detection of myocardial ischemia, since the bulk of the left ventricular myocardium lies beneath it. If only a three-lead electrode system is available, a **modified V5 lead** is obtained by placing the right-arm lead under the right clavicle, the left-arm lead in the V5 position, and the left-leg lead as usual while monitoring lead I.
      5. **A five-lead system** is used (with simultaneous monitoring of leads II and V5) in patients with significant cardiac disease. This combination will provide 80–96% sensitivity for detection of intraoperative ischemic events (V5 alone, 75–80%; II alone, 18–33%).
         a. Most monitors have a **diagnostic** and a **monitor** mode. The diagnostic mode should be used when evaluating ST-segment changes because it filters out less noise (a wider response of 0.05–100 Hz) than the monitor mode (a narrower response of 0.5–100 Hz).
         b. The monitor mode creates a more stable tracing for simple rhythm monitoring.

       c. Calibration of the ECG signal should be checked with the internal calibration button. A 1-mV signal should produce a 1-cm deflection.

       d. Newer monitors now permit continuous analysis and trending of ST-segment changes.

B. Blood pressure

  1. Noninvasive blood pressure measurement involves external pressure applied over a limb with a compression cuff. The cuff is inflated with air to a pressure above systolic to terminate arterial flow and is then slowly deflated. Restoration of flow is detected by auscultation of Korotkoff's sounds, palpation of an arterial pulse, ultrasonic flow detection, or observing changes in the pulsations in the cuff pressure caused by the arterial pulse (oscillotonometry).

    a. Two **sources of error** are common to all these techniques.

      (1) Inappropriate cuff size. A very narrow cuff may produce falsely high measurements, while a very wide cuff may produce falsely low values. The cuff should cover about two-thirds of the upper arm or thigh; that is, the width of the cuff should be 20% greater than the diameter of the limb.

      (2) If the **deflation rate is too rapid,** the measurement may be falsely low, **especially at low heart rates** (recommended rate is 3–5 mm Hg/sec).

    b. Auscultation of Korotkoff's sounds is the most common technique. As the cuff pressure deflates, blood is ejected with turbulent flow. This turbulence creates sounds that can usually be detected by a stethoscope. The sounds continue as the cuff pressure is gradually decreased until the diastolic pressure is reached. At that point, Korotkoff's sounds will change or disappear, as the artery is no longer occluded at any point in the pulse cycle. Perceived **muffling of the sounds** is the standard criteria for the diastolic measurement.

    c. Palpation of the arterial pulse as it first appears distal to a deflating cuff will offer an approximation of the systolic pressure. This value will be lower than that obtained by direct intraarterial measurement.

    d. Doppler ultrasonic flow probes can be used in place of the stethoscope when Korotkoff's sounds are weak or inaudible. This is particularly useful for infants or for low-flow states in adults. An ultrasonic crystal beams a high-frequency signal to the vessel wall. The motion of the vessel wall during systole causes a shift in the frequency of the reflected wave (Doppler principle), which is then converted into an audible signal.

    e. Oscillotonometry is a simple technique for approximating systolic blood pressure and noting trends. As the cuff is deflated, a manometer is observed for a sudden increase in the amplitude of oscillations of the needle as an index to **systolic** blood pressure. This is a useful technique in infants and small children.

   f. Automated devices use periodic cuff inflation and deflation to measure systolic, diastolic, and mean arterial pressures. Typically the cuff is inflated to 170 mm Hg initially, or about 40 mm Hg above the previous systolic measurement, and then deflated linearly in fixed increments of about 3 mm Hg. A microprocessor analyzes the pressure oscillations in the cuff and determines mean pressure to be the average pressure in the cuff at which the maximal oscillation occurs. The diastolic and systolic readings are not always well correlated with invasive measurements and should be interpreted cautiously, especially when severe bradycardia or arrhythmias are present. The cycling time and pressure alarm limits can be set. Motion artifact is rejected by some instruments but will increase the inflation cycle time. External pressure on the cuff will give false readings if sustained or cause the cycling time to be prolonged. Some instruments have a "STAT" mode, which will cycle more rapidly to give an estimate of systolic pressure. Venous congestion may occur if the instrument is set to cycle too frequently; **cycle times less than 2 minutes apart should be avoided for routine monitoring.**

2. Invasive techniques for directly measuring blood pressure require coupling of the intravascular space to an external transducer (usually electronic) through a catheter.

   a. The transducer converts the pressure signal to an electronic signal, which is then amplified and displayed by the monitor. To ensure that the waveform is not distorted, the tubing must be rigid and as short as possible, preferably less than 4 feet (to prevent harmonic amplification). The number of stopcocks should be minimized and the entire system purged of air bubbles. The fluid-filled system must be assembled **aseptically.** A continuous flush device at 3–5 ml/hr at 150 mm Hg (central venous pressure), or 300 mm Hg pressure (artery), or intermittent manual flushing is required to prevent clot formation at the tip of the cannula.

   b. To obtain a true zero, the transducer must be on the same horizontal plane as is the zero point in the cardiovascular system (approximately at the level of the right atrium). This is particularly important in direct measurement of venous pressures.

   c. The internal electrical calibration procedure varies with each type of monitor. The accuracy of the calibration may be confirmed externally by using a mercury manometer.

   d. Periodic recalibration will confirm accuracy.

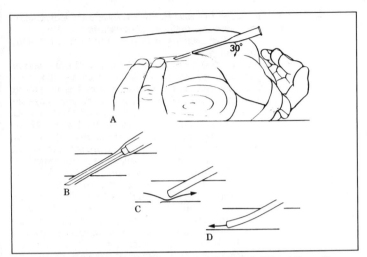

Fig. 10-1. Percutaneous radial artery cannulation. A. Direct threading method. B–D. Transfixing method. The positioning of the hand and forearm is the same for both methods.

Drifting of the baseline may suggest a defective transducer.

- e. **Arterial cannulation**
  - (1) **Indications.** The clinical indications for invasive arterial monitoring include
    - (a) Constant observation when changes in blood pressure may be considered harmful (e.g., intracranial aneurysm, severe carotid or coronary artery disease, induced hypotension).
    - (b) Frequent monitoring of arterial blood gases.
    - (c) The hemodynamically unstable patient.
  - (2) **Location.** The radial artery is most commonly used. Other sites include the ulnar, brachial, axillary, femoral, dorsalis pedis, and superficial temporal arteries. Systolic blood pressure increases with increasing distances from the heart, and the pressure waveform displayed on the monitor narrows.
  - (3) **Radial artery insertion technique**
    - (a) Immobilize the forearm and hand with the wrist hyperextended over a padded arm board (Fig. 10-1). The thumb may be abducted. Palpate the radial artery medial to the head of the radius.
    - (b) After preparing the skin, a 25-gauge needle is used to raise a skin wheal with 1% lidocaine distal to the planned point of entry. A 15-gauge needle skin puncture facilitates passage of the arterial catheter.
    - (c) Select the appropriate-sized catheter (22-

gauge for infants, 20-gauge for larger children, and 18- or 20-gauge for adults).

(d) **Transfixing method.** The catheter is advanced slowly and completely through the artery. Blood will often show in the hub of the needle but may not with the 22-gauge needle. The metal needle is removed from the cannula (keeping it sterile for possible reuse), and the catheter is firmly connected to a T-connector stopcock and flush syringe. The system should allow blood to flow back into the syringe. The catheter is lowered almost parallel to the skin of the wrist and **slowly** withdrawn until blood **pulsates** freely in the system. The catheter is then advanced into the vessel. The catheter should be flushed free of blood and the stopcock turned off until connected to the transducer. A sterile arterial guide wire can be used to aid a difficult catheter insertion.

(e) In the **direct threading technique,** the catheter is advanced slowly until the artery is entered and free flow of blood is observed. The catheter is advanced while rigidly fixing the metal needle. Proximal pressure is applied to occlude the artery while the needle is removed and the flush system is attached.

(f) **Arterial cutdown.** A 1- to 2-cm transverse incision is made over the site of entry into the vessel. A small hemostat can be used to spread the tissue until the artery is found. A suture placed (but not tied) under the artery will stabilize it. The catheter is inserted into the artery as described in **e.** The wound should be closed with interrupted silk sutures.

(g) **Tincture of benzoin** should be used to ensure secure attachment of the catheter and T connector to the skin. The catheter can now be connected to the transducer system.

(h) Never flush the line with more than 3 ml of solution, as retrograde flow has been demonstrated into the cerebral circulation.

(i) A total of 2 ml of blood should be removed to clear the volume in the catheter and T connector prior to taking samples.

3. **Specific considerations with arterial cannulation**

   a. The **Allen's test** has been advocated to assess the relative contribution of the radial and ulnar arteries to blood flow to the hand. However, it does not accurately predict blood flow and is not routinely performed.

   b. **Previous arterial cannulation sites.** Arterial pulsation **proximal** to old arterial cannulation sites should be assessed prior to insertion to confirm that thrombosis has not occurred. Distal pulse may be from ulnar collateral flow. In patients having had cardiac catheterization in one arm, distal pressure may be reduced, and the other arm may need to be used.

c. **Other sites.** For axillary and femoral artery lines, a 2-inch, 18- or 20-gauge catheter is used to enter the vessel (as described in sec. C.7). A 6-inch, 18-gauge catheter is then inserted by Seldinger technique (using a 40-cm, 0.035-inch wire) to prevent dislodgement.

d. **Damped waveform.** One should **verify** adequate blood pressure measurement by another technique. Proximal pressure on the artery, transducer malfunction, and mechanical problems such as air and clot must be ruled out. The catheter should aspirate and flush easily. It may require retaping or replacing with a larger gauge or longer cannula.

4. **Complications** are rare but include thrombosis, distal ischemia, infection, and fistula or aneurysm formation. If the hand or digit appears ischemic, a larger, more proximal vessel should be sought, and the cannula removed as soon as possible.

C. **Central venous pressure (CVP) measurement**
   1. A **central venous catheter** may be employed to
      a. Measure right heart filling pressures as a guide to intravascular volume.
      b. Administer drugs into the central circulation.
      c. Provide access in patients with poor peripheral veins.
      d. Provide a route for long-term parenteral nutrition.
      e. Inject dye for cardiac output determination.
      f. Remove air emboli.
      g. Provide access for transvenous pacing.
   2. **Sites.** The internal jugular vein, subclavian vein, external jugular vein, cephalic vein, axillary vein, and femoral vein may all provide access to the central circulation.
   3. Cannulation of the **right internal jugular vein** (Seldinger technique) (Fig. 10-2).
      a. An oxygen mask is placed, and the patient's head is turned toward the left and *slightly* extended.
      b. Aseptic preparation and draping of the skin should expose the suprasternal notch, clavicle, lower border of the mandible, and lateral border of the sternocleidomastoid muscle.
      c. The midpoint between the mastoid process and the sternal attachment of the sternocleidomastoid muscle is located.
      d. The internal jugular vein can be entered **medial** to the muscle at this point or **lateral** at the apex of the two heads of the sternocleidomastoid muscle. The external jugular vein should be identified to avoid puncture.
      e. The patient is now placed in Trendelenburg position, unless the patient has pulmonary hypertension or congestive heart failure.

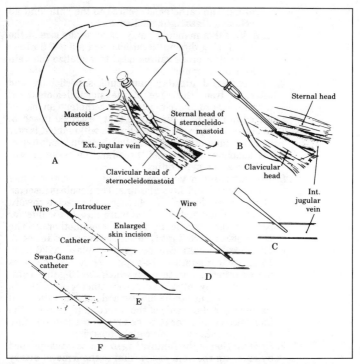

Fig. 10-2. Cannulation of the right internal jugular vein (Seldinger technique). See text for details.

f. The carotid artery is gently palpated, and the skin and deep tissue are infiltrated with 1% lidocaine lateral to the carotid artery. The finder needle (22- or 25-gauge) is advanced lateral to the artery at a 30-degree angle with the skin, pointing toward the ipsilateral nipple until venous blood is aspirated.

g. This needle is removed, and an 18-gauge thin wall (tw) needle (or IV catheter) is inserted at the same angle and depth. Blood should again be easily withdrawn when the vein is entered.

h. The syringe should be loosened, aspiration reconfirmed, and the syringe then removed. A guide wire is advanced through the needle or catheter while the ECG is observed. The wire should pass easily. The tw needle (or catheter) is removed over the guide wire. With countertraction on the skin, the dilator is passed over the wire. The insertion site can be superficially enlarged with a No. 11 blade, and twisting of the dilator may help in advancement. The dilator is withdrawn, and a multilumen catheter is passed over the wire, keeping the distal tip of the wire always visible. The wire is removed, and the infusion ports are flushed with heparinized saline. The catheter is secured to the skin, and an occlusive dressing is applied.

  i. A Valsalva maneuver may increase the size of the vein during difficult locations, and a 5.0–7.5 ultrasound flow probe can be used to visualize the vein prior to venipuncture.

4. The **external jugular vein** runs superficially and laterally from the edge of the sternocleidomastoid muscle toward the clavicle. The catheter can be inserted in a manner similar to that described in sec. **3**. Occlusion of the vein at the clavicle will make it larger and less mobile. The external jugular vein bends to join the subclavian vein, and threading the catheter centrally may be more difficult.

5. The **subclavian vein** crosses under the clavicle just medial to the midclavicular line. The needle is inserted at the outer third of the clavicle and directed toward the sternal notch. It should remain close to the inferior edge of the clavicle to avoid a pneumothorax. The catheter is inserted into the vein as described in sec. **3**.

6. The **basilic vein** can be used to place a 20-inch, 16-gauge catheter. A 14-gauge, $2\frac{1}{2}$-inch catheter is placed into the vein through which the 16-gauge catheter is sterilely introduced. If the catheter is difficult to thread, the arm can be further abducted and the head turned toward the side of the insertion to decrease the incidence of catheter passage up into the jugular vein. A 140-cm guide wire may also be used.

7. Cannulation of the **femoral vein** can be accomplished by entering the vein just medial to the femoral artery (inferior to the inguinal ligament) and proceeding as described in sec. **3**. The leg should be slightly abducted prior to insertion.

8. A **chest x-ray** should be obtained to check the position of the radiopaque catheter and exclude a pneumothorax. Additional verification techniques include the following:

   a. An ECG can be connected by an electrically conductive stopcock to the end of a CVP line filled with normal saline. As the catheter is advanced, the P waves, which are initially deflected downward, become upright as the catheter enters into the right atrium.

   b. The CVP line can be connected to a transducer to observe the pressure waveform as the catheter is advanced. When a right ventricular trace is obtained, the catheter is withdrawn slightly into the superior vena cava.

9. **Waveform**

   a. **Normal.** A CVP trace contains three positive deflections, the a, c, and v waves (Fig. 10-3). Normal CVP is 2–6 mm Hg.

   b. **Abnormal**

      (1) **Cannon a** waves occur with atrioventricular dissociation when right atrial contraction occurs against a closed tricuspid valve.

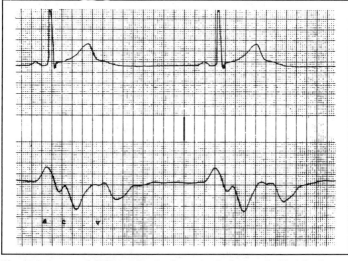

Fig. 10-3. A normal CVP tracing is shown in the bottom half of the figure with its corresponding ECG in the top half. The a, c, and v waves on the venous pressure tracing are labeled. The x descent occurs between the c and v waves, while the y descent occurs after the v wave. (From Kaplan, J. A. *Cardiac Anesthesia* [2nd ed.]. Philadelphia: Saunders, 1987. Vol. 1. P. 186.)

    (2) Tricuspid regurgitation causes retrograde flow through the incompetent valve, producing an increase in right atrial pressure during systole. This is manifested as **abnormal V waves.**
  10. **Complications** of CVP catheter insertion and use include the following:
   a. Arrhythmias. Atrial and ventricular arrhythmias may occur.
   b. Carotid or subclavian artery puncture. Subclavian cannulation may be relatively contraindicated in anticoagulated patients due to inability to compress the vessel.
   c. Pneumothorax, hydrothorax, infection, and **air embolism.**
 D. Pulmonary artery catheters (Swan-Ganz)
  1. **Indications for placement**
   a. Cardiac disease
    (1) Patients with ventricular dysfunction.
    (2) Patients with severe ischemic heart disease.
    (3) Patients with severe valvular heart disease.
    (4) Patients with angina and conduction disease whose ECG may not indicate ischemia (i.e., left bundle branch block, pacing).
    (5) Patients who require pacing intraoperatively.
   b. Noncardiac conditions. Patients with multiorgan dysfunction (sepsis, shock, acute respiratory distress syndrome, and renal failure).

   c. **Surgical.** Certain procedures are associated with profound physiologic changes (e.g., liver or lung transplantation or repair of thoracoabdominal aneurysm).

   d. **Analysis of cardiac output, pulmonary artery (PA) pressure trends, and waveform configurations** can lead to early detection of myocardial or valvular dysfunction, dysrhythmias, and pulmonary hypertension. Large A waves in the wedge position may indicate diminished left ventricular compliance. Similarly, papillary muscle dysfunction and mitral regurgitation may be diagnosed by prominent V waves. Both findings may be present without ECG evidence of ischemia.

2. **Pulmonary artery catheter (PAC) insertion** (Fig. 10-4). The right internal jugular vein is most commonly used because of access from the head of the patient and the lower incidence of pneumothorax, but all the access sites previously mentioned can be used. Most catheters end up in the **right** PA.

   a. Oxygen is supplied by face mask, and the ECG is monitored. The Seldinger technique is used to place a wire into the internal jugular vein as described in sec. **II.C.3.** The dilator/introducer assembly is placed over the wire.

   b. The wire and dilator are removed from the introducer, and the introducer side port is flushed. The patient can now be taken out of Trendelenburg.

   c. The protective sheath (Arrow Cath-Gard or equivalent) is advanced over the PA line, which is then checked for symmetric balloon inflation with 1.5 ml of air. The PA and CVP lumens are flushed with heparinized saline and attached to calibrated pressure transducers through three-way stopcocks. Raising and lowering the distal end of the PA catheter ensure calibration and sensitivity of the transducer prior to insertion.

   d. The catheter has a natural curve that facilitates proper flotation through the heart. The PA line is inserted to 20 cm, and the monitor should confirm a CVP waveform. The balloon is inflated with 1.0–1.5 ml of air, and the PA line is advanced until a right ventricular pressure waveform is seen. This should occur at about 30–35 cm.

   e. The catheter is then advanced until a PA tracing is obtained (about 40–45 cm). Premature ventricular contractions are often encountered.

   f. The PA catheter is inserted until a pulmonary capillary wedge pressure tracing is obtained (about 50–55 cm).

   g. The PA tracing should reappear with deflation of the balloon. If it does not, the line is withdrawn until the PA tracing reappears.

   h. The sterile sheath is connected to the introducer, and an occlusive tape is applied at the sheath's proximal end, allowing play in the catheter (about

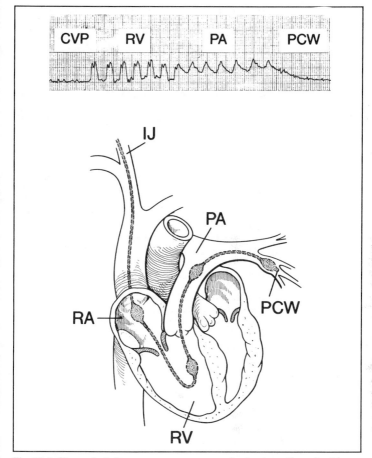

Fig. 10-4. Characteristic pressure waves seen during insertion of a Swan-Ganz catheter.

10 cm). The introducer is secured to the skin and a sterile occlusive dressing applied. The catheter should be secured to the patient's forehead or bed.

i. During PAC insertion, difficulty in passing into the right ventricle and PA may be encountered due to balloon malfunction, valvular lesions, low-flow state, or a dilated right ventricle. The monitoring equipment should be rechecked for calibration and scale. A full 1.5 cc of air in the balloon with slow catheter advancement and large inspirations by the patient to augment stroke volume may be required. The catheter may have to be withdrawn to 20–30 cm, rotated, and readvanced.

3. **Complications**

   a. **Arrhythmias** may occur while the catheter is passing through the ventricle into the pulmonary outflow tract. Lidocaine should always be available, and patients with a history of ventricular ectopy may be given a lidocaine bolus (1 mg/kg) prior to catheter insertion.

b. A transient **right bundle branch block** may occur. In the patient with first-degree block and left bundle branch block, insertion of the PA line may result in complete heart block. Appropriate medications (isoproterenol) and pacing capability (external transcutaneous, transvenous pacer, or Paceport PA catheter) should be available.

c. The balloon should never be kept inflated for an extended period because of the possibility of pulmonary artery rupture or infarction. Balloon inflation should be slow and should stop when the tracing is obtained.

d. The catheter is placed with fluoroscopic visualization when a permanent pacemaker has been placed within the past 3 months, when selective PA placement is necessary as in pneumonectomy, or if a PAC is required in the presence of significant structural abnormalities (Eisenmenger complex).

e. PA lines rarely may knot.

f. Other **complications** as previously described for CVP catheters (see sec. **II.C.10**).

4. Types of PA catheters. These allow for additional injection ports, pacing capability, determination of mixed venous oxygen saturation, and right ventricular ejection fractions. These catheters are often stiffer and may be more difficult to pass. Types include

a. VIP.

b. Paceport.

c. Pacing.

d. Oximetric.

e. Ejection fraction.

5. Cardiac output determination. Cardiac output can be measured by one of three methods:

a. Fick method. This technique uses oxygen consumption and arterial-venous oxygen content differences to determine cardiac output.

b. Dye dilution

(1) This requires injection of a nontoxic dye (indocyanine green) into the central circulation (via a CVP catheter).

(2) The dye is carried to the systemic circulation and the arterial blood continually sampled for the presence of dye and its concentration.

(3) This technique is limited by an inability to perform such measurements repetitively due to increasing background dye concentration.

c. Thermodilution

(1) This is the method used by PACs.

(2) Saline or 5% dextrose in water (10 ml) is injected into the CVP port of the PAC at a lower temper-

ature than blood temperature. This difference in temperature is detected by a thermistor probe at the tip of the PAC and integrated over time to calculate cardiac output.

(3) Potential sources of error:

    (a) Use of the wrong calibration constant will give a false value.

    (b) Lower injectate **volume** than that set for the cardiac output computer will measure a falsely high value.

    (c) Too slow an injection will give a falsely low value.

    (d) Injectate **temperature** does not significantly affect the accuracy of cardiac output determination. Room temperature injectate solution can be used unless the computer is unable to detect a temperature difference between core blood and the injectate, in which case a cooler solution is used.

    (e) Intracardiac shunts render thermodilution cardiac output determination erroneous.

    (f) Respiration affects the reproducibility and accuracy of cardiac output determinations, which are usually obtained at end expiration. At least two determinations should be performed whenever cardiac output is calculated. Some monitors display a temperature dilution curve, which should reveal a quick upstroke and smooth decay.

    (g) Rapid infusion of fluids may alter central temperature measurements.

E. **Transesophageal echocardiography** (TEE) uses a piezoelectric crystal to send and receive ultrasound waves (2.5–10.0 MHz), and the time spent traveling through structures and the intensity of the reflected waves provide information about the function and structure of the imaged organ. Echocardiography is commonly used to image the heart, and advantages of TEE over standard transthoracic echocardiography include

1. Secure transducer position in the esophagus.

2. Continuous monitoring in both awake and anesthetized patients.

3. Excellent image resolution due to the close proximity of the esophageal probe to the heart.

4. Ability to correlate changes in cardiac volumes and wall motion abnormalities with other monitoring devices, including multilead ECG, cardiac output, stroke volume, and filling pressures.

5. Several imaging possibilities exist:

    a. **M-mode** is the standard view, which provides a unidimensional view of structures in a narrow beam. It is used to provide measurement of left ventricular end-diastolic and end-systolic diameter, as well as fractional shortening.

    b. **Two-dimensional mode** is provided by rapidly changing beam direction along a single plane.

Changes in cross-sectional area, as detected by two-dimensional mode, parallel changes in contractility. Wall motion abnormalities are noted with this technique, and ejection fraction can be determined.

   c. **Doppler echocardiography** is used in combination with standard M-mode or two-dimensional echocardiography. The Doppler shift can be used to provide information about the velocity and direction of blood flow and is commonly used to evaluate valvular lesions.

   d. **Other applications of TEE** include monitoring the patient with cardiac disease for cardiac and noncardiac surgery, as a monitor to detect the presence of air emboli, as a diagnostic tool for detecting congenital heart defects, and as a means of evaluating flow limitations after valvular heart surgery.

III. **Ventilation monitoring**

   A. **Precordial or esophageal stethoscopes** allow continuous evaluation of breath sounds; some include a thermistor for temperature measurement.

   B. **Pulse oximetry** (see Chap. 9 for principles).

      1. **Abnormal saturation values** may be caused by problems with the patient or the monitor.

         a. **Patient.** Low oxygen saturation (SaO_2) may be caused by

            (1) Low FiO_2.

            (2) Inadequate ventilation.

            (3) Inadequate perfusion, either of the extremity or due to low-flow states. Hypothermia and cold extremities may cause the oximeter to fail due to vasoconstriction. Keeping the digit warm with a plastic glove may prevent this.

            (4) Abnormal hemoglobins (methemoglobin, carboxyhemoglobin, sulfhemoglobin).

            (5) Injectable dyes (methylene blue, indocyanine green, and indigo carmine).

            (6) Venous congestion.

            (7) The absence of pulsatile flow (e.g., cardiopulmonary bypass), which will result in the monitor falling to the "search" mode.

            (8) Patient movement.

         b. **Monitor.** Low SaO_2 may be caused by

            (1) Defective probe.

            (2) Electrical interference (e.g., electrosurgical unit).

            (3) Overhead infrared light sources, which may be sensed by the probe and potentially cause falsely elevated values (covering the area with an opaque cloth will prevent the problem).

            (4) Defective cable.

            (5) Intrinsic tremors or vibrations in the operating room environment.

   C. **Capnometry.** Capnometers are used in all anesthetizing locations (see Chap. 9 for principles).

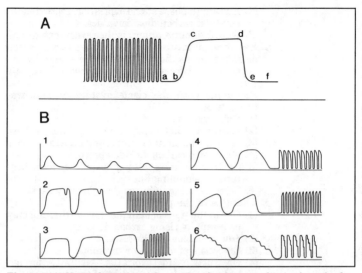

Fig. 10-5. A. Normal capnograph. a = inspiration; b = beginning of exhalation; c = beginning of plateau phase of expiration; d = end expiration; e = ending of steep downstroke with normal inspiration; f = return to zero baseline at end inspiration.
B. Some capnographs that may be seen in practice. 1 = rapidly extinguishing uncharacteristic waveform, compatible with esophageal intubation; 2 = regular dips in end-expiratory plateau, seen in underventilated patients or those recovering from neuromuscular blockade; 3 = upward shift in baseline and topline, seen with rebreathing of carbon dioxide, miscalibration, etc.; 4 = restrictive pulmonary disease; 5 = obstructive pulmonary disease; 6 = cardiogenic oscillations.

1. **Clinical uses** include confirmation of proper endotracheal intubation, assessment of adequate ventilation, and detection of pathologic conditions (malignant hyperthermia, pulmonary embolism). The end-tidal carbon dioxide value is typically several mm Hg below $PaCO_2$ and follows changes fairly well under most conditions. Nevertheless, changes in $\dot{V}/\dot{Q}$ matching, dead space, and pulmonary blood flow can change the end-tidal arterial difference so that end-tidal changes may not accurately reflect the change in $PaCO_2$. In some cases, confirmation of $PaCO_2$ should be performed with arterial blood gases. Also, the end-tidal value itself may be misleading, since a plateau in concentration at the end of expiration is necessary to represent alveolar gas accurately. Display of the waveform is strongly recommended, since it can provide important information.
2. **End-tidal carbon dioxide waveforms** (Fig. 10-5)
   a. **Normal**
      (1) **Carbon dioxide increases** during exhalation as the distal airways empty.

(2) A **plateau** phase at end expiration approximates end-tidal carbon dioxide values.

(3) **Rapid decline** to zero is seen with inspiration.

b. **Esophageal intubation.** An initial pulse of carbon dioxide from swallowed gas may be sensed by the capnometer. However, the waveform will rapidly return to zero.

c. **Problems with the circle system or endotracheal tube**

(1) Disconnection.

(2) Malfunctioning inspiratory or expiratory valves.

(3) Leak in the circuit or sampling system.

(4) Exhausted carbon dioxide absorber.

(5) Obstruction in breathing system, endotracheal tube, or sampling line.

(6) Slow sampling with rapid respiratory rate.

d. **Changes in the patient**

(1) One of the signs of malignant hyperthermia may be a rapidly rising carbon dioxide.

(2) Low perfusion/shock states.

(3) Embolism of air, fat, or thrombus.

(4) Obstruction to expiration—asthma, foreign body, extrinsic compression of the airway.

(5) $\dot{V}/\dot{Q}$ mismatching.

(6) Absorption of carbon dioxide from the peritoneal cavity during laparoscopic procedures.

(7) Reperfusion following release of long-standing tourniquet or arterial clamp.

(8) Early sign of return of neuromuscular function after pharmacologic blockade.

D. **Gas analysis systems** continuously measure anesthetic concentrations and are useful in teaching uptake and distribution, detecting vaporizer malfunction or the presence of residual anesthetic, and detecting air emboli (see Chap. 9 for operating principles). The sampling interval is short to provide sufficient early warning of most untoward events and physiologic changes, but detection of some events such as esophageal intubation (in systems lacking real-time carbon dioxide analysis) may not be sufficiently rapid if long measurement delays are encountered.

Interference between measurements of gases and vapors can cause small errors for some inhalation anesthetics. Aerosols of various beta-2 agonists (e.g., albuterol) can produce falsely high measurements. Measurement errors can also occur if an instrument is not calibrated at the actual working pressure.

IV. **Temperature monitoring**

A. **Indications**

1. **Malignant hyperthermia** is an ever-present danger, and temperature monitoring must be available.

2. **Infants and small children** with a high ratio of body surface area to mass have poor thermal stability and tolerate hypothermia poorly.

3. **Adults** subjected to low ambient temperatures and

large evaporative losses (from burns, exposed peritoneum, transfusion of cold fluids, or extensive irrigation) may become hypothermic.

4. **Cardiopulmonary bypass** with induced hypothermia; rewarming is a particularly hazardous period.
5. The **febrile patient.**
6. The **patient with autonomic dysfunction.**

B. Several **sites** may be used for temperature monitoring, including the skin, axilla, rectum, esophagus, nasopharynx, tympanic membranes, and bladder.

1. **Changes in skin temperature** may not reflect changes in core temperature (skin temperature on the forehead is on average 3–4°C below core temperature).
2. The **axilla** can be used for temperature determination if the probe is secured over the axillary artery and the arm fully adducted to the patient's side. The measured temperature will usually be 1°C lower than core temperature after equilibration.
3. **Rectal** temperatures do not accurately reflect early changes from normal body temperature during anesthesia and should be used only when an alternative is not available. Rectal perforation is a rare complication.
4. **Esophageal** temperature measurements should be recorded in the lower third of the esophagus. Esophageal temperature is an accurate reflection of core and blood temperature.
5. The **nasopharynx** gives an accurate measurement of brain temperature, since it is in close proximity to the carotid artery. The probe can be correctly placed by measuring the distance between the external meatus of the ear and the external nares. The lubricated probe is carefully inserted posterior to that distance. It should be taped to the bridge of the nose and cotton inserted into the nares to prevent skin necrosis during long procedures. Nasopharyngeal probes can cause significant bleeding, especially in pregnant patients (engorged nasal mucosa) and those with coagulopathies. They are relatively contraindicated in patients with head trauma and cerebrospinal fluid rhinorrhea.
6. **Tympanic** membrane temperature measures core temperature by the placement of a special probe near the eardrum, which is in close proximity to the carotid artery. It is very accurate. Perforation of the tympanic membrane has been reported.
7. **If a PA catheter is in place,** core temperature measured by the thermodilution thermistor can be accurately followed.

V. **Neuromuscular blockade monitoring.** See Chap. 12.

VI. **Central nervous system**
   A. **Electroencephalogram.** See Chap. 24.
   B. **Evoked potentials.** See Chap. 24.
   C. **Intracranial pressure monitoring.** See Chap. 24.
   D. **Cerebrospinal fluid pressure.** See Chap. 22.

SUGGESTED READING

Bond, D. M., Champion, L. K., and Nolan, R. Real-time ultrasound imaging aids jugular venipuncture. *Anesth. Analg.* 68:700, 1989.

Bruner, J. M. R. (ed.). *Handbook of Blood Pressure Monitoring.* Littleton, MA: PSG, 1978.

Bruner, J. M. R., and Leonard, P. F. (eds.). *Electricity, Safety, and the Patient.* Chicago: Year Book, 1989.

Clements, F. M., and de Bruijn, N. P. Perioperative evaluation of regional wall motion by transesophageal two-dimensional echocardiography. *Anesth. Analg.* 66:249, 1987.

Denys, B. G., et al. An ultrasound method for safe and rapid central venous access. *N. Engl. J. Med.* 324:566, 1991.

Gravenstein, J. S., and Paulus, D. A. *Monitoring Practice in Clinical Anesthesia* (2nd ed.). Philadelphia: Lippincott, 1987.

Gravenstein, J. S., Paulus, D. A., and Hayes, T. J. (eds.). *Capnography in Clinical Practice.* Boston: Butterworth, 1989.

Gravlee, G. P., and Brockschmidt, J. K. Accuracy of four indirect methods of blood pressure measurement, with hemodynamic correlations. *J. Clin. Monit.* 6:284, 1990.

Kaplan, J. A. Hemodynamic Monitoring. In J. A. Kaplan (ed.), *Cardiac Anesthesia.* New York: Grune & Stratton, 1979. Pp. 179–225.

Legler, D., and Nugent, M. Doppler localization of the internal jugular vein facilitates central venous cannulation. *Anesthesiology* 60:481, 1984.

Smith, J. S., et al. Intraoperative detection of myocardial ischemia in high-risk patients: Electrocardiography versus two-dimensional transesophageal echocardiography. *Circulation* 72:1015, 1985.

Teplick, R., Welch, J. P., and Ford, P. T. Monitoring Devices for Vascular Surgery: Basic Principles, Limitations, and Proper Functioning. In M. Roizen (ed.), *Vascular Anesthesia.* New York: Churchill Livingstone, 1990. Pp. 59–84.

11

Intravenous and Inhalation Anesthetics

Paul Lennon

I. **Pharmacology of intravenous anesthetics**
   A. **Barbiturates** for anesthesia are ultrashort-acting and include thiopental, thiamylal, and methohexital. These medications are used for induction of general anesthesia or as adjuncts to maintenance. Barbiturates are very alkaline (pH > 10) and are usually prepared as dilute solutions (1.0–2.5%) for intravenous (IV) administration.
   1. **Mode of action.** Barbiturates appear to occupy receptors adjacent to gamma-aminobutyric acid (GABA) receptors in the central nervous system and augment the inhibitory tone of GABA.
   2. **Pharmacokinetics.** The redistribution half-lives ($t_{1/2\alpha}$) of these medications are very short (approximately 2–5 minutes) as a result of their high lipid solubility and rapid redistribution into muscle and skin. The elimination half-life ($t_{1/2\beta}$) of thiopental is approximately 12 hours, whereas that of methohexital is 4 hours. Metabolism occurs in the liver to inactive metabolites.
   3. **Pharmacodynamics**
      a. **Central nervous system** (CNS). Barbiturates produce unconsciousness in one arm-to-brain circulation time (approximately 30 seconds). Recovery occurs quickly (approximately 5–10 minutes) as a result of rapid redistribution. Multiple doses or a prolonged infusion may produce prolonged sedation or unconsciousness. In these situations, the longer elimination half-life of thiopental compared with methohexital may be clinically significant. These medications produce no analgesia and may be hyperalgesic in low doses. Barbiturates lead to a dose-dependent decrease in cerebral metabolism and blood flow and, at high doses, may produce an isoelectric electroencephalogram.
      b. **Cardiovascular system.** Barbiturates produce a dose-dependent decrease in arterial blood pressure and cardiac output. Heart rate will often increase via baroreceptor reflexes.
      c. **Respiratory system.** Barbiturates produce a dose-dependent decrease in respiratory rate and tidal volume. Apnea may result for 30–90 seconds after administration.
   4. **Dosage and administration.** The induction dosage of thiopental and thiamylal is 3–5 mg/kg IV. The induction dosage of methohexital is 1–2 mg/kg IV. These dosages should be reduced in sick, elderly, or hypovolemic patients. Rectal administration of methohexital is discussed in Chap. 28.
   5. **Adverse effects**
      a. **Allergy.** Barbiturates should not be administered

to patients with a history of allergy to any barbiturate. Anaphylactic reactions to barbiturates occur rarely.

    b. **Porphyria.** Barbiturates are absolutely contraindicated in patients with acute intermittent porphyria, variegate porphyria, and hereditary coproporphyria. In these patients, barbiturates enhance porphyrin synthesis and may precipitate an acute attack.

    c. **Venous irritation.** Barbiturates may occasionally cause pain at the site of administration. This may be minimized by administering into a flowing IV catheter. The site should be thoroughly inspected for local infiltration prior to administration.

    d. **Tissue damage.** Infiltration or intraarterial administration of a barbiturate may cause severe pain, tissue damage, and necrosis due to its high alkalinity. If intraarterial administration occurs, heparinization and regional sympathetic blockade may be helpful in treatment. Evaluation of IV catheter placement may be accomplished by administration of a "test dose" of thiopental, 25–50 mg IV, immediately prior to administration of the induction dose.

    e. **Myoclonus and hiccoughing** are often associated with the administration of methohexital.

B. Ketamine. An arylcyclohexylamine and a congener of phencyclidine (PCP), ketamine is usually employed as an induction agent. It may be especially useful for intramuscular (IM) inductions in patients in whom IV access is not available (e.g., children).

    1. Mode of action. The mechanism of action of ketamine is not well defined but may include antagonism of the neurotransmitter acetylcholine.

    2. Pharmacokinetics. After IV administration, the $t_{1/2\alpha}$ of ketamine is approximately 10–15 minutes. The $t_{1/2\beta}$ is approximately 3 hours. Metabolism occurs in the liver to multiple metabolites, some of which are active.

    3. Pharmacodynamics

        a. **Central nervous system.** Ketamine is often described as producing a "dissociative" state accompanied by amnesia and analgesia. After an IV induction dose, ketamine produces unconsciousness relatively quickly (30–60 seconds), which may last for 15–20 minutes. After IM administration, the onset of CNS effects is delayed to approximately 5 minutes, with peak effect at approximately 15 minutes. Ketamine increases cerebral blood flow, metabolic rate, and intracranial pressure (ICP).

        b. **Cardiovascular system.** Ketamine tends to produce an increase in heart rate and systemic and pulmonary artery blood pressures. Because of these sympathomimetic effects, ketamine is often employed for induction of general anesthesia in hemodynamically compromised patients. However, if administered in the presence of hypovolemia, autonomic nervous system blockade, or maximal sympathetic nervous system stimulation, ketamine may act as a myocardial depressant.

   c. Respiratory system. Ketamine mildly depresses respiratory rate and tidal volume and has a minimal effect on responsiveness to hypercarbia. Laryngeal protective reflexes tend to be maintained, although the use of an endotracheal tube is not precluded. Ketamine appears to alleviate bronchospasm by a sympathomimetic effect.

4. Dosage and administration. Ketamine is water soluble and may be administered either IV or IM. The usual IV induction dosage of ketamine is 1–2 mg/kg. Intravenous sedative doses may be significantly lower (e.g., 0.2 mg/kg) and must be titrated to the desired effect. The usual IM induction dosage is 5–10 mg/kg, for which concentrated solutions (5%, 10%) are available.

5. Adverse effects

   a. Oral secretions are markedly stimulated by ketamine. Coadministration of an antisialagogue (e.g., glycopyrrolate) may be helpful.

   b. Emotional disturbance. Administration of ketamine may occasionally result in restlessness and agitation during emergence; hallucinations and unpleasant dreams may occur postoperatively. Patient characteristics associated with adverse effects include young age, female sex, and dosages greater than 2 mg/kg. The incidence (up to 30%) of these untoward sequelae may be greatly reduced with coadministration of a benzodiazepine (e.g., midazolam). Alternatives to ketamine should be considered in patients with psychiatric disorders.

   c. Muscle tone. Ketamine may lead to random myoclonic movements, especially in response to stimulation. Muscle tone is often increased.

   d. Central nervous system. Ketamine increases ICP and is relatively contraindicated in patients with head trauma or intracranial hypertension.

   e. Eye movements. Ketamine may lead to nystagmus, diplopia, blepharospasm, and increased intraocular pressure; alternatives should be considered during ophthalmologic surgery.

   f. Anesthetic depth may be difficult to assess. Common signs of anesthetic depth (e.g., respiratory rate, blood pressure, heart rate, eye signs) are less reliable when ketamine is employed.

C. Benzodiazepines. Commonly employed benzodiazepines include midazolam, diazepam, and lorazepam. These medications are often administered for sedation and amnesia or as adjuncts to general anesthetics.

1. Mode of action. Benzodiazepines bind at specific receptors in the CNS and enhance the inhibitory tone of GABA receptors.

2. Pharmacokinetics. Benzodiazepines are metabolized in the liver; active metabolites of diazepam may prolong its clinical effects. The $t_{1/2\beta}$ of midazolam is approximately 2–4 hours. The $t_{1/2\beta}$ of diazepam is approximately 20 hours; the $t_{1/2\beta}$ of lorazepam is approximately 15 hours. Metabolism may be significantly slower in elderly patients or those with hepatic disease. Redistribution, compared with other IV anesthetics, appears to be of less significance.

3. **Pharmacodynamics**
   a. **Central nervous system.** Benzodiazepines produce amnestic, anticonvulsant, hypnotic, muscle-relaxant, and sedative effects in a dose-dependent manner; significant analgesia is not produced. Cerebral blood flow and metabolic rate are reduced. Peak CNS effects occur approximately 2–3 minutes after IV administration of midazolam; this peak occurs later after IV administration of diazepam (4–8 minutes) or lorazepam (20–40 minutes). After IM administration of midazolam, onset is delayed to approximately 10 minutes, and peak CNS effects occur at approximately 45 minutes. Clinical effects of diazepam and lorazepam are significantly more prolonged than those of midazolam. The time to recovery after IV administration of an induction dose of midazolam is approximately 2–4 hours.
   b. **Cardiovascular system.** Benzodiazepines produce a mild systemic vasodilatation and reduction in cardiac output. Heart rate is usually unchanged. However, hemodynamic changes may be pronounced in hemodynamically compromised patients, if rapidly administered in a large dose, or if administered with a narcotic.
   c. **Respiratory system.** With usual sedative doses, benzodiazepines produce a mild dose-dependent decrease in respiratory rate and tidal volume. However, clinical response may be very variable. Respiratory depression may be pronounced if administered with a narcotic, in patients with pulmonary disease, or in debilitated patients.

4. **Dosage and administration.** Diazepam and lorazepam are usually administered IV. Midazolam, a water-soluble benzodiazepine, is administered either IV or IM. Incremental IV sedative doses of benzodiazepines in adults are as follows: midazolam, 0.5–1.0 mg; diazepam, 2.5–5.0 mg; and lorazepam, 0.5 mg (up to 2 mg). The IM dosage of midazolam for sedation is 0.07–0.1 mg/kg. IV induction dosages are as follows: midazolam, 0.15–0.35 mg/kg; diazepam, 0.3–0.4 mg/kg; and lorazepam, 0.04–0.06 mg/kg. These dosages may lead to prolonged sedation postoperatively.

5. **Adverse effects**
   a. **Phlebitis.** Administration of diazepam and, to a lesser extent, lorazepam via a peripheral IV catheter may lead to venous irritation and pain. This effect may be minimized if a large IV catheter and/or a flowing IV catheter is used.
   b. **Variable response.** Patients' clinical response to standard doses of benzodiazepines, especially for

sedation, may be variable and unpredictable. Careful titration, appropriate monitoring, and trained personnel and resuscitative equipment must be available.

   c. **Drug interactions.** Administration of a benzodiazepine to a patient receiving valproate (an anticonvulsant) may precipitate a psychotic episode. CNS depression may be pronounced if a benzodiazepine is administered in the presence of other CNS depressants, especially ethanol.

   d. **Pregnancy and labor.** Administration of diazepam during pregnancy has been associated with birth defects (cleft lip and palate). Benzodiazepines cross the placenta and may lead to a depressed neonate. Benzodiazepines are probably best avoided during pregnancy, especially during the first trimester.

6. **Benzodiazepine antagonist.** Flumazenil is a competitive antagonist for benzodiazepine receptors in the CNS. It has relatively short $t_{1/2\alpha}$ (7–15 minutes) and $t_{1/2\beta}$ (60 minutes) compared with benzodiazepines. Flumazenil is metabolized in the liver to inactive metabolites. After IV administration, reversal of benzodiazepine-induced sedative effects occurs within 2 minutes; peak effects occur at approximately 10 minutes. Administration may need to be repeated later due to its more rapid redistribution and elimination compared with benzodiazepines. For reversal of sedation or unconsciousness due to benzodiazepines, flumazenil should be titrated in IV boluses of 0.3 mg every 30–60 seconds (to a maximum dose of 5 mg). Flumazenil is contraindicated in patients with tricyclic antidepressant overdose and patients receiving benzodiazepines for control of seizures or elevated ICP. Flumazenil should be used cautiously in patients who have had long-term treatment with benzodiazepines.

D. **Etomidate** is an imidazole-containing hypnotic unrelated to other anesthetics; it is most commonly used as an IV induction agent for general anesthesia.

   1. **Mode of action.** Etomidate appears to augment the inhibitory tone of GABA in the CNS.

   2. **Pharmacokinetics.** The $t_{1/2\alpha}$ of etomidate is very short (2–4 minutes). The $t_{1/2\beta}$ is approximately 3 hours. Etomidate is hydrolyzed primarily in the liver to inactive metabolites.

   3. **Pharmacodynamics**

      a. **Central nervous system.** Etomidate produces unconsciousness in approximately one arm-to-brain circulation time (approximately 30 seconds). Recovery occurs quickly (3–5 minutes) due to rapid redistribution. Etomidate does not possess analgesic properties. Cerebral blood flow and metabolism decrease in a dose-dependent manner.

      b. **Cardiovascular system.** Etomidate produces minimal changes in heart rate, blood pressure, and cardiac output; accordingly, etomidate may be a preferred agent for induction of general anesthesia in a hemodynamically compromised patient. Due to its relative lack of either cardiovascular depressant or analgesic properties, tracheal intubation or other significant stimuli may be accompanied by tachycardia and hypertension.

   c. **Respiratory system.** Etomidate produces a dose-dependent decrease in respiratory rate and tidal volume; transient apnea may occur. The respiratory depressant effects of etomidate appear to be less than those of thiopental.

4. **Dosage and administration.** Etomidate is usually dissolved in propylene glycol when supplied for IV administration. An IV induction dosage of etomidate is 0.3 mg/kg.

5. **Adverse effect**

   a. **Myoclonus** may occur after administration, particularly in response to stimulation.

   b. **Nausea and vomiting** may occur with increased frequency in the postoperative period.

   c. **Venous irritation** may be minimized by administration via a flowing IV catheter.

   d. **Adrenal suppression.** Etomidate may suppress adrenal steroid synthesis for up to 24 hours. Although suppression may occur after a single dose, this is of greater significance after multiple doses or use of an infusion.

E. **Propofol** (2,6-diisopropylphenol) is used for induction or maintenance of general anesthesia. It is prepared as a 1% isotonic oil-in-water emulsion, which contains egg lecithin, glycerol, and soybean oil.

   1. **Mode of action.** The mode of action of propofol is not known.

   2. **Pharmacokinetics.** Propofol is rapidly redistributed ($t_{1/2\alpha}$ is 2–4 minutes). The $t_{1/2\beta}$ is approximately 4 hours. Elimination occurs primarily through hepatic metabolism to inactive metabolites.

   3. **Pharmacodynamics**

      a. **Central nervous system.** Propofol rapidly induces unconsciousness (approximately 30–45 seconds). Low doses may produce conscious sedation. Propofol has no analgesic properties. Its pharmacokinetic profile promotes early awakening after a single dose or the termination of an infusion. Cerebral blood flow appears to decrease with administration.

      b. **Cardiovascular system.** Propofol is a cardiovascular depressant; significant decreases in arterial blood pressure and cardiac output occur in a dose-dependent manner similar to that of thiopental. Heart rate is minimally affected.

      c. **Respiratory system.** Propofol produces a dose-dependent decrease in respiratory rate and tidal volume. In addition, the ventilatory response to hypercarbia is diminished. A single induction dose of propofol commonly produces apnea for 30–90 seconds. If used for sedation, appropriate monitoring should be employed, and trained personnel and resuscitative equipment should be available.

4. **Dosage and administration.** Propofol may be diluted, if necessary, only in 5% dextrose in water to a minimum concentration of 0.2%. The usual induction dosage is 2.0–2.5 mg/kg IV. For maintenance of general anesthesia, an initial infusion rate of 0.1–0.2 mg/kg/min may be employed and adjusted accordingly. A dosage of 3–4 mg/kg/hr is often sufficient for sedation. Dosages should be reduced if administered with other anesthetics or in elderly or hemodynamically compromised patients. After opening, propofol should be discarded if not administered within 6 hours (to prevent inadvertent bacterial contamination).

5. **Other effects**

   a. **Allergy.** Propofol should not be administered to patients with a history of allergy to propofol or egg products.

   b. **Lipid disorders.** Propofol is an emulsion and therefore should be used cautiously in patients with disorders of lipid metabolism (e.g., hyperlipidemia, pancreatitis).

   c. **Venous irritation.** The incidence of pain during IV administration of propofol may be as high as 50–70%. This may be reduced by prior administration of narcotics, addition of lidocaine (0.01%) to the induction dose of propofol, administration through a flowing IV catheter, or administration through a large-gauge IV catheter (e.g., 16-gauge) in a large vein (e.g., antecubital).

   d. **Nausea and vomiting** postoperatively may occur less frequently after propofol-based general anesthesia as compared with other methods of general anesthesia.

F. **Narcotics** (opioid agonists). Morphine, meperidine, fentanyl, sufentanil, and alfentanil are the major narcotics used in general anesthesia. Their primary effect is analgesia, and therefore they are used primarily to supplement other anesthetics during induction or maintenance of general anesthesia. In high doses, narcotics are occasionally employed as the sole anesthetic (e.g., cardiac surgery). These narcotics differ primarily in their potency, pharmacokinetics, and side effects.

1. **Mode of action.** Narcotics bind at specific opioid receptors in the brain and spinal cord.

2. **Pharmacokinetics.** After IV administration, narcotics undergo rapid redistribution, and all have large volumes of distribution. Pharmacokinetic data are presented in Table 11-1. Duration of clinical effect is dependent on many factors. For example, although the $t_{1/2\beta}$ of fentanyl is longer than that of morphine, the duration of clinical effect of an IV bolus of morphine may be of a longer duration than that of an equianalgesic dose of fentanyl. This is due to the greater lipid solubility and more rapid redistribution of fenta-

Table 11-1. Narcotic dosages and pharmacokinetics

Narcotic	Dose A	Dose B	Dose C	Dose D	Time to peak CNS effect (min)	$t_{1/2\alpha}$ (min)	$t_{1/2\beta}$ (hr)
Morphine	0.05–2.0 mg/kg	0.2–0.3 mg/kg	1–2 mg/kg		30	9–19	3.0–4.5
Meperidine	0.5–2.0 mg/kg	2–3 mg/kg			15	7–17	3–4
Fentanyl	0.5–2.0 μg/kg	2–8 μg/kg	50–150 μg/kg		5–7	13	4–7
Sufentanil		0.2–0.8 μg/kg	10–30 μg/kg	0.25–1.0 μg/kg/hr	3–4	10–13	2.5
Alfentanil		10–75 μg/kg		0.5–3.0 μg/kg/hr	1–2	10–13	1.5

Dose A: Typical dosages for perioperative analgesia, given in divided IV increments.
Dose B: Typical initial dosages used in nitrous oxide–narcotic–relaxant technique.
Dose C: Dosage range for induction of anesthesia (e.g., cardiac surgery) in patients who will need prolonged postoperative mechanical ventilation.
Dose D: Dosage range for continuous infusion in nitrous oxide–narcotic–relaxant technique.
$t_{1/2\alpha}$ = redistribution half-life; $t_{1/2\beta}$ = elimination half-life.

nyl. Elimination is primarily by the liver and is somewhat dependent on the level of hepatic blood flow and activity of metabolic enzymes. Most narcotics have inactive metabolites that are excreted in the urine.

3. **Pharmacodynamics**

   a. **Central nervous system.** Narcotics produce sedation and analgesia in a dose-dependent manner; euphoria is also common. In large doses, narcotics may produce amnesia and loss of consciousness. As the dosage is increased, minimum alveolar concentration (MAC) may be significantly reduced; however, even with large doses, addition of another anesthetic may be necessary. After IV administration of narcotics, onset of action is within minutes; those narcotics with greater lipid solubility have a more rapid clinical onset. Narcotics decrease cerebral blood flow and metabolic rate. Meperidine, in large doses, may produce CNS excitation and seizures, possibly secondary to the effects of normeperidine, a metabolite.

   b. **Cardiovascular system.** In general, administration of narcotics at normal clinical dosages produces minimal changes in cardiac contractility (except meperidine, which is a direct myocardial depressant). Systemic vascular resistance is usually moderately reduced due to reduced medullary sympathetic outflow. However, systemic resistance may be greatly reduced with the administration of meperidine or morphine due to histamine release; this may be attenuated by slow administration of the narcotic and/or pretreatment with histamine H_1 and H_2 antagonists. In addition, narcotics may markedly enhance the myocardial depressant effects of other anesthetics (e.g., benzodiazepines, volatile inhalation agents). Narcotics (except meperidine) produce bradycardia in a dose-dependent manner by a centrally mediated mechanism; bradycardia may be marked in the presence of beta-adrenergic blockade. Meperidine produces an increase in heart rate, possibly because of its atropine-like structure. The relative hemodynamic stability offered by narcotics often leads to their use as the primary anesthetic in hemodynamically compromised or critically ill patients. However, stability is not always ensured in these patients, and administration of narcotics should be gradual and titrated to desired effect.

   c. **Respiratory system.** Narcotics produce respiratory depression in a dose-dependent manner. Initially, respiratory rate decreases; with larger doses, tidal volume decreases. Ventilatory response to $PaCO_2$ is also diminished. Apnea (with or without unconsciousness) due to respiratory depression may occur with large doses or rapid administration. Apnea or severe impairment of ventilation may also occur secondary to muscle rigidity (see sec. **5.b**). Equianalgesic doses of these narcotics produce similar degrees of respiratory depression. Respiratory depression is accentuated in the presence of other respiratory depressants or preexisting pulmonary disease. Narcotics produce a decrease in the cough reflex in a dose-dependent manner.

4. **Dosage and administration.** Narcotics are usually administered IV, either by bolus or infusion. Appropriate dosages are presented in Table 11-1. These are suggested dosages; clinical dosing must be individualized and based on the patient's underlying condition and clinical response. Greater doses may be required in patients chronically receiving narcotics. Dosage and administration for regional anesthesia are discussed in Chap. 37.

5. **Other effects**
   a. **Pupil size.** Narcotics cause a relatively dose-dependent decrease in pupil size (miosis) by stimulation of the Edinger-Westphal nucleus. Observation of pupil size may be a useful guide in the assessment of narcotic effect.
   b. **Muscle rigidity** may occur with administration of narcotics; its incidence increases with drug potency, dose, rate of administration, and presence of nitrous oxide. Rigidity may be especially pronounced in the chest and abdominal musculature, resulting in the inability to ventilate the patient. This rigidity may be overcome by administration of neuromuscular relaxants or narcotic antagonists. The incidence may be decreased by "pretreatment" with a small dose of a nondepolarizing muscle relaxant.
   c. **Gastrointestinal system.** In general, narcotics produce an increase in the tone and secretions of the gastrointestinal tract and a decrease in motility. Increased tone also occurs in the biliary tract and may result in biliary colic; the incidence may be lower with meperidine.
   d. **Nausea and vomiting** often occur after narcotic administration. This is due to direct stimulation of the chemoreceptor trigger zone.
   e. **Urinary retention** may occur after administration of narcotics. This may be secondary to stimulation of the vesical sphincter and a decrease in awareness of the need to urinate.
   f. **Allergy.** Allergic phenomena have been reported with narcotics but are very rare. Most adverse reactions appear to be predictable, nonallergic, and dose-dependent (e.g., nausea). Patients with a history of an "allergy" to a narcotic should be closely questioned and their medical records examined so as not to exclude these medications unnecessarily.
   g. **Drug interactions.** As previously noted, narcotics may markedly enhance the CNS, cardiovascular, and respiratory effects of other anesthetics. Phenothiazines, monoamine oxidase inhibitors, and tricyclic antidepressants may also markedly enhance the depressant effects of narcotics. Administration

of meperidine to a patient who has received a monoamine oxidase inhibitor may result in delirium and hyperthermia.

6. **Narcotic antagonists** (naloxone). These medications are occasionally used to reverse unanticipated or undesired postoperative narcotic-induced respiratory or CNS depression. The only relatively pure narcotic antagonist available for parenteral administration is naloxone. Narcotic agonist-antagonists are discussed in Chap. 37.

   a. **Mode of action.** Naloxone is a competitive antagonist to narcotics at opioid receptors in the brain and spinal cord.

   b. **Pharmacokinetics.** After IV administration, the $t_{1/2\alpha}$ of naloxone is approximately 1 hour; the $t_{1/2\beta}$ is approximately 1–4 hours. Naloxone is metabolized in the liver.

   c. **Pharmacodynamics.** Naloxone reverses, in a dose-dependent manner, the pharmacologic effects of narcotics (e.g., CNS depression, respiratory depression). After IV administration, peak CNS effects are seen within 1–2 minutes; a significant decline in its clinical effects occurs after 30 minutes. Naloxone may have intrinsic "stimulant" properties, although this does not appear to be of clinical significance. Naloxone crosses the placenta; administration to the mother prior to delivery will decrease the degree of respiratory depression in the neonate secondary to narcotics.

   d. **Dosage and administration.** Naloxone is usually administered IV, although IM administration is also effective. Postoperatively, if needed, naloxone should be titrated every 2–3 minutes in IV boluses of 0.04 mg until the desired effect is attained.

   e. **Adverse effects**
      (1) **Pain.** Naloxone administration, even if cautiously titrated, may lead to the abrupt onset of pain as narcotic analgesia is reversed. This may be accompanied by abrupt hemodynamic changes (e.g., hypertension, tachycardia). Pain management in this situation may be challenging.
      (2) **Cardiac arrest.** Naloxone administration has, in rare cases, precipitated pulmonary edema and cardiac arrest.
      (3) **Renarcotization.** The clinical duration of an IV bolus of naloxone may be significantly less than that of the narcotic(s) previously administered to the patient; this may result in later reappearance of narcotic effects. All patients receiving naloxone require observation for this phenomenon after narcotic reversal.

II. **Pharmacology of inhalation anesthetics.** Inhalation anesthetics are usually administered for maintenance of general anesthesia but are occasionally employed for induction, especially in pediatric patients. General properties of inhalation anesthetics are presented in Table 11-2. Dosages of inhalation

Table 11-2. Properties of inhalation anesthetics

| Anesthetic | Vapor pressure (mm Hg, 20°C) | Partition coefficients | | MAC (%atm; with O₂ only) |
		Blood-gas* (37°C)	Brain-blood (37°C)	
Halothane	243	2.3	2.0	0.74
Enflurane	175	1.8	1.4	1.68
Isoflurane	239	1.4	1.6	1.15
Desflurane	664	0.42	1.3	6.0
Sevoflurane	157	0.69	1.7	2.05
Nitrous oxide	39,000	0.47	1.1	104

MAC = minimal alveolar concentration, which inhibits movement in response to a skin incision in 50% of patients.
* The blood-gas partition coefficient is inversely related to the rate of induction.

anesthetics are expressed as MAC, **the minimal alveolar concentration at one atmosphere at which 50% of patients do not move in response to a surgical stimulus.**

A. Nitrous oxide is a clear, colorless, and odorless gas. It is commonly supplied in pressurized cylinders.

   1. Mode of action. Nitrous oxide appears to produce general anesthesia through interaction with the cellular membranes of the CNS; exact mechanisms are not clear.

   2. Pharmacokinetics. The predominant route of elimination of nitrous oxide is exhalation. Significant biotransformation has not been demonstrated. The uptake and elimination of nitrous oxide are relatively rapid compared with other inhaled anesthetics, primarily as a result of its low blood-gas partition coefficient (0.47). For full discussion, see sec. III.

   3. Pharmacodynamics

   a. Central nervous system. Nitrous oxide produces analgesia in a dose-dependent manner. Concentrations greater than 60% may produce amnesia, although not reliably. Because of its high MAC (104%), sub-MAC concentrations of nitrous oxide are usually combined with other anesthetics to attain surgical anesthesia.

   b. Cardiovascular system. Nitrous oxide is a mild myocardial depressant and a mild sympathetic nervous system agonist. Heart rate and blood pressure are usually unchanged. Nitrous oxide may increase pulmonary vascular resistance in adults.

   c. Respiratory system. Nitrous oxide is a mild respiratory depressant, although less than the volatile anesthetics. Administration of 50–70% nitrous oxide greatly limits the FiO₂ that may be delivered.

   4. Adverse effects

   a. Expansion of closed gas spaces. The predominant constituent in closed gas-containing spaces in the body is nitrogen. Because of the greater solubility of nitrous oxide in blood (by a factor of 31), these spaces will expand as more nitrous oxide diffuses into these spaces than nitrogen diffuses out. Spaces such as a pneumothorax, occluded middle ear, bowel gas, an air embolus, or air in the skull following a pneumoencephalogram will markedly enlarge if nitrous oxide is administered, so it is best avoided in these situations. Nitrous oxide will diffuse into the cuff of an endotracheal tube and may lead to a marked increase in cuff pressure; this pressure should be intermittently assessed and, if necessary, adjusted.

b. **Nausea and vomiting.** Administration of nitrous oxide may increase the incidence of postoperative nausea and vomiting.

c. **Diffusion hypoxia.** After discontinuation of nitrous oxide, its rapid diffusion from the blood into the lung may lead to an alveolar PO_2 dramatically lower than the inspired PO_2, resulting in hypoxia and hypoxemia, especially if breathing room air. This may be avoided by providing oxygen therapy for 3–5 minutes after the discontinuation of nitrous oxide.

d. **Inhibition of tetrahydrofolate synthesis.** Nitrous oxide has been shown to inactivate **methionine synthetase,** a vitamin B_{12}–dependent enzyme necessary for the synthesis of DNA. Nitrous oxide should be used with caution in pregnant patients and those deficient in vitamin B_{12}.

B. **Volatile agents** are liquids whose potent evaporative vapors (in a carrier gas) are employed in inhalation anesthesia. Those in common use today include halothane, enflurane, and isoflurane. Desflurane and sevoflurane are recent additions.

1. **Mode of action.** Volatile agents appear to produce general anesthesia through interaction with the cellular membranes of the CNS; exact mechanisms are not clear.

2. **Pharmacokinetics.** The speed at which a volatile agent is absorbed and excreted (isoflurane > enflurane > halothane) is a function of its blood-gas partition coefficient; a lower solubility will lead to more rapid absorption and excretion (see sec. **III**). Although the predominant route of excretion of volatile agents is through exhalation, these agents also undergo a variable degree of hepatic metabolism (halothane 15%, enflurane 2–5%, isoflurane < 0.2%).

3. **Pharmacodynamics**

a. **Central nervous system.** Volatile agents may produce unconsciousness and amnesia at relatively low inspired concentrations (25% MAC). At higher doses, further generalized CNS depression occurs. At high inspired concentrations (> 2%), enflurane can produce electroencephalogram epileptiform activity. Volatile agents tend to produce decreased amplitude and increased latency of somatosensory evoked potentials. Volatile agents increase cerebral blood flow (halothane > enflurane > isoflurane) and decrease cerebral metabolic rate (isoflurane > enflurane > halothane).

b. Cardiovascular system. Volatile agents produce dose-dependent myocardial depression (halothane > enflurane > isoflurane) and systemic vasodilatation (isoflurane > enflurane > halothane). Heart rate tends to be unchanged, although isoflurane administration may lead to an increase in heart rate. Volatile agents sensitize the myocardium to the arrhythmogenic effects of catecholamines (halothane > enflurane > isoflurane), which is of particular concern during infiltration of epinephrine-containing solutions or the administration of sympathomimetic agents. With halothane, subcutaneous infiltration with epinephrine should not exceed 2 µg/kg/20 min. In a subgroup of patients with coronary artery disease, isoflurane may contribute to myocardial ischemia; the clinical significance of this is not clear (see Chap. 23).

c. Respiratory system. Volatile agents produce dose-dependent respiratory depression with a decrease in tidal volume, an increase in respiratory rate, and an elevation in $PaCO_2$. The degree of respiratory depression differs among agents (halothane > isoflurane > enflurane). Equipotent doses of volatile agents possess similar bronchodilator potency. However, these agents may also be airway irritants (isoflurane > enflurane > halothane) and, during light levels of anesthesia, may precipitate coughing, laryngospasm, or bronchospasm, particularly in patients who smoke or have asthma. The lesser pungency of halothane may make it more amenable as an inhalation induction agent.

d. Muscular system. Volatile agents produce a dose-dependent decrease in muscle tone, often enhancing surgical conditions. Administration of a volatile agent may precipitate malignant hyperthermia in a susceptible patient (see Chap. 18).

e. Liver. Volatile agents tend to cause a decrease in hepatic perfusion; this decrease is greatest with halothane, intermediate with enflurane, and least with isoflurane. Rarely, a patient may develop hepatitis secondary to exposure to a volatile agent, most notably halothane ("halothane hepatitis") (see Chap. 5).

f. Renal system. Volatile agents decrease renal blood flow through either a decrease in mean arterial blood pressure or an increase in renal vascular resistance. Fluoride ion, a product of enflurane metabolism, is nephrotoxic; its low serum levels even during prolonged enflurane administration are of unclear clinical significance (see Chap. 4).

4. Desflurane and sevoflurane. Uptake of desflurane or sevoflurane, due to their lower blood-gas partition coefficients, occurs more rapidly than with other volatile agents. Likewise, emergence after their use is faster. Metabolism of desflurane appears to be minimal. Metabolism of sevoflurane generates fluoride ion; although significant serum levels are measurable, levels do not appear to attain the threshold necessary for renal dysfunction. Desflurane and sevoflurane are myocardial depressants with hemodynamic effects similar to those of isoflurane. Desflurane and sevoflurane produce dose-dependent respiratory depression similar to that of other volatile agents. Desflurane appears to have greater airway irritant properties than isoflurane; sevoflurane appears to have minimal airway irritant properties.

III. **Inhalation anesthetic uptake, distribution, and elimination.** An inhalation anesthetic is usually delivered at a given concentration by a vaporizer into a circuit. However, when an anesthetic is initially introduced into a circuit or its delivered concentration is increased, many factors ultimately determine the partial pressure of the anesthetic in various tissues.

A. **Inspired anesthetic concentration.** An anesthesia circuit in which rebreathing occurs (i.e., semi-open, semi-closed, or closed) may produce an inspired anesthetic concentration significantly less than that initially delivered into the circuit due to the following factors:

1. **Circuit size** relative to fresh gas inflow rate. Until equilibration occurs throughout the circuit, the inspired anesthetic concentration will be less than that delivered. Equilibration of the circuit (and the functional residual capacity) occurs more quickly at higher fresh gas flows and with smaller circuits.

2. **Fresh gas inflow rate.** A decrease in the fresh gas inflow rate will increase the amount of rebreathing. Increased rebreathing will add anesthetic-depleted exhaled gas to the inspiratory limb of the circuit and diminish the concentration of inspired anesthetic.

3. **Solubility in circuit components.** The inspired anesthetic concentration will be decreased by uptake of the agent by tubing and soda lime until full equilibration occurs. In general, the more fat soluble an anesthetic is, the more pronounced this effect will be.

B. **Alveolar anesthetic concentration.** The alveolar anesthetic concentration (F_A) may differ significantly from the inspired anesthetic concentration (F_I) The rate of rise of the ratio of these two concentrations (F_A/F_I) determines the speed of induction of general anesthesia. Two opposing processes, anesthetic delivery to and uptake from alveoli, determine the F_A/F_I at a given time after administration of an inhalation anesthetic.

1. **Increased anesthetic delivery** to the alveoli will lead to an increase in the rate of rise of F_A/F_I. Delivery to the alveoli, in an anesthesia circuit other than a closed system, may be altered by the following factors:

a. **Alveolar ventilation.** Increased ventilation, without alteration of other processes that affect anesthetic delivery or uptake, increases F_A/F_I (Fig. 11-1).

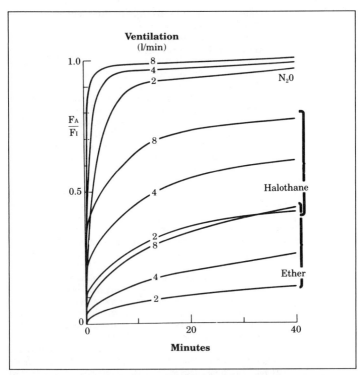

Fig. 11-1. The ratio of alveolar to inspired gas concentrations (FA/FI) as a function of time with varying minute ventilation. At constant cardiac output, increasing minute ventilation increases the alveolar rate of rise of anesthetic concentration. This effect is more marked with anesthetics with higher blood solubility (e.g., ether), decreasing correspondingly with lower solubility (e.g., nitrous oxide). (From E. I. Eger, *Anesthetic Uptake and Action.* Baltimore: Williams & Wilkins, 1974.)

This effect is more pronounced with the more blood-soluble agents (i.e., higher blood-gas partition coefficient; see Table 11-2).

b. **Concentration effect.** Uptake of anesthetic from alveoli by blood concentrates the anesthetic remaining in the alveoli and increases the input of additional anesthetic into alveoli via augmentation of inspired volume. The net effect of these two processes is an increase in the rate of rise of an anesthetic's alveolar concentration as its inspired concentration is increased.

c. **The second gas effect.** When two inhalation anesthetics are administered together, uptake by blood of large volumes of a "first" gas (e.g., nitrous oxide) increases both the alveolar concentration of a "second" gas (e.g., isoflurane) and the input of additional "second" gas into alveoli via augmentation of inspired volume.

2. **Anesthetic is taken up from alveoli by blood.** Multiple factors can lead to increased uptake, thereby decreasing the rate of rise in alveolar anesthetic concentration (and the speed of induction).

   a. **Cardiac output.** An increase in cardiac output (and pulmonary blood flow) will increase anesthetic uptake and decrease the rate of rise in alveolar concentration. Conversely, a decrease in cardiac output will have the opposite effect. This effect of cardiac output is pronounced with nonrebreathing circuits or highly soluble anesthetics. It is also accentuated early in the course of anesthetic administration.

   b. **Anesthetic solubility.** Increasing anesthetic solubility in blood increases uptake, thereby slowing the rate of rise of F_A/F_I (see Fig. 11-1). Solubility of halogenated volatile anesthetics in blood is increased somewhat with hypothermia and hyperlipidemia.

   c. **Gradient between alveolar and venous blood.** The uptake of anesthetic by blood perfusing the lung will increase (and the rate of rise of F_A/F_I will decrease) as the gradient between the partial pressure of anesthetic between the alveoli and blood increases. This gradient will be particularly large early in the course of anesthetic administration.

C. The partial pressure of an inhalation anesthetic in arterial blood usually approximates its alveolar pressure. However, the arterial partial pressure may be significantly less when marked ventilation-perfusion abnormalities (e.g., shunt) are present, especially with less-soluble anesthetics (e.g., nitrous oxide). The rate of equilibration of anesthetic partial pressure between blood and a particular organ system is dependent on the following factors:

1. **Tissue blood flow.** Equilibration occurs more rapidly in tissues receiving increased perfusion. The most highly perfused organ systems receive approximately 75% of cardiac output; these include the brain, kidney, heart, liver, and endocrine glands and are referred to as the **vessel-rich group.** The remainder of the cardiac output perfuses predominantly muscle and fat.

2. **Tissue solubility.** For a given arterial anesthetic partial pressure, anesthetic agents with a high tissue solubility are slower to equilibrate. Solubilities of anesthetic agents differ among tissues. Blood-brain partition coefficients of inhalation agents are shown in Table 11-2.

3. **Gradient between arterial blood and tissue.** Until equilibration is reached between the anesthetic partial pressure in the blood and a particular tissue, a gradient exists that leads to uptake of anesthetic by the tissue. The rate of uptake will decrease as the gradient decreases.

D. Elimination. After discontinuation, inhalation anesthetics are eliminated from the body by the following routes:
1. **Exhalation.** This is the predominant route of elimination. After discontinuation, an anesthetic's tissue and alveolar partial pressures decrease by the same processes (although reversed) by which they increased when the anesthetic was introduced.
2. **Metabolism.** Inhalation anesthetics may eventually undergo varying degrees of hepatic metabolism (see sec. **II.B.2**). While anesthetizing concentrations of an agent are present (e.g., induction, maintenance), metabolism probably has little effect on the alveolar concentration due to saturation of hepatic enzymes. After discontinuation of the anesthetic, metabolism may contribute to the decrease in the alveolar concentration; however, the effect is not clinically significant.
3. **Anesthetic loss.** Inhalation anesthetics can be lost from the body both percutaneously and through visceral membranes; these losses are probably negligible.

SUGGESTED READING

Barash, P. G., Cullen, B. F., and Stoelting R. K. *Clinical Anesthesia*. Philadelphia: Lippincott, 1989.

Eger, E. I. *Anesthetic Uptake and Action*. Baltimore: Williams & Wilkins, 1974.

Gilman, A. G., et al. *Goodman and Gilman's The Pharmacologic Basis of Therapeutics*. New York: Pergamon, 1990.

Johnston, R. R., Eger, E. I., and Wilson, C. A. A comparative interaction of epinephrine with enflurane, isoflurane, and halothane in man. *Anesth. Analg.* 55:709, 1976.

Miller, R. D. *Anesthesia*. New York: Churchill Livingstone, 1990.

Philbin, D. M., et al. Fentanyl and sufentanil anesthesia revisited: How much is enough? *Anesthesiology* 73:5, 1990.

White, P. F., Way, W. L., and Trevor, A. J. Ketamine: Its pharmacology and therapeutic uses. *Anesthesiology* 56:119, 1982.

12

Neuromuscular Blockade

George Shorten

I. Neuromuscular transmission

A. A typical motor neuron comprises a cell body with a prominent nucleus, many dendrites, and a single myelinated axon. Many axons from other neurons converge on the dendrites and the cell body. These axodendritic and axosomatic synapses mediate such functions as pre- and postsynaptic inhibition and presynaptic facilitation. The axon of a motor neuron loses its myelin sheath as it approaches the neuromuscular junction and ends in a number of synaptic knobs or terminal buttons. Within the axoplasm of these knobs are vessels containing the neurotransmitter **acetylcholine** (ACh) (Fig. 12-1).

B. The necessary substrates for ACh synthesis are **choline** and **acetate.** Both are transported into the axoplasm from the nearby extracellular fluid, the latter stored in the mitochondria of the nerve terminal as **acetylcoenzyme A** (CoA). Other molecules used in the synthesis and storage of ACh are made in the cell body and transported to the nerve ending. The main enzyme that catalyzes the synthesis of ACh in the nerve ending is **choline-*O*-acetyltransferase.** ACh is stored in the cytoplasm until some is transported into vesicles and moved into position for release. The function of the remaining "nonvesicular" ACh is unclear. The vesicles are arranged in triangular arrays, the apex of which comprises a thickened portion of membrane known as the "active zone." The sites of vesicular discharge lie on either side of these active zones, aligned exactly opposite the "shoulders" of convolutions on the postjunctional membrane. The postjunctional nicotinic receptors are concentrated on these shoulders.

C. The current understanding of the physiology of neuromuscular transmission favors the **"quantal theory."** In response to a nerve action potential, voltage-dependent calcium channels open, and calcium ions rapidly enter the nerve ending, combining with calmodulin. The calmodulin-Ca^{2+} complex causes the vesicular membrane to fuse with that of the nerve ending, thus discharging "packets" or quanta of ACh into the synaptic cleft. The amount of transmitter released is determined both by the change in concentration in intracellular calcium and by the duration of the calcium influx. Nonquantal release of ACh also takes place, but its mechanism and function are poorly understood.

D. Fast rates of stimulation require that the nerve increase its stores of releasable ACh, a process known as **mobilization.** Mobilization includes choline transport, synthesis of CoA, and movement of vesicles to the release site. Under normal conditions, nerves are able to mobilize transmitter rapidly enough to replace that which has been released. In the presence of *d*-tubocurarine (dTC), mobilization of transmitter is impaired, ACh output

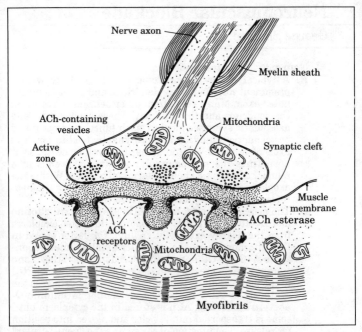

Fig. 12-1. The neuromuscular junction.

cannot keep pace with demands, and the muscle response fades.

E. **Released ACh** diffuses across the synaptic cleft and binds to nicotinic cholinergic receptors. These receptors comprise five subunits, two of which are identical and contain the ACh binding sites. When ACh binds to both these sites, a conformational change is produced in a receptor-associated protein, resulting in the opening of a cationic channel. Sodium (Na^+) and calcium (Ca^{2+}) ions move inward, and potassium (K^+) ions move outward, producing a change in the transmembrane potential known as the end-plate potential (EPP). If this EPP exceeds the firing threshold for the adjacent muscle, an action potential results that is propagated throughout the muscle membrane and initiates the contractile process. The magnitude of a muscle contraction in response to nerve stimulation is not dependent on the size of the action potential (being an all-or-none process), but on the number of muscle fibers stimulated. Normally a large margin of safety exists, since both the amount of ACh released and the number of receptors present at the end plate are far greater than the minimum that are necessary for muscle contraction.

F. **Membrane repolarization** is achieved once ACh diffuses away from its receptor to be broken down by the enzyme acetylcholinesterase, present in the synaptic cleft.

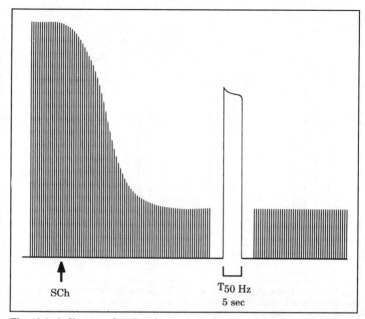

Fig. 12-2. A diagram showing the response to succinylcholine infusion at the arrow. During the beginning of the steady state block, tetanus at 50 Hz showed no fade or posttetanic potentiation.

II. **Types of neuromuscular blockade.** There are classically three types of neuromuscular blockade: depolarizing, nondepolarizing, and phase II.

A. **Depolarizing blockade** occurs when drugs mimic the action of the neurotransmitter ACh. Succinylcholine (SCh), like ACh, is a quaternary amine. It binds and activates the ACh receptor, which leads to depolarization of the end plate and adjacent muscle membrane. Because SCh is not degraded as quickly as ACh, end-plate depolarization persists and leads to accommodation or inexcitability of the muscle membrane adjacent to the junctional membrane. This perijunctional membrane accommodation explains the profound muscle relaxation in the presence of an EPP below the threshold that normally triggers a muscle action potential.

1. **Depolarizing blockade** (Figs. 12-2 and 12-3) is characterized by
   a. Muscle fasciculation followed by relaxation.
   b. Absence of fade following tetanic or train-of-four (TOF) stimulation.
   c. Absence of posttetanic potentiation.
   d. Potentiation of the block by anticholinesterases.
   e. Antagonism of the block by nondepolarizing relaxants.

2. Depolarizing blockade from SCh **ends** when the molecule diffuses from the receptor and is broken down to

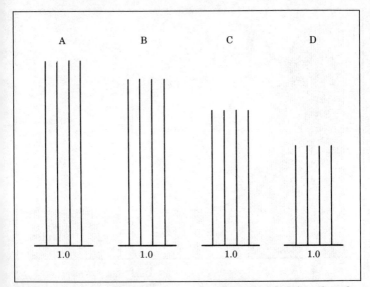

Fig. 12-3. The train-of-four response at A prior to the administration of a depolarizing relaxant. Responses B, C, and D show a decrease in the amplitude of the train-of-four response with no change in the T4 ratio (i.e., no fade).

choline and succinic acid in two stages. First, SCh is hydrolyzed by plasma cholinesterase to choline and succinylmonocholine (a depolarizing agent with about 1/20 the potency of the dicholine). Second, and much more slowly, succinylmonocholine is converted to choline and succinic acid by both plasma cholinesterase and acetylcholinesterase.

3. The **clinical pharmacology** of SCh is summarized in Table 12-1.

4. **Side effects.** In general, the side effects of **depolarizing relaxants** like SCh are related to their ability to mimic the action of ACh at ACh receptors (both nicotinic and muscarinic) in other tissues.

   a. **Muscle pains** following SCh occur more frequently in women and in ambulatory patients after minor surgical procedures. The incidence of myalgias may be reduced by administering a small dose of nondepolarizing relaxant (e.g., 3 mg of tubocurarine) 3 minutes prior to SCh or by pretreatment with lidocaine (2 mg/kg) or diazepam (0.05 mg/kg). None of these techniques completely eliminates the possibility of a patient's suffering from post-SCh myalgia. If pretreating for a rapid sequence induction, the dose of SCh is increased to 1.5 mg/kg. Pretreatment with a nondepolarizing relaxant may cause diplopia, weakness, and a decreased vital capacity, and awake patients should be warned of this.

Table 12-1. Comparative clinical pharmacology of relaxants[a,b]

Drug	ED_{95}[c] (mg/kg IV)	Intubating dose[d] (mg/kg IV bolus)	Time to intubation[e] (min)	Time to 25% recovery[f] (min)	Elimination
Succinylcholine (SCh)[g]	0.25	1	1	5–10	Breakdown by plasma cholinesterase
Pancuronium	0.07	0.08–0.1	3–5	80–100	70–80% renal, 15–20% biliary excretion and liver metabolism
Vecuronium	0.06	0.1–0.12	2–3	25–30	10–20% renal, 80% biliary excretion and hepatic metabolism
d-Tubocurarine (dTC)	0.51	0.5–0.6	3–5	80–100	70% renal, 15–20% biliary excretion, which increases in renal failure
Metocurine	0.28	0.3–0.4	3–5	80–100	80–100% renal
Atracurium	0.25	0.4–0.5	2–3	25–30	Ester hydrolysis independent of plasma cholinesterase and Hofmann elimination (pH and temperature dependent)
Gallamine	3.0	3.0–4.0	3–5	80–100	100% renal
Pancuronium and dTC	0.02 + 0.15	0.02 + 0.15	3–5	40–60	
Pancuronium and metocurine	0.02 + 0.07	0.02 + 0.07	3–5	40–60	
Pipecuronium	0.05–0.06	0.07–0.085	5	47–124	Mainly excreted in the urine and to a lesser extent in the bile
Doxacurium	0.03	0.05–0.08	4–5	100–160	Excreted unchanged in urine and bile
Mivacurium	0.09	0.15–0.25	1.5–2.0	16–20	Hydrolysis by plasma cholinesterase

[a] All doses were determined under balanced (nitrous oxide–narcotic) technique.

[b] There is a large variability in patient response to all relaxants, especially at the extremes of age. Therefore, patients should be monitored as described in sec. IV.

[c] An ED_{95} dose of relaxant gives adequate surgical relaxation with nitrous oxide–narcotic anesthesia.

[d] All relaxants are potentiated by potent inhalation anesthetics. In general, relaxant doses should be reduced by 40% with halothane, 50–60% with enflurane and isoflurane.

[e] For rapid sequence inductions with nondepolarizers, onset time can be reduced by using a "priming" dose 3–5 minutes prior to the full dose. These doses for 90-second onset time are atracurium, 0.06–0.08 mg/kg; vecuronium, 0.01 mg/kg, then 0.5–0.6 mg/kg; pancuronium, 0.015 mg/kg, then 0.15–0.2 mg/kg. As always, resuscitation equipment should be available when pretreating with a nondepolarizer. Patients should be informed that they may experience diplopia, drooping of the eyelids, and difficulty swallowing but should be assured that the ability to breathe will be maintained or supported. No nondepolarizer has as reliable or rapid an onset as does SCh.

[f] Maintenance doses to be given when the twitch height reaches 25% of control are generally 20–25% of the initial dose.

[g] SCh can be given as a continuous drip of a dilution of 1 gm/500 ml of normal saline or 5% D/W at 2–4 mg/min with the aid of a blockade monitor.

[h] Both pancuronium and vecuronium have active liver metabolites.

[i] Laudanosine, a metabolite of atracurium, is metabolized by the liver and eliminated through the kidneys.

    b. Ganglionic stimulation. SCh may increase heart rate and blood pressure in adults or cause bradycardia in children or adults receiving a second dose of SCh. Pretreatment with atropine is most successful if given intravenously immediately prior to SCh.

    c. Hyperkalemia. SCh normally causes the serum K^+ level to increase 0.5–1.0 mEq/L, but K^+ may significantly rise in patients with burns, upper and lower motor neuron disease, trauma, prolonged bed rest, muscle diseases, and closed head injuries due to proliferation of extrajunctional ACh receptors. In burned patients, the time of greatest risk is from 2 weeks to 6 months after the burn has been sustained, although it is advisable to avoid the use of SCh in burned patients except in the first 24 hours for 2 years after the injury.

    d. A transient increase in intraocular pressure occurs following an intubating dose of SCh due to contraction of the extraocular muscles. The use of SCh in open eye injuries is controversial (see Chap. 25 for full discussion).

    e. Increased intragastric pressure after SCh administration results from fasciculation of abdominal muscles. This averages 15–20 mm Hg in an adult but does not occur to a significant extent in infants and children. It can be attenuated by pretreatment with a nondepolarizing relaxant (e.g., 3 mg of dTC).

    f. SCh produces a mild, short-lived rise in **cerebral blood flow** and **intracranial pressure.**

    g. Phase II block occurs with repeated or continuous administration of SCh in dosages of 5–6 mg/kg in conjunction with halothane and enflurane and 8–12 mg/kg with nitrous oxide–narcotic anesthesia. The mechanism is not clear but may be due to a conformational change in the receptor. Phase II blockade is **characterized** by

        (1) Tetanic or TOF fade.

        (2) Tachyphylaxis.

        (3) Post-tetanic facilitation.

        (4) Partial or complete reversal with anticholinesterases.

    h. Prolonged blockade may be caused by low plasma cholinesterase levels, drug-induced inhibition of cholinesterase activity, or genetically atypical enzyme.

        (1) Decreased levels are seen in the last trimester of pregnancy; with liver disease, starvation, carcinomas, hypothyroidism, burn patients, shock, uremia, and cardiac failure; and following therapeutic radiation.

        (2) Inhibition of plasma cholinesterase occurs with the use of echothiophate eye drops, anticholinesterases, phenelzine (a monoamine oxidase inhibitor), and organophosphate compounds (insecticides and nerve gases). Serum cholines-

terase levels are not usually altered following hemodialysis.

(3) **Heterozygous atypical plasma cholinesterase** occurs in 4% of the general population, while the incidence of homozygous atypical cholinesterase enzyme is 1/2800. These patients demonstrate prolonged neuromuscular blockade and respiratory insufficiency for 2–3 hours after SCh administration. Plasma cholinesterase is evaluated by laboratory assays that yield dibucaine and fluoride numbers. **Normal plasma cholinesterase is 80% inhibited in vitro by the local anesthetic, dibucaine (i.e., dibucaine number 80), and the homozygous atypical plasma cholinesterase is only 20% inhibited (dibucaine number 20).** A range of dibucaine numbers from 30 to 65 occurs in heterozygotes. Other individuals sensitive to SCh may have an abnormal enzyme called the fluoride-resistant enzyme (with a mean dibucaine number of 34) or a silent gene with complete absence of plasma cholinesterase (dibucaine number 0).

i. **Triggering of malignant hyperthermia.** Failure of the masseter to relax or generalized myotonia after SCh should alert one to this possibility (see Chap. 18).

B. **Nondepolarizing blockade** is classically attributed to a pure, reversible competition between antagonist molecules and ACh for occupancy of the ACh binding site.

1. **Other mechanisms**

a. **Ion channel blockade.** Classic nondepolarizing agents such as gallamine and tubocurarine have a great capacity to block open ion channels as well as a high affinity for the ACh receptor binding sites. Open channel blockade is more likely to occur during rapid stimulation of the muscle. This phenomenon is termed **use dependence.**

b. Blockade of the entrance to closed ion channels.

c. Binding to another "allosteric" site on the receptor that renders it unresponsive to ACh.

d. **Desensitization** produced by long duration of exposure of the ACh receptor to an agonist.

e. Interference with presynaptic ACh mobilization or Ca^{2+} influx. The commonly used nondepolarizing relaxants probably mediate these prejunctional effects by binding to cholinergic receptors on the nerve ending.

f. Alteration of the lipid environment of the ACh receptor, thus changing channel properties.

2. Nondepolarizing blockade (Figs. 12-4 and 12-5) is **characterized** by

a. Absence of fasciculations.

b. Fade during tetanic and TOF stimulation.

c. Post-tetanic potentiation.

d. Antagonism of block by depolarizing agents and anticholinesterases.

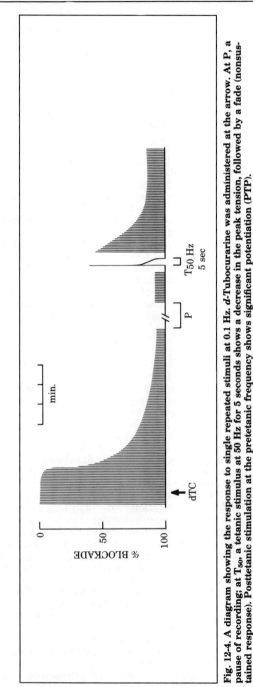

Fig. 12-4. A diagram showing the response to single repeated stimuli at 0.1 Hz. *d*-Tubocurarine was administered at the arrow. At P, a pause of recording; at T₅₀, a tetanic stimulus at 50 Hz for 5 seconds shows a decrease in the peak tension, followed by a fade (nonsustained response). Posttetanic stimulation at the pretetanic frequency shows significant potentiation (PTP).

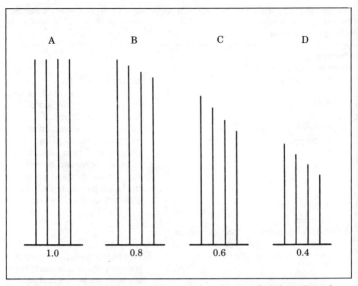

Fig. 12-5. The train-of-four response at A is prior to administration of a nondepolarizing relaxant. Responses B, C, and D show the progressive decrease in twitch height and T4 ratio (fade).

    e. Potentiation of block by other nondepolarizing agents.

3. Nondepolarizing muscle relaxants are quaternary ammonium compounds and include two major categories: **steroid derivatives** (pancuronium, vecuronium, and pipecuronium) and **benzylisoquinolines** (tubocurarine, metocurine, atracurium, doxacurium, and mivacurium).

    a. **Combinations** of pancuronium with either tubocurarine or metocurine act synergistically, as does the combination of atracurium with vecuronium. Agents of similar chemical structure, such as tubocurarine and metocurine, when combined do not demonstrate synergism.

    b. Two new long-acting agents, **pipecuronium,** a steroid derivative, and **doxacurium,** a benzylisoquinoline, have recently become available. Their main advantage is the absence of significant cardiovascular effects. Their likely use will be in long cardiovascular cases in which hemodynamic stability is particularly important.

    c. **Mivacurium,** a benzylisoquinoline compound, is rapidly broken down by plasma cholinesterase and thus is noncumulative. It only demonstrates significant cardiovascular side effects and histamine release in doses twofold greater than ED_{95} (i.e., > 0.15 mg/kg). It is likely that the noncumulative properties of mivacurium will make it useful for adminis-

Table 12-2. Location and function of nicotinic and muscarinic receptors

Type of receptor	Function
Nicotinic	
Neuromuscular junction	
Presynaptic	Maintains ACh release at high-frequency stimulation
Postsynaptic	Initiates depolarization of muscle membrane
Autonomic ganglia cell bodies—both sympathetic and parasympathetic	Initiates depolarization of ganglion cell, leading to generalized sympathetic effects (increased vessel wall tone, increased sweating) and parasympathetic effects listed below
Muscarinic	
Peripheral postganglionic parasympathetic nerve endings	
Heart (via vagus nerve)	Slows sinus node, lowers atrial conduction, lowers atrioventricular node conduction
Smooth muscles at bronchi and bronchioles	Bronchoconstriction
Gastrointestinal	Raises tone
Genitourinary	Raises bladder tone, lowers sphincter tone
Eye	Miosis
Secretory glands	Stimulates salivary, tracheobronchial, lacrimal, digestive, and exocrine sweat glands

tration by infusion and that the rapidity of spontaneous recovery may make reversal unnecessary.

    d. With the availability of newer noncumulative relaxants and dedicated syringe pumps, nondepolarizing relaxants are now commonly administered by infusion. Of the currently used relaxants, the duration of action of **atracurium** is least affected by the magnitude or frequency of the dose. One of the breakdown products of atracurium, laudanosine, is a tertiary amine that can cross the blood-brain barrier. In high doses, laudanosine has produced convulsions in animals. Even after prolonged infusion of atracurium in humans, laudanosine concentrations are considerably less than those that produce convulsions.

  4. The **clinical pharmacology** of the nondepolarizing relaxants is summarized in Table 12-1.

  5. The **side effects** of the nondepolarizing relaxants stem from antagonism of ACh at cholinergic receptors. These relaxants vary in their antinicotinic and antimuscarinic effects. Table 12-2 reviews the site and function of cholinergic receptors.

Table 12-3. Cardiovascular side effects of relaxants

Drugs	Histamine release[a]	Ganglionic effects	Vagolytic activity	Sympathetic stimulation
Succinylcholine	+	Stimulates	0	0
Pancuronium	0	0	+	+
Vecuronium	0	0	0	0
d-Tubocurarine	+ +	Blocks	0	0
Metocurine	+	Weak block	0	0
Atracurium	+[b]	0	0	0
Gallamine	0	0	+ +	+
Mivacurium	+	0	0	0
Pancuronium	0	0	0	0
Doxacurium	0	0	0	0

[a] Histamine release is dose and rate dependent and therefore less pronounced if drugs are given slowly.
[b] At doses > 0.5 mg/kg.

6. The **cardiovascular side effects** of nondepolarizing relaxants are summarized in Table 12-3. Hypotension following a high dose of atracurium (0.8 mg/kg) is prevented if the drug is administered slowly (i.e., over 30 seconds) but not by priming or pretreatment with antihistamines.

C. The cardiovascular side effects and metabolism of relaxants are major determinants in selecting the **best relaxant** for a particular clinical situation. For example, the rapid onset and short duration of SCh make it ideal for intubation of the patient with a full stomach and for short procedures like rigid bronchoscopy. Atracurium is metabolized in the plasma (by pH and temperature-dependent degradation and nonspecific ester hydrolysis), which makes it an ideal relaxant for use in renal or liver failure and for short procedures, particularly when SCh is contraindicated. The vagolytic effect of pancuronium and gallamine is useful in situations in which an elevated heart rate is desirable (e.g., in pediatric cases) and to counterbalance the vagotonic effects of high-dose fentanyl. Histamine release from dTC administration can significantly contribute to hypotension, and its increased biliary clearance in renal failure makes it a reasonable choice in such patients. The minimal histamine-releasing properties of metocurine and the lack of cardiovascular effects of vecuronium make them ideal when hemodynamic perturbations are not well tolerated (e.g., in coronary artery disease).

III. Reversal of neuromuscular blockade

A. **Recovery from succinylcholine**

1. Recovery of muscle function and strength after SCh-induced depolarizing blockade occurs in 10–15 minutes and does not require antagonism. Patients with atypical or altered plasma cholinesterase will have a greatly prolonged duration of blockade.

2. Reversal of **phase II blockade** occurs spontaneously

within 10–15 minutes in approximately 50% of patients. The remainder have prolonged responses. It is advisable to allow these patients to recover spontaneously for 20–25 minutes after turning off the SCh infusion. After this period, reversal with an anticholinesterase agent may be attempted if a plateau in recovery (as judged by blockade monitoring) is reached. Earlier reversal could worsen the block.

B. **Nondepolarizing blockade** spontaneously reverses when the relaxants diffuse from their sites of action. Reversal can be accelerated by administering agents that inhibit acetylcholinesterase, thereby increasing the ACh available to compete with the relaxants for their binding sites. Other drugs like 4-aminopyridine increase the release of ACh presynaptically; however, only the anticholinesterases are in widespread clinical use. The latter may act presynaptically by increasing the mobilization and/or release of ACh and also by direct depolarization of the postjunctional membrane.

C. **Anticholinesterases.** The three principal drugs are edrophonium, neostigmine, and pyridostigmine. Both neostigmine and pyridostigmine bind covalently with acetylcholinesterase, while edrophonium only binds electrostatically. This accounts for edrophonium's shorter duration of action. Like ACh, all three have muscarinic as well as nicotinic effects. Muscarinic stimulation leads to salivation, bradycardia, tearing, miosis, and bronchoconstriction. Administration of an anticholinergic drug (e.g., atropine or glycopyrrolate) prior to the anticholinesterase will minimize muscarinic receptor stimulation. Nausea and vomiting occur more frequently when neuromuscular blockade is reversed with neostigmine and atropine than when spontaneous recovery is allowed to occur. Table 12-4 summarizes the clinical pharmacology of these three relaxant antagonists.

D. **Time to adequate reversal** is related to the degree of spontaneous recovery prior to the administration of the reversal agent; it will thus take longer from a deeper block. Reversal should not be attempted unless at least one response to TOF stimulation is present. Factors normally influencing ease of reversibility include the relaxant used, the mode of administration (i.e., single bolus, repeated boluses, or infusion), depth of blockade, the use of inhalation agents, and the choice of reversal agent. Clinical evidence of adequate neuromuscular recovery should include adequate ventilation and oxygenation, sustained grip strength, the ability to sustain head lift or movement of an extremity without fade, and the absence of discoordinated muscle activity. Factors to be considered if nondepolarizing neuromuscular blockade is abnormally prolonged or resistant to reversal are listed in Table 12-5. If residual weakness is present after attempted reversal, the endotracheal tube should be left in place to provide adequate ventilation and airway protection. Patients should be transferred to the postanesthesia or intensive care unit. Attempts to reverse a deep or

Table 12-4. Clinical pharmacology of reversal drugs

Drugs	Dosage	Time to peak antagonism (min)	Duration of antagonism (min)	Excretion pattern[a]	Dosage of atropine required[b] (μg/kg)
Edrophonium	0.5–1.0 mg/kg	1	40–65	70% renal 30% hepatic	7–10
Neostigmine	0.03–0.06 mg/kg up to 5 mg	7	55–75	50% renal 50% hepatic	15–30
Pyridostigmine	0.25 mg/kg	10–13	80–130	75% renal 25% hepatic	15–20

[a] The increased duration during renal failure exceeds the increased durations of pancuronium and curare, and so there is no "recurarization."
[b] Dosage of glycopyrrolate = ½ dosage of atropine. The onset time of atropine is much faster than that of glycopyrrolate, and it peaks in a little over a minute compared to 4–5 minutes for glycopyrrolate. Therefore, glycopyrrolate is a good choice with pyridostigmine, which has a longer time to peak antagonism. However, glycopyrrolate should be given at least 3 minutes before edrophonium. There appears to be less tachycardia, fewer arrhythmias, and a greater secretory drying effect with glycopyrrolate.

Table 12-5. Clinical assessment of blockade

Evoked response (by blockade monitor)	Clinical correlate
95% suppression of single twitch at 0.15–0.1 Hz	Adequate intubating conditions
90% suppression of single twitch; train-of-four count of 1 twitch	Surgical relaxation with nitrous oxide–narcotic anesthesia
75% suppression of single twitch; train-of-four count of 3 twitches	Adequate relaxation with inhalation agents
25% single-twitch suppression	Decreased vital capacity
Train-of-four ratio > 0.75; sustained tetanus at 50 Hz for 5 seconds	Head lift for 5 seconds; vital capacity $= 15$–20 ml/kg; inspiratory force $= -25$ cm H_2O; effective cough
Train-of-four ratio $= 1.0$	Normal expiratory flow rate, vital capacity, and inspiratory force

resistant block with excessive doses of neostigmine may increase the degree of residual weakness, that is, neostigmine-induced block.

IV. **Monitoring neuromuscular function**

    A. There are several **reasons to monitor** neuromuscular function under anesthesia:

        1. As an objective addition to clinical assessment in determining degree of relaxation during surgery and degree of recovery before extubation.

        2. To facilitate timing of intubation.

        3. To titrate dosage according to patient response.

        4. To monitor for the development of phase II block.

        5. To permit early recognition of patients with abnormal plasma cholinesterase.

    B. The **peripheral nerve stimulators** in use today employ various patterns of stimulation: single-twitch, tetanus, TOF, and double-burst stimulation as well as the "post-tetanic count." The adductor pollicis response to ulnar nerve stimulation at the wrist is most often used, since it is easily accessible and results are not complicated by direct muscle activation. Cutaneous electrodes are placed at the wrist over the ulnar nerve and attached to a battery-driven pulse generator, which delivers a graded impulse of electrical current at a specified frequency. Evoked muscle tension can be estimated by feeling for thumb adduction or measured using a strain gauge attached to the thumb. The response to nerve stimulation may also be quantified by analyzing the integrated electromyogram (EMG) of the muscle. Following the administration of a muscle relaxant, the developed tension and twitch height decrease with the onset of neuromuscular blockade. Since the diaphragm is more resistant to the action of nondepolarizing muscle relaxants than is the adductor pollicis, monitoring the degree of recovery in the latter prior to extubation provides an added margin of safety. If the ulnar nerve is unavailable, other sites may be used (e.g., facial nerve).

C. The relationship between the response to various patterns of stimulation and clinical criteria (Table 12-5) is as follows:

1. **Single twitch.** A supramaximal stimulus lasting 0.2 msec at a frequency of 0.1 Hz is generally used. The control height of muscle twitch is determined prior to administration of the muscle relaxant, and then the degree of blockade can be assessed by comparing subsequent twitch height to that of control. A supramaximal stimulus ensures recruitment of all muscle fibers, and a short duration, like 0.2 msec, prevents repetitive nerve firing. Stimulus frequency affects twitch height and degree of fade, and 0.1 Hz is chosen because at that frequency 95% twitch depression corresponds to satisfactory intubating conditions and adequate surgical relaxation. This frequency is great enough to stress the neuromuscular junction and thus demonstrate fade during incomplete block, but not great enough to elicit posttetanic potentiation, which would compromise subsequent measurements. It is not a sensitive measure of onset or recovery from blockade, since 75% of receptors must be blocked before twitch height begins to decrease and at control height approximately 75% of receptors are still occupied.

2. **Tetanic stimulus.** Tetanic nerve stimulation frequencies vary from 50–200 Hz. **During depolarizing blockade, the peak tension is reduced but sustained over time; that is, there is no fade. With nondepolarizing block and phase II block, the peak tension is also reduced but tetanic fade is demonstrated.** Tetanic fade is a prejunctional phenomenon due to the effects of curare-like drugs on mobilization of ACh during high-frequency stimulation. A tetanic stimulus at 50 Hz for 5 seconds is clinically useful, since a sustained tension at this frequency corresponds to that achieved with maximum voluntary effort. However, tetanic stimuli are painful and can speed recovery in the stimulated muscle, thus misleading the observer with respect to the degree of recovery in important respiratory and airway muscles.

3. **Posttetanic single twitch** is the resumption of single-twitch stimulation 6–10 seconds after a tetanic stimulus. An increase in twitch after a tetanus is known as posttetanic potentiation (PTP) and can be explained by increased mobilization and synthesis of ACh during and after tetanic stimulation during partial curarization. **Both nondepolarizing and phase II blockade will exhibit PTP; depolarizing blockade will not.** A normal muscle will show no PTP by EMG but may exhibit mechanical PTP due to a change in the contractile response in the muscle. The presence of electromyographic PTP is indicative of residual nondepolarizing blockade.

4. **Train-of-four (TOF).** Four supramaximal stimuli at a

frequency of 2 Hz are repeated at intervals of no less than 10 seconds apart. Responses at this frequency show fade during partial curarization. During nondepolarizing neuromuscular blockade, elimination of the fourth response corresponds to 75% depression of the first response when compared to control. Likewise, disappearance of the third, second, and first responses correspond to 80%, 90%, and 100% of the first twitch respectively. The ratio of the height of the fourth to the first twitch (the "TOF ratio") correlates with the degree of clinical recovery. A TOF ratio of 0.75 indicates that the single twitch has returned to control and that a 50-Hz tetanus for 5 seconds will be fully sustained. This level of recovery correlates with adequate clinical recovery. TOF is the most useful method for clinical monitoring, since it does not require a control height, it is not as painful as tetanic stimuli, and it does not induce changes in subsequent recovery. It is a good measure of relaxation in the range of blockade required for surgical relaxation (75–90%) and is useful in assessing recovery from blockade (Fig. 12-6). It is not helpful in quantifying the degree of depolarizing blockade because no fade will be evident. However, TOF monitoring may be used to detect fade, signifying the onset of phase II blockade during continuous or repeated administration of SCh.

5. **Posttetanic count.** Intense nondepolarizing blockade may be quantified by applying a 50-Hz tetanus for 5 seconds and observing the response thereafter to single-twitch stimulation starting 3 seconds after the tetanus. The number of responses detectable is predictive of the time before spontaneous recovery will occur.

6. **Double-burst stimulation (DBS).** Residual curarization is present if the response to the second of two short 50-Hz tetani separated by 750 msec is less than the first. It has been suggested that fade in response to DBS is more easily detected than fade in response to TOF stimulation.

V. **Neuromuscular disorders influencing the response to muscle-relaxant drugs**

A. **Myasthenia gravis (MG)**

1. MG is an autoimmune disease with a prevalence in the general population of 1/20,000. It is most common in young adult females.

2. Antibodies to the ACh receptor are detectable in the serum of 90% of MG patients but may be absent in those with early ocular presentations. Anti-acetylcholinesterase receptor (AChR) antibody titers correlate poorly with clinical signs but may be useful predictors of sensitivity to nondepolarizing muscle relaxants. Thymomas may be found in 10% of MG patients, and thymic hyperplasia is very common.

3. The **presentation** of MG often involves the gradual onset of pharyngeal or ocular weakness (although any muscle group may be affected), which becomes worse with exercise.

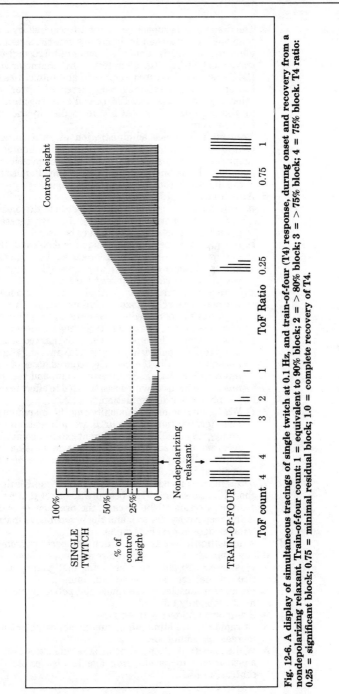

Fig. 12-6. A display of simultaneous tracings of single twitch at 0.1 Hz, and train-of-four (T4) response, during onset and recovery from a nondepolarizing relaxant. Train-of-four count: 1 = equivalent to 90% block; 2 = >80% block; 3 = >75% block; 4 = 75% block. T4 ratio: 0.25 = significant block; 0.75 = minimal residual block; 1.0 = complete recovery of T4.

4. The **diagnosis** is supported by the clinical history and confirmed by transiently improved muscle strength following administration of edrophonium (10 mg) intravenously (the "Tensilon test"), by characteristic EMG findings (decreased amplitude and rate of rise of the end-plate potential, causing increased "jitter" or "blocking" on single-fiber EMG), and most specifically by the presence of anti-AChR antibodies in the patient's serum.

5. **Treatment** includes administration of anticholinesterases (e.g., pyridostigmine), corticosteroids, immunosuppressive drugs such as azathioprine or cyclophosphamide, plasmapheresis, and thymectomy. Remission of the disease is common after thymectomy.

6. **Anesthetic considerations**

   a. Anticholinesterase medications should be discontinued on the morning of surgery. In severe cases, preoperative plasmapheresis may be useful.

   b. If a regional anesthetic technique is employed, the skeletal muscle relaxation produced by regional anesthesia may exacerbate any underlying muscle weakness and cause respiratory insufficiency.

   c. With general anesthesia, a decision must be made as to whether muscle-relaxant administration is necessary. For many procedures, volatile agents provide adequate muscle relaxation (including transcervical thymectomy). These patients exhibit marked sensitivity to nondepolarizing muscle relaxants and slight resistance to SCh. If necessary, reduced doses of the intermediate-acting agents atracurium and vecuronium may be used, with doses titrated to effect using peripheral nerve stimulation.

   d. While neuromuscular monitoring is mandatory, misinterpretation may occur. Since different muscle groups may be affected to different extents, complete recovery of the adductor pollicis does not necessarily imply full recovery either of the muscles of the upper airway or of ventilation.

7. After major procedures, **postoperative ventilation** should be considered. The best predictors of this need are the duration of the disease, the presence of coexisting respiratory disease, and the preoperative maintenance dose of pyridostigmine.

B. The **myasthenic syndrome** (Eaton-Lambert syndrome) differs from MG in the following respects:

   1. It is associated with an underlying malignancy (particularly oat-cell carcinoma of the lung).

   2. Peripheral muscles of the limbs and pelvic girdle are most commonly affected.

   3. Symptoms improve with exercise.

   4. At rapid rates of stimulation, muscle action potentials increase in amplitude.

   5. While sensitivity to nondepolarizing relaxants exists, a sensitivity to depolarizing agents also exists (in contrast to MG).

6. The **etiology** of the condition is prejunctional, not postjunctional as in MG. Decreased quantal release of ACh from the motor nerve ending in response to nerve stimulation is responsible for the muscle weakness.

7. The therapeutic response to anticholinesterases is unpredictable.

C. The **muscular dystrophies** are a group of inherited myopathies characterized by progressive weakness without evidence of abnormal carbohydrate or lipid storage in muscle fibers. **Duchenne's** (pseudohypertrophic) **muscular dystrophy** is the most common and most severe. Transmitted as X-linked recessive, presentation occurs in early childhood with progressive limb weakness. Kyphoscoliosis and hip and knee contractures are common. Clinical cardiomyopathy and mitral regurgitation due to papillary muscle dysfunction are rare, although electrocardiographic changes are present in 60–90% of patients. Diaphragmatic function is preserved, but total lung capacity and residual volume are reduced, and patients have recurrent pulmonary infections. Malignant hyperthermia occurs with increased incidence in these patients, and SCh should be avoided because of the potential hyperkalemic response and life-threatening cardiac arrhythmias. While sensitivity to nondepolarizing agents is likely in Duchenne-type proximal muscle atrophy, neuromuscular monitoring is mandatory if they are used.

D. **Myotonic syndromes** are characterized by a defect in muscle relaxation and persistent contraction of skeletal muscles when stimulated. This results from a failure to return cytoplasmic calcium to the sarcoplasmic reticulum when the stimulus is discontinued. The most important of these are **myotonia dystrophica** (characterized by weakness, myotonia, cataracts, mental retardation, frontal balding, cardiomyopathy, and endocrine dysfunction), **myotonia congenita** (which is manifest at birth and is nonprogressive), and **paramyotonia** (in which myotonia only occurs on exposure to cold). Sustained skeletal muscle contraction may follow the administration of SCh. This will not be relieved either by administering a nondepolarizing agent or by increasing depth of anesthesia. Intravenous quinidine (300–600 mg) or warming the patient may help to relieve the myotonia. Neostigmine does not appear to produce a myotonic response. The response to nondepolarizing muscle relaxants is normal, and the association between the myotonic syndromes and malignant hyperthermia is controversial.

E. **Familial periodic paralyses** are characterized by intermittent episodes of profound skeletal muscle weakness with sparing of the bulbar musculature only. The episodes may be associated with hyper-, normo-, or hypokalemic variants. Abnormal potassium flux can cause hyper- or hypopolarization of resting skeletal muscle cells. Thus potassium influx will hyperpolarize cell membranes, rendering them less sensitive to SCh and more sensitive to nondepolarizing agents. When necessary, it is reasonable to administer muscle relaxants in small initial doses with neuromuscular monitoring to quantify their effect. SCh has produced a myotonic response in these patients.

SUGGESTED READING

Agoston, S., and Bowman, W. C. (eds.). *Monographs in Anesthesiology: Muscle Relaxants.* New York: Elsevier, 1990.

Ali, H. H. Monitoring of neuromuscular function. *Semin. Anesth.* 3:280, 1984.

Ali, H. H., and Savarese, J. J. Monitoring of neuromuscular function. *Anesthesiology* 45:216, 1976.

Ali, H. H., and Savarese, J. J. Neuromuscular Blockade. In R. R. Atia (ed.), *Practical Anesthetic Pharmacology.* New York: Appleton-Century-Crofts, 1978. Pp. 36–58.

Basta, S. J., et al. Clinical pharmacology of doxacurium chloride, a new long-acting nondepolarizing muscle relaxant. *Anesthesiology* 69:478, 1988.

Dreyer, F. Acetylcholine receptor. *Br. J. Anaesth.* 54:115, 1982.

Larijani, G. E., et al. Clinical pharmacology of pipecuronium bromide. *Anesth. Analg.* 68:734, 1989.

Miller, R. D. (ed.). *Anesthesia.* New York: Churchill Livingstone, 1986. Pp. 835–943.

Savarese, J. J., et al. The clinical neuromuscular pharmacology of mivacurium chloride (BW 1090U): A short-acting nondepolarizing ester neuromuscular blocking drug. *Anesthesiology* 68:723, 1988.

13

Airway Evaluation and Management

Robert Gaiser

I. **Anatomy**
  A. The **upper airway** is that portion above the vocal cords.
    1. The **nasal passages** consist of the septum, turbinates, and adenoids.
    2. The **oral cavity** includes the dentition and tongue.
    3. The **pharynx** consists of the tonsils, uvula, and epiglottis.
    4. **Glottis.**
  B. The **lower airway** includes structures below the vocal cords.
    1. The **vocal cords** are the narrowest part of the airway in the adult and the limiting factor for endotracheal tube (ETT) size.
    2. The **larynx** is located at the level of the fourth through sixth cervical vertebrae. It is an intricate structure composed of cartilage, ligaments, and muscles.
      a. **Functions**
        (1) Airway protection.
        (2) Respiration.
        (3) Phonation.
      b. There are nine **cartilages** in the larynx.
        (1) Unpaired: thyroid, cricoid, and epiglottis.
        (2) Paired: arytenoid, corniculate, and cuneiform.
    3. The **cricoid** is the only complete cartilaginous ring found in the respiratory system and is inferior to the thyroid cartilage. It is the narrowest part of the airway in the pediatric patient.
    4. The **cricothyroid membrane** connects the thyroid cartilage and cricoid ring. It measures 0.9 cm × 3.0 cm in the adult and is quite thin with no major vessels in the midline.
    5. The **trachea** is a fibromuscular tube, approximately 10–12 cm in length with a diameter of approximately 20 mm in the adult. It is supported by 20 U-shaped cartilages. It enters the chest cavity at the superior mediastinum and bifurcates (at the sternal angle) at the lower border of the fourth thoracic vertebra.
    6. The **carina** marks the division of the trachea into the right and left main stem bronchi. The right is 2.5 cm long with a 25-degree take-off angle, and the left is 5 cm long with a take-off angle of 45 degrees.
  C. The **laryngeal muscles** can be divided into two groups:
    1. Muscles that open and close the glottis: lateral cricoarytenoid, posterior cricoarytenoid, and transverse arytenoid.
    2. Muscles that control the tension of the vocal ligaments: cricothyroid, vocalis, and thyroarytenoid.
  D. **Innervation**
    1. **Sensory**

   a. The **glossopharyngeal nerve** (ninth cranial nerve) supplies the posterior third of the tongue and the oropharynx from its junction with the nasopharynx to include the pharyngeal surfaces of the soft palate, epiglottis, and the fauces, to the junction of the pharynx and esophagus.
   b. The **superior laryngeal nerve,** a branch of the vagus nerve, supplies the mucosa from the epiglottis to and including the vocal cords.
   c. The **recurrent laryngeal nerve,** a branch of the vagus nerve, supplies the mucosa below the vocal cords to the trachea.

2. **Motor**
   a. The external branch of the superior laryngeal nerve supplies the cricothyroid muscle.
   b. The recurrent laryngeal nerve supplies all the intrinsic muscles of the larynx except the cricothyroid.

II. Evaluation
A. History
1. Particular importance should be placed on diseases that may affect the airway.
   a. **Arthritis** may lead to markedly decreased neck mobility. In **rheumatoid arthritis,** cervical spine instability is common. Atlantoaxial subluxation and consequent separation of the atlantoodontoid articulation may result in protrusion of the odontoid process into the foramen magnum with impingement on the spinal cord. Synovitis of the temporomandibular joint may lead to marked limitation of mandibular motion. The arytenoids can also be involved.
   b. **Infection** of the floor of the mouth, salivary glands, tonsils, or pharyngeal abscess may result in pain, edema, and trismus with limited mouth opening.
   c. **Tumors** may obstruct the airway or cause extrinsic compression and tracheal deviation.
   d. **Morbidly obese** individuals may have a history of sleep apnea from hypertrophied tonsils and adenoids.
   e. **Trauma.** A history of trauma may require investigation of potential cervical spine injury, basilar skull fracture, or intracranial injury (see Chap. 32).
   f. **Burns.** See Chap. 32.
   g. **Trisomy 21** (Down's syndrome) patients may have atlantoaxial instability and macroglossia.
   h. **Scleroderma** may result in decreased mandibular motion and narrowing of the oral aperture due to taut skin.
   i. **Acromegaly.** Excess growth hormone may cause mandibular hypertrophy with overgrowth and enlargement of the tongue and epiglottis. The glottic opening may be narrowed due to enlargement of the vocal cords.
   j. **Dwarfism** may be associated with atlantoaxial instability and potentially difficult airway manage-

ment secondary to hypoplasia of the mandible (micrognathia).

- **k. Congenital anomalies.** A variety of congenital syndromes may complicate airway management, particularly patients with craniofacial abnormalities such as Pierre Robin syndrome or Treacher Collins syndrome. These are reviewed in the Suggested Reading list.

2. If old medical records are available, **prior anesthesia records should be reviewed** for the ease of intubation and ventilation (number of attempts, ability to mask ventilate, type of laryngoscope blade used, use of stylet, or any other modifications of technique).

3. **Specific symptoms** related to airway compromise should be determined, including hoarseness, stridor, wheezing, dysphagia, dyspnea, and positional airway obstruction.

4. **Previous head/neck surgery or radiation** may require further evaluation.

B. **Physical examination**

1. Obvious, specific findings that may indicate a **difficult airway** include
   - **a.** Inability to open mouth.
   - **b.** Poor cervical spine mobility.
   - **c.** Receding chin (micrognathia).
   - **d.** Prominent incisors.
   - **e.** Short, muscular neck.
   - **f.** Morbid obesity.

2. **Injuries** to the face, neck, or chest must be evaluated to assess their contribution to airway compromise.

3. General signs of **acute airway compromise** include agitation, anxiety, changes in respiratory rate and pattern, and tachycardia.

4. **Head and neck examination**
   - **a. Nose.** The patency of the nares or the presence of a deviated septum should be determined by occluding one and then the other nostril and asking the patient which side permits easier breathing. This is especially important should nasotracheal intubation be required.
   - **b. Mouth**
     - (1) **Mouth opening.** Patients should be able to open their mouths at least 3 finger breadths.
     - (2) **Teeth.** Poor dentition may increase the risk of dental damage and dislodgement during airway manipulation. Loose teeth must be identified preoperatively and protected with a plastic dental guard or occasionally removed by an oral surgeon.
     - (3) **Tongue.** Macroglossia is seen in a variety of congenital syndromes.
   - **c. Neck**
     - (1) If the thyromental distance (the distance from the lower border of the mandible to the thyroid notch with the neck fully extended) is less than

3–4 finger breadths, there may be difficulty with visualization of the trachea.

(2) **Cervical spine mobility.** Patients should be able to touch their chin to their chest and extend their neck as far posteriorly as possible.

(3) The presence of **a healed or patent tracheostomy stoma** may be a clue to subglottic stenosis.

5. **Airway classification.** The **Mallampati classification** is based on the hypothesis that when the base of the tongue is disproportionately large, the tongue overshadows the larynx, resulting in difficult exposure of the latter during laryngoscopy. Assessment is made with the patient sitting upright, with the head in the neutral position, the mouth open as wide as possible, and the tongue protruded maximally.

a. **Class I.** Faucial pillars, soft palate, and uvula are visible.

b. **Class II.** Faucial pillars and soft palate may be seen, but uvula is masked by the base of the tongue.

c. **Class III.** Only soft palate is visible. Intubation is predicted to be difficult in patients with class III airways.

C. **Laboratory studies.** In most patients a careful history and physical examination will be all that is needed to evaluate an airway properly. Useful adjuncts may include the following:

1. **Laryngoscopy** (direct, indirect, and fiberoptic) will provide information regarding the hypopharynx, laryngeal inlet, and vocal cord function. It can be performed in a conscious patient using topical anesthesia or a nerve block.

2. **The chest radiograph** may reveal tracheal deviation or narrowing.

3. **Tracheal tomograms.**

4. **Cervical spine films** are important in trauma cases and should be done whenever there is an injury above the clavicle.

5. The **computed tomography (CT) scan** can further delineate masses obstructing the airway.

6. **Pulmonary function tests** and flow volume loops can help determine the degree and site of airway obstruction (see Chap. 3).

7. **Baseline arterial blood gases** may indicate those patients who are chronically hypoxic and those who are carbon dioxide retainers.

III. **Basic airway management**

A. **Mask airway**

1. **Indications**

a. To provide **inhalation anesthesia** for short operative procedures in patients not at risk for regurgitation of gastric contents.

b. To **preoxygenate** (denitrogenate) a patient as a prelude to endotracheal intubation.

c. To assist or control **ventilation** as part of initial resuscitation.

2. **Technique** involves the placement of a face mask and maintenance of a patent airway.

   a. A **mask** is selected to provide a snug seal around the bridge of the nose, cheeks, and mouth. Clear plastic masks have a less noxious odor and allow for observation of the lips (for color) and mouth (for secretions or vomitus).

   b. **Mask placement.** The mask is held in the left hand so that the little finger is at the angle of the mandible, the third and fourth fingers are along the mandible, and the index finger and thumb are placed on the mask. The right hand is available to control the reservoir bag. If the patient is large, two hands may be required to maintain a good mask fit, necessitating an assistant to control the bag. Head straps may be used to assist mask fit.

   c. **Edentulous patients** may present a problem when attempting to achieve an adequate seal with the face mask due to collapse of mandible to maxilla distance, usually maintained by teeth. An oral airway should correct this problem, and the cheeks may be compressed against the mask to decrease leaks. Two hands may be required to do this.

   d. **Ventilation** is assessed and may be assisted or controlled.

   e. **Airway obstruction** may be recognized by stridor, a high-pitched crowing sound, and a "rocking" motion of the chest and abdomen. In addition, there will be no respiratory excursions in the reservoir bag.

   f. Maneuvers to maintain **airway patency** include the following:

     (1) **Neck extension.**

     (2) **Jaw thrust,** by placing the fingers under the angles of the mandible and lifting forward.

     (3) An **oral airway** can maintain upper airway patency in patients who have airway obstruction from their tongue and soft palate but may not be well tolerated if they have an intact gag reflex. Complications from use of oral airways include vomiting, laryngospasm, and dental trauma. If the airway is too short, it may compress the tongue, producing complete obstruction.

     (4) A **nasal airway** helps maintain upper airway patency in a patient with minimal to moderate obstruction and is well tolerated by awake or sedated patients with an intact gag reflex. Nasal airways can cause epistaxis and are usually avoided in patients who are anticoagulated.

   g. **Complications.** With a mask airway technique, aspiration is a possibility, as the airway is not protected, laryngospasm may occur, and two hands may be required.

B. The **laryngeal mask** comes in four sizes: 1 (< 6.5 kg) and 2 (6.5–25.0 kg) for pediatrics, and 3 and 4 for adults (Fig. 13-1). It is inserted into the hypopharynx in its anatomic position and then passed downward behind the larynx,

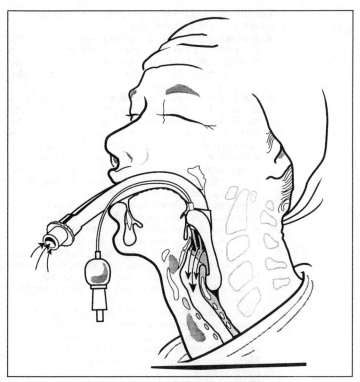

Fig. 13-1. Laryngeal mask (Courtesy of Dr. A. I. J. Brain).

sealing the glottic opening, and enabling ventilation after inflation of the cuff. A slight but unmistakable bulging of the tissues overlying the larynx serves to indicate the mask is in position. It allows positive-pressure ventilation, can support an airway when the trachea cannot be visualized and intubated with standard techniques, and may be used as a guide for placement of an ETT (a 6-mm ID ETT will pass through a No. 3 and No. 4 laryngeal mask). There may be occasional difficulty in obtaining a good seal. The laryngeal mask does not protect against regurgitation and pulmonary aspiration and requires anesthesia for placement (e.g., by topical, regional, or general anesthesia).

IV. **Intubation**

A. **Orotracheal intubation**

1. **Indications.** Endotracheal intubation is required to provide a patent airway when patients are at risk for aspiration, when airway maintenance by mask is difficult, and for prolonged controlled ventilation. It may also be required for specific surgical procedures (e.g., head/neck, intrathoracic, or intraabdominal).

2. **Technique.** Intubation is usually performed with a

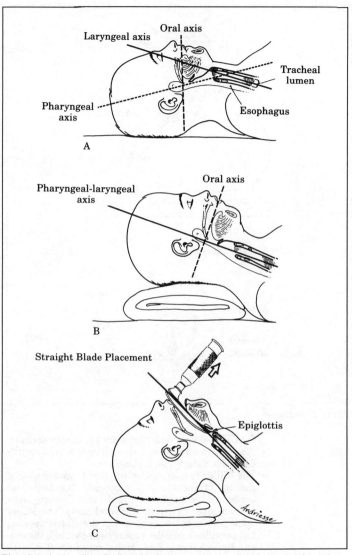

Fig. 13-2. Anatomic relations for laryngoscopy and endotracheal intubation.

laryngoscope (Fig. 13-2). The Macintosh and Miller blades are most commonly used.

a. The **Macintosh** is a curved blade whose tip is inserted into the vallecula (the space between the base of the tongue and the pharyngeal surface of the epiglottis) (Fig. 13-2D). It provides a good view of the oro- and hypopharynx, thus allowing more room

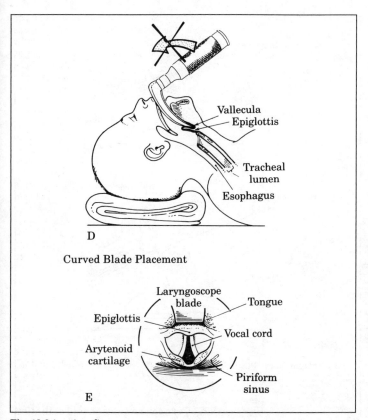

D

Curved Blade Placement

E

Fig. 13-2 (continued)

for ETT passage with diminished epiglottic trauma.
Size ranges vary from 1–4, with most adults requiring a Macintosh No. 3 blade.

b. The **Miller** is a straight blade that is passed so that
the tip of the blade lies beneath the laryngeal
surface of the epiglottis (Fig. 13-2C). The epiglottis
is then lifted to expose the vocal cords. The Miller
blade allows better exposure of the glottic opening
but provides a smaller passageway through the oro-
and hypopharynx. Size ranges vary from 0–3, with
most adults requiring a Miller No. 2 or No. 3 blade.

c. The patient should be positioned with the head
elevated approximately 10 cm, with pads placed
under the occiput and the jaw lifted forward. This
can be accomplished by placing two folded blankets
under the head so that it is in the *sniffing position*.
This position aligns the oral, pharyngeal, and laryngeal axes so that the pathway from the lips to the
glottis is most nearly in a straight line (Fig. 13-2A
and B).

d. The laryngoscope is held in the left hand near the junction between the handle and blade. After opening the mouth with a scissoring motion of the right hand, the laryngoscope is inserted into the right side of the patient's mouth to avoid the incisor teeth while sweeping the tongue to the left. The lips should not be pinched between the blade and teeth. The blade is then advanced toward the midline until the epiglottis comes into view. The tongue and pharyngeal soft tissues are then lifted to expose the glottic opening. The laryngoscope should be used to lift (Fig. 13-2C) rather than act as a lever (Fig. 13-2D) to prevent damage to the maxillary incisors or gingiva.

e. An appropriate **ETT size** depends on the patient's age, body habitus, and type of surgery. A 7.0-mm ETT is used for most women and an 8.0-mm ETT for most men. The ETT is held in the right hand as one would hold a pencil and advanced through the oral cavity from the right corner of the mouth, and then through the vocal cords. The anatomic view for visualization with a Macintosh laryngoscope is seen in Figure 13-2E. If visualization of the glottic opening is incomplete, it may be necessary to use the epiglottis as a landmark immediately beneath which a styletted ETT is passed into the trachea. External cricoid pressure may also aid in visualization. The proximal end of the ETT cuff is placed just below the vocal cords, and the marking on the tube is noted in relation to the patient's incisors (or lips). The cuff is inflated just to the point of obtaining a seal in the presence of 20–30 cm H_2O positive-pressure ventilation.

f. Verification of proper endotracheal intubation can be confirmed by the **detection of end-tidal carbon dioxide** and auscultation over both lung fields and the stomach. If breath sounds are heard on the right only, a right main stem intubation has occurred (more commonly), and the ETT should be withdrawn until breath sounds are heard bilaterally. Listening for breath sounds high in each axilla will usually avoid the examiner's being misled by breath sounds transmitted from the opposite lung or stomach.

g. The tube should then be securely fastened to the cheeks with tape, occasionally using benzoin.

3. Complications of orotracheal intubation include injury of the lips or tongue, dental injuries, pharyngeal/tracheal mucosal trauma, tracheal tears, avulsion of arytenoid cartilages, and vocal cord damage.

B. Nasotracheal intubation

1. Indications. Nasotracheal intubation may be required in patients undergoing an intraoral procedure or requiring long-term intubation, as it provides greater patient comfort and less potential for tube kinking. This technique minimizes cervical spine manipulation, of particular concern in patients with an unstable cervical spine (see Chap. 32).

2. **Contraindications.** Basilar skull fractures, especially of the ethmoid bone, nasal fractures, chronic epistaxis, coagulopathy, and nasal polyps are relative contraindications to nasal intubation.

3. **Technique.** The nasal mucosa is anesthetized and vasoconstricted with a 4% cocaine solution or a phenylephrine-lidocaine mixture using cotton-tipped pledgets. If both nares are patent, the right naris is preferred because the bevel of most tracheal tubes, when introduced through the right naris, will face the flat nasal septum, reducing damage to the turbinates. The inferior turbinates interfere with passage and limit the size of the ETT. Usually a 6.0- to 6.5-mm ETT is used for women and a 7.0- to 7.5-mm ETT for men. After passage through the naris into the pharynx, the tube is advanced through the glottic opening. Passage under direct vision using a laryngoscope and Magill forceps may be required.

4. **Complications**
   a. These are similar to those described for orotracheal intubation (see sec. **A.3**).
   b. In addition, one may see nasal hemorrhage, submucosal dissection, and dislodgement of enlarged tonsils and adenoids.
   c. Infection of the frontal and maxillary sinuses and bacteremia may be seen.

C. **Awake intubation**
   1. **Indications.** Awake oral or nasal intubation should be considered when there is
      a. A difficult intubation anticipated in a patient at risk for aspiration.
      b. Uncertainty about the ability to ventilate or intubate following induction of general anesthesia (e.g., morbidly obese patients).
      c. A need to assess neurologic function after intubation or positioning for surgery (e.g., patient with an unstable cervical spine).

   2. **Technique**
      a. To perform an **awake intubation,** a 4% lidocaine gargle, followed by a lidocaine spray or nebulizer is used to decrease upper airway sensation. Specific nerve blocks include the following:
         (1) **Superior laryngeal nerve.** A 25-gauge needle is directed toward the greater cornu of the hyoid bone and walked off in a caudal direction until inserted in the thyrohyoid membrane. After negative aspiration, 2 ml of 2% lidocaine is injected bilaterally.
         (2) The **recurrent laryngeal nerve** can be blocked by a transtracheal approach. A 25-gauge needle is inserted through the cricothyroid membrane in the midline, and after aspiration of air to confirm placement within the tracheal lumen, 2

ml of 2% lidocaine is injected, and the needle is withdrawn. The patient will cough when local anesthetic is injected, aiding in proximal anesthetic spread. This block is usually not performed in the patient with a full stomach because of the risk for aspiration.

b. Awake oral laryngoscopy often allows one to assess the airway. Sedatives such as midazolam, propofol, and fentanyl may be used in addition to the nerve blocks described above.

c. Awake nasal intubation may be performed after adequate topical anesthesia and regional airway blocks.

(1) Incremental doses of sedatives are useful adjuncts.

(2) A well-lubricated ETT is passed into the nasopharynx with gentle pressure.

(3) Deep, resonant breath sounds may be noted as the tube is advanced toward the glottis. An exaggerated sniffing position may be useful.

(4) Successful intubation is noted when the patient is unable to phonate, breath sounds are noted with ventilation, and carbon dioxide is noted on the capnograph.

3. Complications are as previously described in sec. **A.3.**

D. The **light wand** consists of a malleable lighted stylet over which an ETT can be passed blindly into the trachea. To insert, the operating room lights are dimmed, and the light wand is advanced following the curve of the tongue. A glow noted in the lateral neck indicates that the tip of the ETT lies in the piriform fossa. If the tip enters the esophagus, there is a marked diminution in the light's brightness. When the tip is correctly positioned in the trachea, a marked glow is noted in the anterior neck. At this point, the ETT is slid off in the same manner as a standard stylet.

E. Fiberoptic intubation. The flexible fiberoptic laryngoscope consists of glass fibers that are bound together to provide a flexible unit for the transmission of light and images. The fiberoptic bundle is fragile, and excessive bending can result in damage to the visual elements. The working channel can be used to administer topical anesthetics and deliver supplemental oxygen and suction. In general, this channel works best for the delivery of supplemental oxygen, and at flow rates of 10–15 L/min, it tends to keep the visual elements clear of secretions. The visual field often becomes limited as the fiberoptic bronchoscope nears the glottic opening, as secretions, blood, or fogging of the lens may obscure the view. Immersion of the tip of the fiberoptic scope in warm water or silicone helps to prevent fogging, as does high oxygen flow.

1. Standard equipment for fiberoptic intubation includes

a. An oral bite block.

b. An Ovassapian airway.

   c. Topical anesthetics.
   d. Suction.
   e. A fiberoptic scope with light source.
2. **Indications**
   a. The flexible fiberoptic laryngoscope can be used in both awake and anesthetized patients to evaluate and intubate their airways. It can be used for both nasal and oral endotracheal intubation and should be used as a first option in an anticipated difficult airway rather than as a "last resort."
   b. Initial fiberoptic intubation is recommended for patients with known or suspected cervical spine pathology, head and neck tumors, morbid obesity, and known prior or suspected ventilation or intubation difficulty.
3. **Technique.** An ETT is styletted over the fiberoptic scope, oxygen tubing is attached to the suction port, and the control lever is grasped with the right hand while the scope is advanced or maneuvered with the left hand. An oral Ovassapian airway is helpful and well tolerated for oral attempts. It is important to keep the fiberoptic scope in the midline when advancing it to prevent entering the piriform fossa. The tip of the scope is positioned anteriorly when in the hypopharynx and advanced toward the epiglottis. If mucosa or secretions impair the view, the scope should be retracted or removed to clean the tip and reinserted in the midline. As the scope slides beneath the epiglottis, the vocal cords will be seen. The scope is advanced with the tip in a neutral position until tracheal rings are noted. If topical anesthesia is adequate, the patient will tolerate this with no coughing. The scope is stabilized, and the ETT is advanced over it and into the trachea. If there is resistance to passage, the ETT may need to be turned 180 degrees in the counterclockwise direction to prevent contact with the anterior commissure and allow passage through the vocal cords.

F. **Retrograde tracheal intubation**
   1. **Indications.** This technique is performed when previously described techniques have been unsuccessful. It is performed in a conscious patient who is ventilating with a stable airway.
   2. **Technique.** The cricothyroid membrane is identified and punctured in the midline with an 18-gauge IV catheter (Fig. 13-3). An 80-cm, 0.025-inch guide wire is introduced and directed cephalad. A laryngoscope is used to visualize and retrieve the wire. An ETT is passed over the wire, which serves as a guide through the vocal cords.

V. **Emergency airway techniques**
   A. **Percutaneous needle cricothyroidotomy** involves the placement of a 14-gauge catheter or 7.5 Fr introducer through the cricothyroid membrane into the trachea. Oxygen can be administered by connecting the breathing circuit to a 3-mm ID ETT adapter inserted directly into the IV catheter or to a 7.5-mm ID ETT adapter inserted into a

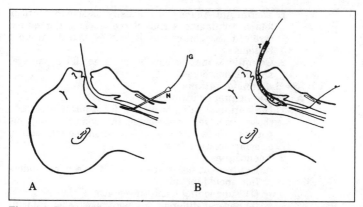

Fig. 13-3. Retrograde technique for tracheal intubation. A. A needle (*N*) has been inserted cephalad into the cricothyroid membrane and the guide wire (*G*) is delivered through the mouth. B. The needle has been removed and an endotracheal tube (*T*) is placed over the guide wire and advanced into the trachea, the two ends of the guide carefully followed. (From P. Barriott and B. Riou. Retrograde technique for tracheal intubation in trauma patients. *Crit. Care Med.* 16:713, 1988.)

3-ml syringe barrel and connected to the IV catheter. Once in place, the catheter must be carefully secured to the neck because dislodgement during ventilation may lead to severe barotrauma, massive emphysema of the neck and anterior chest, and loss of the airway.

1. Oxygenation, but not ventilation, can be achieved through the catheter at rates of 10–12 L/min. This is a temporary maneuver and is absolutely contraindicated in cases of complete upper airway obstruction, as severe barotrauma may result.

2. Some ventilation may be achieved with jet ventilation by pressing the oxygen flush valve for 1 second and allowing for passive exhalation over 2–3 seconds.

3. **Complications** include tissue emphysema, barotrauma, and pneumothorax. Furthermore, the airway is not "protected," and aspiration is a possibility.

B. **Cricothyroidotomy** is a simple, rapid, and safe method for upper airway obstruction. With the neck extended, a transverse incision is made in the cricothyroid membrane in the midline. The handle of the scalpel is used to separate the tissues separating the cartilages until a tracheostomy tube or endotracheal tube is inserted.

C. **Rigid bronchoscopy** may be necessary to support an airway obstructed by a foreign body, traumatic disruption, stenosis, or mediastinal mass. It is important to have a range of scope sizes available (including pediatric sizes), and an inhalation induction with spontaneous ventilation is required.

D. **Tracheostomy** may be performed under local anesthesia prior to the induction of general anesthesia for a patient with a particularly difficult airway.

1. **Technique.** An incision is usually made in the third or fourth cartilaginous ring of the trachea. It requires careful dissection of vessels, nerves, and the thyroid isthmus.
2. **Complications** include hemorrhage, false passage, and pneumothorax.

VI. **Special considerations**

A. **Rapid sequence induction**

1. **Indications.** Patients at risk for aspiration include those who have recently eaten (full stomach), pregnant patients, those with bowel obstruction, morbid obesity, or symptomatic reflux.

2. **Technique**

a. **Equipment** necessary for a rapid sequence induction should include
   (1) Functioning tonsil-tip suction.
   (2) Several different laryngoscope blades (Macintosh/Miller).
   (3) Several styletted ETTs, including one size smaller than normal.
   (4) An assistant who can perform cricoid pressure.

b. The patient is **preoxygenated** using high flow rates of 100% oxygen for 3–5 minutes (denitrogenation). Four full vital capacity breaths of 100% oxygen achieve the same results when time is of the essence.

c. With the IV administration of an induction agent (e.g., thiopental, propofol, or ketamine) and succinylcholine, an assistant employs the Sellick maneuver by placing firm downward pressure on the cricoid cartilage, effectively compressing and occluding the esophagus. This maneuver will prevent passive regurgitation of gastric contents into the trachea, will limit gastric inflation during mask ventilation, and may bring the vocal cords into better view by displacing them posteriorly. It will not prevent active vomiting.

d. **There should be no attempt to ventilate the patient by mask.** Intubation can usually be performed within 30–60 seconds. **Cricoid pressure is maintained until proper verification of successful endotracheal intubation.**

e. If intubation attempts are unsuccessful, cricoid pressure should be maintained continuously during all subsequent intubation maneuvers, while mask ventilation with 100% oxygen is administered.

B. **Endotracheal tube changes.** Occasionally an ETT must be changed in a patient with a difficult airway, usually because of a cuff leak.

1. The oropharynx is suctioned and the patient is ventilated with 100% oxygen by Ambu bag.

2. A tracheal tube changer is placed through the ETT and into the distal trachea. The old ETT is slid off the changer, and a new ETT is passed over the changer into the trachea. Alternatively, the patient can be reintubated by using a fiberoptic bronchoscope. An

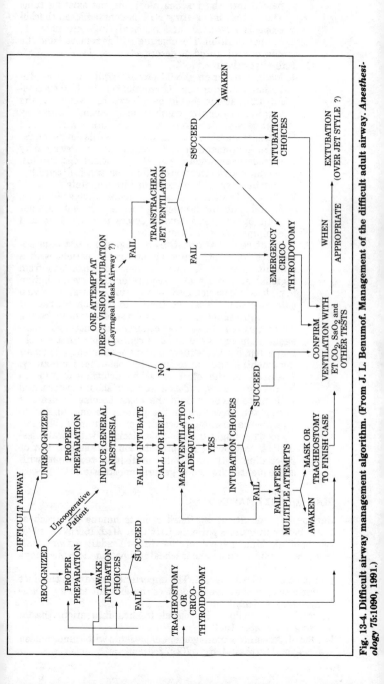

Fig. 13-4. Difficult airway management algorithm. (From J. L. Benumof. Management of the difficult adult airway. *Anesthesiology* 75:1090, 1991.)

ETT is placed over the bronchoscope, and the scope is passed into the trachea alongside the existing tube. The cuff of the existing ETT is deflated, the bronchoscope is advanced, and tracheal rings are noted to confirm position. The existing ETT is removed and the new one advanced as described in sec. **IV.E.**

C. **Failed intubation**
   1. Mask ventilation should proceed while another intubation technique (e.g., fiberoptic) is tried. If unsuccessful, the patient should be allowed to awaken. If the surgical procedure prohibits delay (such as an emergent cesarean section), mask ventilation with cricoid pressure should continue. If mask ventilation is impossible, placement of a laryngeal mask airway may provide adequate oxygen. If the patient desaturates, percutaneous cricothyroidotomy or surgical cricothyroidotomy should be performed immediately.
   2. The key to success is careful preoperative evaluation, formulating and proceeding with a plan that does not limit options, and having access to extra help and equipment (Fig. 13-4).

D. **Role of regional anesthesia.** Regional anesthesia appears to be an attractive option for the patient with a difficult airway. However, serious complications from regional anesthesia may require emergency intubation (e.g., loss of consciousness and seizure from an intravascular injection of local anesthetic). In addition, the patient may require supplementation with sedatives or narcotics, which may result in airway compromise. Successful management includes the use of a continuous catheter technique, test doses, frequent patient assessment, and small incremental volumes to limit the potential for toxicity. Adequacy of the block must be determined prior to beginning surgery, and a backup plan should be discussed with the surgeon should the block become inadequate during the procedure or the patient become unable to tolerate the position, procedure, or duration of the operation. This might include field blockade with local anesthetics, postponing the procedure until another day, or proceeding with an awake intubation technique with subsequent induction of general anesthesia.

SUGGESTED READING

Barriot, P., and Riou, B. Retrograde technique for tracheal intubation in trauma patients. *Crit. Care Med.* 16(7):712, 1988.

Benumof, J. Management of the difficult adult airway with special emphasis on awake tracheal intubation. *Anesthesiology* 75(6):1087, 1991.

Benumof, J., and Scheller, M. The importance of transtracheal jet ventilation in the management of the difficult airway. *Anesthesiology* 71:769, 1989.

Butler, F., and Cirillo, A. Retrograde tracheal intubation. *Anesth. Analg.* 39(4):333, 1960.

Donlon, J. Anesthetic management of patients with compromised airways. *Anesthesiol. Rev.* 7(2):22, 1980.

Ellis, P., et al. Guided orotracheal intubation in the operating room using a lighted stylet: A comparison with direct laryngoscopic technique. *Anesthesiology* 64:823, 1986.

Grande, C., Stene, J., and Bernhard, W. Airway management: Considerations in the trauma patient. *Crit. Care Clin.* 6(1):37, 1991.

Heath, M., and Allagain, J. Intubation through the laryngeal mask. *Anaesthesia* 46:545, 1991.

Jones, A., and Pelton, D. An index of syndromes and their anaesthetic implications. *Can. Anaesth. Soc. J.* 23(2):207, 1976.

King, T., and Adams, A. Failed tracheal intubation. *Br. J. Anaesth.* 65:400, 1990.

Malan, T., and Johnson, M. The difficult airway in obstetric anaesthesia: Techniques for airway management and the role of regional anesthesia. *J. Clin. Anesth.* 1(2):104, 1988.

Mallampati, S., et al. A clinical sign to predict difficult tracheal intubation: A prospective study. *Can. Anaesth. Soc. J.* 32(4):429, 1985.

Wilson, M., et al. Predicting difficult intubation. *Br. J. Anaesth.* 61:211, 1988.

14

Administration of General Anesthesia

Paul Lennon

The goals of general anesthesia are to provide amnesia, analgesia, and optimal surgical conditions, with the health and safety of the patient as the primary concern.

I. **Preoperative preparation.** The anesthesiologist assumes responsibility for the patient when the preoperative medication is administered. An unstable patient should be accompanied by an anesthesiologist during transport to the operating room.

A. The **preoperative evaluation** may have been conducted any time from minutes to weeks prior to the time of surgery. The medical record should be reviewed for additional information, laboratory data, consultant notes, interim changes in the patient's condition (e.g., recent episode of angina), and time and dose of the premedication. The patient's NPO status should be confirmed.

B. **Intravenous access.** The appropriate size and number of IV catheters placed are determined by the patient's medical condition and the nature of the surgery. A single, well-functioning 18- or 20-gauge catheter is often sufficient for a healthy patient undergoing routine surgery. At least one 14- or 16-gauge catheter is preferred if the need for rapid volume or blood product infusion is anticipated. IV catheters are usually placed in the hand, forearm, or antecubital space after subcutaneous infiltration with 1–2 ml of 1% lidocaine. IV cannulation may be difficult in presurgical patients because of anxiety, obesity, multiple prior IVs, or low intravascular volume. Occasionally, a small-gauge IV catheter (20- or 22-gauge) is placed prior to induction with later placement of one or more larger catheters. All IV catheters should be securely taped and labeled. If a patient arrives with an IV catheter in place, its function should be assured, the site inspected, and the catheter securely taped. The type of IV solution and tubing may need to be changed.

C. **Anxiety.** During this time, the patient may be very anxious. This is managed most effectively by conversing with and reassuring the patient. When appropriate, a benzodiazepine (e.g., midazolam, 0.5- to 1.0-mg IV increments) or a narcotic (e.g., fentanyl, 25-μg IV increments) may be administered. These dosages must be individualized to the patient's age and medical condition. Appropriate monitoring should be employed and resuscitative equipment available.

D. **Intravascular volume.** It is not uncommon for preoperative patients to be hypovolemic. Common causes include prolonged NPO status (especially children), prolonged severe illness, hemorrhage, fever, vomiting, diuretic use, and preoperative bowel preparations. Many anesthetics are systemic vasodilators and myocardial depressants. Their administration can lead to marked hypotension, particularly when fluid deficits have not been replaced.

E. Monitoring. Standard monitoring and appropriate invasive monitoring (e.g., arterial line) for induction should be in place. Monitoring that is not required for induction may be placed afterward. For further discussion, see Chap. 10.

II. Induction involves the transition from an awake, conscious patient with intact protective reflexes to an unconscious patient who is entirely dependent on the anesthesiologist. Airway maintenance and hemodynamic stability are critical components of this period.

A. Positioning. The patient is usually supine with extremities resting comfortably on padded surfaces in neutral anatomic position. The head should rest comfortably on a soft but firm support (e.g., folded blankets, foam headrest) and be slightly raised.

B. Environment. Patient comfort is of the utmost importance. Shivering should be avoided by the use of warm blankets and/or warming of the room. Noise in the room must be minimized, and nonessential discussion should cease.

C. Techniques

1. **Intravenous** induction is most commonly performed and usually is preceded by the administration of oxygen by a mask placed gently on the patient's face. Patients who express a fear of masks may have this deferred until intravenous sedation has had some effect. A potent, short-acting hypnotic (thiopental, 2–4 mg/kg, or propofol, 1–2.5 mg/kg) is then administered intravenously. Inhalation agents are administered with the loss of eyelid reflex. The patient may continue to breathe spontaneously or need assistance. If intubation is to be performed, a muscle relaxant is given to facilitate laryngoscopy, but **the ability to ventilate the patient must be confirmed prior to muscle-relaxant administration.**

2. **Inhalation induction** is employed to maintain spontaneous ventilation (compromised airway) and to defer the placement of an IV catheter (pediatrics). With this induction, the classic "stages" of general anesthesia can be seen (Table 14-1).

3. **Intramuscular induction** using ketamine and **rectal induction** using methohexital are most commonly performed in children and are discussed in Chap. 28.

D. Airway management. During induction, the patient's airway is of critical importance and may need to be assisted with oral or nasopharyngeal airways (see Chap. 13).

E. Laryngoscopy and **intubation** may be associated with a profound sympathetic response including hypertension and tachycardia. These responses may be modified by administering narcotics, lidocaine, beta blockers, or further hypnotic intravenously prior to intubation.

F. Regional anesthesia. If a combination of regional and

Table 14-1. The stages of general anesthesia

The "stages" or planes of anesthesia were defined by Guedel after careful observation of patient responses during induction with diethyl ether. Induction with modern anesthetic agents is sufficiently rapid that these descriptions of individual stages are often not applicable or appreciated. However, modification of these categories still provides useful terminology to describe progression from the awake to the anesthetized state.

Stage I: Amnesia	This period begins with induction of anesthesia and continues to loss of consciousness. The threshold of pain perception is not lowered during stage I.
Stage II: Delirium	This period is characterized by uninhibited excitation and potentially injurious responses to noxious stimuli, including vomiting, laryngospasm, hypertension, tachycardia, and uncontrolled movement. The pupils are often dilated, gaze may be divergent, respiration is frequently irregular, and breath holding is common. Desirable induction drugs accelerate transition through this stage.
Stage III: Surgical anesthesia	In this target depth for anesthesia, the gaze is central, pupils are constricted, and respirations are regular. Anesthesia is considered sufficient when painful stimulation does not elicit somatic reflexes or deleterious autonomic responses (e.g., hypertension, tachycardia).
Stage IV: Overdosage	Commonly referred to as "too deep," this stage is marked by shallow or absent respirations, dilated and nonreactive pupils, and hypotension that may progress to circulatory failure. Anesthesia should be lightened immediately.

general anesthesia is planned, induction of regional anesthesia (e.g., epidural anesthesia) is often begun first to confirm the effectiveness of the technique. Induction of general anesthesia may then require some modification (e.g., a patient with a high sensory level may be more sensitive to the hypotensive effects of induction agents) such as having a vasopressor readily available.

G. **Positioning for surgery.** Usually a patient is positioned for the surgical procedure after induction of general anesthesia. Movement of a supine patient into another position (e.g., sitting position) may be accompanied by hemodynamic instability (e.g., hypotension) due to the lack of intact compensatory hemodynamic reflexes. Positioning should occur at a controlled pace with frequent assessment of the patient's condition. Close attention to the patient's airway and ventilation during this period is imperative. Patients with a positional neurologic deficit may, after an "awake intubation" (see Chap. 13), be assisted to their surgical position prior to induction.

III. **Maintenance**

  A. This **interval of time** begins when a patient is at an adequate depth of anesthesia for the start of surgery and continues until the time surgical anesthesia is no longer necessary. While physiologic changes associated with anesthesia during this time may not be as abrupt or as large as those that occur during induction and emergence, many surgical maneuvers can be associated with dramatic hemodynamic disturbances (i.e., vena cava compression, cardiac compression).

  B. **Depth of anesthesia** must be constantly assessed by observing the responses to surgical stimulation and anticipating changes that may occur. Responses may be **somatic** (movement, coughing, breath holding) or **autonomic** (tachycardia, hypertension, mydriasis, sweating, or tearing). Somatic responses are markedly attenuated or abolished by the administration of muscle relaxants; autonomic responses can be altered by regional anesthesia and autonomic blocking drugs (beta blockers) and may be due to causes other than surgical stimulation (e.g., hypoxia, hypercarbia, hypovolemia). Evaluating the level of anesthesia is an integration of many clinical observations, judgment, and experience, used to respond appropriately to the clinical situation.

  C. **Methods**

    1. In a **pure inhalation technique,** the concentration of the volatile anesthetic is titrated to patient movement (if muscle relaxants are not used), blood pressure (which decreases with increasing depth), and ventilation (respiratory rate increases and tidal volume decreases with increasing depth). Nitrous oxide, if used, is adjusted to ensure adequate oxygenation. This technique allows for spontaneous ventilation and rapid emergence.

    2. In a **nitrous oxide–narcotic–relaxant technique** ("balanced"), specific drugs are used to provide the separate components of general anesthesia. Nitrous oxide 65–70% is combined with narcotics, which are given as a loading dose early in the operation and then titrated to the patient's heart rate and blood pressure in response to surgical stimulation. An estimate of the total narcotic requirement should be calculated and large doses avoided near the termination of surgery to prevent a delayed emergence. Ventilation is controlled because of respiratory depression secondary to the narcotics and the need for muscle relaxants with most surgical procedures. This technique minimizes myocardial depression and is the technique of choice for patients susceptible to malignant hyperthermia. Depending on the nitrous oxide concentration, patient's age, and physical status, however, awareness during surgery is of concern.

    3. **Total intravenous anesthesia** employs the continuous infusion or repeated boluses of one or more short-

acting IV anesthetics (e.g., alfentanil, propofol) with or without a muscle relaxant. The infusion is discontinued a sufficient interval of time before the end of surgery. This interval (e.g., propofol—5 minutes, alfentanil—20 minutes) is dependent on the duration of action of the IV anesthetic. This technique is particularly useful in situations where ventilation is interrupted (e.g., bronchoscopy, laser airway surgery) and allows for rapid emergence.

4. **Combinations** of the above methods are often employed. A low concentration of a volatile anesthetic (e.g., isoflurane 0.3–0.5%) is often added to a nitrous oxide–narcotic–relaxant technique to ensure amnesia. Nitrous oxide is frequently used in conjunction with IV anesthetics. Multiple anesthetics reduce the need for, as well as the potential toxicity of, a large dose of a single anesthetic. However, adverse medication reactions (or interactions) increase with the number of anesthetics administered.

D. **Ventilation** of the patient during general anesthesia may be either spontaneous, assisted, or controlled.

1. **Spontaneous or assisted ventilation.** A patient may breathe spontaneously with or without assistance, via either a mask or an endotracheal tube (ETT). However, respiratory function may be significantly compromised intraoperatively by the patient's medical condition, position, external pressure on the thorax, surgical maneuvers (e.g., peritoneal insufflation, open chest, surgical packing), or medications (e.g., muscle relaxants). Most general anesthetics depress respiration in a dose-dependent manner, and therefore hypoventilation and a decreased tidal volume often occur with a mild to moderate rise in $PaCO_2$. Spontaneous or assisted ventilation allows for the ability to assess the depth of anesthesia by observation of respiratory rate and pattern.

2. **Controlled ventilation.** Although a mask may be used, an ETT and mechanical ventilator are employed if ventilation is controlled for a significant period of time. Initial ventilator settings usually consist of a tidal volume of 10–15 ml/kg and a respiratory rate of 8–10 breaths/min. Peak inspiratory pressures should be noted and kept at less than 50 cm H_2O (for further details, see Chaps. 9 and 35).

3. **Assessment.** Adequacy of ventilation is confirmed by continual observation of the patient, including auscultation of breath sounds and inspection of the anesthesia machine (e.g., reservoir breathing bag, ventilator bellows, peak inspiratory pressure) and monitors (e.g., capnograph, pulse oximeter). Arterial blood gas analysis and adjustments in the patient's ventilation may be required intraoperatively. If mechanical ventilation is inadequate, manual ventilation with 100% oxygen by the reservoir breathing bag should be employed until the problem is corrected.

E. **Intravenous fluids.** Intraoperative IV fluid therapy is required, particularly if surgery is of significant duration or magnitude.

1. **Preoperative fluid deficits.** Most patients are NPO for at least 8 hours prior to surgery. The amount of fluid usually lost by an adult (at rest) per hour, known as **maintenance fluid,** is calculated at 60 ml plus 1 ml/kg (for each kilogram greater than 20). Therefore, a healthy 50-kg adult who has fasted for 8 hours has a "fluid deficit" of $(60 + 30) \times 8$ ml $= 720$ ml. In general, at least half of this deficit should be corrected prior to induction; the remainder should be corrected intraoperatively.

2. **Intraoperative IV fluid requirements**

   a. **Maintenance fluid requirements** continue intraoperatively, as in sec. 1. In some instances (e.g., hand surgery), this may be the major component of the fluid requirement.

   b. **"Third space losses"** constitute fluid requirements due to tissue edema from surgical trauma and evaporative losses at the surgical site. These may be substantial and depend on the site and extent of surgery. They range from 3–5 ml/kg/hr (mastectomy) up to 15–20 ml/kg/hr (abdominal aortic aneurysm).

   c. **Blood loss** may be difficult to estimate. The amount present in the suction canisters should be frequently noted, taking into consideration the presence of other fluids (e.g., irrigation, ascites). Used surgical sponges should be checked by the anesthesiologist and may be weighed in pediatric operations. Blood lost on the surgical field (e.g., surgical drapes) and on the floor should be estimated. If blood loss is substantial, monitoring serial hematocrits is warranted.

3. **Replacement of deficits.** Fluids should be administered IV to correct the patient's estimated deficit. Trends in heart rate, blood pressure, and urine output may serve as a guide to intravascular volume replacement. Measurement of central venous pressure or pulmonary artery occlusion pressure may be necessary.

   a. **Crystalloid solutions** are used to replace maintenance fluid requirements and "third space losses." The IV solution should optimally be a relatively isotonic balanced salt solution (e.g., Lactated Ringer's). Blood loss may also be replaced with a balanced salt solution. Crystalloid, due to its relative lack of sequestration in the intravascular space, should be administered in a 3 : 1 ratio of volume to estimated blood loss. With continued blood loss, this ratio may need to be increased. IV glucose administration is not necessary unless specifically indicated (e.g., insulin-dependent diabetes mellitus, hepatic disease); preferably, therapy should be guided by serum or finger-stick glucose measurement.

   b. **Colloid solutions** (e.g., packed red blood cells, albumin 5%, hydroxyethyl starch 6%) may be used to replace blood loss or restore intravascular volume. To replace blood loss, colloid solutions should be administered in an approximately 1 : 1 ratio of volume to estimated blood loss (see Chap. 33).

   c. **Blood transfusion** is discussed in Chap. 33.

F. **Regional anesthesia.** If regional anesthesia is also employed, the patient's general anesthetic requirement is markedly reduced and may only be needed to provide unconsciousness and amnesia and attenuate stimuli from airway manipulation (e.g., ETT). An increase in the general anesthetic requirement usually indicates the need for reinforcement of the regional anesthetic.

IV. **Emergence from general anesthesia.** During this period of time, the patient makes the transition from an unconscious state to an awake state in which vital reflexes return to the patient (e.g., airway protection).

A. **Goals.** Patients should be awake and responsive to diminish risk for airway obstruction or pulmonary aspiration. This will also facilitate immediate neurologic assessment. In patients with cardiovascular disease, hemodynamics should be controlled.

B. **Technique.** The degree of surgical stimulation diminishes as the procedure nears completion. Appropriate anesthetic depth should be maintained. Residual muscle relaxation should be reversed, and the patient should be allowed to breathe spontaneously. The presence of an ETT and associated airway manipulations may be very irritating to a patient emerging from general anesthesia. Lidocaine (0.5–1.0 mg/kg IV) can be given to suppress coughing but may prolong emergence.

C. **Positioning.** If the patient's position was changed after induction, the patient is usually returned to the supine position. However, if the anesthesiologist is confident that the patient can maintain and protect the airway, the patient may be extubated in that position. A method for quickly returning the patient to the supine position must be available.

D. **Environment.** The operating room should be warmed, blankets placed on the patient, and noise and conversation minimized.

E. **Pain management.** The presence of moderate to severe pain on emergence can lead to a very tumultuous awakening. Analgesic requirements should be estimated and administered prior to awakening. A regional block or infiltration of the site with local anesthetic may be employed.

F. **Mask ventilation.** At the time of emergence, a patient who has been mask ventilated should spontaneously breathe oxygen (100%) by mask. A period of light anesthesia occurs prior to regaining consciousness. Stimulation (especially of the airway) during this period may precipitate laryngospasm and is best avoided. The patient should not be moved from the operating room table until protective airway reflexes have returned and the patient is awake, following verbal commands, and is adequately oxygenating and ventilating.

G. **Extubation.** A patient who has had an ETT placed is usually extubated either after awakening from anesthesia (**awake extubation**) or while still significantly anesthetized near the conclusion of surgery (**deep extubation**). Patients who usually remain intubated postoperatively include those with respiratory failure, delayed awakening, or marked hemodynamic instability. Also included are patients whose airway may be significantly jeopardized if extubated (e.g., extensive oral surgery) and patients who have just undergone an especially prolonged, invasive surgical procedure.

1. **Awake extubation** is indicated in patients with full stomachs, patients who are difficult to mask ventilate or intubate, patients with possible glottic edema (e.g., prolonged head-down position), and patients who have just undergone tracheal or maxillofacial surgery.

   a. **Criteria.** The patient must be able to maintain and protect the airway. In addition, prior to extubation, the patient must be awake, follow simple verbal commands (e.g., squeeze hand), be hemodynamically stable, and spontaneously breathe with acceptable oxygenation and ventilation. Residual muscle relaxation must be adequately reversed as assessed by clinical criteria and a peripheral nerve stimulator.

   b. **Technique.** The patient breathes 100% oxygen, and the oropharynx is suctioned. Mild positive pressure is applied via the ETT (to prevent inadvertent aspiration of oropharyngeal secretions), the cuff is deflated, and the ETT is removed. Oxygen (100%) is administered by mask while the adequacy of ventilation is assessed. Pulse oximetry is useful at this time. This is a critical moment; the anesthesiologist's attention should remain focused primarily on the patient while observing the patient's ability to ventilate, oxygenate, and protect the airway.

2. **Deep extubation** avoids coughing and straining that may be undesirable with certain procedures (e.g., middle-ear surgery, transurethral resection of the prostate, open-eye procedures, or abdominal or inguinal herniorrhaphy). Extubation under deep anesthesia may also be useful following anesthesia for asthmatic patients.

   a. **Criteria.** Anesthetic depth must be sufficient to avoid untoward responses (e.g., coughing, laryngospasm) to airway stimulation. If needed, anesthesia may be deepened with either a small dose of an IV hypnotic anesthetic or inhalation of a high concentration of a volatile agent. Residual muscle relaxation should be adequately reversed, and preferably ventilation should be either spontaneous or assisted. Relative contraindications to deep extubation are noted at the beginning of sec. G.

   b. **Technique.** All necessary airway equipment and medications should be readily available for replacement of the ETT. Surgical positioning must allow unrestricted access to the head for airway management. The oropharynx is suctioned, the ETT cuff is deflated, and the ETT is removed. Inhalation anesthesia is continued by mask until emergence is desired.

H. Agitation. Severe agitation is occasionally seen on emergence from general anesthesia, especially in adolescents. Physiologic causes (pain, hypoxia, hypercarbia, airway obstruction, and full bladder) must be excluded. Reassurance may be sufficient. Pain, a common reason for agitation, may be treated with **cautious** titration of a narcotic (e.g., fentanyl, 25-μg IV increments; morphine, 2-mg IV increments).

I. Delayed awakening. On occasion, a patient will not awaken within an expected period of time after the administration of general anesthesia. Ventilatory support and airway protection should be continued, and etiologies should be investigated (see Chap. 34).

V. Transport. Following surgery and general anesthesia, a patient is transported by the anesthesiologist to either a postanesthesia care unit (PACU) or an intensive care unit (ICU). Supplemental oxygen should be available, and the patient's airway, ventilation, and overall condition continually observed. Placing the patient in the lateral position may discourage aspiration and upper airway obstruction. If the patient is hemodynamically unstable or requires IV vasoactive agents, monitoring of the arterial blood pressure and electrocardiogram is essential. Medications and airway equipment should accompany the anesthesiologist, especially if the patient is unstable or if transport involves travel over a significant distance. Upon transfer of responsibility for patient care in the PACU or ICU, the anesthesiologist should provide a concise but thorough summary of the patient's past medical history, intraoperative course, and current postoperative condition and therapy.

VI. Postoperative visit. A postoperative evaluation of the patient should be performed by the anesthesiologist within 24–48 hours and documented in the patient's medical record. The patient's general condition includes a review of the medical record, discussion, and examination of the patient. The patient's perspective of his or her perioperative course is very informative. Specific complications such as nausea, sore throat, dental injury, nerve injury, ocular injury, pneumonia, or change in mental status should be ascertained. Complications that require further therapy (e.g., epidural blood patch) or consultations (e.g., neurologist) should be addressed.

SUGGESTED READING

Barash, P. G., Cullen, B. F., and Stoelting R. K. *Clinical Anesthesia*. Philadelphia: Lippincott, 1989.

Denlinger, J. K. Prolonged Emergence and Failure to Regain Consciousness. In F. K. Orkin and L. H. Cooperman (eds.), *Complications in Anesthesiology*. Philadelphia: Lippincott, 1983. Pp. 368–378.

15

Local Anesthetics

Bobbie Jean Sweitzer

I. General principles
A. Chemistry.
Local anesthetics are weak bases whose structure consists of an aromatic moiety connected to a substituted amine through an ester or amide linkage. The pK_a values of local anesthetics are near physiologic pH; thus, in vivo, both charged and uncharged forms are present to a significant degree. The degree of ionization is important because the uncharged form is most lipid soluble and able to gain access to the axon. The clinical differences between the ester and amide local anesthetics involve their potential for producing adverse effects and the mechanisms by which they are metabolized.

1. **Esters.** Procaine, cocaine, chloroprocaine, and tetracaine.
2. **Amides.** Lidocaine, mepivacaine, bupivacaine, etidocaine, and ropivacaine.

B. Commercial preparations
1. Commercially available solutions of local anesthetics are supplied at an acidic **pH** to enhance chemical stability. Plain solutions are usually adjusted to a pH of 6, while those containing a vasoconstrictor are adjusted to a pH of 4 because of the lability of catecholamine molecules at alkaline pH. Lower pH values, by decreasing the proportion of molecules in the uncharged form, result in a slower onset time of anesthesia.
2. Antimicrobial preservatives are added to multidose vials. Only preservative-free solutions should be used in spinal, epidural, or caudal anesthesia to prevent potentially neurotoxic effects.

C. Mechanism of action
1. Local anesthetics block nerve conduction by **impairing propagation of the action potential** in axons. They have no effect on the resting or threshold potentials but decrease the rate of rise of the action potential such that the threshold potential is not reached.
2. Local anesthetics **interact directly with specific receptors** on the Na^+ channel, inhibiting Na^+ ion influx. The anesthetic molecule must traverse the cell membrane through passive nonionic diffusion of the molecule in the uncharged state and then bind to the sodium channel in the charged state.
3. **Physiochemical factors** of the local anesthetics affect neural blockade.
   a. **Lipid solubility** increases the **potency,** as local anesthetics more easily cross nerve membranes.
   b. **Protein binding.** Agents with a high degree of protein binding will have a prolonged **duration** of effect.
   c. **pK_a** determines **speed of onset** of neural blockade.

Table 15-1. Classification of nerve fibers

Fiber type	Myelin	Diameter (microns)	Function
A-α	+ +	6–22	Motor efferent, proprioception afferent
A-β	+ +	6–22	Motor efferent, proprioception afferent
A-γ	+ +	3–6	Muscle spindle efferent
A-δ	+ +	1–4	Pain, temperature, touch afferent
B	+	< 3	Preganglionic autonomic
C	−	0.3–1.3	Pain, temperature, touch afferent, postganglionic autonomic

pK_a is the pH at which 50% of the local anesthetic is in the charged form and 50% uncharged. Agents with a lower pK_a value will have a faster onset because a greater fraction of the molecules will exist in the uncharged form and thus will more easily diffuse across nerve membranes.

4. Differential blockade of nerve fibers

   a. Peripheral nerves are classified according to size and function (Table 15-1). Thin nerve fibers are more easily blocked than thick ones. However, myelinated fibers are more readily blocked than unmyelinated ones because of the need to produce blockade only at the nodes of Ranvier.

   b. By careful selection of an appropriate agent and concentration, it is possible selectively to block pain and temperature sensation (A-delta and C fibers) in the absence of significant motor blockade (A-alpha fibers).

   c. Differential blockade is a reflection of the arrangement of the fibers within the peripheral nerve; the outermost layer is blocked first with a concentration gradient toward the center.

5. Sequence of clinical anesthesia. Neural blockade of peripheral nerves usually progresses in the following order:

   a. Sympathetic block with peripheral vasodilation and skin temperature elevation.

   b. Loss of pain and temperature sensation.

   c. Loss of proprioception.

   d. Loss of touch and pressure sensation.

   e. Motor paralysis.

6. Metabolism of local anesthetics

   a. Esters. The ester linkage is readily cleaved by plasma cholinesterase. The half-life of esters in the circulation is very short (about 1 minute). The degradation product of ester metabolism is *p*-aminobenzoic acid.

   b. Amides. The amide linkage is cleaved through initial *N*-dealkylation followed by hydrolysis, which occurs primarily in the liver. Patients with severe hepatic disease may be more susceptible to adverse reactions from amide local anesthetics. The elimination half-life for amide local anesthetics is approximately 2–3 hours.

7. Pathophysiologic factors

    a. A decrease in cardiac output reduces the volume of distribution and plasma clearance of local anesthetics, increasing plasma concentration and the potential for toxicity.

    b. Hepatic disease (see sec. **6.b**).

    c. Renal disease has minimal effect.

    d. Patients with reduced cholinesterase activity (newborn, pregnant) may have an increased potential for toxicity.

II. Clinical uses of local anesthetics. The choice of local anesthetic must take into consideration the duration of surgery, regional technique used, surgical requirements, the potential for local or systemic toxicity, and any metabolic constraints (Table 15-2).

A. Esters

    1. Procaine (Novocain)

        a. Fast onset, short duration, low potency, and low toxicity.

        b. Used for local infiltration and for spinal anesthesia when very short duration is desired.

    2. Chloroprocaine (Nesacaine)

        a. Very rapid onset, short duration, low potency, and very low toxicity.

        b. Very rapid hydrolysis by plasma cholinesterase accounts for its low toxicity and short duration.

        c. Used for local infiltration, nerve blocks, and epidural anesthesia.

        d. The bisulfite preservative formerly associated with neurologic deficits from inadvertent subarachnoid injection has been removed.

    3. Tetracaine (Pontocaine)

        a. Slow onset, very long duration, high potency, and moderate toxicity.

        b. Used primarily for spinal anesthesia.

        c. Produces motor blockade and sensory blockade of similar duration and intensity.

        d. It is commercially supplied as a 1% isobaric solution or as tetracaine crystals, 20 mg/ampule.

            (1) A **hyperbaric** solution is prepared by mixing equal volumes of the 1% solution with 10% dextrose.

            (2) An **isobaric** solution is prepared by mixing equal volumes of the 1% solution with cerebrospinal fluid (CSF) obtained at the time of lumbar puncture. Alternatively, 4 ml of CSF may be used to dissolve 20 mg of tetracaine crystals.

            (3) A **hypobaric** solution is prepared by dissolving 20 mg of tetracaine crystals in 20 ml of sterile, preservative-free water.

B. Amides

    1. Lidocaine (Xylocaine)

        a. Rapid onset, moderate duration, moderate potency, and moderate toxicity.

Table 15-2. Local anesthetic agents

Anesthetic technique	Anesthetic	Concentration (%)	Duration (hr)	Duration (hr) with epinephrine	Dose range (ml; 70-kg patient)
Peripheral nerve block	Lidocaine	1–2	1.5–3.0	2–4	40–50
	Mepivacaine	1–2	3–5	3–5	40–50
	Bupivacaine	0.25–0.5	6–12	6–12	40–50
	Etidocaine	1.0–1.5	6–12	6–12	40–50
Epidural and caudal	Chloroprocaine	2–3	0.25–0.5	0.5–1	20–30
	Lidocaine	1–2	0.5–1.0	0.75–1.5	20–30
	Mepivacaine	1–2	0.75–1.0	1–2	20–30
	Bupivacaine	0.25–0.75	1.5–3.0	2–4	20–30
	Etidocaine	0.5–1.5	1.5–3.0	2–4	20–30
Local infiltration	Procaine	0.5–1.0	0.25–0.5	0.5–1.5	1–60
	Lidocaine	0.5–1.0	0.5–2.0	1–3	1–50
	Mepivacaine	0.5–1.0	0.5–2.0	1–3	1–50
	Bupivacaine	0.25–0.5	2–4	4–8	1–45
Spinal	Lidocaine (hyperbaric)	5	0.75–1.5	0.75–1.5	60 mg (1.2 ml)
	Lidocaine (isobaric)	2	1–2	1–2	60 mg (3 ml)
	Bupivacaine (hyperbaric)	0.75	2–4	2–4	9 mg (1.2 ml)
	Bupivacaine (isobaric)	0.5	2–4	2–4	15 mg (3 ml)
	Tetracaine (hyperbaric)	0.5	2–3	3–5	12 mg (2.4 ml)
	Tetracaine (isobaric)	0.5	3–5	5–8	15 mg (3 ml)
	Tetracaine (hypobaric)	0.1	3–5	5–8	10 mg (10 ml)

      b. The most frequently used local anesthetic for all types of regional anesthesia.

  2. Mepivacaine (Carbocaine)

      a. Moderate onset, duration, potency, and toxicity.

      b. Used for local infiltration, nerve blocks, and epidural anesthesia.

  3. Bupivacaine (Marcaine, Sensorcaine)

      a. Slow onset, very long duration, high potency, and high toxicity.

      b. Frequently used for all types of local and regional anesthesia when prolonged duration is desired.

      c. Sensory blockade is of greater intensity and duration than motor blockade.

      d. Inadvertent intravascular injection may result in cardiac arrest remarkably resistant to therapy, especially in pregnant patients.

  4. Etidocaine (Duranest)

      a. Rapid onset, very long duration, high potency, and moderate toxicity.

      b. Used in nerve blocks and epidural anesthesia.

      c. Produces motor blockades in excess of the accompanying sensory blockade. The 1.5% concentration is necessary for epidural anesthesia in intraabdominal procedures.

  5. Ropivacaine

      a. Slow onset, long duration, high potency, and moderate toxicity.

      b. Produces sensory blockade in excess of motor blockade.

      c. Currently an investigational agent. It will probably be used in a similar manner to bupivacaine with much less cardiac toxicity.

C. Combinations of local anesthetics. Mixtures of local anesthetics potentially provide the best characteristics of the individual agents. A chloroprocaine-bupivacaine or lidocaine-bupivacaine mixture is reported to produce a block with rapid onset and long duration. The systemic toxicity of combinations appears to be merely additive. Despite the potential benefit of combinations, the neural blockade produced by mixtures is unpredictable and the clinical utility is in question.

D. Adjuvants

  1. Epinephrine

      a. Epinephrine may be added to local anesthetics to

        (1) Prolong the duration of anesthesia. This varies with the type of regional block and concentration of local anesthetic.

        (2) Decrease systemic toxicity by decreasing the rate of absorption, thus minimizing peak blood levels of local anesthetics.

        (3) Increase intensity of the block.

        (4) Decrease surgical bleeding.

        (5) Assist in the evaluation of a test dose.

      b. Clinical applications

        (1) Using plain solutions and adding epinephrine (1:200,000) just prior to administration permit

the use of a solution with high pH and may speed onset of the block. A 1:200,000 dilution is achieved by adding 0.1 ml of 1:1000 epinephrine (with a TB syringe) to 20 ml of local anesthetic solution.

(2) The maximum dose of epinephrine should probably not exceed 10 $\mu g \cdot kg^{-1}$ in pediatric patients or 200–250 μg in adults.

(3) Epinephrine should not be used in peripheral nerve blocks in areas with poor collateral blood flow (e.g., digits, penis, toes) or in IV regional techniques. Caution is advised in patients with severe coronary artery disease, arrhythmias, uncontrolled hypertension, hyperthyroidism, and uteroplacental insufficiency.

2. Phenylephrine has been shown to have similar effects to epinephrine without any particular advantages. Five milligrams of phenylephrine is added to solutions of local anesthetics to prolong spinal anesthesia.

3. Sodium bicarbonate. Addition of sodium bicarbonate to local anesthetic solutions raises the pH and increases the concentration of nonionized-free base. The increased percentage of nonionized drug will increase the rate of diffusion and speed the onset of neural blockade. Typically, 1 mEq of sodium bicarbonate is added to each 10 ml of lidocaine or mepivacaine; only 0.1 mEq of sodium bicarbonate may be added to each 10 ml of bupivacaine to avoid precipitation.

III. Toxicity (Table 15-3)

A. Allergic reactions. True allergic reactions to local anesthetics are rare. It is important to differentiate these from common, nonallergic responses such as syncope and vasovagal reaction.

1. Ester-type local anesthetics may cause allergic reactions due to the metabolite *p*-aminobenzoic acid. In addition, these anesthetics may produce allergic reactions in persons sensitive to sulfonamides or thiazide diuretics.

2. Amide-type local anesthetics are essentially devoid of allergic potential. Anesthetic solutions containing methylparaben as the preservative may produce an allergic reaction in someone sensitive to *p*-aminobenzoic acid.

3. Local hypersensitivity reactions may manifest as local erythema, urticaria, edema, or dermatitis.

4. Systemic hypersensitivity reactions are rare and present as generalized erythema, urticaria, edema, bronchoconstriction, hypotension, or cardiovascular collapse.

5. Treatment is symptomatic and supportive (see Chap. 18).

B. Local toxicity. Tissue toxicity is rare. Neurotoxicity can occur secondary to unintentional subarachnoid injection of large volumes or high concentrations of local anesthetics or chemical contamination of a solution.

Table 15-3. Relative toxicity of local anesthetics

| Agent | Approximate potency ratios[a] | | Maximum recommended doses[b] | |
	Spinal anesthetic potency	CNS toxicity	Plain solution (mg)	Epinephrine-containing (mg)
Procaine	1	1	400	600
Chloroprocaine	1	1	800	1000
Lidocaine	2	3	300	500
Mepivacaine		2	300	500
Etidocaine		6	300	400
Bupivacaine	14	12	175	225
Tetracaine	10	8	100[c]	200

[a] Potency ratios and equivalent doses depend on the method of anesthesia used.

[b] Maximum dose as recommended by the manufacturer in the United States for peripheral nerve blocks in 70-kg individuals.

[c] Tetracaine is used only for spinal anesthesia, primarily because of its toxic potential. When used at the recommended doses for spinal anesthesia, CNS and cardiovascular toxicity are unlikely.

C. **Systemic toxicity** usually results from either accidental intravascular injection or overdose.

1. **Accidental intravascular injection** most commonly occurs during nerve blockade in areas with large blood vessels (e.g., axillary or vertebral artery and epidural vein). This can be minimized by the following maneuvers:

    a. Aspiration prior to injection.

    b. Use of epinephrine-containing solutions for test dose.

    c. Use of small incremental volumes in establishing the block.

    d. Use of proper technique during IV regional anesthesia (see Chap. 17).

2. **Central nervous system (CNS) toxicity**

    a. **Clinical features** of CNS toxicity include light-headedness, tinnitus, metallic taste, visual disturbance, and numbness of the tongue and lip. These may progress to muscle twitching, loss of consciousness, grand mal seizure, and coma.

    b. CNS toxicity is **exacerbated** by hypercarbia, hypoxia, and acidosis.

    c. **Treatment.** At the first sign of toxicity, oxygen should be administered. If seizure activity interferes with ventilation or is prolonged, anticonvulsant treatment is indicated with either benzodiazepines (e.g., midazolam, 1–2 mg) or barbiturates (e.g., thiopental, 50–200 mg). Succinylcholine can be given to facilitate intubation. This abolishes muscular activity and decreases the risk of metabolic acidosis, but neuronal seizure activity continues, and cerebral metabolism and oxygen requirements remain elevated with a risk of cerebral ischemia.

3. **Cardiovascular toxicity.** The cardiovascular system is more resistant than the CNS to toxic effects, but cardiovascular toxicity may be severe and difficult to treat.

    a. **Clinical features.** Cardiovascular toxicity is manifested by decreased ventricular contractility, decreased conduction, and loss of peripheral vasomotor tone, which may lead to cardiovascular collapse.

    b. The **intravascular injection of bupivacaine or etidocaine** may result in cardiovascular collapse, often refractory to therapy because of the high degree of tissue binding displayed by these agents.

    c. **Treatment**

       (1) Oxygen must be administered and the circulation supported with volume replacement and vasopressors, including inotropes as necessary. Advanced cardiac life support should be performed if indicated (see Chap. 36).

       (2) Ventricular tachycardia should be treated by cardioversion. Local anesthetic-induced cardiac arrhythmias are difficult to treat but subside over time if the patient can be hemodynamically maintained.

(3) Bretylium may be more effective than lidocaine for ventricular arrhythmias associated with intravascular injections of bupivacaine, and very large doses of epinephrine may be necessary for successful resuscitation.

(4) Prolonged administration of cardiopulmonary resuscitation may be required until the cardiotoxic effects subside with drug redistribution.

SUGGESTED READING

Barash, P. G., Cullen, B. F., and Stoelting, R. K. *Clinical Anesthesia*. Philadelphia: Lippincott, 1989.

Cousins, M. J., and Bridenbaugh, P. O. *Neural Blockade in Clinical Anesthesia and Management of Pain*. Philadelphia: Lippincott, 1988.

Covino, B. G., and Vassallo, H. G. *Local Anesthesia: Mechanisms of Action and Clinical Use*. New York: Grune & Stratton, 1976.

Reiz, S., and Nath, S. Cardiotoxicity of local anaesthetic agents. *Br. J. Anaesth.* 58:736, 1986.

Strichartz, G. R., and Covino, B. G. Pharmacology of Local Anesthetic Drugs. In R. D. Miller (ed.), *Anesthesia*. New York: Churchill Livingstone, 1990. Pp. 437–470.

16

Spinal, Epidural, and Caudal Anesthesia

Rowan Molnar

I. General considerations

A. The **preoperative assessment** of the patient for regional anesthesia is the same as that for general anesthesia. The details of the procedure to be performed, including its anticipated length, patient position, expected blood loss, and degree of muscle relaxation required, should all be taken into account in selecting the appropriateness of a regional technique.

B. The **physical examination** should document any specific neurologic deficits. The area where the block is to be administered should be inspected for potential difficulties or pathology.

C. A **history of bleeding** as well as a review of the **current medication regimen** may indicate a need for additional bleeding studies.

D. Patients should be provided with a **detailed explanation of the planned procedure.** In addition, they should be reassured that additional sedation and anesthesia can be given during the operation and that general anesthesia is an option should the block fail or the operation become more prolonged or extensive than originally thought.

E. For all regional techniques, patients should receive standard monitoring (see Chap. 10) and have an IV in place. In addition, oxygen, equipment for positive-pressure ventilation and intubation, and drugs to provide hemodynamic support must be available.

II. Segmental level required for surgery

A. A knowledge of the sensory, motor, and autonomic distribution of spinal nerves will help the anesthesiologist determine the correct segmental level required for a particular operative procedure, as well as predict the potential physiologic effects of producing a block to that level. Fig. 16-1 illustrates the dermatomal distribution of the spinal nerves.

B. Afferent autonomic nerves innervate visceral sensation and viscerosomatic reflexes at spinal segmental levels much higher than would be predicted from skin dermatomes.

C. Table 16-1 provides some minimal suggested levels for common surgical procedures.

III. Contraindications to peridural anesthesia

A. **Absolute**
   1. Lack of patient consent.
   2. Localized infection at skin puncture site.
   3. Generalized sepsis (e.g., septicemia, bacteremia).
   4. Coagulopathy.
   5. Allergy to that specific class of local anesthetic agent.
   6. Raised intracranial pressure.

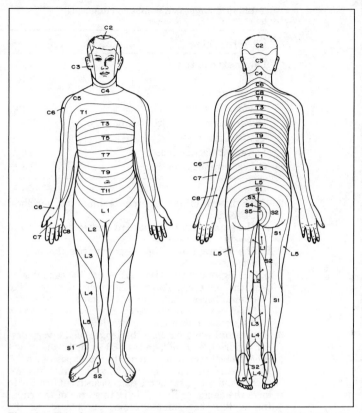

Fig. 16-1. Skin dermatomes corresponding to respective sensory innervation by spinal nerves.

    B. Relative
        1. Localized infection peripheral to regional technique site.
        2. Hypovolemia.
        3. Central nervous system disease.
        4. Chronic back pain.
        5. Patients taking platelet-inhibiting drugs, including aspirin, dipyridamole, and nonsteroidal antiinflammatory agents.
IV. Spinal anesthesia involves the administration of local anesthetic into the subarachnoid space. The technique is the simplest for blocking spinal nerves and provides excellent operating conditions for suitable procedures.
    A. Anatomy
        1. The **spinal canal** extends from the foramen magnum to the sacral hiatus. The boundaries of the bony canal are the vertebral body anteriorly, the pedicles laterally, and the spinous processes and laminae posteriorly (Fig. 16-2).

Table 16-1. Suggested minimum cutaneous levels for spinal anesthesia

Operative site	Level
Lower extremities	T12
Hip	T10
Vagina/uterus	T10
Bladder/prostate	T10
Lower extremities with tourniquet	T8
Testis/ovaries	T8
Lower intraabdominal	T6
Other intraabdominal	T4

2. Three **interlaminar ligaments** bind the vertebral processes together:
   a. The **supraspinous ligament** connects the apices of the spinous processes.
   b. The **interspinous ligament** connects the spinous processes.
   c. The **ligamentum flavum** connects the caudal edge of the vertebrae above to the cephalad edge of the lamina below. This ligament is composed of elastic fibers and is easily recognized by its increased resistance to passage of a needle.
3. The **spinal cord** extends the length of the vertebral canal during fetal life, ends at L3 at birth, and moves progressively cephalad to reach the adult position of L1 by 2 years of age. The conus medullaris, lumbar, sacral, and coccygeal nerve roots branch out distally to form the cauda equina. It is in this area of the canal (below L2) that spinal needles are placed, as the mobility of the nerves reduces the danger of trauma from the needle.
4. The spinal cord is invested in three **meninges:**
   a. The **pia mater.**
   b. The **dura mater,** which is a tough, fibrous sheath running longitudinally the entire length of the spinal cord and is tethered caudally at S2.
   c. The **arachnoid,** which lies between the pia and dura mater.
5. The **subarachnoid space** lies between the pia mater and the arachnoid and extends from the attachment of the dura at S2 to the cerebral ventricles above. The space contains the spinal cord, nerves, cerebrospinal fluid, and blood vessels that supply the cord.
6. **Cerebrospinal fluid** (CSF) is a clear, colorless fluid that fills the subarachnoid space. The total volume of CSF is 100–150 ml, while the volume in the spinal subarachnoid space is 25–35 ml. CSF is continuously formed at a rate of 450 ml/day by secretion or ultrafiltration of plasma from the choroid arterial plexuses located in the lateral, third, and fourth ventricles. CSF is reabsorbed into the bloodstream through the arach-

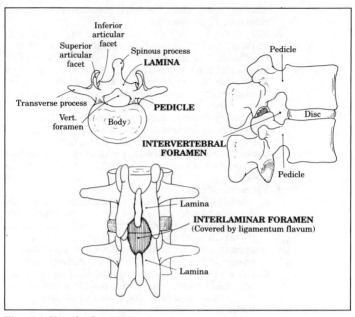

Fig. 16-2. Vertebral anatomy.

noid villi and granulations that protrude through dura to lie in contact with the endothelium of the cerebral venous sinuses. The specific gravity of CSF ranges from 1.003–1.009 at 37°C.

B. Physiology

1. **Neural blockade.** Smaller C fibers conveying autonomic impulses are more easily blocked than the larger sensory and motor fibers. As a result, the level of autonomic blockade extends above the level of the sensory blockade by two to three segments (e.g., sensory block to T3 is associated with complete blockade of the autonomic nervous system). Similarly, fibers conveying sensation are more easily blocked than the larger motor fibers so that sensory blockade will extend above the level of motor blockade.

2. **Cardiovascular.** Hypotension is directly proportional to the degree of sympathetic blockade produced. Sympathetic blockade results in dilatation of arteries and venous capacitance vessels, leading to decreased systemic vascular resistance and decreased venous return. If the block is below T4, increased baroreceptor activity leads to an increase in activity to the cardiac sympathetic fibers and vasoconstriction of the upper extremities. Blockade above T4 interrupts cardiac sympathetic fibers leading to bradycardia, decreased cardiac output, and a further decrease in blood pressure. These changes are more marked in patients who are hypo-

volemic, are elderly, or have obstruction to venous return (e.g., pregnancy).

3. **Respiratory.** Low spinal anesthesia has no effect on ventilation. With ascending height of the block into the thoracic area, there is a progressive, ascending intercostal muscle paralysis. This has little effect on ventilation in the supine surgical patient who still has diaphragmatic ventilation mediated by the phrenic nerve. However, ventilation in patients with poor respiratory reserve, such as the morbidly obese, may be profoundly impaired. Both intercostal and abdominal muscle paralysis decrease the efficiency of the patient to cough effectively, which may be important in patients with chronic obstructive pulmonary disease.

4. **Visceral effects**
   a. **Bladder.** Sacral blockade results in an atonic bladder able to retain large volumes of urine. Blockade of sympathetic efferents (T5–L1) results in an increase in sphincter tone, producing retention. A urinary catheter should be placed if anesthesia or analgesia is maintained for a prolonged period.
   b. **Intestine.** Visceral sympathetic blockade (T5–L1) produced by spinal anesthesia results in contraction of the small and large intestine due to parasympathetic predominance.

5. **Renal.** Spinal anesthesia produces a 5–10% decrease in glomerular filtration rate and effective renal plasma flow, which is of little clinical significance. This change is markedly increased in hypovolemia.

6. **Neuroendocrine.** The neuroendocrine or "stress" response to surgery is a complex hormonal and metabolic cascade mediated by both neural and humoral pathways that increases the body's metabolic rate, mobilizes energy stores, and retains water and electrolytes. This response may adversely alter postoperative outcome, particularly in compromised patients. Spinal anesthesia to T5 inhibits part of the neural component of the stress response through its blockade of sympathetic afferents to the adrenal medulla, as well as blockade of sympathetic and somatic pathways mediating pain. Other components of the stress response are not impaired. Vagal afferent fibers from upper abdominal viscera are not blocked and can stimulate release of hypothalamic and pituitary hormones, such as antidiuretic hormone and adrenocorticotropic hormone. Blood loss and infection can also cause the central release of humoral factors. Spinal blockade abolishes the increase in blood glucose seen during surgery under general anesthesia. Normal glucose tolerance and insulin release are seen.

7. **Thermoregulation.** Vasodilatation in the lower limbs predisposes to hypothermia, particularly if the legs are left uncovered.

C. **Technique**
   1. **Spinal needle.** Spinal anesthesia is achieved most

commonly with 22- or 25-gauge, 3½-inch Quincke Point needles, although smaller ones (27-gauge) are available. The 22-gauge needle is more rigid and is more easily directed and inserted. A higher incidence of postdural puncture headache is seen with this needle. The 25-gauge needle is much more pliable and easily bent, often requiring a 19-gauge, 1½-inch introducer needle for insertion. It is associated with a very low incidence of postdural puncture headache (as low as 1%). Newer needles such as the "Sprotte" and "Whitacre" points feature a pencil-point design with the opening of the lumen on the side. These needles may reduce the incidence of postdural puncture headache by producing a splitting rather than a cutting of the dural fibers on insertion.

2. **Patient position.** The lateral decubitus, prone, and sitting positions are all commonly used for administration of spinal anesthesia.

   a. In the **lateral** position, the patient is placed with the affected side up if a hypobaric technique is to be used and with the affected side down if a hyperbaric technique is to be used. The spine is horizontal and parallel to the edge of the table. The knees are drawn up toward the chest and the chin flexed downward onto the chest to obtain maximal flexion of the spine.

   b. The **sitting** position is useful for low spinal blocks required in certain gynecologic and urologic procedures and is commonly used in obese patients to assist in identification of the midline. It is used in conjunction with hyperbaric anesthetics. The head and shoulders are flexed downward onto the trunk with the arms resting on a Mayo stand. The feet should be supported on a stool, and the patient's back should be close to the edge of the table. An assistant should be available to stabilize the patient, and the patient should not be oversedated.

   c. The **prone** position is used in conjunction with hypobaric anesthesia for procedures on the rectum, perineum, and anus. The jackknife position can be used for both administration of spinal anesthesia and surgery.

3. **Approaches**

   a. A line connecting the upper borders of the iliac crests crosses the spinous process of L4 or the L3–L4 interspace. The L2–L3, L3–L4, or L4–L5 interspaces are commonly used for spinal anesthesia.

   b. A large skin area is prepared with an appropriate antiseptic solution. Care must be taken to avoid contamination of the spinal kit with antiseptic solution, which is potentially neurotoxic.

   c. The stylet is checked to ascertain its correct fit within the needle.

   d. Local infiltration with 1% lidocaine is then performed at the intended spinal puncture site with a 25-gauge needle.

(1) **Midline.** The spinal needle (or introducer) is placed through the skin wheal into the interspinous ligament. The needle should be in the same plane as the spinous processes with a slight cephalad angulation toward the interlaminar space.

(2) **Paramedian.** This approach is useful in patients who cannot be adequately flexed due to pain or whose ligaments of the interspinous space may be ossified. The spinal needle is placed 1.5 cm lateral to the center of the selected interspace. The needle is aimed medially and slightly cephalad and passed lateral to the supraspinous ligament. If the lamina is contacted, the needle is redirected and walked off in a medial and cephalad direction.

(3) **Needle placement.** The needle is inserted so that its bevel is parallel to the fibers that run longitudinally to reduce the incidence of postdural puncture headache. The needle is advanced until increased resistance is felt as it passes through the ligamentum flavum. As the needle is advanced beyond this ligament, a sudden loss of resistance is felt as the needle "pops" through the dura.

(4) The stylet is removed and correct placement confirmed by free flow of CSF into the hub of the needle. If flow of CSF is sluggish, the hub is rotated in 90-degree increments until good flow is established. Careful aspiration of the needle may be required if a 25-gauge needle is used or the CSF pressure is low. To avoid plugging of the needle's lumen with tissue, the stylet should always be in place when the needle is advanced. Paresthesia occurring with placement of the needle requires immediate withdrawal and repositioning.

(5) **Administration of anesthetic.** The syringe containing the predetermined dose of local anesthetic is connected to the needle. Aspiration of CSF into the syringe can be seen to have a birefringent effect if dextrose is used, as for hyperbaric techniques, and confirms free flow. The drug is then slowly injected. Reaspiration of CSF at the end of injection confirms that the needle point is still within the subarachnoid space. The needle is then removed and the patient gently repositioned in the desired position.

e. **Blood pressure, pulse, and respiratory function** are closely monitored (every 60–90 seconds) for 10–15 minutes. The ascending anesthetic level is determined using pinprick or alcohol. Fixation of local anesthetic level takes approximately 20 minutes.

f. **Continuous spinal anesthesia** allows for the level

Table 16-2. Drugs and dosages for hyperbaric spinal anesthesia

	Level (mg)*			Duration (min)
Drug	T10	T8	T6	
Tetracaine	10	12	14	90–120
Bupivacaine	7.5	9.0	10.5	90–120
Lidocaine	50	60	70	30–90

* Doses are based on a 66-inch patient. An additional 2 mg of tetracaine, 10 mg of lidocaine, or 1.5 mg of bupivacaine should be added or subtracted for each 6 inches in height above or below 66 inches.

of sensory blockade to be titrated using small aliquots of drug. With this technique, a high sympathetic block can be avoided (of particular concern in the compromised patient). The duration of anesthesia can be extended for long surgical procedures by repeat administration of drug. An epidural kit (with a 17-gauge needle and 20-gauge catheter) should be used. The catheter is threaded through the needle and advanced 2–4 cm past the tip of the needle. Stimulation of nerve roots by the catheter tip is very painful, and thus the catheter should be advanced no further than this. Neurotoxicity from hyperbaric local anesthetic solutions in glucose injected through specialized small-bore spinal catheters (26–32 gauge) has been reported, possibly due to the development of very high concentrations of local anesthetic around the nerves of the cauda equina. Therefore, these small-bore catheters should not be used for continuous spinal anesthesia.

D. **Determinants of level of spinal blockade**
   1. **Drug dose.** The anesthetic level varies directly with the dose of agent used.
   2. **Drug volume.** The greater the volume of the injected drug, the further that drug will spread within the CSF. This is especially so when hyperbaric solutions are used.
   3. **Turbulence of CSF.** Turbulence created within the CSF during or after injection will increase spread of the drug and the level obtained. Turbulence is created by rapid injection, barbotage (the repeated aspiration then reinjection of small amounts of CSF mixed with drug), coughing, and excessive patient movement.
   4. **Baricity of local anesthetic.** Local anesthetic solutions can be described as hyperbaric, hypobaric, or isobaric in relation to the baricity of CSF.
      a. **Hyperbaric** solutions are typically prepared by mixing the drug with dextrose. They flow to the most dependent part of the CSF column due to gravity (Table 16–2).
      b. **Hypobaric** solutions are prepared by mixing the drug with sterile water. They flow to the highest part of the CSF column.

    c. Isobaric solutions supposedly have the advantage of a predictable spread through the CSF that is independent of patient position. Increasing the dose of an isobaric anesthetic has more of an effect on the duration of anesthesia than on the dermatomal spread. Patient positioning can be altered to confine or increase the spread of these mixtures.

  5. Increased intraabdominal pressure. Pregnancy, obesity, ascites, or abdominal tumors decrease flow within the inferior vena cava. This increases flow through the epidural venous plexus, reducing the volume of CSF within the vertebral column, causing injected local anesthetic to spread further.

  6. Spinal curvatures. The lumbar lordosis and thoracic kyphosis influence the spread of hyperbaric solutions. Drug injected above L3 while the patient is in the lateral position will spread cephalad, where it is limited by the thoracic curvature at T4 (Fig. 16–3).

E. Determinants of duration of spinal blockade

  1. Drugs and dose. Characteristic duration is specific for each drug (see Chap. 15).

  2. Vasoconstrictors. The addition of epinephrine, 0.2 mg. (0.2 ml of 1:1000), or phenylephrine, 2–5 mg, has been shown to prolong the duration of spinal anesthesia by tetracaine by up to 50%. The epinephrine should be added to the solution immediately before use, otherwise the onset of anesthesia may be slower. This effect of epinephrine has not been demonstrated with bupivacaine.

F. Complications

  1. Acute

    a. Hypotension is a common complication of spinal anesthesia and may be profound in the hypovolemic patient. Intravenous administration of 500–1000 ml of lactated Ringer's solution prior to performing the block will decrease the incidence of hypotension. Oxygen by mask should be available. Leg elevation, ephedrine (5–10 mg IV bolus), or a phenylephrine infusion may be necessary. Bradycardia can result from blockade of cardiac sympathetic fibers and may be treated with IV atropine, 0.4–1.2 mg. Patients with impaired cardiac reserve require care in administering large volumes of IV fluid, as the translocation of fluid from the peripheral to central circulation that occurs during recession of the block and return of systemic vascular tone may lead to volume overload and pulmonary edema.

    b. Paresthesia. During placement of the spinal needle or injection of anesthetic, direct trauma to a spinal nerve or intraneural injection may occur.

    c. Blood tap. Puncture of an epidural vein during needle insertion may result in either blood or a mixture of blood and CSF emerging from the spinal needle. If the fluid does not rapidly clear, the needle should be withdrawn and reinserted.

    d. Dyspnea is a common complaint with high spinal

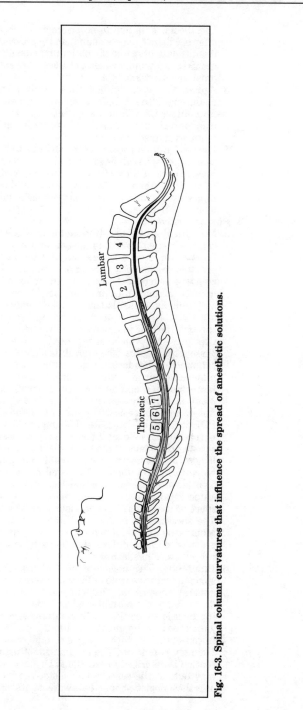

Fig. 16-3. Spinal column curvatures that influence the spread of anesthetic solutions.

anesthesia. It is due to proprioceptive blockade of afferent fibers from abdominal and chest wall movement. Reassurance of the patient may be all that is required, although evidence of adequate ventilation must be ascertained.

e. **Apnea** can occur either as a result of reduced medullary blood flow from severe hypotension, or from direct C3–C5 blockade ("total spinal"), inhibiting phrenic nerve function. Ventilatory support is required immediately.

f. **Nausea and vomiting** are usually due to hypotension or unopposed vagal stimulation. Treatment involves restoration of blood pressure, oxygen administration, and IV atropine. Care should be taken in giving the antiemetic droperidol, as it may augment the hypotension.

2. **Postoperative**

a. **Postdural puncture headache** is characteristically worsened by sitting upright and improved by lying down. It is a severe occipital headache that radiates to the posterior cervical region. With increasing severity it becomes circumferential and may be accompanied by tinnitus, blurred vision, and diplopia. Onset is usually 24–48 hours postoperatively. It is due to a continued leak of CSF through the hole in the dura mater, resulting in low CSF pressure, which causes traction on meningeal vessels and nerves. The overall incidence of postdural puncture headache is approximately 5–10% but may be higher in younger patients, with the use of larger needles, and after multiple attempts. Treatment is initially conservative with bed rest, IV fluids, and analgesics. The use of caffeine (300 mg PO) or caffeine benzoate (500 mg in 500 ml of normal saline IV over 2 hours) has also been advocated at this stage. If the headache is severe or lasts longer than 24 hours, an **epidural blood patch** can be performed. A total of 10–15 ml of the patient's own blood is drawn in a sterile manner from the antecubital vein and is injected into the epidural space at the point of the previous lumbar puncture. The success rate is 95% with the first treatment. Meningitis and arachnoiditis are rare but must be considered in the differential diagnosis of a postdural puncture headache.

b. **Backache.** The incidence of backache following spinal anesthesia is no different from that following general anesthesia. The suggested mechanism is flattening of the normal lumbar lordotic curve during muscle relaxation, with resultant stretching of joint capsules, ligaments, and muscles. Treatment is conservative, with analgesics and reassurance.

c. **Urinary retention.** The mechanism of urinary retention is described in sec. B.4.a. Urinary retention may outlast the sensory and motor blockade. The anesthesiologist should be aware of its presence, particularly if the patient has preexisting urinary obstructive symptoms or if large volumes of IV fluids have been administered during surgery.

d. Neurologic impairment following spinal anesthesia is exceptionally rare, although it is often foremost in the patient's mind. Neurologic damage may be direct, due to needle trauma; toxic, due to introduction of chemicals, viruses, or bacteria; or ischemic, due to vascular compromise from compression by an extradural hematoma. Direct nerve trauma from surgical procedures or improper positioning of the patient may also occur. Neurologic impairment should be evaluated by a neurologist early in the postoperative period, as prompt diagnosis and treatment are essential to improving outcome.

e. Infection following spinal anesthesia is exceedingly rare. Meningitis, arachnoiditis, and epidural abscess can result. Possible etiologies include chemical contamination and viral or bacterial infection. Early consultation with a neurologist is essential for prompt diagnosis and treatment.

V. Epidural anesthesia is achieved by introduction of local anesthetic solutions into the epidural space.

A. Anatomy. The epidural space extends from the base of the skull to the sacrococcygeal membrane. Posteriorly it is bounded by the ligamentum flavum, the anterior surfaces of the laminae, and the articular processes. Anteriorly it is bounded by the posterior longitudinal ligament covering the vertebral bodies and intervertebral disks. Laterally it is bounded by intervertebral foraminae and the pedicles. It has direct communications with the paravertebral space. It contains fat and lymphatic tissue, as well as epidural veins, which are most prominent in the lateral part of the space. The veins have no valves and directly communicate with the intracranial veins. The veins also communicate with the thoracic and abdominal veins through the intervertebral foraminae and with the pelvic veins through the sacral venous plexus. The space is widest in the midline and tapers off laterally. In the lumbar region it is 5–6 mm wide in the midline, while in the midthoracic region the space is 3–5 mm wide.

B. Physiology

1. Neural blockade. Local anesthetic placed in the epidural space acts directly on the spinal nerve roots located in the lateral part of the space. These nerve roots are covered by the dural sheath, and local anesthetic gains access to the CSF by uptake through the dura. The onset of the block is slower than with spinal anesthesia, and the intensity of the sensory and motor block is less. Anesthesia develops in a segmental manner, and selective blockade can be achieved.

2. Cardiovascular. Hypotension from sympathetic blockade is similar to that described for spinal anesthesia (see sec. **IV.B.2**). In addition, the large doses of local anesthetic used may be absorbed into the systemic circulation, leading to myocardial depression. Epinephrine used with the local anesthetics may also be absorbed, producing systemic effects such as tachycardia and hypertension.

3. The other physiologic changes seen are similar to those described for spinal anesthesia (see sec. **IV.B**).

4. Epidural anesthesia has been shown to reduce venous thrombosis and subsequent pulmonary embolism in orthopedic surgery. This is probably due to increased lower limb perfusion. Furthermore, a decreased coagulation tendency, decreased platelet aggregation, and improved fibrinolytic function have been shown during epidural anesthesia.

C. **Technique**

1. **Epidural needles.** Most commonly the 17-gauge Tuohy or Weiss needle is used for identification of the epidural space. This needle is styletted, has a blunt leading edge with a lateral opening, and has a thin wall to allow passage of a 20-gauge catheter. A 22-gauge needle is frequently used for a "single-dose" technique.

2. **Patient position.** Patients can be positioned for epidural anesthesia in either the sitting or lateral positions. The same considerations apply as for spinal anesthesia (see sec. **IV.C.2**).

3. **Approaches.** Whether from a midline or paramedian approach, the needle should enter the **epidural space** in the midline, as the space is widest here and there is a decreased risk of puncturing epidural veins, spinal arteries, or spinal nerve roots, all of which lie in the lateral part of the epidural space. Palpation of landmarks, skin preparation, and draping are as described for spinal anesthesia (see sec. **IV.C.3**).

a. **Lumbar.** A long, 25-gauge needle is used for superficial and deep infiltration of local anesthetic into the supraspinous and interspinous ligaments. This needle also assists in defining the direction in which the epidural needle should be inserted. A 15-gauge needle can be used to make a skin puncture to facilitate epidural needle passage. The epidural needle is advanced through the supraspinous and interspinous ligaments in a slightly cephalad direction, until it comes to lie within the "rubbery" ligamentum flavum.

(1) **Loss of resistance technique.** The stylet is removed and a lubricated syringe containing approximately 3 cc of air or saline is firmly attached to the needle hub. Constant pressure is applied to the plunger of the syringe as the needle is advanced slowly. When the bevel enters the epidural space, there is a marked "loss of resistance" to plunger displacement.

(2) **Hanging drop technique** relies on the principle that a drop of fluid placed on the hub of the epidural needle (once the ligamentum flavum has been entered) will retract into the needle as

the tip of the needle is advanced into the epidural space. This negative pressure is provided by "tenting" of the dura by the needle tip but may be altered by transmitted changes in intraabdominal and intrathoracic pressure (e.g., pregnancy, obesity). Drop retraction only occurs 80% of the time, so if a change in compliance is felt while advancing through the ligamentum flavum, it should be checked by "loss of resistance."

b. **Thoracic** epidural anesthesia provides upper abdominal and thoracic anesthesia with a smaller dose of local anesthetic. Postoperative analgesia can be produced without lower extremity blockade. While the technique is the same as for lumbar placement, the thoracic vertebral spinous processes are much more sharply angulated downward such that the tip of the superior spinous process overlies the lamina of the vertebra below, and the epidural needle should be directed in a more cephalad direction. In addition, there is a risk of producing trauma to the underlying spinal cord if dural puncture occurs.

c. **Placement of catheter.** An epidural catheter allows for repeated injection of local anesthetic for prolonged procedures and provides a route for postoperative analgesia.

(1) A 20-gauge radiopaque catheter with 1-cm graduations is threaded through the epidural needle, whose bevel is pointing in a cephalad direction. If the catheter contains a wire stylet, it should be withdrawn 1–2 cm to decrease the incidence of paresthesia and dural or venous puncture.

(2) The catheter is advanced 2–5 cm into the epidural space. The patient may experience an abrupt paresthesia, which is usually transient. If it is sustained, the catheter must be repositioned. The catheter must not be withdrawn through the needle, as this may shear the catheter tip. If the catheter must be withdrawn, the catheter and needle are removed together.

(3) The distance from the surface of the patient's back to a mark on the catheter is measured (the graduated glass syringe is useful for this purpose).

(4) The needle is carefully withdrawn over the catheter and the distance from the patient's back to the mark on the catheter is again measured. If the catheter was advanced, it is withdrawn to leave 2–3 cm in the epidural space.

(5) Epidural catheters to be used for postoperative analgesia can be tunneled subcutaneously through a 2-inch, 18-gauge catheter, inserted beside an exiting epidural catheter and running lateral. Tunneling of catheters has been reported to provide better fixation and less displacement in the postoperative period as well as decreasing

local infection of the catheter and epidural space. The catheter is fitted with an adapter to allow attachment of a syringe. Gentle aspiration is performed to check for blood or CSF return, and the catheter is then securely taped to the patient's back using a large, clean, reinforced dressing.

   d. **Test dose.** A test dose of local anesthetic agent is given either through the needle if a single-dose technique is employed or through the catheter. A test dose consists of 3 ml of local anesthetic and 1:200,000 epinephrine. This should have little effect in the epidural space. If it has been placed into the CSF, neurologic manifestations of a spinal block will occur rapidly. If the solution has been injected into an epidural vein, a 20–30% increase in heart rate will be seen.

   e. **Injection of anesthetic.** The anesthetic solution should be administered in 3- to 5-ml increments every 3–5 minutes until the total dose has been given. With each injection, aspiration is performed to ensure continued catheter or needle placement within the epidural space.

D. **Determinants of level of epidural blockade**

   1. **Volume of local anesthetic.** For the induction of epidural blockade, a maximum dose of 1.6 ml of local anesthetic per segment should be used.

   2. **Age.** The volume of local anesthetic should be reduced by 50% in the elderly and neonates. Stenosis of intervertebral foraminae in the elderly reduces the lateral paravertebral spread of injected drug, allowing for more cephalad spread.

   3. **Pregnancy.** A reduction in dose of 30% is made in pregnant women. Not only are neurons in pregnancy more sensitive to the effects of local anesthetic, but inferior vena cava compression increases blood flow through the epidural venous plexus, reducing the potential volume of the epidural space.

   4. **Speed of injection.** Rapid injection into the epidural space produces a less reliable block than does a slow, steady injection at approximately 0.5 ml/sec. Rapid injection of drug has the potentially hazardous effect of dramatically increasing pressure within the epidural space. Such a rise in pressure can produce headache, raised intracranial pressure, and spinal cord ischemia by decreasing spinal cord blood flow.

   5. **Position.** The position of the patient has a slight effect on the level of epidural blockade. Patients sitting upright have greater caudad spread of blockade, while patients positioned laterally have a higher level of block on the dependent side.

   6. **Spread of epidural blockade.** Onset of blockade occurs first and is most dense at the level of injection. Spread of blockade occurs faster in a cephalad than a caudad direction. This is most likely due to the relative difference in size between the large lower lumbar and

sacral nerve roots compared to the smaller thoracic nerve roots. There is often anesthetic sparing of the L5–S1 nerve root because of its large size and, thus, relative resistance to anesthetic penetration. Spread is greatest at 20–30 minutes.

E. **Determinants of onset and duration of epidural blockade**

1. **Selection of drug.** See Chap. 15.

2. **Addition of epinephrine.** Epinephrine, added in a concentration of 1:200,000, diminishes the systemic uptake and plasma levels of local anesthetic, as well as prolonging the duration of action. This effect is more marked with the short-acting agents such as lidocaine where prolongation is 50%. It is not as marked with the longer-acting agents such as bupivacaine. Commercially premixed local anesthetic solutions are buffered at a low pH. This slows the onset of block by reducing the amount of local anesthetic base available for penetration of nerves. This can be avoided by adding epinephrine to the solution immediately before use.

3. **Addition of opioid.** The addition of fentanyl, 50–100 μg, to the local anesthetic solution shortens the onset, increases the level, and prolongs the duration of the block. Fentanyl is thought to produce this effect by having a selective action at the substantia gelatinosa of the dorsal horn of the spinal cord to modulate pain transmission. This action is synergistic with the actions of the local anesthetic drug.

4. **pH adjustment of solution.** The addition of sodium bicarbonate to the local anesthetic solution in a ratio of 1 ml of 8.4% sodium bicarbonate to each 10 ml of lidocaine (0.1 ml for each 10 ml of bupivacaine) has been shown to decrease the onset time for blockade. It is thought that this effect is due to an increased amount of local anesthetic base, and thus more drug crosses axonal membranes.

F. **Complications**

1. **Acute**

a. **Dural puncture.** Unintentional dural puncture occurs in 1% of epidural injections performed. If this occurs, the anesthesiologist has a number of options depending on anesthetic requirements for the case. A conversion to spinal anesthesia can be made by injection of an appropriate amount of anesthetic into the CSF. Continuous spinal anesthesia can be performed by insertion of the epidural catheter into the subarachnoid space through the needle. If epidural anesthesia is required (e.g., for postoperative analgesia), the catheter should be repositioned at an interspace above the one punctured so that the tip of the epidural catheter lies well away from the site of dural puncture. The possibility of spinal anesthesia with injection of the epidural catheter should be considered.

b. **Catheter complications**

(1) Inability to thread the epidural catheter is a

common difficulty. This is usually a result of the epidural needle being inserted in the lateral part of the epidural space rather than in the midline or the bevel of the needle being at too acute an angle to the epidural space for the catheter to emerge. It can also be due to the bevel of the needle being only partially through the ligamentum flavum when loss of resistance is found. In the latter case, cautious advancement of the needle 1 mm into the epidural space may facilitate catheter insertion. The catheter and needle should be withdrawn together and repositioned if resistance occurs.

(2) The catheter can be inserted into an epidural vein such that blood can be aspirated from the catheter or tachycardia is noted with the test dose. The catheter should be gently withdrawn until blood can no longer be aspirated and then retested. Significant withdrawal should prompt removal and reinsertion.

(3) Catheters can break off or become knotted within the epidural space. In the absence of infection, a retained catheter is no more reactive than a surgical suture. The patient should be informed of the problem and reassured. The complications of surgical exploration and removal of the catheter are greater than conservative management.

c. **Unintentional subarachnoid injection.** The injection of a large volume of local anesthetic into the subarachnoid space can produce total spinal anesthesia. Treatment is similar to that described for spinal complications (see sec. **IV.F**).

d. **Intravascular injection** of local anesthetic into an epidural vein causes central nervous system and cardiovascular toxicity and may result in convulsions and cardiopulmonary arrest. Resistant ventricular fibrillation with IV bupivacaine 0.75% has been described (see Chap. 15).

e. **Local anesthetic overdose.** Systemic local anesthetic toxicity is possible with epidural anesthesia, where relatively large amounts of drug are used as compared to spinal anesthesia.

f. **Direct spinal cord injury** is possible if the epidural injection is above L2. The onset of a unilateral paresthesia during needle insertion signifies lateral entry into the epidural space. Further injection or insertion of a catheter at this point may produce trauma to a nerve root. Small feeder arteries to the anterior spinal artery also run in this area as they pass through the intervertebral foramen. Trauma to these arteries may result in anterior spinal cord ischemia or an epidural hematoma.

g. **Bloody tap.** Perforation of an epidural vein by the needle will result in blood emerging from the end. The needle should be removed and repositioned. It is preferable to reposition the needle at a different interspace, as the presence of blood in the original space will make it difficult to determine correct needle placement.

2. **Postoperative**
   a. **Postdural puncture headache.** If the dura is punctured with a 17-gauge epidural needle, there is a 75% chance of a young patient's developing a postdural puncture headache. Management is the same as that described under spinal anesthesia (see sec. **IV.F.2.a**).
   b. **Infection.** Epidural abscess is an extremely rare complication of epidural anesthesia. The source of infection in the majority of cases is from hematogenous spread to the epidural space from an infection in another area. Infection can also arise from contamination during insertion, contamination of an indwelling catheter used for postoperative pain relief, or a cutaneous infection at the insertion site. The patient presents with fever, severe back pain, and localized back tenderness. Progression to nerve root pain and paralysis then occurs. Initial laboratory investigations reveal a leukocytosis and a lumbar puncture suggestive of a parameningeal infection. Definitive diagnosis is with myelography or magnetic resonance imaging (MRI). Treatment includes urgent decompression laminectomy and antibiotics. Good neurologic recovery is associated with rapid diagnosis and treatment.
   c. **Epidural hematoma** is an extremely rare complication of epidural anesthesia. Trauma to epidural veins in the presence of a coagulopathy may result in a large epidural hematoma. The patient presents with severe back pain and persistent neurologic deficit after epidural anesthesia. Rapid diagnosis is required with computed tomography scan or MRI. Urgent decompression laminectomy is required to preserve neurologic function.

VI. **Caudal anesthesia**
   A. **Anatomy.** The caudal space is an extension of the epidural space. The sacral hiatus is formed by the failure of the laminae of S5 to fuse. The hiatus is bound laterally by the sacral cornua, which are the inferior articulating processes of S5. The sacrococcygeal membrane is a thin layer of fibrous tissue that covers the sacral hiatus. The caudal canal contains the sacral nerves, the sacral venous plexus, the filum terminale, and the dural sac, which usually ends at the lower border of S2. In neonates the dural sac may extend to S4.
   B. **Physiology.** The physiology of caudal anesthesia is similar to that described for epidural anesthesia (see sec. **V.B**).
   C. **Technique**
      1. Caudal epidural anesthesia is performed with the patient in the lateral, prone, or jackknife position.
      2. The sacral cornua are palpated. If they are difficult to

palpate directly, the location of the sacral hiatus can be estimated by measuring 5 cm from the tip of the coccyx in the midline.

3. Skin preparation and draping are as described for spinal anesthesia (see sec. **IV.C.3**).

4. A skin wheal is raised with 1% lidocaine between the sacral cornua.

5. A 22-gauge spinal needle is inserted at an angle of 70–80 degrees to the skin. The needle is advanced through the sacrococcygeal membrane when a characteristic "pop" is felt. One should avoid attempting to thread the needle up the caudal canal, as this increases the likelihood of puncturing an epidural vein.

6. The stylet is withdrawn and the hub of the needle inspected for passive CSF or blood flow. The needle can then be aspirated as a further check. The needle should be repositioned if either blood or CSF appears.

7. A test dose of 3 ml of local anesthetic solution with epinephrine (1:200,000) is given, similar to that for lumbar epidural anesthesia (see sec. **V.C.3.d**), and the patient is observed for signs of subarachnoid or IV injection. As the caudal canal has a rich epidural venous plexus, IV injections are frequently seen and can occur even though blood cannot be aspirated from the needle.

8. A caudal catheter can be placed in a manner analogous to that for lumbar epidural anesthesia using a 17-gauge Tuohy needle and catheter (see sec. **V.C.3.a**). In this way the catheter can be used for postoperative analgesia. This technique is particularly valuable in pediatric patients.

9. The level, onset, and duration for caudal anesthesia follow the same principles outlined for epidural anesthesia (see secs. **V.D** and **E**). The extent of caudal block is less predictable than other epidural techniques because of the variability in content and volume of the caudal canal, as well as the amount of local anesthetic solution that leaks out the sacral foramina. To obtain sacral anesthesia, a volume of 10–15 ml should be sufficient.

D. Complications. The complications of caudal anesthesia are similar to those of epidural anesthesia (see sec. **V.F**).

SUGGESTED READING

Cousins, M. J., and Bridenbaugh, P. O. *Neural Blockade in Clinical Anaesthesia and Management of Pain.* Philadelphia: Lippincott, 1988.

Jarvis, A. P., Greenwalt, J. W., and Fagraeus, L. Intravenous caffeine for post dural puncture headache. *Reg. Anaesth.* 11:42, 1986.

Modig, J., et al. Thromboembolism after total hip replacement: Role of epidural and general anesthesia. *Anesth. Analg.* 62:174, 1983.

Moore, D. C. *Regional Block: A Handbook for Use in the Clinical*

Practice of Medicine and Surgery (4th ed.). Springfield, IL: Thomas, 1981.

Rao, T. L. K., and El-Etr, A. A. Anticoagulation following placement of epidural and subarachnoid catheters: An evaluation of neurologic sequelae. *Anesthesiology* 55:618, 1981.

Rigler, M. L., et al. Cauda equina syndrome after continuous spinal anesthesia. *Anesth. Analg.* 72:275, 1991.

Vandam, L. D. Complications of Spinal and Epidural Anaesthesia. In F. K. Orkin and L. H. Cooperman (eds.), *Complications of Anesthesiology*. Philadelphia: Lippincott, 1983.

17

Regional Anesthesia

Conor O'Neill

I. General considerations

A. **Peripheral nerve blockade** requires identifying a nerve as precisely as possible and depositing an appropriate volume of local anesthetic near it. It can provide anesthesia for many surgical procedures without significant disruption of autonomic function.

B. The **preoperative assessment, preparation of the patient,** and **degree of monitoring** are the same as for central neuraxial blockade (see Chap. 16). Preoperative medication may be prescribed, although nerve blocks may require a higher degree of cooperation (especially when eliciting paresthesias) than spinal or epidural anesthesia.

C. All blocks should be performed with **strict sterile technique** (i.e., sterile equipment, preparation of the skin with an antiseptic solution, and appropriate sterile draping). Prior to inserting any block needle, a skin wheal should be raised with local anesthetic.

II. Equipment

A. **Needles used for nerve blockade**

1. To decrease the possibility of nerve damage, a block needle should be of the minimum diameter possible, preferably 22-gauge.

2. A B-bevel (19-degree angle) or short bevel (45-degree angle) is superior to the standard A-bevel.

3. Upper extremity blocks are usually best performed with a 1½-inch needle, while many lower extremity blocks require needle lengths of 2 to 3½ inches.

B. **Nerve stimulators** designed for regional anesthesia deliver a current of 0.1–10.0 mA at a frequency of 1 pulse/sec. Insulated needles provide the best results, although uninsulated needles may be used as well.

C. Many blocks require depositing **a large volume of local anesthetic in a single injection.** This may be most easily accomplished by connecting a large-volume syringe to the block needle with sterile extension tubing, which will ensure stable needle position during aspiration and injection.

D. **Catheter techniques** for continuous blockade of various nerves are best accomplished with commercially available kits.

III. Nerve localization techniques

A. A **paresthesia** can be elicited by contacting a nerve with a needle. Disadvantages to this technique are patient discomfort during the paresthesia and possibly a higher incidence of postanesthetic neuropathy.

B. **Electrical stimulation** of a mixed nerve produces a motor response.

1. A **ground electrode** is attached to the patient, and the positive lead of the stimulator is connected to it.

The negative terminal of the stimulator is attached to the needle.

2. The **nerve stimulator** is set at an initial current of 2–3 mA and the needle moved toward the nerve until a motor response in the desired muscle group occurs. Twitches may also arise from local muscle stimulation and should be differentiated from those due to nerve stimulation. Regardless of its origin, if a twitch is uncomfortable the current should be reduced. After eliciting the desired twitch, the needle position and stimulator output are adjusted to produce the maximum twitch at the lowest output. When the current required for a response is 0.5–1.0 mA, the needle is close to the nerve and the local anesthetic may be injected.

3. An **advantage** of this technique is that it may be used on patients who are unable to report paresthesias reliably, whether from altered mental status, from oversedation, or following induction of general anesthesia. Patient discomfort related to paresthesia is avoided, and the incidence of postanesthetic neuropathies may be diminished.

4. The major **disadvantage** of a nerve stimulator technique is the need for specialized equipment at an increased cost.

C. **Infiltration** without precise localization will reliably block many nerves due to their consistent relationship to palpable anatomic landmarks.

IV. **Contraindications.** Absolute contraindications to regional anesthesia include lack of patient consent and when nerve blockade would hinder the proposed surgery. Relative contraindications include coagulopathy, infection at the skin entry site, and the presence of neurologic disease such as multiple sclerosis or polio.

V. **Complications common to all nerve blocks**
A. **Reactions to local anesthetics** consist of intravascular injection, overdose, and allergic responses. Test doses and intermittent aspiration during injection may help prevent intravascular injection, and benzodiazepine premedication may ameliorate the central nervous system toxicity of local anesthetics.

B. **Nerve damage** is a rare complication that may result from needle trauma or from intraneural injection. Patient reports of pain during injection may be due to intraneural injection. This may be difficult to differentiate from **pressure paresthesia,** a paresthesia that is potentiated on injection. However, if the pain is severe or does not subside after the first few milliliters of local anesthetic, the needle should be repositioned before continuing.

C. **Hematomas** may result from arterial puncture but usually resolve without residua.

VI. **Regional anesthesia of the head and neck. Cervical plexus block** is the most commonly used regional anesthetic technique of the head and neck.

A. **Anatomy** (Fig. 17–1). The cervical plexus lies in the paravertebral region of the upper four cervical vertebrae,

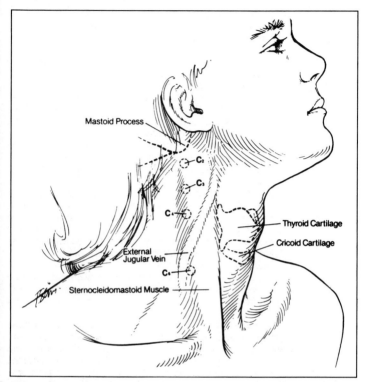

Fig. 17-1. External landmarks for cervical plexus blockade. (From P. P. Raj, *Clinical Practice of Regional Anesthesia*. New York: Churchill Livingstone, 1991.)

where it is formed from the ventral rami of the C1–C4 spinal nerve roots. It is deep to the sternocleidomastoid muscle and anterior to the middle scalene muscle, in continuity with the nerve roots forming the brachial plexus (see sec. **VII.A**). The plexus has two sets of branches: superficial and deep. The superficial branches pierce the cervical fascia anteriorly, just posterior to the sternocleidomastoid, and supply the skin of the back of the head, side of the neck, and anterior and lateral shoulder. The deep branches supply the muscles and other deep structures of the neck, as well as forming the phrenic nerve.

B. Indications. Superficial cervical plexus block produces cutaneous anesthesia only and is useful for superficial procedures on the neck and shoulder. Deep cervical plexus block is a paravertebral block of the C1–C4 nerve roots that form the plexus, thus anesthetizing both the deep and superficial branches. Common indications for deep cervical plexus block are

1. Cervical lymph node biopsy/excision.
2. Carotid endarterectomy.

3. Thyroid operations.
4. **Tracheostomy** (when combined with topical airway anesthesia).

C. **Techniques**
1. For a **superficial block,** 10 ml of local anesthetic is injected subcutaneously along the posterior border of the sternocleidomastoid.
2. For a **deep block,** the patient is positioned supine with the neck slightly extended and the head turned toward the opposite side. A line is drawn connecting the tip of the mastoid process and Chassaignac's tubercle (the most prominent of the cervical transverse processes, located at the level of the cricoid cartilage). A second line is drawn 1 cm posterior to the first line. The C2 transverse process can be palpated 1–2 cm caudad to the mastoid process, with the C3 and C4 processes lying at 1.5-cm intervals along the second line. At each level, a 22-gauge, 5-cm needle is inserted perpendicular to the skin with caudad angulation. It is advanced 1.5–3.0 cm until the transverse process is contacted. After careful aspiration for CSF or blood, 10 ml of solution is injected at each transverse process.

D. **Complications.** A variety of complications are possible with deep cervical plexus block, owing to the close proximity of the needle to a variety of important neural and vascular structures.
1. **Phrenic nerve block** is the most common complication. This block should be used cautiously in patients with diminished pulmonary reserve. Bilateral deep cervical plexus block will lead to phrenic and recurrent laryngeal nerve blockade. Due to the risk of respiratory dysfunction, bilateral blockade is rarely performed.
2. **Subarachnoid injection** resulting in total spinal anesthesia.
3. **Epidural injection** with resultant bilateral cervical epidural anesthesia.
4. **Vertebral artery injection** causing CNS toxicity with very small doses of local anesthetic.
5. **Recurrent laryngeal nerve block** causing hoarseness and vocal cord dysfunction.
6. **Cervical sympathetic nerve block** leading to Horner's syndrome.

VII. **Regional anesthesia of the upper extremity**
A. **Anatomy**
1. With the exception of the skin over the shoulder and medial arm, the upper extremity is innervated entirely by the brachial plexus. The skin over the shoulder is supplied by the cervical plexus, while the skin over the medial arm is supplied by the intercostobrachial nerve, a branch of the T2 spinal nerve.
2. The **brachial plexus** is formed from the anterior roots of the spinal nerves emanating from C5–C8 and T1, with frequent contributions from C4 and T2. Each root travels laterally in the trough of its cervical transverse process and then is directed toward the first rib where it fuses with the other four roots to form the three

trunks of the plexus. The roots are sandwiched between the anterior and middle scalene muscles, the fasciae of which form a sheath that envelops the plexus. This sheath encloses the plexus through its course, providing a closed potential space for the injection of local anesthetics.

3. The trunks pass over the first rib through the space between the anterior and middle scalene muscles, in association with the subclavian artery, which is invested by the same fascial sheath. The roots and trunks give off several branches, which innervate the neck, shoulder girdle, and chest wall. Stimulating these nerves as they exit the plexus proximally cannot be relied on for plexus localization.

4. As the trunks pass over the first rib and under the clavicle, they reorganize to form the three cords of the plexus. The cords descend into the axilla where each gives off one major branch, in addition to several minor branches, before becoming a major terminal nerve of the upper extremity. Branches of the lateral and medial cords form the median nerve. The lateral cord gives off a branch that forms the musculocutaneous nerve, while the posterior cord gives rise to the axillary and radial nerves. The medial cord also forms the ulnar nerve and medial antebrachial and brachial cutaneous nerves. In the axilla, the median nerve lies lateral to the axillary artery, the radial nerve posterior, and the ulnar nerve medial. The axillary and musculocutaneous nerves exit the sheath high up in the axilla, the musculocutaneous nerve traveling through the substance of the coracobrachialis muscle before becoming subcutaneous below the elbow (Fig. 17–2).

5. The cutaneous distribution of the nerves of the plexus is summarized in Fig. 17–3. The median cutaneous nerves of the arm and forearm are minor branches of the medial cord.

6. The major **motor functions** of the five nerves are as follows:
   a. **Axillary.** Shoulder abduction.
   b. **Musculocutaneous.** Elbow flexion.
   c. **Radial.** Elbow, wrist, and finger extension.
   d. **Median.** Wrist and finger flexion.
   e. **Ulnar.** Wrist and finger flexion.

B. Indications
   1. **Brachial plexus blockade** anesthetizes the upper extremity with the exception of the skin over the shoulder and medial arm. The preferred approach to the plexus depends on the surgical site.
      a. The **interscalene approach** blocks the cervical plexus in addition to the brachial plexus, thereby anesthetizing the skin over the shoulder. The ulnar nerve is frequently spared. This approach is most useful for shoulder surgery. It is less useful for forearm and hand operations, unless accompanied by an ulnar nerve block.

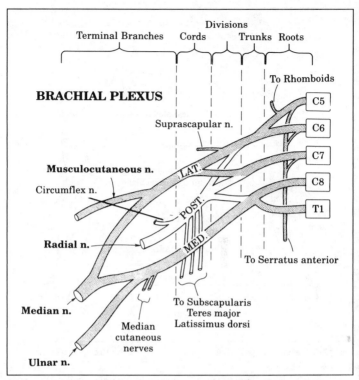

BRACHIAL PLEXUS

Divisions

Terminal Branches   Cords   Trunks   Roots

To Rhomboids

C5

C6

Suprascapular n.

C7

Musculocutaneous n.   LAT.

C8

Circumflex n.   POST.

T1

Radial n.   MED.

To Serratus anterior

Median n.

To Subscapularis
Teres major
Latissimus dorsi

Median
cutaneous
nerves

Ulnar n.

Fig. 17-2. Diagram of the brachial plexus and peripheral nerve formation.

    b. The **supraclavicular approach** anesthetizes the entire plexus, owing to its compact nature at the point of injection and the fact that none of the nerves has yet left the plexus.

    c. The **axillary approach** is the most popular because of its ease and safety. Since the musculocutaneous and median cutaneous nerves of the arm exit the sheath more proximally, they are not blocked by this approach, making it unreliable for operations proximal to the elbow.

  2. The **intercostobrachial nerve** must be blocked in addition to the plexus for procedures involving the medial arm or utilizing a tourniquet.

  3. **Blockade of an individual peripheral nerve** may be useful when limited anesthesia is required or a plexus block is incomplete. The musculocutaneous nerve may be blocked at the axilla or the elbow, while each of the other major terminal nerves may be blocked at either the elbow or the wrist.

C. Techniques

  1. Interscalene (Fig. 17–4)

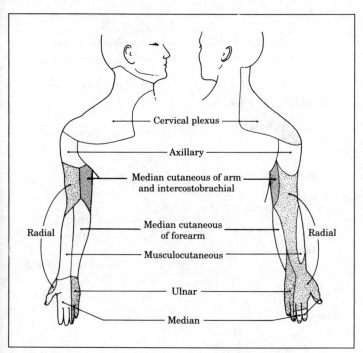

Fig. 17-3. Cutaneous peripheral nerve supply of the upper extremity.

a. The patient is positioned supine with the head turned slightly away from the side to be blocked.

b. The lateral border of the sternocleidomastoid is identified by having the patient lift his or her head off the bed. The anterior scalene muscle lies below the posterior edge of the sternocleidomastoid. By rolling the fingers posteriorly over the anterior scalene muscle, a groove will be felt between the anterior and middle scalenes. The intersection of this groove with a transverse plane at the level of the cricoid cartilage is the point at which the needle should enter the skin. As the scalenes are accessory muscles of respiration, asking the patient to take slow deep breaths while palpating for the groove may assist in locating it. Additionally, the external jugular vein frequently crosses the groove at the level of C6 and may be a useful landmark.

c. A 1½-inch needle is advanced into the groove, perpendicular to the skin in all directions. Stimulation of the plexus will result in a paresthesia or muscle twitch below the shoulder. Paresthesia or twitches confined to the shoulder may result from suprascapular or cervical plexus stimulation and do not reliably localize the plexus. Despite being accurately placed in the groove, the needle will some-

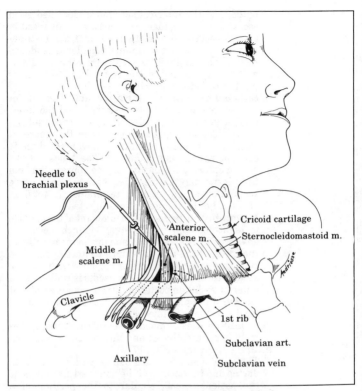

Fig. 17-4. Interscalene approach to brachial plexus block.

times contact the cervical transverse process without stimulating the plexus. If that is the case, withdrawing the needle slightly and then injecting will result in an adequate block.

   d. A volume of **30–40 ml** of anesthetic should be injected.

   e. If digital pressure is held distal to the injection site, cervical plexus block will accompany the brachial plexus block.

   f. Complications are identical to those of the cervical plexus block (see sec. **VI.D**).

2. The **supraclavicular block** provides anesthesia of the brachial plexus at the level of the nerve trunks and produces reliable anesthesia of the elbow, forearm, and hand. Three approaches will be described; for each, the patient is placed in the supine position and the head turned to the contralateral side. With each of these techniques, it is generally safe to direct the needle laterally, but medial direction should be avoided to avoid entering the cupola of the lung.

   a. Parascalene approach. The clavicle and lateral border of the sternocleidomastoid muscle are palpated, and the interscalene groove identified as in sec. **C.1.b.** A 22-gauge, 4-cm needle is advanced in an anteroposterior direction. Using a nerve stimulator or paresthesia technique, the plexus is identified. If the first rib is contracted, the needle is withdrawn and redirected. A total of 20–30 ml of local anesthetic is injected.

b. Subclavian perivascular approach. The patient is prepared as previously described, and the interscalene groove is identified. The pulse of the subclavian artery is palpated inferiorly in this space. A 22-gauge, 1½-inch needle is advanced directly caudad, not mesiad or dorsad. The "click" of the needle entering the plexus may be appreciated, and the plexus may be identified with either a nerve stimulator or paresthesia technique. A total of 20–30 ml of local anesthetic is injected.

c. Plumb-bob approach. The midpoint of the clavicle is identified and a 22-gauge, 1½-inch needle is advanced in a caudad direction in a plane parallel to that of the head and neck until contacting the first rib. If a paresthesia or motor response with a nerve stimulator is not elicited, the needle is walked in an anterior and then posterior direction across the first rib. Once the plexus has been located, 25–40 ml of local anesthetic is injected.

d. Complications common to each of these approaches include pneumothorax and intravascular injection.

3. Axillary approach (Fig. 17–5)

a. The patient is positioned supine with the arm abducted and the dorsum of the hand resting alongside the patient's head, similar to the position of a military salute.

b. The axillary artery is palpated and fixed at its most proximal location in the axilla. If the artery is difficult to palpate, moving the patient's hand laterally or reducing the degree of abduction at the shoulder may be helpful.

c. A 23-gauge needle is advanced through the skin just superior to the palpating fingertip, directing the needle toward the apex of the axilla. Localization of one of the nerves of the plexus by either paresthesia or nerve stimulation confirms that the needle tip is within the plexus sheath, and 40–50 ml of local anesthetic may be injected.

d. If the axillary artery is penetrated, the needle should be advanced until it is just through the posterior wall of the artery, as evidenced by an inability to aspirate blood, and the local anesthetic injected.

e. Frequently, as the sheath is penetrated, a prominent pop will be appreciated. If this occurs and the needle is observed to pulsate in synchrony with the pulse, the needle is within the sheath and the anesthetic may be injected.

f. At this point, while continuing to hold distal pres-

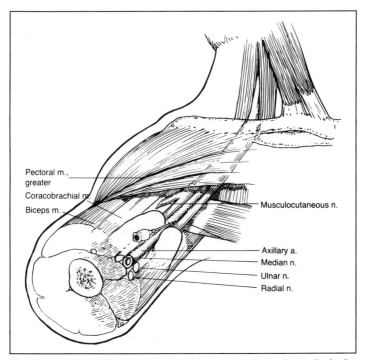

Fig. 17-5. Axillary block. The arm is abducted at right angles to the body. Distal digital pressure is maintained during needle placement and injection of local anesthetic. (From R. D. Miller, *Anesthesia* [3rd ed.] New York: Churchill Livingstone, 1991.)

sure on the upper arm, the needle is redirected so that the tip of the needle is just superior to the artery and perpendicular to the skin in all planes. The needle is advanced until the humerus is contacted and then swung through a 30-degree arc superiorly, and 5 ml of local anesthetic can be injected in a fanwise manner. This will block the musculocutaneous nerve in its course through the coracobrachialis muscle.

g. After blocking the musculocutaneous and intercostobrachialis nerves, the needle should be withdrawn and the patient's arm replaced at his or her side.

h. Digital pressure should be continued for a period of 3–5 minutes after the needle is withdrawn.

i. The most common **complication** specific to the axillary approach is injection of local anesthetic into the axillary artery.

4. Intercostobrachial nerve block requires subcutaneous injection of 5 ml of local anesthetic, beginning directly inferior to the axillary artery and extending to the inferior border of the axilla.

5. Ulnar nerve block

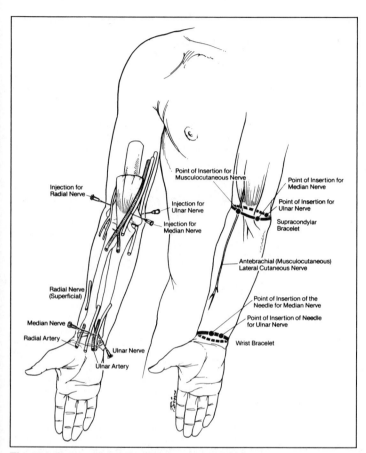

Fig. 17-6. Deep anatomy for elbow and wrist block of musculocutaneous, radial, ulnar, and median nerves. (From P. P. Raj, *Clinical Practice of Regional Anesthesia.* New York: Churchill Livingstone, 1991.)

    a. Elbow. The ulnar groove in the medial epicondyle is located, and 5–10 ml of local anesthetic is injected 3–5 cm proximal to the groove in a fanwise fashion.

    b. Wrist (Fig. 17-6). The ulnar nerve is just lateral to the flexor carpi ulnaris tendon at the level of the ulnar styloid process. The needle is inserted perpendicular to the skin, just lateral to the tendon, to pierce the deep fascia. A total of 3–6 ml of solution is injected.

6. Median nerve block

    a. Elbow (Fig. 17-6). The median nerve is just medial to the brachial artery. The artery is palpated 1–2 cm proximal to the elbow crease, and 3–5 ml of anesthetic is injected just medial to it in a fanwise fashion.

    b. Wrist (Fig. 17-6). The median nerve lies between

the palmaris longus tendon and the flexor carpi radialis tendon, 2–3 cm proximal to the wrist crease. The needle is inserted perpendicular to the skin close to the lateral border of the palmaris longus, to pierce the deep fascia. A total of 3–5 ml of anesthetic is injected.

7. **Radial nerve block**
   a. **Elbow** (Fig. 17–6). The radial nerve lies lateral to the biceps tendon, medial to the brachioradialis muscle, at the level of the lateral epicondyle of the humerus. The needle is inserted 1–2 cm lateral to the tendon and advanced until the lateral epicondyle is contacted. A total of 3–5 ml of anesthetic is injected.
   b. **Wrist.** The radial nerve divides into its terminal branches, which lie in the superficial fascia. A total of 5–10 ml of local anesthetic is injected subcutaneously, extending from the radial artery anteriorly to the extensor carpi radialis posteriorly, beginning just proximal to the wrist.

8. **Musculocutaneous nerve block.** The musculocutaneous nerve may be blocked in the axilla, as decribed in sec. **3.** Its terminal cutaneous component is blocked concomitantly with the radial nerve block at the elbow.

9. **Intravenous regional anesthesia (Bier block).** IV administration of local anesthetic distal to a tourniquet is a simple way to anesthetize an extremity.
   a. A 20- to 22-gauge IV catheter is placed in the operative extremity as distally as possible and capped off with a heparin-lock device. A pneumatic double tourniquet is applied proximally and the extremity exsanguinated by elevating it and wrapping it distally to proximally with an Esmarch's bandage.
   b. Both tourniquet cuffs should be checked, and the proximal cuff inflated to 150 mm Hg greater than systolic pressure. Absence of pulses after inflation ensures arterial occlusion.
   c. Local anesthetic is injected, with anesthesia ensuing in less than 5 minutes. Tourniquet pain generally becomes unbearable by 1 hour and is the limiting factor for the success of this technique. When the patient complains of pain, the distal tourniquet that overlies anesthetized skin should be inflated and the proximal tourniquet released. Some advocate changing cuffs at 45 minutes, before the onset of pain.
   d. Average drug doses are 50 ml of 0.5% lidocaine for an arm and 100 ml of 0.25% lidocaine for a leg. No vasoconstrictors should be used.
   e. A toxic reaction to the local anesthetic is the major **complication** associated with IV regional anesthesia. It may occur during injection if the tourniquet fails or with tourniquet deflation, particularly with an inflation time of less than 25 minutes. Careful attention to drug dosage and to the adequacy of

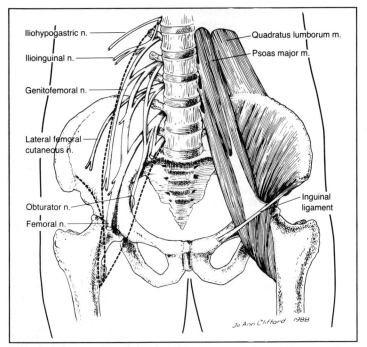

Fig. 17-7. The lumbar plexus lies in the psoas compartment between the psoas major and quadratus lumborum. (From R. D. Miller, *Anesthesia* [3rd ed.] New York: Churchill Livingstone, 1991.)

vascular occlusion will minimize the risk of a local anesthetic reaction. If the tourniquet is deflated before 25 minutes, the patient should be observed closely for evidence of toxicity.

VIII. **Regional anesthesia of the lower extremity**

   A. **Anatomy.** There are two major plexi that innervate the lower extremity: the lumbar plexus and the sacral plexus.

   1. The **lumbar plexus** (Fig. 17-7) is formed within the substance of the psoas muscle from the anterior rami of the L1–L4 spinal nerves, with a variable contribution from the twelfth thoracic nerve. The most cephalad nerves of the plexus are the iliohypogastric, ilioinguinal, and genitofemoral nerves. These nerves pierce the abdominal musculature anteriorly before supplying the skin of the hip and groin. The remainder of the lower abdomen is supplied by intercostal nerves. The three caudal nerves of the lumber plexus are the lateral femoral cutaneous, femoral, and obturator nerves.

   a. The **lateral femoral cutaneous (LFC) nerve** passes under the lateral end of the inguinal ligament and is a pure sensory nerve to the lateral thigh and buttock.

   b. The **femoral nerve** passes under the inguinal ligament just lateral to the femoral artery and supplies the muscles and skin of the anterior thigh, as well as the knee and hip joints. The saphenous nerve is the cutaneous termination of the femoral nerve, supplying the skin of the medial leg and foot. It is the only nerve of the lumbar plexus that innervates the lower extremity below the knee.

c. The **obturator nerve** exits from the pelvis through the obturator canal of the ischium, supplying the adductor muscles of the thigh, the hip and knee joints, and a variable portion of the skin of the medial thigh.

2. The **sacral plexus** is formed from the ventral rami of the fourth and fifth lumbar nerves and the first, second, and third sacral nerves. The two major nerves of the sacral plexus are the sciatic nerve and the posterior cutaneous nerve of the thigh.

a. The **posterior cutaneous nerve of the thigh** travels with the sciatic nerve in its proximal extent and supplies the skin of the posterior thigh. Techniques for blocking the sciatic nerve will also block the posterior cutaneous nerve of the thigh concomitantly.

b. The **sciatic nerve** passes out of the pelvis through the greater sciatic foramen, becomes superficial at the lower border of the gluteus maximus, descends along the medial aspect of the femur, and becomes superficial again at the popliteal fossa. There it divides into the tibial nerve and the common peroneal nerve.

(1) The **tibial nerve** travels down the posterior calf and passes under the medial malleolus before dividing into its terminal branches. It supplies the skin of the medial and plantar foot and causes plantar flexion.

(2) The **common peroneal nerve** winds around the head of the fibula before dividing into the superficial and deep peroneal nerves.

(a) The **superficial peroneal nerve** is a sensory nerve that passes down the lateral calf, dividing into its terminal branches just medial to the lateral malleolus supplying the anterior foot.

(b) The **deep peroneal nerve** enters the foot just lateral to the anterior tibial artery, lying at the superior border of the malleolus, in between the anterior tibialis tendon and the extensor hallucis longus tendon. While primarily a motor nerve causing dorsiflexion of the foot, it also sends a sensory branch to the web space between the first and second toes.

(3) The **sural nerve** is a sensory nerve formed from branches of the common peroneal and tibial nerves. It passes under the lateral malleolus, supplying the lateral foot.

B. **Indications.** In contrast to the upper extremity, anesthetizing the entire lower extremity requires blocking components of both the lumbar and sacral plexuses. In part because multiple injections may be required, lower extremity blocks have been unpopular with many clinicians. However, they are useful when limited anesthesia is required (making a single injection feasible) or when a regional technique is preferable, but a central neuraxis block is contraindicated. In addition, many of these blocks may be used as adjuncts to general anesthesia to provide postoperative analgesia.

1. While **low abdominal operations** may be performed with combined lumbar plexus block and intercostal nerve blocks, this is rarely done. However, an ilioinguinal-iliohypogastric (IL/IH) block is a simple and very useful block, providing excellent analgesia for groin operations (e.g., hernia repair).

2. **Hip operations** require anesthesia of the entire lumbar plexus with the exception of the IL and IH nerves. This is most easily accomplished with a lumbar plexus block (psoas block).

3. **Major thigh operations** (e.g., placement of a femoral rod) require anesthesia of the lateral femoral cutaneous, femoral, obturator, and sciatic nerves. Obturator nerve block may be difficult to perform. Alternatively, these operations may be performed with a lumbar plexus (psoas) block.

4. **Operations limited to the anterior thigh,** for example, muscle biopsies in patients susceptible to malignant hyperthermia, may be done with a combined LFC-femoral block. The nerves may be blocked separately or together with a "3 in 1" block (see sec. **C.2**). Alone, an LFC block gives excellent analgesia for skin graft donor sites. An isolated femoral nerve block is particularly useful for providing postoperative analgesia for femoral shaft fractures or as the sole anesthetic for quadricepsplasty or repair of a patellar fracture.

5. For **tourniquet pain,** a combined LFC-femoral nerve block, in concert with a sciatic block, will usually provide adequate analgesia. This is because the area of skin that the obturator nerve supplies is generally small.

6. **Open operations on the knee** require anesthesia of the LFC, femoral, obturator, and sciatic nerves, most easily accomplished with a combined psoas-sciatic block. For knee arthroscopy, combined "3 in 1" and femoral-sciatic nerve blocks provide adequate anesthesia.

7. **Operations distal to the knee** require sciatic block as well as block of the saphenous component of the femoral nerve. The branches of the sciatic nerve can be blocked with multiple injections at the ankle or with a single injection in the popliteal fossa. The latter is particularly useful when cellulitis is present at the ankle. Ankle block will provide reliable anesthesia for transmetatarsal and toe amputations.

C. **Techniques.** Although paresthesias may be used for nerve localization in the lower extremity, in general a nerve stimulator is more accurate.

1. **Lumbar plexus block** (psoas block)
   a. Local anesthetic deposited into the substance of the psoas muscle will be confined by its fascia and will anesthetize the entire plexus.
   b. The patient is placed in the lateral position, hips flexed, with the surgical side uppermost. A 22-gauge, 3½-inch spinal needle is inserted perpendicular to the skin at a point 3 cm cephalad to a line connecting the iliac crests and 4–5 cm lateral to the midline. If the transverse process of L4 is contacted, the needle is redirected cephalad. The plexus is localized using a nerve stimulator, correct placement being confirmed by a quadriceps twitch (any twitch resulting in patellar movement). A volume of 30–40 ml is injected.
   c. Epidural blockade is a complication of this approach, occurring with an incidence of approximately 10%.

2. **"3 in 1" block**
   a. The three branches of the lumbar plexus can be blocked with a single injection.
   b. With the patient in the supine position, a 2½- to 3-inch needle is inserted just caudad to the inguinal ligament, lateral to the femoral artery. The needle is directed cephalad at an angle of 45 degrees until a quadriceps twitch or paresthesia is elicited. While distal pressure is maintained, 30–40 ml of local anesthetic is injected, theoretically forcing the anesthetic more proximally onto lumbar nerve roots.

3. **Ilioinguinal-iliohypogastric nerve block.** A 1½-inch needle is inserted perpendicular to the skin 3 cm medial to the anterior superior iliac spine (ASIS). The ASIS is contacted, and 10–15 ml of local anesthetic is injected during needle withdrawal to the skin.

4. **LFC nerve block.** A 1½-inch needle is inserted 1.5 cm caudad and 1.5 cm medial to the ASIS. It is directed in a slightly lateral and cephalad direction to strike the iliac bone medially just below the ASIS, where 5–10 ml of local anesthetic is deposited.

5. **Femoral nerve block** is carried out identically to the "3 in 1" block (see sec. 2), with the exception that the needle is directed perpendicular to the skin, rather than at a 45-degree angle. A volume of 15–20 ml of local anesthetic will suffice.

6. **Obturator nerve block.** In the supine position, the pubic tubercle is identified, and a 3-inch needle is inserted 1.5 cm caudal and 1.5 cm lateral to the tubercle. After contact with the bone, the needle is withdrawn and redirected slightly lateral and caudal while advancing 2–3 cm into the obturator foramen. After aspiration, 20 ml of local anesthetic is injected while fanning lateral.

7. **Sciatic nerve block**

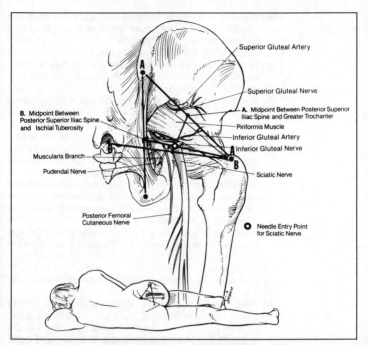

Fig. 17-8. Technique of the posterior approach to the sciatic nerve with the patient in the Sims' position. Line *A-A* joins the posterior superior iliac spine to the greater trochanter. At its midpoint a perpendicular line is dropped. This line joins the line drawn perpendicularly from midpoint of line *B-B* between sacral hiatus and greater trochanter. Some prefer a perpendicular line drawn from the midpoint of the line connecting posterior superior iliac spine and ischial tuberosity. This line meets the perpendicular line drawn from *A-A*. (From P. P. Raj, *Clinical Practice of Regional Anesthesia.* New York: Churchill Livingstone, 1991.)

a. **Indications**
   (1) **Surgery of the leg** when blocked proximally in combination with femoral nerve blockade.
   (2) **Surgery of the knee** when combined with blockade of the femoral, LFC, and obturator nerves.
   (3) **Foot and ankle surgery** when combined with saphenous nerve (femoral) blockade.

b. **Classic posterior approach.** The patient is placed in the Sims' position (the lateral decubitus position with the leg to be blocked uppermost and flexed at the hip and knee [Fig. 17-8]). The posterior superior iliac spine and greater trochanter are identified, and a straight line is drawn connecting the two. At its midpoint, a perpendicular line is drawn inferiorly for 3–4 cm. A 3½-inch, 22-gauge needle is inserted perpendicularly to the skin 3 cm below the midpoint and connected to the nerve stimulator at an initial current of 2.5 mA. The needle is advanced to a depth of approximately 3 cm to elicit a motor response in the sciatic distribution (contraction of hamstring or gastrocnemius, foot dorsi- or plantar flexion) or paresthesia in the leg or foot. If buttock contraction is observed, the inferior or superior gluteal nerves are being stimulated, and the needle is simply redirected. When an appropriate motor response is noted, the stimulus current is decreased in stepwise fashion to determine the threshold for stimulation. The needle is advanced in depth or changed in angle of approach until the goal of a stimulus threshold less than 1.0 mA is reached. After a test dose, 40 ml of local anesthetic is injected with incremental aspiration every 5 ml.

c. **Lithotomy approach.** With the patient supine, the lower extremity is flexed as far as possible at the hip and supported by stirrups or an assistant. The midpoint of a line between the greater trochanter and the ischial tuberosity is located. A 3½-inch needle attached to a nerve stimulator is inserted perpendicular to the skin at this point and advanced until a motor response is seen, indicating sciatic nerve stimulation. Then, 20–30 ml of local anesthetic is injected.

d. **Sciatic block at the knee** (Fig. 17–9). With the patient prone, the knee is flexed 30 degrees. This outlines the borders of the popliteal fossa, which is bounded by the knee crease inferiorly, the long head of the biceps femoris laterally, and the superimposed tendons of the semimembranosus and semitendinosus muscles medially. A vertical line is drawn on the skin dividing the fossa into two equilateral triangles. A needle is inserted 6 cm superior to the knee crease, 1 cm lateral to the line bisecting the fossa. The nerve is localized with a nerve stimulator, and 30–40 ml of local anesthetic is deposited.

8. **Saphenous nerve block.** The saphenous nerve (femoral) can be blocked at the ankle (see sec. **9**) or at the knee. At the knee, 10 ml of local anesthetic is injected in the deep subcutaneous tissue, extending from the medial surface of the tibial condyle to the superimposed tendons of the semimembranosus and semitendinosus muscles.

9. **Ankle block** (Fig. 17–10)

a. The five nerves supplying the foot can be blocked at the ankle. The foot is elevated by a pillow to provide easy access to both sides of the ankle.

b. At the superior border of the malleoli, the **deep peroneal nerve** is situated between the anterior tibialis tendon and the extensor hallucis longus tendon, which are easily palpable with dorsiflexion of the foot and extension of the great toe. A 1½-inch needle is inserted just lateral to the anterior tibial artery between the two tendons until the tibia is contacted, then withdrawn while depositing 5–10 ml of local anesthetic.

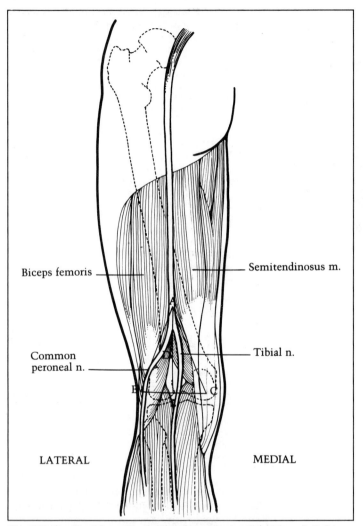

Fig. 17-9. Popliteal fossa block. The two major trunks of the sciatic bifurcate in the popliteal fossa 7 to 10 cm above the knee. A triangle is drawn using the heads of the biceps femoris and the semitendinosus muscles and the skin crease of the knee; a long needle is inserted 1 cm lateral to a point 6 cm cephalad on the line from the skin crease that bisects this triangle. (From M. F. Mulroy, *Regional Anesthesia*. Boston: Little, Brown, 1989.)

c. A 10-ml volume of local anesthetic is then injected subcutaneously across the anterior surface of the tibia, from malleolus to malleolus. This will block the **superficial peroneal nerve** laterally and the **saphenous nerve** medially.

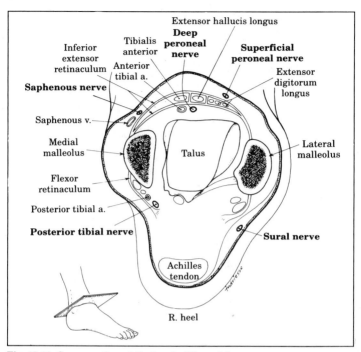

Fig. 17-10. Cross section at the level of the ankle.

    d. To block the **posterior tibial nerve,** the needle is
inserted posterior to the medial malleolus, directed
toward the inferior border of the posterior tibial
artery. A paresthesia may be noted in the sole of the
foot. The needle is withdrawn 1 cm from the point of
bony contact, and 5–10 ml of local anesthetic is
injected in a fan-shaped area.

    e. The **sural nerve** is blocked by inserting the needle
midway between the Achilles tendon and the lateral
malleolus, directed toward the posterior surface of
the lateral malleolus. Bone is contacted, the needle
is withdrawn, and 5 ml of local anesthetic is injected.

D. Complications include epidural blockade with potential
sympathetic block accompanying lumbar plexus block,
intravascular injection, inadvertent arterial puncture,
and neural trauma (particularly if a paresthesia technique was performed).

SUGGESTED READING

Cousins, M. J., and Bridenbaugh, P. O. *Neural Blockade in
Clinical Anesthesia and Management of Pain* (2nd ed.). Philadelphia: Lippincott, 1988.

Lanz, E., et al. The extent of blockade following various techniques of brachial plexus block. *Anesth. Analg.* 62:55, 1983.

Miller, R. D. *Anesthesia* (3rd ed.). New York: Churchill Livingstone, 1991.

Parkinson, S. K., et al. Extent of blockade with various approaches to the lumbar plexus. *Anesth. Analg.* 68:243, 1989.

Raj, P. P. *Clinical Practice of Regional Anesthesia.* New York: Churchill Livingstone, 1991.

Rorie, D. K., et al. Assessment of block of the sciatic nerve in the popliteal fossa. *Anesth. Analg.* 59:371, 1980.

Scott, D. B. *Techniques of Regional Anesthesia.* Norwalk, CT: Appleton and Lange, 1989.

Vongvises, P., and Panijayanond, T. A parascalene technique of brachial plexus anesthesia. *Anesth. Analg.* 58:267, 1979.

Wildsmith, J. A. W., and Armitage, E. N. *Principles and Practice of Regional Anesthesia.* Edinburgh: Churchill Livingstone, 1987.

Winnie, A. P. *Plexus Anesthesia,* vol. 1. Philadelphia: Saunders, 1990.

Winnie, A. P., and Collins, V. J. The subclavian perivascular technique of brachial plexus anesthesia. *Anesthesiology* 25(3):353, 1964.

18

Intraanesthetic Problems

Douglas Raines, Bobby Su-Pen Chang, and
Onofrio Patafio

I. **Common problems**
  A. **Hypotension** is a significant decrease of arterial blood
     pressure below the patient's normal range. It may be due
     to a decrease in cardiac function (contractility), systemic
     vascular resistance, or venous return.
     1. **Contractility**
        a. Most anesthetic agents, including inhalation
           agents, barbiturates, and benzodiazepines (see
           Chap. 11), cause a dose-dependent, direct myocar-
           dial depression. **Opiates** are not myocardial depres-
           sants when used in the usual clinical doses.
        b. **Cardiac medications** such as beta antagonists,
           calcium channel blockers, and lidocaine are myocar-
           dial depressants.
        c. **Cardiac dysfunction** may occur with myocardial
           ischemia or infarction, hypocalcemia, severe acido-
           sis or alkalosis, hypothermia less than 32°C, cor
           pulmonale, vagal reflexes, and systemic toxicity
           from local anesthetics (particularly bupivacaine).
     2. **Decreased systemic vascular resistance (SVR)**
        a. **Isoflurane,** and to a lesser extent halothane and
           enflurane, produce a decrease in SVR.
        b. **Opiates** produce loss of vascular tone by reducing
           sympathetic nervous system outflow. Morphine can
           release histamine with resultant vasodilation.
        c. Large doses of **benzodiazepines** may decrease
           SVR, partially when administered with opiates.
        d. A decrease in SVR can be seen with many of the
           drugs used during anesthesia.
           (1) **Direct vasodilators** (nitroprusside, nitroglyc-
               erin, hydralazine).
           (2) **Alpha-adrenergic blockers** (droperidol, chlor-
               promazine, phentolamine, labetalol).
           (3) **Histamine releasers** (curare).
           (4) **Ganglionic inhibitors** (trimethaphan).
           (5) **Calcium channel blockers.**
           (6) **ACE inhibitors.**
        e. **Sympathetic blockade** occurs frequently during
           spinal and epidural anesthesia.
        f. **Septic shock** causes release of vasoactive sub-
           stances that mediate hypotension.
        g. **Vasoactive metabolites** (e.g., bowel manipulation,
           tourniquet release) may cause hypotension.
        h. **Allergic reactions** (see sec. II.I) may cause pro-
           found hypotension.
     3. **Inadequate venous return**
        a. **Hypovolemia** may result from blood loss, insensi-
           ble evaporative losses, preoperative deficits (e.g.,
           NPO status, vomiting, diarrhea, nasogastric tube

suction, enteric drains, and bowel preparations), polyuria (secondary to diuretics, diabetes mellitus, diabetes insipidus, postobstructive diuresis), and adrenal insufficiency.

b. Caval compression may result from surgical maneuvers or a gravid uterus.

c. Increased venous capacitance may occur with sympathetic blockade from ganglionic blockers and regional anesthesia, vasodilators (nitroglycerin), histamine-releasing medications, and induction agents (e.g., barbiturates and propofol).

d. Increased right atrial pressure from increased intrathoracic pressure during ventilation with large tidal volumes and positive end-expiratory pressure (PEEP) will impair venous return. Other etiologies include pulmonary hypertension, right ventricular diastolic dysfunction from ischemia, volume overload, valvular heart disease, pneumothorax, and cardiac tamponade.

4. Arrhythmias

a. Tachyarrhythmias result in hypotension from decreased diastolic filling time.

b. Atrial fibrillation, atrial flutter, and **junctional rhythms** cause hypotension from loss of the atrial contribution to diastolic filling. This is particularly pronounced in patients with valvular heart disease or diastolic dysfunction, where atrial contraction accounts for greater than 30% of end-diastolic volume.

c. Bradyarrhythmias may cause hypotension if preload reserve is inadequate to maintain a compensatory increase in stroke volume.

5. Treatment should be directed toward correcting the underlying cause and may include

a. Decreasing anesthetic depth.

b. Volume expansion to improve cardiac filling.

c. Repositioning the patient in the Trendelenburg posture to increase venous return.

d. Vasopressor support to increase vascular resistance or decrease venous capacitance (e.g., phenylephrine) and increase stroke volume (e.g., dopamine).

e. Correction of mechanical causes such as placement of a chest tube for pneumothorax, reducing or eliminating PEEP, changing from mechanical ventilation to hand ventilation, or relieving obstruction of the vena cava (e.g., left uterine displacement for a pregnant patient).

f. Cardiac ischemia or arrhythmias should be treated.

g. Vagolytic drugs should be administered to increase heart rate, and cardiac pacing is useful for heart block.

B. Hypertension

1. Etiologies

a. Catecholamine excess, which may be seen with inadequate anesthesia (especially during laryngoscopy, intubation, and emergence); hypoxia; hypercarbia; patient anxiety, fear, or pain during a regional anesthetic; and prolonged tourniquet use.

b. **Preexisting disease** (e.g., essential hypertension).

c. **Increased intracranial pressure.**

d. **Systemic absorption of vasoconstrictors** such as epinephrine, phenylephrine, and cocaine.

e. **Aortic cross-clamping.**

f. **Rebound hypertension** from discontinuation of clonidine, beta blockers, or alpha-methyldopa.

g. **Drug-drug interactions.** Tricyclic antidepressants and monoamine oxidase inhibitors given with ephedrine may cause an exaggerated hypertensive response.

h. **Bladder distention** can cause hypertension.

i. **Hypervolemia.**

j. **Administration of indigo carmine dye** (via an alpha-adrenergic effect).

2. **Treatment** is directed toward correcting the underlying cause and may include

a. Improving oxygenation and ventilatory abnormalities.

b. Increasing depth of anesthesia.

c. Sedating an anxious patient or emptying a full bladder.

d. **Medications.** For further discussion, see Chap. 19.

(1) **Beta antagonists**

(a) Labetalol, 5- to 10-mg increments IV.

(b) Propranolol, 0.5- to 1.0-mg increments IV.

(c) Esmolol, 5- to 10-mg increments IV.

(2) **Vasodilators**

(a) Hydralazine, 5–20 mg IV.

(b) Nitroglycerin infusion starting at 20 μg/min IV and increasing until desired effect.

(c) Nitroprusside infusion, 20 μg/min IV and titrating to effect.

(d) Trimethaphan infusion, 1 mg/min IV and titrating to effect.

C. **Arrhythmias**

1. **Sinus bradycardia** is a heart rate less than 60 beats/min. Unless there is severe underlying heart disease, hemodynamic changes are minimal. With slow ventricular rates, atrial and ventricular ectopic escape beats or rhythms occur more commonly.

a. **Etiologies**

(1) **Hypoxia.**

(2) **Intrinsic cardiac disease** such as sick sinus syndrome, complete (third-degree) heart block, and acute myocardial infarction (MI) (particularly inferior wall MI).

(3) **Medications** such as succinylcholine (especially in young children), anticholinesterases, beta antagonists, calcium channel blockers, digoxin, and narcotics.

(4) **Increased vagal tone** occurs with traction on the peritoneum or spermatic cord, the oculocardiac reflex, direct pressure on the vagus nerve or

carotid sinus during neck or intrathoracic surgery, centrally mediated vagal response from anxiety or pain, and Valsalva maneuvers.

(5) **Increased intracranial pressure.**

b. **Treatment**

(1) Verify adequate oxygenation and ventilation.

(2) **Bradycardia due to increased vagal tone** requires discontinuation of the provocative stimulus. Atropine (0.4–0.8 mg IV) may be needed.

(3) In patients with **intrinsic cardiac disease,** treatment should proceed with atropine (0.4–0.8 mg IV), chronotropes (e.g., ephedrine, isoproterenol), and cardiac pacing.

2. **Sinus tachycardia** is a heart rate greater than 100 beats/min. The rate is regular and rarely exceeds 160 beats/min.

a. **Etiologies** include catecholamine excess, hypercarbia, hypoxia, hypotension, hypovolemia, medications (e.g., pancuronium, atropine, ephedrine), fever, MI, pulmonary embolism, malignant hyperthermia, pheochromocytoma, and thyrotoxicosis.

b. **Treatment** should be directed toward correcting the underlying cause and may include

(1) Correcting oxygenation and ventilatory abnormalities.

(2) Increasing the depth of anesthesia.

(3) Optimizing intravascular volume.

(4) **Medications** such as narcotics and beta antagonists. High-risk patients with coronary artery disease should be treated with beta antagonists to control heart rate while the cause is being determined.

3. **Heart block**

a. **First-degree atrioventricular (AV) block** is prolongation of the P–R interval for 0.2 msec or longer. In first-degree block, every atrial pulse is transmitted to the ventricle.

b. **Second-degree AV block** can be divided into two types: Mobitz 1 (Wenckebach) and Mobitz 2.

(1) **Mobitz 1** usually occurs when a conduction defect is in the AV node and is manifested by a progressive P–R prolongation culminating in a nonconducted P wave. It is generally benign.

(2) **Mobitz 2** is a block in or distal to the AV node with a constant P–R interval. It is more likely to progress to third-degree block.

c. **Third-degree heart block** is usually due to lesions distal to the His bundle and is characterized by the complete absence of AV conduction. Usually a slow ventricular rate is seen (< 45/min). P waves occur regularly but are independent of QRS complexes (AV dissociation).

4. **Treatment**

a. **First-degree heart block** does not require specific treatment in the absence of severe bradycardia or hypotension.

   b. Second-degree heart block
   - (1) **Mobitz 1** requires treatment only if bradycardia, congestive heart failure, or bundle branch block occurs. Transvenous pacing may be necessary, particularly during inferior MIs.
   - (2) **Mobitz 2** may require temporary pacemaker insertion.
   c. Third-degree heart block requires pacemaker insertion.
   d. Useful **medications** include atropine and isoproterenol.
   e. External transcutaneous pacing is an additional option.
D. **Supraventricular tachycardias** originate at or above the bundle of His, and the resulting QRS complexes are narrow except during aberrant conduction.
   1. **Premature atrial contractions** (PACs) occur when ectopic foci in the atria fire before the next expected impulse from the sinus node. The P wave of a PAC characteristically looks different from preceding P waves, and the P–R interval may vary from normal. Early PACs may cause aberrant QRS complexes or be nonconducted to the ventricle, if the latter is still in a refractory period. PACs are common and benign and usually require no treatment.
   2. **Junctional or atrioventricular nodal rhythms** are characterized by absent or abnormal P waves and normal QRS complexes. Although they may indicate ischemic cardiac disease, junctional rhythms are commonly seen in normal individuals receiving inhalation anesthesia. In the patient whose cardiac output depends heavily on the contribution from atrial contraction, stroke volume and blood pressure may decline precipitously. Treatment should include the following:
      a. Reduction of anesthetic depth.
      b. Increasing intravascular volume.
      c. Atropine in increments of 0.2 mg IV may convert a slow junctional rhythm to sinus rhythm, particularly if secondary to a vagal mechanism.
      d. Propranolol in increments of 0.25 mg IV may be used.
      e. If the arrhythmia is associated with hypotension, increasing the blood pressure with vasopressors (e.g., ephedrine or norepinephrine) may be required.
      f. If necessary, atrial pacing may be instituted to restore atrial contraction.
   3. **Atrial fibrillation** is an irregular rhythm with an atrial rate of 350–600 beats/min and a variable ventricular response. It may be seen with myocardial ischemia, mitral valvular disease, hyperthyroidism, excessive sympathetic stimulation, or digitalis toxicity, following pneumonectomy, or when the heart has been manipulated. Treatment is based on the hemodynamic status.
      a. Rapid ventricular rate with **stable hemodynamics** can be treated with propranolol (0.5-mg increments

IV), esmolol (5- to 10-mg increments), or verapamil (5- to 10-mg increments).

b. Rapid ventricular rate with **unstable hemodynamics** requires synchronized cardioversion starting with 25–50 joules.

4. **Atrial flutter** is an irregular rhythm with an atrial rate of 250–350 beats/min and a characteristic sawtooth configuration. It is seen in patients with underlying heart disease (i.e., rheumatic heart disease and mitral stenosis). A 1:1 or 2:1 block will result in a rapid ventricular rate (usually 150 beats/min). Treatment includes digoxin (if digitalis toxicity is not a likely cause), propranolol, esmolol, verapamil, or cardioversion.

5. **Paroxysmal supraventricular tachycardia** is a tachyarrhythmia (atrial and ventricular rates of 150–250 beats/min) with reentry usually through the AV node. This rhythm may be associated with Wolff-Parkinson-White syndrome, thyrotoxicosis, or mitral valve prolapse. Patients without heart disease may develop this due to stress, caffeine, or excess catecholamines. Treatment includes carotid sinus massage, verapamil, propanolol, digoxin, edrophonium, or phenylephrine. Cardioversion may be required for the hemodynamically unstable patient.

E. **Ventricular arrhythmias**
1. **Premature ventricular contractions** (PVCs) are bizarre, widened QRS complexes. When coupled alternately with normal beats, ventricular bigeminy exists. PVCs are occasionally seen in normal individuals. Under anesthesia they frequently occur during states of catecholamine excess, hypoxia, or hypercarbia. They may also signify myocardial ischemia or infarction, digitalis toxicity, or hypokalemia. PVCs require therapy when they are **multifocal, occur in runs, increase in frequency,** or **land on or near the preceding T wave** (R-on-T phenomenon); these situations may precede the development of ventricular tachycardia, ventricular fibrillation, and cardiac arrest. Treatment in an otherwise healthy individual includes increasing alveolar ventilation, improving oxygenation, and deepening anesthesia. Patients with coronary artery disease who continue to have ventricular irritability should be given lidocaine, 1 mg/kg IV, followed by a lidocaine infusion at 1–2 mg/min. Refractory ventricular ectopy may require further treatment (see Chap. 36).

2. **Ventricular tachycardia** is a dangerous widecomplex tachyarrhythmia at a rate of 150–250 beats/min. Lidocaine and cardioversion are the first-line therapy (see Chap. 36 for treatment).

3. **Ventricular fibrillation** is chaotic ventricular activity resulting in ineffective ventricular contractions. Defibrillation and cardiopulmonary resuscitation (CPR) are required (see Chap. 36 for treatment).

4. **Ventricular preexcitation. Wolff-Parkinson-White**

syndrome is due to an accessory pathway connecting the atria and ventricle. The most common mechanism is characterized by antegrade conduction through the normal AV conduction system and retrograde conduction through the accessory pathway. Characteristic electrocardiographic (ECG) findings include a short P–R interval, a wide QRS complex, and a slurred delta wave at the onset of the QRS. Tachyarrhythmias are common. Treatment involves administration of verapamil or cardioversion. These patients are at high risk for ventricular fibrillation.

F. Hypoxia results when oxygen delivery to the tissues is insufficient to meet their metabolic demands.

1. Intraoperative etiologies

a. Inadequate oxygen supply

(1) Empty reserve oxygen tanks with loss of the main pipeline supply.

(2) A tank containing something other than oxygen connected to the oxygen yoke.

(3) An oxygen flowmeter that is leaking or not turned to a sufficient flow.

(4) Breathing system disconnection.

(5) Large leaks in the anesthesia machine, ventilator, carbon dioxide absorber, or breathing circuit or around the endotracheal tube.

(6) Obstructed endotracheal tube.

(7) Malpositioned intubation (e.g., esophageal).

b. Hypoventilation (see sec. **G**).

c. Ventilation-perfusion inequalities are seen in atelectasis, pneumonia, pulmonary edema, and other parenchymal pathologic states. Other causes include compression from packs and retractors and endobronchial intubation.

d. Reduction in oxygen-carrying capacity. Oxygen-carrying capacity is reduced with shock, anemia, methemoglobinemia, and hemoglobinopathies.

e. A left shift of the hemoglobin-oxygen dissociation curve results from hypothermia, decreased 2, 3-diphosphoglycerate concentration, alkalosis, and hypocarbia.

f. Right-to-left cardiac shunt.

g. Shock from any cause produces inadequate tissue perfusion.

2. Treatment

a. If the patient is being mechanically ventilated, **ventilation by hand** with 100% oxygen should be begun to assess pulmonary compliance. **Breath sounds** should be evaluated, the surgical field checked for mechanical pressure on the airway, **the endotracheal tube** examined for obstruction or dislodgement, and adequate movement of the chest wall or diaphragm confirmed.

b. Blood or secretions should be suctioned and the endotracheal tube replaced if necessary.

c. The breathing circuit, ventilator, and anesthesia

machine should be checked for a **leak.** If present, ventilation should be started with 100% oxygen via an alternate source such as an Ambu self-inflating bag until the problem is rectified.

d. Adequate oxygen delivery to the patient should be confirmed with an in-line oxygen analyzer.

e. **Tissue hypoperfusion** and **shock** from any cause will lead to hypoxia and must be properly treated.

f. **Right-to-left shunting** may occur with conditions such as ventricular septal defects, tetralogy of Fallot, pulmonary atresia, or patent ductus arteriosus in a stressed neonate, particularly when pulmonary vascular resistance is elevated. Hypoxia and hypercarbia must be prevented and adequate ventilation restored.

G. **Hypercarbia** is due either to inadequate ventilation or to increased carbon dioxide production.

1. **Inadequate ventilation**

a. **Central depression** of the medullary respiratory center can be caused by narcotics, barbiturates, benzodiazepines, and volatile agents. Controlled ventilation may be required.

b. **Neuromuscular depression** may be seen with high spinal and epidural anesthesia, phrenic nerve paralysis, and muscle relaxants.

c. **Inadequate ventilation settings** during controlled ventilation.

d. **Increased airway resistance** may occur with bronchospasm and decreased pulmonary compliance.

e. **Pulmonary etiologies** include main stem intubation, upper airway obstruction, congestive heart failure, and hemo- or pneumothorax.

f. **Rebreathing** of exhaled gases may occur from an exhausted carbon dioxide absorber, inspiratory or expiratory valve failure, or inadequate fresh gas flows in nonrebreathing systems.

g. Primary central nervous system (CNS) pathology (tumor, ischemia, edema) may compromise ventilation.

2. **Increased carbon dioxide production** results from exogenous carbon dioxide (e.g., absorption of carbon dioxide from insufflation during laparoscopy), reperfusion, total parenteral nutrition, hypermetabolic states (e.g., malignant hyperthermia), and acid-base abnormalities.

3. **Treatment**

a. **CNS depressants.** Relative **overdose of sedating premedication** may cause respiratory depression. This is particularly true for the elderly and patients with significant multisystem pathology. Patients may require a spectrum of interventions from verbal and physical stimuli to pharmacologic reversal (e.g., naloxone and flumazenil) or assisted ventilation and endotracheal intubation.

b. **Inadequate ventilation**

(1) Hypercarbia may occur if ventilator settings during **controlled ventilation** are inadequate. Most anesthesia machine ventilators have settings to adjust the rate, tidal volume, PEEP, and I:E ratio.

(2) Hypercarbia may occur in the setting of a general anesthetic when ventilation is spontaneous. This is particularly true when high concentrations of volatile anesthetic are used or when IV narcotics are administered.

c. **Increased airway resistance.** Intrinsic airway disease, foreign bodies, or mechanical irritation may cause **bronchoconstriction** and increased airway resistance.

(1) The endotracheal tube position should be checked and withdrawn slightly to avoid endobronchial placement or carinal stimulation.

(2) Foreign material such as blood or pus should be suctioned until clear.

(3) A trial of inhaled sympathomimetic is a reasonable first option, followed by IV sympathomimetic or methylxanthine (see sec. **II.B.4.c**).

d. **Rebreathing of carbon dioxide** can occur with either dysfunction of the inspiratory or expiratory flow valves or exhaustion of the carbon dioxide absorbent.

(1) Increasing the rate of fresh gas flow will minimize rebreathing as a temporizing measure.

(2) Leaking valves should be replaced or exhausted carbon dioxide absorbent changed.

e. Carbon dioxide production may be increased in certain states.

(1) The diagnosis of **malignant hyperthermia** must always be considered, particularly in a patient with concurrent unexplained tachycardia (see sec. **II.H**).

(2) **Sepsis** is a common cause of hypercarbia, particularly in patients with lung disease. Minute ventilation should be increased and appropriate antibiotics administered.

(3) Hypercarbia is commonly seen during **surgical procedures** such as with carbon dioxide laparoscopy, aortic reperfusion after cross-clamp release, or limb reperfusion after use of a tourniquet. This is easily corrected by a brief period of increased minute ventilation.

H. **Urine output** is normally 0.5–1.0 ml/kg/hr.

1. **Low urine output** (oliguria) is less than 20 ml/hr. Prerenal, intrarenal, and postrenal causes are described in Chap. 4.

a. Treatment includes ruling out mechanical causes (e.g., malpositioned or kinked Foley catheter).

b. Hypotension should be corrected to improve renal perfusion pressure.

c. Volume status should be assessed. A fluid bolus of 250 ml of crystalloid may be given if hypovolemia is suspected. If oliguria persists, a central venous pressure line may be required to help guide further fluid management. Patients with reduced ventricular function may require placement of a pulmonary artery catheter.

d. If oliguria persists, renal blood flow can be increased with

(1) Dopamine infusion, 1–2 μg/kg/min (minimal beta-1 or alpha effect).

(2) Mannitol, 12.5–25.0 gm IV.

(3) Lasix, 2–20 mg IV.

e. Intraoperative diuretics may be required to preserve urine output in patients on chronic diuretic therapy.

2. **Anuria** is a rare occurrence in the perioperative period. Mechanical causes including ureteral damage or transection must be excluded (as in sec. **1.a**), and hemodynamic instability must be treated.

3. **High urine output** may occur in response to vigorous fluid administration, but other causes must be considered including hyperglycemia, nephrogenic diabetes insipidus, exogenous diuretics, and theophylline. High urine output is not a problem unless associated with hypovolemia or electrolyte abnormalities. Treatment should be directed at the underlying cause.

I. **Hypothermia** is a common problem in the operative period.

1. **Heat loss** may occur from any of the following mechanisms:

a. **Radiation** accounts for 60% of heat loss. Radiant heat loss is dependent on cutaneous blood flow and exposed body surface area.

b. **Evaporation** accounts for 20% of heat loss. Heat loss occurs from the energy needed to vaporize liquid from mucosal and serosal surfaces, skin, and lungs. Evaporative loss is dependent on exposed surface area and the relative humidity of ambient gas.

c. **Conduction** is the heat transfer from a warm to a cool object. This accounts for 5% of heat loss and is proportional to the area exposed, difference in temperature, and thermal conductivity.

d. **Convection** is the loss of heat by conduction to a moving gas and accounts for 15% of heat loss. The high air flow in the operating room (10–15 room volume changes per hour) results in significant heat loss.

2. **Pediatric patients** are particularly susceptible to intraoperative hypothermia (see Chap. 28).

3. **Geriatric patients** are also more prone to hypothermia (see Chap. 26).

4. **Anesthetic effects.** Volatile anesthetics impair the thermoregulatory center located in the posterior hypothalamus and predispose to heat loss due to their vasodilatory properties. Narcotics will reduce the vasoconstriction mechanism for heat conservation because of their sympatholytic properties. Muscle relaxants

reduce muscle tone and prevent shivering. Regional anesthesia produces sympathetic blockade, muscle relaxation, and sensory blockade of thermal receptors inhibiting compensatory responses.

5. **Hypothermia** is associated with a number of physiologic changes.

   a. **Cardiovascular.** Increased SVR, ventricular arrhythmias, and myocardial depression may occur.

   b. **Metabolic.** Decreased metabolic rate, decreased tissue perfusion leading to metabolic acidosis, and hyperglycemia (from catecholamine response) may occur.

   c. **Pulmonary.** Increased pulmonary vascular resistance and decreased hypoxic pulmonary vasoconstriction occur.

   d. **Hematologic.** Increased blood viscosity, leftward shift of the hemoglobin dissociation curve, impaired coagulation, and thrombocytopenia occur.

   e. **Neurologic.** Decreased cerebral blood flow, increased cerebrovascular resistance, decreased minimum alveolar concentration, delayed emergence from anesthesia, drowsiness, and confusion may occur.

   f. **Drug disposition.** Decreased hepatic blood flow and metabolism coupled with decreased renal blood flow and clearance result in decreased anesthetic requirement.

   g. **Shivering** can increase heat production by 100–300%. However there is a concomitant increase in oxygen consumption up to 500% and increased production of carbon dioxide.

   h. **Renal.** Cold diuresis secondary to impaired sodium resorption and decreased renal blood flow may lead to hypovolemia.

6. **Prevention and treatment of hypothermia**

   a. **Maintain or raise ambient temperature.** All anesthetized patients will become hypothermic if room temperature is below 21°C.

   b. **Covering exposed surfaces** will minimize conductive and convective losses (i.e., use a blanket or a plastic bag over the arms and head).

   c. **Warming IV fluids and blood during transfusion** is essential in cases requiring large fluid replacement (see Chap. 14).

   d. **Heated humidifiers** added to the anesthetic circuit will warm and humidify inspired gas, minimizing evaporative loss from the lungs. The temperature of inspired gas must be monitored and kept below 105°F, otherwise there is potential for scalding of the airway. Alternatively, "artificial noses" (passive heat and moisture exchangers) can be placed between the endotracheal tube and breathing circuit. These are high surface area hydroscopic membrane filters that trap the warmth and humidity of expired air.

   e. Use of **closed or low-flow semiclosed circuit**

anesthesia will also decrease evaporative losses. This will provide rebreathing of gases that have been warmed and humidified by previous transit through the lungs.

   f. **Warming blankets** placed beneath the patient can raise body temperature by conduction from warm water pumped through the blanket. This method is most effective in children less than 10 kg. The temperature should be kept below 40°C to avoid burns. Forced air exchange blankets provide both insulation and active cutaneous warming.

   g. **Radiant warmers** and **heating lamps** warm patients by infrared radiation and are only useful for infants. The warming lamps should be kept at least 70 cm from the patient to avoid burns.

   h. Use of **warm irrigation solutions** will reduce heat loss.

J. Hyperthermia is a rise in temperature of 2°C/hr or 0.5°C/15 min. It is rare for a patient to become hyperthermic as a result of maneuvers to conserve body heat in the operating room. Since a decrease in temperature during anesthesia is usually the rule, any rise in temperature must be investigated. Hyperthermia and its accompanying hypermetabolic state produce an increase in oxygen consumption, cardiac work, glucose demand, metabolic acidosis, and compensatory minute ventilation. Sweating and vasodilatation will result in decreased intravascular volume and venous return. Extreme temperatures higher than 42.2°C may cause CNS damage.

  1. Etiologies

    a. **Malignant hyperthermia** must be considered during any perioperative temperature increase (see sec. **II.H**).

    b. **Hypermetabolic states** such as sepsis, infection, thyrotoxicosis, pheochromocytoma, and transfusion reactions may cause hyperthermia.

    c. **Injury** to the hypothalamic thermoregulatory center from anoxia, edema, trauma, or tumor may affect temperature set points in the hypothalamus.

    d. **Neuroleptic malignant syndrome** from neuroleptics such as phenothiazines is a rare cause in this setting.

    e. **Sympathomimetics** such as monoamine oxidase inhibitors, amphetamines, cocaine, and tricyclic antidepressants may produce a hypermetabolic state. Anticholinergics, such as atropine and glycopyrrolate, may also promote unopposed sympathetic vasoconstriction and suppress sweating.

  2. Treatment. Extreme hyperthermia can be treated by cooling exposed body surfaces (skin) or by performing internal lavage (stomach, bladder, bowel, and peritoneum) using cold saline, ice, cooling blankets, and reduced ambient temperature. Volatile liquids such as alcohol and freon applied to the skin will promote evaporative heat loss. Conductive heat loss can be increased with vasodilators such as nitroprusside and nitroglycerin. Centrally active agents such as aspirin and acetaminophen can be given by nasogastric tube or through the rectum. If malignant hyperthermia is suspected, dantrolene treatment must be initiated.

K. **Sweating** (diaphoresis) may occur in response to the sympathetic discharge caused by anxiety, pain, hypercarbia, or noxious stimuli in the presence of inadequate anesthesia. It may also be seen in conjunction with bradycardia, nausea, and hypotension as part of a generalized vagal reaction or as a thermoregulatory response to hyperthermia.

II. Life-threatening problems

A. Laryngospasm

1. Laryngospasm is most commonly caused by an **irritative stimulus to the airway** during a light plane of anesthesia. Common noxious stimuli that may elicit this reflex include secretions, vomitus, blood, inhalation of pungent volatile anesthetics, oropharyngeal or nasopharyngeal airway placement, laryngoscopy, painful peripheral stimuli, and peritoneal traction during light anesthesia.

2. **Reflex closure of the vocal cords,** causing partial or total glottic obstruction, may be manifested in less severe cases by crowing respirations or stridor and, when complete, by a "rocking" obstructed pattern of breathing. In this situation, the abdominal wall rises with contraction of the diaphragm during inspiration, but because air entry is blocked, the chest sinks or fails to expand. During expiration, the abdomen falls as the diaphragm relaxes, and the chest returns to its original position. With complete obstruction, the anesthesiologist will not be able to ventilate the patient.

3. The hypoxia, hypercarbia, and acidosis that result will cause hypertension and tachycardia. Hypotension, bradycardia, and ventricular arrhythmias leading to cardiac arrest will ensue unless airway patency is restored within minutes. Children, because of their small functional residual capacity and relatively high oxygen consumption, are particularly prone to these complications.

4. **Treatment.** Deepening the anesthetic level and removing the stimulus (e.g., by suction, withdrawal of an artificial airway, or stopping peripheral stimulation) while administering 100% oxygen may be adequate to relieve laryngospasm. If laryngospasm is not relieved, continuous positive pressure on the airway with a good mask fit may "break" the spasm, and if not, a small dose of succinylcholine (e.g., 10–20 mg in an adult) will relax the striated muscles of the larynx. The patient should be ventilated with 100% oxygen, and either the anesthetic level should be deepened before the noxious stimulation is resumed or the patient may be allowed to awaken if laryngospasm has occurred during emergence.

B. Bronchospasm

1. **Reflex bronchiolar constriction** may be centrally

mediated, as in asthma, or it may be a local response to airway irritation. Bronchospasm is common in anaphylactoid drug and blood transfusion reactions, as well as in cigarette smokers and those with chronic bronchitis. Like laryngospasm, bronchospasm may be elicited by noxious stimuli such as secretions or endotracheal intubation.

2. Bronchospasm can be detected by characteristic wheezing (usually more pronounced on expiration) and is associated with tachypnea and dyspnea in the awake patient. An anesthetized patient may be difficult to ventilate due to diminished compliance. The marked increase in airway pressures required for ventilation may cause air trapping, hypoxemia, impaired venous return, and decreased cardiac output.

3. **Histamine-releasing drugs** (e.g., morphine, *d*-tubocurarine, atracurium, or metocurine) and **beta-adrenergic antagonists** may exacerbate bronchoconstriction.

4. **Treatment**
   a. The endotracheal tube's position should be checked and withdrawn slightly, as **carinal** stimulation is a potential cause.
   b. **Deepening the anesthetic level** will frequently reverse bronchospasm that is secondary to "light anesthesia." This can usually be accomplished with an inhalation agent, but an intravenous agent may be necessary when ventilation is significantly impaired. Ketamine has the advantage of causing bronchodilatation by releasing endogenous catecholamines, but propofol or barbiturates are acceptable choices. If oxygenation is impaired, the inspired oxygen concentration should be increased.
   c. **Inhaled bronchodilators** have limited systemic absorption, which may minimize cardiovascular side effects. Nebulized forms may contain large particles, which deposit to a large extent in tubing and upper airways. Metered dose inhalers (MDI) are effective when properly used. Specific agents include
      (1) **Beta-adrenergic agonists,** which stimulate beta-2 receptors on bronchial smooth muscle, producing bronchodilatation.
         (a) **Isoetharine** (Bronkosol, 0.5 ml/2.5 ml of saline q3–4h) has the lowest beta-2 selectivity.
         (b) **Albuterol** (Proventil or Ventolin-MDI, 2 puffs q3–4h, or nebulizer with 0.3 ml/2–3 ml of saline q4–6h) is more beta-2 selective.
         (c) **Metaproterenol** (Alupent-MDI, 2 puffs q3–4h, or nebulizer with 0.3 ml/2.5 ml of saline q4–6h) is more selective than isoetharine and less than albuterol.
      (2) **Steroids. Beclomethasone** (Vanceril-MDI, 2 puffs q6h) is an inhaled corticosteroid useful in chronic bronchial asthma. It is not effective in acute exacerbations. Little systemic absorption

occurs, thus avoiding systemic side effects such as adrenal suppression.

    d. Intravenous agents

      (1) Sympathomimetics. Stimulation of beta-2 receptors in the lung activates adenylate cyclase, increasing intracellular levels of cyclic adenosine monophosphate (cAMP), which produces bronchial smooth muscle relaxation.

        (a) Epinephrine is a powerful bronchodilator. At low dose (0.25–1.0 μg/min), beta-2 effects predominate, with an increase in heart rate due to beta-1 stimulation. At higher doses, alpha effects become predominant, with large increases in systolic blood pressure.

        (b) Isoproterenol is a nonselective beta agonist that produces tachycardia in a dose-dependent manner and to a greater extent than low-dose epinephrine.

        (c) Terbutaline sulfate (0.25 mg SQ, which may be repeated in 15 minutes but no more than 0.5 mg total in a 4 hour period, is a relatively selective beta-2 agonist, although it may produce tachycardia in some patients.

      (2) Methylxanthines (aminophylline, 5 mg/kg/30 min IV load, then 0.5–1.0 mg/kg/hr). The mechanism of action of theophylline is controversial but is most likely due to endogenous catecholamine release. It also increases intracellular cAMP concentration through inhibition of phosphodiesterase, producing bronchodilatation. Although widely used in both acute and chronic reactive airway disease, this drug has a very narrow therapeutic-toxic ratio, and metabolism can be altered in many circumstances (e.g., increased by smoking and decreased by some antibiotics, age, liver disease, and anesthetics). Manifestations of toxicity include nausea, vomiting, headache, restlessness, irritability, hypotension, tachycardia, arrhythmias, and seizures.

      (3) Corticosteroids. IV glucocorticoids (methylprednisolone [Solu-Medrol], 30–60 mg IV q6h) are useful in acute asthmatic exacerbations, as they decrease inflammation and inhibit histamine release and arachidonic acid metabolism. Beneficial effects may take hours, however, and should be used to supplement the effects of sympathomimetics.

    e. Adequate hydration and humidification of inspired gases will minimize inspissation of secretions and facilitate ventilation. However, ultrasonic aerosols are irritating and may increase airway resistance.

C. Aspiration. General anesthesia causes a depression of airway reflexes that predisposes patients to aspiration. Aspiration of gastric contents from vomiting or regurgitation may cause bronchospasm, hypoxemia, atelectasis, tachypnea, tachycardia, and hypotension. The severity of symptoms depends on the volume and pH of the gastric material aspirated. An aspirate with a pH less than 2.5 in a volume greater than 0.4 cc/kg is associated with increased morbidity. Conditions that predispose to aspiration include gastric outlet obstruction, small-bowel obstruction, symptomatic hiatal hernia, pregnancy, severe obesity, and recent food ingestion.

1. If vomiting or regurgitation occurs in an **anesthetized patient whose airway is not protected by an endotracheal tube,** the patient should be placed in Trendelenburg position to minimize passive flow of gastric contents into the trachea, the head should be turned to the side, the upper airway suctioned, and an endotracheal tube placed. Suctioning the endotracheal tube prior to instituting positive-pressure ventilation avoids forcing gastric contents into the distal airways. Evidence of significant aspiration includes wheezing, decreased lung compliance, and hypoxemia. Arterial blood gases and a chest x-ray should be obtained, but radiographic evidence of infiltrates may be delayed. Bronchodilators such as aminophylline or beta agonists may be useful.

2. Aspiration of **solid foreign bodies** such as teeth and food may require bronchoscopy and lavage.

3. Aspiration of **blood,** unless of large volume, is usually clinically benign.

4. **Antibiotics** are not routinely administered unless signs of bacterial infection develop.

5. **Sputum** Gram's stain and cultures should be done daily.

6. The use of high-dose **steroids** for the treatment of aspiration remains controversial and is usually not advised.

7. If **significant aspiration** has occurred, it is imperative that close postoperative observation in an intensive care unit be undertaken. This includes pulse oximetry, arterial blood gases, and repeat chest x-rays. Intubation and mechanical ventilation may be necessary.

D. **Pneumothorax**

1. **Etiologies.** A pneumothorax is the accumulation of gas within the pleural space. It may occur in a number of situations:

a. Spontaneous rupture of blebs and bullae.

b. Blunt or penetrating chest trauma.

c. Surgical entrance into the pleural space during thoracic, upper abdominal, or retroperitoneal surgery, tracheostomy, or surgery of the chest wall or neck.

d. As a complication of procedures such as subclavian or internal jugular vein catheter placement, thoracentesis, pericardiocentesis, and intercostal nerve blockade.

e. During positive-pressure ventilation using high pressures and volumes, causing barotrauma and alveolar rupture. Patients with chronic obstructive pulmonary disease are at particularly high risk.

   f. Malfunction of chest tubes.

2. **Physiologic effects** of pneumothoraces are largely a function of the gas volume and the rate of expansion. Small pneumothoraces may have no significant cardiopulmonary effect, while larger ones may result in significant lung collapse and hypoxemia. A **tension pneumothorax** occurs when there is a one-way leak into the pleural space, causing a significant increase in intrapleural pressure. This can result in compression of major blood vessels and mediastinal shift with hypotension and a reduction in cardiac output.

3. The **diagnosis** of pneumothorax can be difficult to make. Signs of pneumothorax include wheezing, decreased breath sounds, a reduction in lung compliance, an increase in peak inspiratory pressure, and hypoxemia. Hypotension reflects the presence of a tension pneumothorax.

4. **Treatment. Nitrous oxide should be discontinued,** and the patient should be ventilated with 100% oxygen. Tension pneumothoraces require immediate evacuation. A large-bore catheter (14- to 16-gauge) on a 10-ml syringe is inserted at the second or third intercostal space in the midclavicular line and aspirated to confirm the presence of air. A chest tube is then placed at the eighth intercostal space in the posterior axillary line.

E. **Myocardial ischemia**

1. **Etiology.** Myocardial ischemia is the result of an imbalance between myocardial oxygen supply and consumption and, if untreated, may lead to myocardial infarction.

2. **Clinical features**

   a. In the awake patient, myocardial ischemia may manifest as chest pain. However, asymptomatic ischemia is common in the perioperative period, particularly in diabetic patients. In patients under general anesthesia, hemodynamic instability and ECG changes may occur with ischemia.

   b. ECG changes such as ST-segment depression greater than 1 mm or T-wave inversion may indicate subendocardial ischemia. ST-segment elevation is seen with transmural myocardial ischemia. ST-segment changes may also be seen with electrolyte abnormalities. Lead V_5 is the most sensitive lead for detecting ischemia (see Chap. 10).

   c. Other indicators of ischemia include

      (1) Hypotension.

      (2) Changes in central filling pressures or cardiac output as detected with a pulmonary artery catheter.

      (3) Regional wall motion abnormalities as detected with transesophageal echocardiography.

3. **Treatment**

   a. Hypoxemia and anemia should be corrected to maximize myocardial oxygen delivery.

b. Nitroglycerin (starting at 0.5 μg/kg/min IV or 0.15 mg SL) reduces ventricular diastolic pressure and volume through venodilation and leads to a decrease in myocardial oxygen demand. Additionally, nitroglycerin can improve oxygen delivery by coronary artery dilatation.

c. Beta-adrenergic antagonists (propranolol in 0.5- to 1.0-mg increments IV or esmolol in 5- to 10-mg increments IV) decrease myocardial oxygen consumption by decreasing heart rate and contractility.

d. Myocardial ischemia occurring in the setting of hypotension may require a vasopressor such as phenylephrine (10–30 μg/min) or norepinephrine (1–5 μg/min) to improve myocardial perfusion pressure. Anesthetic depth may need to be decreased and intravascular volume optimized.

e. When myocardial ischemia results in a significant reduction in cardiac output and hypotension (cardiogenic shock), positive inotropes such as dopamine (5–20 μg/kg/min) or norepinephrine (5–15 μg/min) are indicated. Insertion of a pulmonary artery catheter is required to assess ventricular function and response to therapy.

f. Intraaortic balloon counterpulsation may ultimately be required to augment cardiac output (see Chap. 23).

F. Pulmonary embolism is the obstruction of pulmonary blood flow by thrombus, air, fat, or amniotic fluid.

1. Thromboemboli most commonly arise from the deep venous system of the pelvis and lower extremities. Predisposing factors for the development of thrombi are stasis, hypercoagulability, and vascular wall abnormalities. Associated conditions include pregnancy, trauma, carcinoma, prolonged bed rest, and vasculitis.

a. Physical findings are fairly nonspecific and include tachypnea and tachycardia, dyspnea, rales, bronchospasm, and fever.

b. Laboratory studies. The ECG reveals a nonspecific tachycardia unless embolization is severe, in which case **right-axis deviation, right bundle branch block,** and **anterior T-wave changes** may be seen. The chest x-ray may be unremarkable unless pulmonary infarction has occurred. Blood gases typically reveal hypoxemia. With a large embolism, the end-tidal carbon dioxide will be decreased. In spontaneously breathing patients, hypocapnia and respiratory alkalosis may result from the increased respiratory rate. Definitive diagnosis requires a pulmonary angiogram.

c. Intraoperative treatment of a suspected pulmonary embolism is supportive. Oxygenation is optimized. Intraoperative heparinization or thrombolytic therapy is usually not an option due to the risk of hemorrhage. In patients who are severely hypoxic or hypotensive, cardiopulmonary bypass and pulmonary embolectomy may be considered.

2. **Air embolism** occurs during entrainment of air into a vein or venous sinus. It occurs most commonly during intracranial surgery in the sitting position, where dural venous sinuses are stented open by supporting soft tissues. Air embolism may also occur during liver transplantation, open cardiac procedures, and insufflation associated with laparoscopy.

   a. **Early indicators** include (in order of decreasing sensitivity) transesophageal echocardiography, precordial Doppler over the right atrium, a decrease in end-tidal carbon dioxide, and an increase in end-tidal nitrogen.

   b. **Late indicators** include elevation of central venous pressure, hypoxemia, hypotension, ventricular ectopy, and a "mill-wheel murmur."

   c. When air embolism is suspected, **treatment** begins with limiting the entrainment of additional air by flooding the surgical field with saline or repositioning the patient so that venous pressure is increased. If a central venous catheter is in place, it should be aspirated in an attempt to remove air. **Nitrous oxide should be discontinued** to avoid enlarging the size of bubbles within the circulation. Fluid and vasopressors are used to maintain blood pressure.

   d. The use of PEEP in the setting of air embolism is controversial. It will limit the entrainment of air by raising central venous pressure but at the expense of venous return and possibly cardiac output.

3. **Fat embolism** occurs after trauma or surgery involving the long bones, pelvis, or ribs.

   a. **Clinical features.** Initial signs and symptoms are related to mechanical obstruction of the pulmonary circulation and are similar to those found with thromboembolism. The release of free fatty acids may lead to diminished mental status, worsening hypoxemia, fat globules in the urine, and petechial hemorrhages.

   b. **Treatment** is supportive, with the administration of supplemental oxygen and ventilation as necessary.

4. **Amniotic fluid emboli.** See Chap. 29.

G. **Cardiac tamponade.** Accumulation of blood or other fluid within the pericardial sac may prevent adequate ventricular filling and result in a reduction in stroke volume and cardiac output. When the accumulation is rapid, cardiovascular collapse may occur within minutes.

1. Cardiac tamponade may be **associated** with

   a. Chest trauma.

   b. Cardiac or thoracic surgery.

   c. Pericardial tumor.

   d. Pericarditis (acute viral, pyogenic, uremic, or postradiation).

   e. Myocardial perforation by a central venous or pulmonary artery catheter.

   f. Aortic dissection.

2. **Clinical features** include tachycardia, hypotension,

jugular venous distention, muffled heart sounds, and a decrease in pulse pressure. An ECG may reveal electrical alternans and diffusely low voltage. A paradoxical pulse (greater than 10 mm Hg inspiratory decrease in systolic blood pressure) may also be appreciated. There is equalization of right and left heart pressures as reflected in identical central venous, right ventricular, pulmonary artery, and pulmonary capillary wedge pressures. Chest x-ray findings may include an enlarged cardiac silhouette. An echocardiogram is diagnostic.

3. The **treatment** of a hemodynamically unstable patient with suspected cardiac tamponade is **pericardiocentesis.** Intravascular volume should be augmented and vasopressors administered to maintain blood pressure. A long needle (i.e., 22-gauge spinal needle) is inserted between the xiphoid process and the left costal margin and directed toward the left shoulder. If the precordial lead of the ECG is attached to the needle, an injury current (ST-segment elevation) will be observed when the needle contacts the epicardium. The needle should be withdrawn slightly and aspirated. Complications of pericardiocentesis include pneumothorax, coronary artery laceration, and myocardial perforation.

H. Malignant hyperthermia

1. **Etiology.** Malignant hyperthermia is a hypermetabolic syndrome occurring in genetically susceptible patients after exposure to an anesthetic triggering agent. Triggering anesthetics include halothane, enflurane, isoflurane, desflurane, sevoflurane, and succinylcholine. The syndrome is thought to be due to a reduction in the reuptake of Ca^{2+} by the sarcoplasmic reticulum necessary for termination of muscle contraction. Consequently, muscle contraction is sustained, resulting in signs of hypermetabolism, including tachycardia, acidosis, hypercarbia, hypoxemia, and hyperthermia. The first signs of malignant hyperthermia usually occur in the operating room but may be delayed until the patient reaches the postanesthesia care unit or even the postoperative floor.

2. **Clinical features**
   a. Unexplained tachycardia.
   b. Hypercarbia or tachypnea in the spontaneously breathing patient.
   c. Acidosis.
   d. Muscle rigidity even in the presence of neuromuscular blockade. Masseter spasm after giving succinylcholine is associated with malignant hyperthermia. However, not all patients who develop masseter spasm will develop malignant hyperthermia.
   e. Hypoxemia.
   f. Ventricular arrhythmias.
   g. Hyperkalemia.
   h. Fever is a late sign.
   i. Myoglobinuria.

    j. The presence of a large difference between mixed venous and arterial carbon dioxide confirms the diagnosis of malignant hyperthermia.

3. Treatment

  a. Discontinue all anesthetics, and hyperventilate with 100% **oxygen.** Surgery should be concluded as quickly as possible and the anesthesia machine changed when feasible. It is prudent to summon help early in a suspected case of malignant hyperthermia.

  b. Administer **dantrolene** (Dantrium), 2.5 mg/kg IV initially and repeated to a total of 10 mg/kg or more if signs of malignant hyperthermia persist. It is the only known specific treatment for malignant hyperthermia. Its efficacy is due to its ability to inhibit Ca^{2+} release from the sarcoplasmic reticulum. Each ampule contains 20 mg of dantrolene and 3 gm of mannitol and should be reconstituted with 50 ml of sterile water.

  c. Sodium bicarbonate administration should be guided by arterial blood gases.

  d. Hyperkalemia may be corrected with insulin and glucose. However, hypokalemia may occur as the attack is brought under control. Calcium is avoided.

  e. Arrhythmias generally subside with resolution of the hypermetabolic phase of malignant hyperthermia. Persistent arrhythmias can be treated with procainamide.

  f. Hyperthermia is treated by a variety of methods. These include the use of refrigerated IV fluids, gastric, rectal, and bladder lavage with cold saline, and surface cooling with ice. When hyperthermia is profound, extracorporeal cooling can be used. Cooling should be stopped when body temperature reaches 38°C to avoid hypothermia. Shivering can be prevented by maintaining neuromuscular blockade using a nondepolarizing neuromuscular blocker. This reduces oxygen consumption while improving ventilatory control.

  g. Urine output should be maintained at 2 ml/kg/min to avoid renal tubular damage from myoglobin. This is done by maintaining adequate central filling pressures and administering furosemide or mannitol.

  h. Recrudescence, disseminated intravascular coagulation, and acute tubular necrosis may occur following an acute episode of malignant hyperthermia. Therefore, dantrolene therapy should be continued (1 mg/kg IV or PO q6h) and observation maintained in an intensive care unit for 48–72 hours after an episode of malignant hyperthermia.

4. Anesthesia for malignant hyperthermia–susceptible patients

  a. A family history of anesthetic problems suggesting susceptibility, such as unexplained fevers or death during anesthesia, should be sought in every patient.

b. Malignant hyperthermia may be triggered in susceptible patients who have had previous uneventful exposures to triggering agents.

c. Pretreatment with dantrolene is generally not recommended for malignant hyperthermia–susceptible patients. However, a malignant hyperthermia cart or other dantrolene supply should be present in the operating room.

d. The anesthesia machine should be prepared by changing the carbon dioxide absorbent and fresh gas tubing, disconnecting the vaporizers, using a disposable breathing circuit, and flushing the machine with oxygen at a rate of 10 L/min for 5 minutes.

e. Local or regional anesthesia should be considered, but general anesthesia with nontriggering agents is acceptable. Safe drugs for induction and maintenance of general anesthesia include barbiturates, propofol, benzodiazepines, narcotics, and nitrous oxide. Nondepolarizing neuromuscular blockers may be used and safely reversed.

f. Close monitoring for early signs of malignant hyperthermia such as unexplained hypercarbia or tachycardia is crucial.

5. Associated syndromes. An increased risk of malignant hyperthermia has been reported in association with a number of disorders. In many of these cases, the association is not well established. However, patients with the following disorders should be treated as though they are susceptible to malignant hyperthermia.

a. Duchenne muscular dystrophy and other muscular dystrophies.

b. King-Denborough syndrome, characterized by dwarfism, mental retardation, and musculoskeletal abnormalities.

c. Central core disease, a rare myopathy.

d. Neuroleptic malignant syndrome (NMS) is associated with the administration of neuroleptic drugs and shares many of the features of malignant hyperthermia.

(1) Clinical features. NMS typically develops over 24–72 hours and is clinically similar to malignant hyperthermia, presenting as a hypermetabolic episode consisting of hyperthermia, autonomic nervous system instability, pronounced muscle rigidity, and rhabdomyolysis. Creatine kinase and hepatic transaminases are often increased, and mortality approaches 30%.

(2) Treatment of NMS is with dantrolene, although benzodiazepines, dopamine antagonists like bromocriptine, and nondepolarizing muscle relaxants will also decrease muscle rigidity.

(3) Anesthetic implications

(a) The exact relationship between NMS and malignant hyperthermia is unclear. However, some patients with a history of NMS may be clinically at risk for malignant hyperthermia, and a conservative approach may be warranted (e.g., avoidance of known triggering agents).

(b) Patients with NMS must be appropriately monitored for malignant hyperthermia during all anesthetics (e.g., temperature, end-tidal carbon dioxide). They should *not* be pretreated with dantrolene.

I. Anaphylactic and anaphylactoid reactions

1. **Anaphylaxis is a life-threatening allergic reaction.** It is initiated by antigen binding to IgE antibodies on the surface of mast cells and basophils, causing release of pharmacologically active substances. These include histamine, leukotrienes, prostaglandins, kinins, platelet-activating factor, and chemotactic factors of anaphylaxis.

2. **Anaphylactoid reactions** are clinically similar to anaphylactic reactions, but they are *not* mediated by IgE and do not require prior sensitization to an antigen.

3. **Clinical features** of anaphylactic or anaphylactoid reactions include
   a. Urticaria and flushing.
   b. Bronchospasm or airway edema leading to respiratory compromise or collapse.
   c. Hypotension and shock due to peripheral vasodilatation and increased capillary permeability.
   d. Pulmonary edema.

4. **Treatment**
   a. In the presence of circulatory collapse, discontinue anesthetic agents.
   b. Administer 100% oxygen. Assess the need to intubate and ventilate.
   c. Treat hypotension with intravascular volume expansion using a balanced salt solution, colloid, or both.
   d. Give **epinephrine,** 50–100 μg IV. For overt cardiovascular collapse, epinephrine, 0.5–1.0 mg IV, is indicated, followed by an infusion if hypotension persists. Other catecholamines such as norepinephrine or isoproterenol may be useful.
   e. **Steroids** (hydrocortisone, 250 mg–1.0 gm IV, or methylprednisolone, 1–2 gm IV).
   f. **Histamine antagonists** (diphenhydramine, 0.5–1.0 mg/kg IV) may be useful as second-line therapy.

5. **Prophylaxis for drug hypersensitivity reactions**
   a. **H_1 antagonists.** Diphenhydramine (0.5–1.0 mg/kg) the night before and morning of exposure.
   b. **H_2 antagonists.** Cimetidine (150–300 mg) or ranitidine (1–2 mg/kg) the night before and morning of exposure.
   c. **Corticosteroids.** Prednisone (1 mg/kg or 50 mg for adults) q6h for 4 doses prior to exposure.

J. Fire and electrical hazards in the operating room

1. **Fire in the operating room** is a rare event that requires the presence of an ignition source, fuel, and oxidizing agent (see Chap. 25).
   a. Lasers and electrocautery devices are the most common ignition sources.
   b. Fuels include alcohol, solvents, sheets and drapes, and plastic or rubber materials (including endotracheal tubes). Unlike diethyl ether and cyclopropane, modern inhalation anesthetics are not fuels.
   c. **Oxygen is by far the most common oxidizing agent,** although nitrous oxide will also support combustion. Materials that are only marginally combustible in air can produce a massive flame in the presence of high oxygen concentration. Therefore supplemental oxygen should only be administered when medically indicated.
   d. **Fire extinguishers** should be readily available in all anesthetizing locations. Carbon dioxide or Halon fire extinguishers offer the advantage of efficacy against a variety of fires without producing the particulate contamination seen with dry chemical extinguishers. During an electrical fire, it is important to remember to unplug the electrical source.
2. **Electrical safety**
   a. The electrical injury that occurs when a current passes through intact skin is known as **macroshock.** It may result in a thermal injury, or it may disrupt normal physiologic function and cause cardiac or respiratory arrest. An alternating current of 60 cycles/sec will barely be perceptible at a current of 1 mA. A current of 10–20 mA results in a sustained muscular contraction referred to as the "let go current." At this current, a person is unable to let go of an electrical wire. Currents exceeding 100 mA may result in ventricular fibrillation.
   b. Conventional electrical circuits are grounded. They consist of three wires referred to as "hot," "neutral," and "ground." The danger of such circuits is that contact between the hot wire and an instrument's metal case (fault) can cause shock if a person contacts the case and ground. Fortunately, an intact ground wire provides a low-resistance pathway for current flow, which significantly reduces the current that passes through the case. An added measure of safety is provided by utilizing an **ungrounded electrical circuit in the operating room.** This system utilizes an isolation transformer that isolates the power from ground. In such a system, an individual would have to contact both conductors simultaneously to be at risk of a shock. **In an ungrounded electrical circuit, a single fault does not result in shock hazard or power disruption.** A single fault simply converts an ungrounded system into a grounded system. All equipment will continue to function normally. The integrity of the circuit is monitored with a line isolation

monitor. It alarms when a single fault capable of producing a "ground-seeking current" of more than 5 mA occurs. When this occurs, the offending piece of equipment should be sought out and removed, since a second fault may result in a shock hazard.

c. **Microshock** occurs when current passes directly to the heart. Commonly used guide wires and pacing wires provide electrical conduits to the heart. Ventricular fibrillation can be produced by as little as 100 μA of current applied to the myocardium. This is well below the 5 mA required before a line isolation monitor alarms. Therefore, **line isolation monitors do not protect a patient from microshock.** To minimize the likelihood of microshock, all equipment should be properly grounded with a three-prong plug, and connections to the patient should be electrically isolated. Battery operation does not ensure electrical isolation.

d. **Burns** from electrosurgical units (Bovie) may result from poor contact between the dispersive electrode (grounding pad) and the patient, since electrical power dissipation is proportional to the resistance at the skin. Under such conditions, anything that is grounded may provide an alternate pathway for current to flow, resulting in burns at sites distant from the dispersive electrode. The risk of burn can be minimized by ensuring that the electrode gel is adequate, that the dispersive electrode is placed near the surgical site, and that the patient is insulated from possible alternative pathways for current flow.

SUGGESTED READING

Barash, P. G., Cullen, B. F., and Stoelting, R. K. *Clinical Anesthesia.* Philadelphia: Lippincott, 1989.

Beebe, J. J., and Sessler, D. I. Preparation of anesthesia machines for patients susceptible to malignant hyperthermia. *Anesthesiology* 69:395, 1988.

Bruner, J. M. R., and Leonard, P. F. *Electricity, Safety and the Patient.* Chicago: Year Book, 1989.

Gravenstein, N. *Manual of Complications During Anesthesia.* Philadelphia: Lippincott, 1991.

Holdcroft, A. *Body Temperature Control in Anaesthesia, Surgery and Intensive Care.* London: Bailliere Tindall, 1980.

Jones, D. E., and Ryan, J. F. Treatment of the Acute Hyperthermic Crisis, Malignant Hyperthermia. In B. A. Britt (ed.), *Malignant Hyperthermia.* Boston: Martinus Nijhoff, 1987. P. 397.

Kallos, T., Lampe, K. F., and Orkin, F. K. Pulmonary Aspiration of Gastric Contents. In F. K. Orkin and L. H. Cooperman (eds.), *Complications in Anesthesiology.* Philadelphia: Lippincott, 1983. P. 152.

Levy, J. H. Allergic reactions during anesthesia. *J. Clin. Anesth.* 1(1):44, 1988.

Miller, R. D. *Anesthesia.* New York: Churchill Livingstone, 1990.

Orkin, F., and Cooperman, L. *Complications in Anesthesiology*. Philadelphia: Lippincott, 1983.

Stoelting, R. K., Dierdorf, S. F., and McCammon, R. L. *Anesthesia and Co-Existing Disease*. New York: Churchill Livingstone, 1988.

19

Perioperative Hemodynamic Control

Mansoor Husain

I. **Blood flow. Systemic blood pressure** is routinely monitored as a reflection of adequate local tissue perfusion. This is because pressure is clinically much easier to measure than flow. However, organs require an adequate blood flow rather than a minimal blood pressure to meet their metabolic needs.

Organ blood flow = (mean arterial pressure [MAP] − organ venous pressure) / organ vascular resistance

MAP = cardiac output × systemic vascular resistance (SVR)

Cardiac output, in turn, is influenced by heart rate, preload, afterload, and myocardial compliance and contractility. These variables are separate yet intimately interdependent and controlled by autonomic nervous system and humoral control mechanisms.

II. **Autoregulation.** The ability of an organ or vascular bed to maintain adequate blood flow despite varying blood pressure is termed autoregulation. Metabolic regulation controls about 75% of all local blood flow in the body. Organs have differing ability (autoregulatory reserve) to increase or decrease their vascular resistance to provide tight coupling between metabolic demand and organ blood flow. In general, anesthetics inhibit autoregulation, making organ perfusion pressure-dependent. The most important of these organs are the brain, kidneys, heart, and lungs (see appropriate chapters for detailed discussions on each).

III. **Adrenergic receptor physiology.** Adrenergic receptors can be distinguished by their response to a series of catecholamines. Receptors that demonstrate an order of potency such that norepinephrine > epinephrine > isoproterenol are termed **alpha receptors.** Those receptors that respond with an order of potency isoproterenol > epinephrine > norepinephrine are termed **beta receptors.** Receptors that interact exclusively with dopamine are termed **dopaminergic.** Adrenergic receptors can be further subdivided based on their pharmacology and anatomic location.

   A. **Alpha-1 receptors** are located postsynaptically in vascular smooth muscle and also in the smooth muscle of the coronary arteries, uterus, skin, intestinal mucosa, and splanchnic bed. Activation causes arteriolar and venous constriction and relaxation of the intestinal tract. Postsynaptic cardiac alpha-1 receptors increase inotropy and decrease heart rate.

   B. **Alpha-2 receptors**
      1. **Presynaptic** alpha-2 receptors are located within the central nervous system (CNS). Activation causes inhibition of norepinephrine release and a decrease in sympathetic outflow leading to hypotension and bradycardia.

   2. Postsynaptic alpha-2 receptors are located both peripherally in vascular smooth muscle and within the CNS. Activation of peripheral postsynaptic alpha-2 receptors causes vasoconstriction and a hypertensive (pressor) response. Activation of the central receptors is associated with analgesia and an anesthesia-sparing effect.

C. **Beta-1 receptors** are located in the myocardium, the sinoatrial node, the ventricular conduction system, and adipose tissue. Activation causes an increase in inotropy, chronotropy, myocardial conduction velocity, and lipolysis.

D. **Beta-2 receptors** are located in vascular, bronchial, and uterine smooth muscle and the smooth muscle in skin. Stimulation leads to vasodilation, bronchodilation, and uterine relaxation. Beta-2 receptor activation also promotes gluconeogenesis, insulin release, and potassium uptake by cells.

E. **Dopaminergic receptors**
   1. **Dopaminergic-1 receptors** are located postsynaptically on renal and mesenteric vascular smooth muscle and mediate vasodilation.
   2. **Dopaminergic-2 receptors** are presynaptic and inhibit norepinephrine release.

F. **Receptor regulation.** There is an inverse relationship between receptor number and the concentration of circulating adrenergic agonist and the duration of exposure to that agonist. This is termed **receptor up and down regulation.** Sudden cessation of beta-blockade therapy may be associated with rebound hypertension and tachycardia with resulting myocardial ischemia. This is a result of beta-receptor proliferation (up regulation) and consequent hypersensitivity to endogenous catecholamines.

IV. **Adrenergic pharmacology** (Table 19-1)
A. **Alpha agonists**
   1. **Phenylephrine** is a direct-acting alpha-1 agonist at normal clinical doses with some beta-receptor activity at extremely high concentrations. Phenylephrine causes both arterial and venous vasoconstriction. This dual action leads to an increase in venous return (preload) and mean arterial blood pressure (afterload). Phenylephrine maintains cardiac output in patients with a normal heart but may decrease cardiac performance in an ischemic heart. Phenylephrine has a short duration of action that makes it easily titratable.
   2. **Methoxamine** is a pure alpha-1 receptor agonist. It is rarely used in clinical practice today. It has a long duration of action that makes it difficult to titrate.
B. **Beta agonists. Isoproterenol** is a direct-acting beta-adrenergic agonist. It causes an increase in heart rate and contractility while reducing SVR. It is also a pulmonary vasodilator and a powerful bronchodilator.
   1. **Indications**
      a. Hemodynamically significant, atropine-resistant bradycardia.

Table 19-1. Drug dosages of commonly used vasopressors and inotropes

Drug name (Trade name)	IV bolus	IV infusion	Dose	Adrenergic effects		
				Alpha	Beta	DA
Phenylephrine (Neo-Synephrine)	50–100 μg	a. 10 mg/250 ml b. 40 μg/ml c. 0.1–20.0 μg/kg/min d. 5–10 min		++++		
Isoproterenol (Isuprel)	0.4 mg	a. 1μg/250 ml b. 4 μg/ml c. 0.15 μg/kg/min to desired effect d. 5–10 min			++++	
Epinephrine (Adrenalin)	20–100 μ (hypotension); .5–1 mg (cardiac arrest)	a. 1 mg/250 ml b. 4 μg/ml c. 0.5–4.00 μg/kg/min d. 1–2 min	Low High	+ +++	++ ++++	
Norepinephrine (Levophed)	NR	a. 4 mg/250 ml b. 16 μg/ml c. 1–30 μg/kg/min d. 1–2 min	Low High	++ ++++	+ ++	
Dopamine (Inotropin)	NR	a. 200 mg/250 ml b. 800 μg/ml c. 2–10 μg/kg/min d. 5–10 min	Low High	 ++	 ++	+++ +++
Dobutamine (Dobutrex)	NR	a. 250 mg/250 ml b. 1000 μg/ml c. 2–30 μg/kg/min d. 5–10 min		+	+++	
Ephedrine	5–10 mg	NR 5–10 min duration		++	++	
Amrinone	NR	0.75 mg/kg IV loading dose, then 5–10 μg/kg/min; 2.5–12.0 hr duration	Nonsympathomimetic			

a = mix in 5% D/W; b = concentration; c = IV dosage range; d = duration; DA = dopaminergic; NR = not recommended.

      b. Pulmonary hypertension and right heart failure.

      c. Atrioventricular block until temporary pacing can be instituted.

      d. Low cardiac output states requiring fast heart rates (pediatric patients who have a fixed stroke volume, cardiac transplant recipients).

      e. Status asthmaticus.

      f. Beta-blockade overdose.

    2. Continuous electrocardiographic (ECG) **monitoring** is recommended with IV administration, which may be through a peripheral IV.

    3. Side effects include vasodilation, hypotension, and tachydysrhythmias.

C. Mixed agonists

    1. Epinephrine is a direct-acting alpha- and beta-receptor agonist produced by the adrenal medulla.

      a. Indications

        (1) Cardiac arrest.

        (2) Anaphylaxis.

        (3) Bronchospasm.

        (4) Cardiogenic shock.

        (5) Massive hemorrhage.

        (6) Prolongation of regional anesthesia.

      b. Clinical effect with epinephrine is the sum total of its alpha- and beta-receptor activation on various tissue beds, with beta effects predominating at lower doses. Epinephrine increases myocardial contractility and heart rate at all doses. At lower doses, epinephrine causes bronchodilation, vasodilation, increased cardiac output, and tachycardia. As the dose of epinephrine increases, alpha effects predominate, and stroke volume may fall as SVR (afterload) increases. Significant tachycardia, dysrhythmias, and myocardial ischemia may limit the usefulness of epinephrine in the clinical setting. Volatile anesthetics (especially halothane) can sensitize the myocardium to circulating catecholamines to produce potentially life-threatening dysrhythmias. Epinephrine should be administered through a central IV, as severe tissue necrosis can occur if extravasated.

    2. Norepinephrine is the neurotransmitter of the sympathetic nervous system. Norepinephrine is a potent alpha- and beta-receptor agonist with alpha effects predominating at lower doses and having minimal effect on beta-2 receptors as compared with epinephrine. An infusion of norepinephrine increases systolic and diastolic blood pressure, while cardiac output remains the same or decreases as SVR (afterload) increases. Myocardial performance may increase, however, if the increased blood pressure leads to an increase in coronary blood flow. Norepinephrine increases the vascular resistance of most organs, thereby diminishing organ blood flow despite increases in MAP. Norepinephrine is useful in the setting of hypotension that is associated with mild myocardial depression. As with most vasoactive drugs, ECG and invasive monitoring are recommended to follow clinical effectiveness.

3. **Dopamine** is the immediate precursor of norepinephrine and produces a dose-related combination of alpha-, beta-, and dopamine-receptor effects. At lower doses (approximately < 4 µg/kg/min), renal and splanchnic vessel dopamine receptors are primarily activated, resulting in increased renal blood flow, glomerular filtration, and sodium (Na^+) excretion. As the concentration of dopamine is increased, beta effects become apparent, leading to increases in myocardial contractility, heart rate, and arterial blood pressure. At high doses (> 10 µg/kg/min), alpha-1 effects predominate, leading to marked increases in arterial and venous blood pressure and decreases in renal blood flow. Dopamine also contributes indirect effects by causing release of norepinephrine from nerve terminals. Dopamine is commonly used in low doses for the therapy of oliguria accompanying low-output states. Dopamine may also be indicated in states of shock associated with a failing myocardium. Tachycardia (often seen even at lower doses), increased myocardial oxygen consumption, and profound vasoconstriction frequently limit the clinical usefulness of dopamine.

4. **Dobutamine** is a synthetic catecholamine that has beta-1, beta-2, and alpha-1 adrenergic receptor activity. Dobutamine is a mixture of stereoisomers; the L(−)-isomer stimulates alpha-1 receptors and the D(+)-isomer has beta-1 and beta-2 receptor activity. Dobutamine increases myocardial contractility through its effect on cardiac alpha-1 and beta-1 receptors. In the peripheral vasculature, dobutamine is a vasodilator, as its beta-2 effect overshadows its alpha-1 properties. Dobutamine may cause a small increase in heart rate secondary to the positive chronotropic effects of beta-1 activation by the D(+)-isomer. Dobutamine is a useful agent for the treatment of low-output states caused by myocardial dysfunction secondary to acute infarction, cardiomyopathy, or myocardial depression following cardiac surgery. Hemodynamic effects of dobutamine are similar to those of a combination of dopamine and nitroprusside. Dobutamine typically increases cardiac output with a decrease in SVR and minimal effect on arterial blood pressure and heart rate. Pulmonary vascular resistance (PVR) decreases, making dobutamine beneficial for patients with right heart failure. Systemic hypotension (dobutamine is an inotrope, not a pressor), increased myocardial oxygen consumption, and dysrhythmias are the most common side effects.

5. **Ephedrine** is a plant-derived, noncatecholamine, adrenergic agonist. Ephedrine causes the release of norepinephrine and other endogenous catecholamines stored within nerve terminals. Ephedrine is also a weak direct alpha- and beta-adrenergic receptor ago-

nist. Tachyphylaxis limits ephedrine use to bolus administration for the temporary treatment of hypotension associated with hypovolemia, regional anesthesia, myocardial depression due to anesthetic overdose, or bradycardia.

D. Nonadrenergic sympathomimetic agents. Amrinone and milrinone are synthetic, noncatecholamine, nonglycosidic, bipyridine derivatives. They act by inhibiting the enzyme phosphodiesterase-III, thereby increasing cyclic adenosine monophosphate levels and causing increased contractility and peripheral vasodilation. Their action is **independent** of adrenergic receptors, and as such their effect is **additive** to that of adrenergic agents.

1. **Amrinone** produces a dose-dependent improvement in cardiac index, left ventricular work index, and ejection fraction, while heart rate and MAP remain constant. Time to peak effect is about 5 minutes, and elimination occurs by the liver with an elimination half-life of 5–12 hours depending on the severity of cardiac disease. Side effects are uncommon and include dose-dependent but reversible hypotension, thrombocytopenia, liver function test abnormalities, fever, and gastrointestinal distress.

2. **Milrinone** is a derivative of amrinone and shares the same hemodynamic profile. Milrinone is 20 times more potent than amrinone but does not have many of the side effects associated with its parent compound. Milrinone has not as yet been approved by the Federal Drug Administration for clinical use in this country.

V. Beta-adrenergic antagonists (Table 19–2)

A. Propranolol is a nonselective, beta-1 and beta-2 adrenergic receptor antagonist available in both IV and PO form. Propranolol is the prototype beta-adrenergic antagonist against which other drugs in this class are judged. Propranolol is highly lipophilic, is almost entirely absorbed after oral administration, and undergoes up to 75% first-pass clearance by the liver. Hemodynamic effects of propranolol and other beta-adrenergic antagonists are secondary to a reduction of cardiac output and suppression of the renin-angiotensin system. Beta-adrenergic antagonists can be distinguished by their **relative** beta-1 selectivity, their intrinsic sympathomimetic activity, and their pharmacologic half-lives.

B. Esmolol is a selective beta-1 adrenergic receptor antagonist that contains an ester linkage in its molecular structure. Esmolol is metabolized rapidly by an esterase located in the cytoplasm of red blood cells. Esmolol has a time to peak effect of 5 minutes and an elimination half-life of 9 minutes. Esmolol is valuable perioperatively because it can be administered IV, has a fast onset, has a very short duration of action, and can be given to patients with asthma, chronic obstructive pulmonary disease, or myocardial dysfunction. The red blood cell esterase is different from plasma pseudocholinesterase and is not affected by anticholinesterases. Rapid administration of esmolol in large boluses has been associated with severe

Table 19-2. Beta-adrenergic antagonists

Drug name (trade name)	Beta-1 selectivity	Bioavailability	Beta half-life*	Elimination	ISA	Usual PO dose	IV dose
Propranolol (Inderal)	0	33%	3–4 hr	H	0	10–20 mg bid-qid	0.5–1.0 mg increment
Metoprolol (Lopressor)	++	50%	3–4 hr	H	0	50 mg qd	5–25 mg increment
Atenelol (Tenormin)	++	55%	6–9 hr	R (85%)	0	50 mg qd	NR
Nadolol (Corgard)	0	20%	14–24 hr	R (75%)	0	40 mg qd	NR
Pindolol (Visken)	0	90%	3–4 hr	H (60%) R (40%)	+	5 mg bid	NR
Timolol (Blocadren)	0	75%	4–5 hr	H (80%) R (20%)	0	5–15 mg qd-bid	NR
Labetalol (Trandate, Normodyne)	0	25%	3–8 hr	H	0	100 mg bid	5–10 mg boluses
Esmolol (Brevibloc)	++	—	9 min	Red blood cell esterase	0	—	10–20 mg bolus; 0.25–0.5 mg/kg load, then 50–200 µg/kg/min

ISA = intrinsic sympathomimetic activity; H = hepatic elimination; R = renal elimination; NR = not recommended.
* Beta half-life may not be predictive of clinical duration of action.

hypotension and cardiac depression leading to cardiac arrest in some situations.

C. **Labetalol** is a mixed alpha- and beta-adrenergic receptor antagonist with a ratio of beta- to alpha-adrenergic receptor blockade of 3 : 1 when given PO and 7 : 1 when administered IV. Labetalol is available in both IV and PO form. Labetalol decreases PVR, blunts the reflex increase in heart rate, and minimally affects cardiac output. Labetalol is useful intraoperatively to blunt the sympathetic response to tracheal intubation and to control hypertensive episodes. Labetalol is also used in the management of patients with pheochromocytomas and the clonidine withdrawal syndrome. Labetalol does not increase intracranial pressure in patients with intracranial hypertension.

VI. Vasodilators (Table 19-3)

A. **Sodium nitroprusside** is a direct-acting vasodilator that acts on arterial and venous vascular smooth muscle.

1. The **mechanism of action** of sodium nitroprusside is common to all nitrates. The nitroso moiety decomposes to release nitric oxide. Nitric oxide is an unstable, short-lived compound that activates guanylate cyclase. This results in an increase in the concentration of cyclic guanosine monophosphate, which causes smooth muscle relaxation.

2. The **hemodynamic effects** of sodium nitroprusside are principally afterload reduction by arterial vasodilation and some preload reduction by increasing venous capacitance. These effects typically cause a reflex increase in heart rate and myocardial contractility, an increase in cardiac output, and marked decreases in SVR and PVR. Sodium nitroprusside dilates cerebral blood vessels and should be used with caution in patients with decreased intracranial compliance.

3. Sodium nitroprusside dilates all vascular beds equally, increasing overall blood flow. However, a **vascular steal phenomenon** may be created where blood flow to an ischemic region that is maximally vasodilated may be shunted to nonischemic regions that can vasodilate further. This is especially important in the coronary vasculature, where ischemia may be exacerbated with the use of sodium nitroprusside even though overall myocardial oxygen consumption has been reduced by afterload reduction.

4. Sodium nitroprusside is useful **perioperatively** because it has a fast onset time (1–2 min), and its effect is dissipated within 2 minutes of discontinuation.

5. **Cyanide toxicity.** An aqueous solution of sodium nitroprusside undergoes photodecomposition that inactivates the compound but does not release cyanide ion. In vivo, sodium nitroprusside reacts nonenzymatically with the sulfhydryl groups in hemoglobin to release five cyanide radicals per molecule. Cyanide ion is converted to thiocyanate by tissue and liver rhodanase and excreted in urine. Thiocyanate has a half-life of 4 days and will accumulate in the presence of renal

Table 19-3. Vasodilator drugs

Drug Name (trade name)	IV push	IV infusion	Mechanism of action
Nitroglycerin	50–100 µg	a. 50 mg/250 ml b. 200 µg/ml c. 0.1 µg/kg/min d. 4 min	Venous vasodilator
Nitroprusside (Nipride)	NR	a. 50 mg/250 ml b. 200 µg/ml c. 0.2 µg/kg/ml and titrate up d. 4 min	Arterial greater than venous vasodilation
Hydralazine (Apresoline)	2.5–5.0 mg IV q15min 20–40 mg IV q4–6 h	NR	Direct-acting vascular smooth muscle dilation
Phentolamine (Regitine)	1–5 mg IV	a. 10 mg/250 ml b. 40 µg/ml c. 1–2 µg/kg/min and titrate up d. 5–10 min	Alpha-receptor blockade
Trimethaphan	0.5–2.0 mg IV; start with 1-mg bolus	a. 500 mg/500 ml b. 1 mg/ml c. 0.5–6.0 mg/min d. 5–10 min	Ganglionic blockade and histamine release
Labetalol (Normodyne or Trandate)	2.5–5.0 mg IV q5 min	a. 200 mg/250 ml b. 0.6 mg/ml c. 1–5 mg/min d. 15 min	Alpha- and beta-receptor agonist
Prostaglandin E₁	NR	a. 1–2 mg/250 ml b. 4–8 µg/ml c. 0.05 µg/kg/min and titrate up d. 1 min	Direct vasodilator via prostaglandin receptors in vascular smooth muscle

a = mix in 5% D/W; b = concentration; c = IV dosage range; d = duration; NR = not recommended.

failure. The cyanide ion binds to intracellular cytochrome oxidase and disrupts the electron transport chain, which can lead to cell hypoxia and death even in the face of adequate PO_2.

   a. Clinical features. Tachyphylaxis, metabolic acidosis, and elevated mixed venous oxygen are early signs of cyanide toxicity, which typically occurs when more than 1 mg/kg has been administered within 2.5 hours and when the blood concentration of cyanide ion is greater than 100 µg/dl. Symptoms of cyanide toxicity include fatigue, nausea, muscle spasm, angina, and mental confusion.

   b. Treatment. Cyanide toxicity is treated by discontinuation of sodium nitroprusside and the administration of 100% oxygen and sodium thiosulfate, 150 mg/kg dissolved in 50 ml of water, over 15 minutes. Severe cyanide toxicity (base deficit > 10 mEq, hemodynamic instability) may require the additional administration of amyl nitrate (by inhalation or direct injection into the anesthesia circuit) or sodium nitrate, 5 mg/kg IV over 5 minutes. These two compounds create methemoglobin, which will bind to the cyanide ion and form inactive cyanmethemoglobin.

B. Nitroglycerin is a potent venodilator that also relaxes arterial, pulmonary, ureteral, uterine, gastrointestinal, and bronchial smooth muscle. Nitroglycerin has a greater effect on venous capacitance than on arteriolar tone; nitroglycerin's major mechanism of decreasing MAP is reduction of venous return.

   1. Indications. Nitroglycerin is useful for treating congestive heart failure and myocardial ischemia by increasing coronary flow and improving left ventricular performance. Nitroglycerin increases venous capacitance, decreases venous return (preload), and consequently decreases ventricular end-diastolic volume. By the law of Laplace, tension = pressure × radius. A decrease in end-diastolic volume is associated with a decrease in pressure and size (radius) and subsequently a decrease in ventricular wall tension (stress), which reduces myocardial oxygen consumption.

   2. Reflex tachycardia frequently occurs and must be treated with beta blockade to avoid increasing myocardial consumption and negating nitroglycerin's beneficial effects.

   3. Tolerance develops with continuous infusion, and doses have to be increased to achieve the same hemodynamic and antianginal effects.

   4. Complications. Nitroglycerin is metabolized by the liver and has no known toxicity in the clinical dose range. Extremely high doses and prolonged continuous use produce methemoglobin. Nitroglycerin produces cerebral vasodilation and should be used with caution in patients with low intracranial compliance.

C. Hydralazine is a direct-acting arterial vasodilator whose action is independent of adrenergic or cholinergic receptors. Hydralazine decreases MAP by a reduction in arteriolar tone and vascular resistance of the coronary, cerebral, renal, uterine, and splanchnic systems. This helps preserve blood flow to these organs. The vasodilation induced by hydralazine triggers a reflex increase in heart rate and causes activation of the renin-angiotensin system. These effects can be attenuated by the concomitant use of a beta blocker. Intraoperatively, hydralazine is administered in IV bolus fashion to treat hypertensive emergencies or to augment other hypotensive agents. The time to peak effect of IV hydralazine is 15–20 minutes with an elimination half-life of 4 hours. Hydralazine is metabolized through acetylation by the liver. Long-term use has been associated with a lupus-like syndrome, skin rash, drug fever, pancytopenia, and peripheral neuropathy.

D. Phentolamine is a short-acting selective alpha-adrenergic receptor antagonist that causes predominantly arterial and some venous vasodilation. Phentolamine is used mainly for states of norepinephrine excess (e.g., pheochromocytoma), as an adjuvant for induced hypotension, and for infiltration into skin where norepinephrine has been accidentally extravasated (5–10 mg diluted in 10 ml of saline). Reflex tachycardia is common, and beta blockade is recommended to blunt this response.

E. Trimethaphan decreases MAP through ganglionic blockade and also by some direct vasodilator and histamine-releasing properties. It has a fast onset (1–2 minutes) and short duration of action (5–10 minutes) and can reduce MAP without decreasing cardiac output or causing reflex tachycardia. Trimethaphan does not activate the renin-angiotensin system and increases intracranial pressure much less than sodium nitroprusside. Disadvantages include tachyphylaxis with continued use, histamine release with high doses, and the side effects of ganglionic blockade such as mydriasis and cycloplegia. Mydriasis may be extreme, so trimethaphan is contraindicated in patients with known narrow-angle glaucoma and relatively contraindicated where pupil size serves as an indicator of the patient's neurologic status.

F. Calcium channel antagonists alter calcium flux across cell membranes, and cause varying degrees of arterial vasodilation with minimal effect on venous capacitance. They decrease vascular resistance of peripheral organs and cause coronary artery vasodilation. They are also myocardial depressants and affect atrioventricular conduction.

    1. Verapamil is a papaverine derivative. It has the highest electrophysiologic potency of the calcium channel antagonists. Verapamil is the drug of choice for supraventricular tachydysrhythmia (SVT). Verapamil can also control the ventricular rate in atrial flutter and atrial fibrillation (5–10 mg IV bolus, 1–2 mg in an unstable patient) when there is no aberrant pathway (e.g., the Wolff-Parkinson-White [WPW] syndrome). Verapamil is a powerful myocardial depressant and should be used with caution in the hypotensive patient or the patient with impaired left ventricular function.

2. **Diltiazem** is a selective coronary vasodilator that has much lower electrophysiologic and peripheral vasodilating effects as compared to verapamil. Diltiazem causes a slight decrease in heart rate with little or no effect on myocardial contractility. Diltiazem is the most common calcium channel antagonist for chronic therapy of myocardial ischemia.

3. **Nifedipine** is a potent peripheral and coronary artery vasodilator. Nifedipine has the least effect on atrioventricular conduction and myocardial contractility. Nifedipine is not available in IV form, is light sensitive, and is administered either PO or SL.

G. **Prostaglandin E_1 (PGE_1)** is a stable metabolite of arachidonic acid and causes peripheral and pulmonary vasodilation via prostaglandin receptors located in vascular smooth muscle. It is used to dilate the ductus arteriosus in neonates and infants with ductal-dependent congenital heart disease (e.g., transposition of the great arteries). PGE_1 is also used to treat refractory pulmonary hypertension after mitral valve replacement and in patients with severe right heart failure. This is usually in conjunction with norepinephrine infusion via a left atrial line to counteract PGE_1's powerful systemic vasodilating effects. PGE_1 is metabolized in the lung and is almost completely eliminated during its first passage.

H. **Adenosine** inhibits norepinephrine release and has been used in clinical trials to induce hypotension in humans. Adenosine dilates cerebral blood vessels, impairs autoregulation, and is metabolized to uric acid. More recently, adenosine's ability to slow conduction through the atrioventricular node has led to its use in diagnosing and treating SVTs, including those with an aberrant pathway (e.g., WPW syndrome). A dose of 6 mg IV is administered while the ECG is continuously monitored. The dose is usually doubled to a maximum of 12 mg or until effect. Asystole is brief (< 1 minute), with resumption of sinus rhythm or the original dysrhythmia.

VII. **Cholinergic physiology. Acetylcholine (ACh)** is the neurotransmitter of the parasympathetic nervous system. Acetylcholinesterase and plasma pseudocholinesterase are the enzymes responsible for the efficient and complete metabolism of ACh. ACh interacts with all cholinergic receptors. However, cholinergic receptors can be further classified as muscarinic and nicotinic depending on their affinity for atropine and nicotine respectively. Stimulation of muscarinic receptors leads to a decrease in heart rate; an increase in gastrointestinal motility and in gastric, pancreatic, bronchial, and salivary secretions; an increase in ureteral and bladder smooth muscle tone; and constriction of the sphincter muscle of the iris. Atropine, glycopyrrolate, and scopolamine are muscarinic receptor antagonists that are used in anesthesia primarily to reduce salivary and respiratory secretions and to counteract bradycardia due to vagal stimulation and the side effects of anesthetic drugs.

VIII. Drug dosage calculations. Drug dosages frequently require conversion between units of measurement before bolus or continuous infusion administration to the patient.

A. A drug concentration expressed as Z% contains

Z mg/dl = Z g/100 ml = (10 × Z) g/L = (10 × Z) mg/ml

Example: A 2.5% solution of sodium thiopental is equivalent to 25 g/L or 25 mg/ml.

B. A drug concentration expressed as a ratio is converted as follows:

1:1000 = 1 g/1000 ml = 1 mg/ml

1:10,000 = 1 g/10,000 ml = 0.1 mg/ml

1:1,000,000 = 1 g/1,000,000 ml = 1 μg/ml

C. Continuous drug infusions are calculated based on a simple formula:

Z mg/250 ml = Z μg/min at an infusion rate of 15 ml/hr or 15 drops/min

Standard drug mixes in use at the Massachusetts General Hospital are shown in Table 19-1. The desired rate of infusion for any drug is easily calculated as either a fraction or multiple of 15 ml/hr or 15 drops/min. For example, an 80-kg patient needs dopamine at 5 μg/kg/min:

5 × 80 = 400

400/200 (number of milligrams in 250-ml solution) × 15 ml/hr = 30 ml/hr.

X. Induced hypotension

A. Indications

1. When control of bleeding improves operating conditions and facilitates surgical technique (e.g., middle ear microsurgery, cerebral aneurysm clipping, plastic surgery) or reduces or eliminates the need for blood transfusion (e.g., orthopedic surgery, patients with rare blood groups, religious constraints).

2. When reduction in MAP decreases the risk of vessel rupture (e.g., aortic dissection, resection of intracranial aneurysms, arteriovenous malformation surgery).

B. Contraindications

1. Vascular insufficiency to brain, heart, or kidneys.

2. Cardiac instability (unless afterload reduction improves performance).

3. Uncontrolled hypertension.

4. Anemia.

5. Hypovolemia.

6. Inexperience of the anesthesiologist.

C. Anesthetic considerations

1. Hypotension is not synonymous with inadequate local tissue perfusion so long as organ vascular resistance falls in parallel with MAP.

2. An MAP of 50–60 mm Hg in young healthy patients and an MAP of 60–70 mm Hg in suitable older patients will usually provide a relatively bloodless field (most surgical bleeding is venous in origin).

3. Myocardial ischemia necessitates abandoning hypotensive techniques.
4. Patients should be positioned with the operative site uppermost.
5. Hypotensive techniques abolish normal compensatory mechanisms. Therefore, careful **volume replacement** is essential.
6. Controlled ventilation is always indicated during induced hypotension. Positive airway pressure diminishes venous return and potentiates induced hypotension.

D. Preparation
1. Generous premedication will decrease excessive circulating catecholamines.
2. In addition to standard monitoring, a Foley catheter, separate IV with an infusion pump for drug administration, and an arterial catheter should be placed. A central venous pressure monitor may be required if large blood loss is expected.
3. Resuscitation drugs including calcium chloride, inotropes, and pressors should be available.

E. Methods
1. **Preganglionic blockade** is produced by either a high spinal or epidural anesthesia. Concurrent endotracheal intubation and general anesthesia are usually necessary because of the hypotension and respiratory difficulty associated with the high sympathetic block. Significant bradycardia may occur secondary to unopposed vagal activity.
2. **Ganglionic blockade** is produced with trimethaphan (see sec **VI.E**). Total dose should not exceed 1000 mg. Usual dosage is 0.5–6.0 mg/min. Duration varies from 10–30 minutes, though effects may persist for 60 minutes after discontinuation.
3. **Myocardial depression** may be produced by high inspired concentrations of inhalation anesthetics.
4. **Peripheral vasodilation** may be produced with
   a. **Sodium nitroprusside,** which increases the activity of the renin-angiotensin system. This can be attenuated by treatment with propranolol or captopril. Sodium nitroprusside may be combined with trimethaphan (250 mg of trimethaphan + 25 mg of sodium nitroprusside in 500 ml of 5% dextrose in water, with the infusion starting at 0.1 ml/min).
   b. **Nitroglycerin** is the preferred agent in patients with coronary artery disease.
   c. **Labetalol.**

F. Reversal of hypotension
1. Blood pressure should be allowed to normalize prior to closure to facilitate hemostasis.
2. If hypotension persists and immediate reversal is necessary in **spite of adequate volume repletion,** ephedrine (5–10 mg IV), phenylephrine (titrated to desired blood pressure), or calcium chloride in increments of 250 mg IV may be given.

G. Complications

1. Cerebral ischemia, thrombosis, or edema.
2. Acute renal failure.
3. Myocardial infarction, congestive heart failure, and cardiac arrest.
4. Reactive hemorrhage with hematoma formation.

SUGGESTED READING

Durrett, L. R., and Lawson, N. W. Autonomic Nervous System Physiology and Pharmacology. In P. G. Barash, B. F. Cullen, and R. K. Stoelting (eds.), *Clinical Anesthesia*. New York: Lippincott, 1989.

Fahmy, N. R. Deliberate Hypotension. In M. C. Rogers (ed.), *Current Practice of Anesthesiology*. Philadelphia: B. C. Decker, 1988. Pp. 117–120.

Gilman, A. G., et al. *The Pharmacologic Basis of Therapeutics*. New York: Macmillan, 1989.

Larach, D. R., and Kofke, W. A. Cardiovascular Drugs. In W. A. Kofke and J. H. Levy (eds.), *Postoperative Critical Care Procedures of the Massachusetts General Hospital*. Boston: Little, Brown, 1986. Pp. 464–522.

20

Anesthesia for Abdominal Surgery

Adam Sapirstein

I. **Preanesthetic considerations**
   A. **Assessment of preoperative fluid status** is fundamental, as surgical pathology may cause derangements in volume homeostasis (e.g., colon cancer).
      1. **History of fluid losses**
         a. **Bleeding from gastrointestinal sources** such as ulcers, neoplasms, esophageal varices, diverticuli, angiodysplasia, or hemorrhoids.
         b. **Emesis or gastric drainage,** which may lead to significant losses, particularly in patients with bowel obstruction. Patients should be questioned as to the quantity, quality (presence of blood), and frequency of emesis.
         c. **Diarrhea,** which may result from intestinal disease, infection, or cathartic bowel preparations. This can cause the loss of 1–2 liters of extracellular fluid.
         d. **Sequestration of fluid** in the bowel lumen and interstitium due to ileus or peritonitis.
         e. **Fever,** which causes insensible fluid loss.
      2. **Evidence of hypovolemia on physical examination.** Postural changes in vital signs may reveal mild to moderate hypovolemia, and severe hypovolemia will cause tachycardia and hypotension. Dryness of the mucous membranes, decreased skin turgor, decreased skin temperature, and mottling may indicate decreased peripheral perfusion secondary to hypovolemia.
      3. **Laboratory analysis** including hematocrit, serum osmolality, blood urea nitrogen–creatinine ratio, electrolyte concentrations, and urine output is useful in estimating volume deficits.
   B. **Metabolic and hematologic derangements** occur frequently in patients undergoing emergency abdominal surgery. Hypokalemic metabolic alkalosis may be seen in patients with large gastric losses. Large diarrheal losses or septicemia can cause metabolic acidosis, and sepsis can cause coagulopathy from disseminated intravascular coagulation.
   C. **A history of previous abdominal surgery,** intraabdominal infection, radiation therapy, or steroid use can contribute to the difficulty, length, and fluid loss of an operation.
II. **Anesthetic techniques.** Choice of technique will be determined by factors relating to the patient, operative procedure, anesthesiologist, and surgeon.
   A. **General anesthesia** is the most commonly employed technique.
      1. **Advantages**
         a. The ability to protect the airway and ensure adequate ventilation.

      b. Rapid induction and controllable depth and duration.

  2. Disadvantage. Loss of airway reflexes creates a risk of aspiration during both routine and emergency surgery.

B. Regional anesthetic techniques for abdominal surgery include spinal, epidural, caudal, and nerve blocks.

  1. Lower abdominal procedures (e.g., inguinal hernia repair) can usually be performed with regional anesthesia techniques that produce a sensory level to T4–T6.

    a. Epidural anesthesia is usually performed with a continuous catheter technique. A "single-dose" technique can be used when the duration of surgery is 1–3 hours.

    b. Spinal anesthesia can be performed using a single-dose or continuous catheter technique.

    c. Nerve blocks can also be performed to provide anesthesia for abdominal surgery.

      (1) Bilateral blockade of T8–T12 intercostal nerves provides somatic sensory anesthesia, while celiac block provides visceral anesthesia for procedures such as cholecystectomy.

      (2) Blockade of the ilioinguinal, iliohypogastric, and genitofemoral nerves produces a field block that is satisfactory for herniorrhaphy. These nerve blocks are easily performed by the anesthesiologist but may require direct supplementation of spermatic cord structures by the surgeon.

  2. Regional anesthesia alone is usually unsuitable for **upper abdominal surgery.**

    a. Anesthesia with a spinal or epidural block for upper abdominal procedures (above the umbilicus) may require a sensory level to T2–T4. High thoracic levels produce paralysis of the intercostal muscles such that deep breathing is impaired, and patients often complain of dyspnea even though minute ventilation is maintained. Intraperitoneal air or high abdominal exploration produces a dull pain referred to as a C5 distribution (usually over the shoulders).

    b. Celiac plexus blockade incompletely blocks upper abdominal sensation, and visceral traction is poorly tolerated.

  3. Advantages

    a. Maintenance of the patient's ability to communicate symptoms such as chest pain.

    b. Maintenance of airway reflexes.

    c. Profound muscle relaxation and bowel contraction, which provide optimal surgical exposure.

    d. Increased blood flow to the bowel from complete sympathectomy.

    e. Postoperative analgesia from continuous techniques.

  4. Disadvantages

    a. Toxicity from local anesthetic if inadvertent IV injection occurs.

      b. Patients must be cooperative for institution of the block and positioning during the operation.

      c. Possible failure of technique necessitating conversion to general anesthesia intraoperatively.

      d. Regional nerve blockade may be contraindicated in the patient with an abnormal bleeding profile or localized infection at the site.

      e. Sympathectomy leading to venodilation and bradycardia may precipitate profound hypotension. Unopposed parasympathetic action leads to bowel contraction and more rapid transit times. Contracted bowel may make anastomotic construction more difficult. This can be reversed with glycopyrrolate, 0.2–0.4 mg IV.

      f. High-level blocks may compromise pulmonary function.

C. Combined technique includes the use of epidural with general anesthesia. Patients with impaired pulmonary or cardiovascular function may benefit from the sympathectomy and analgesia that a combined technique provide.

  1. Advantages

      a. Epidural anesthesia reduces the requirement for general anesthesia, minimizing some of the myocardial and central nervous system depression.

      b. Combined techniques may be particularly useful in reducing postoperative ventilatory depression after upper abdominal surgery. Epidural analgesia leads to improvement in lung function, as measured by spirometry and arterial blood gases. Improvement in postoperative functional residual capacity (FRC) has the theoretic advantage of reducing pulmonary complications.

  2. Disadvantages

      a. In addition to the disadvantages listed in sec. **B.4,** the combined technique requires sound clinical judgment to manage the hemodynamic changes of both a general and regional anesthetic. Sympathectomy produced by regional anesthesia can potentiate hypovolemia, and the differentiation between regional anesthesia–induced hypotension and hypotension from other causes may be difficult.

      b. Additional time for epidural catheter placement and testing is added to preparation time.

D. Local field block can be performed by the anesthesiologist or surgeon for more superficial procedures such as ventral herniorrhaphy and gastrostomy. Such blocks require technical expertise and a cooperative patient.

III. Management of anesthesia

  A. Standard **monitors** are used as described in Chap. 10.

  B. Induction of anesthesia should be conducted as described in Chap. 14. Conditions that require **rapid sequence induction** are often encountered in abdominal surgery. Patients who are described as having a "full stomach" and thus require rapid sequence induction include

    1. Trauma victims in whom gastric emptying is

delayed. If the time interval between the patient's last oral intake and the accident is less than 8 hours, the patient should be considered to have a full stomach.

2. Patients with **evidence of bowel obstruction.**
3. Patients with **symptomatic hiatal hernias.**
4. Patients in the second or third trimester of **pregnancy.**
5. **Significantly obese** patients.
6. Patients with **ascites.**

C. **Maintenance of anesthesia**

1. **Fluid management** requires proper replacement of deficits and ongoing losses and administration of maintenance fluids.

   a. **Surgical bleeding** should be estimated by observing the field and the suction traps and by weighing sponges. Blood under drapes or within the bowel may be impossible to estimate with accuracy.

   b. **Edema of the bowel and its mesentery** can result from direct trauma to the capillary endothelium. Bowel manipulation and intestinal pathology can cause endothelial damage and lead to sequestration.

   c. **Evaporative loss** from peritoneal surfaces can be profound and is directly related to the area exposed. Fluid replacement is guided by clinical judgment and invasive monitoring. A rough estimate of 7–15 ml/kg/hr may be required.

   d. **Ascitic fluid** is usually drained abruptly with surgical entry into the peritoneum. Rapid drainage results in decreased intraabdominal pressure and may cause acute hypotension. Replacement of ascitic fluid by the peritoneum will occur and is a source of fluid loss.

   e. **Nasogastric and other enteric drainage** should be quantified and replaced.

2. **Muscle relaxation** is required for all but the most superficial of intraperitoneal operations. The degree of relaxation becomes critical at the time of abdominal closure, as bowel distention, edema, or organ transplantation may increase the volume of abdominal contents. Prior to closure, the degree of muscle relaxation should be adequate to facilitate the procedure while still permitting reversal of the relaxant for extubation.

   a. **Titrating relaxants** to obtain a single twitch by train-of-four monitoring should allow reversibility of the relaxant. The patient and surgical field must also be observed for signs of neuromuscular recovery.

   b. The **potent inhalation agents** block myoneural conduction and are synergistic with the relaxants. Therefore, increasing the concentration of these drugs can increase the degree of muscle relaxation.

   c. **Flexing the operating table** may decrease tension on transverse abdominal and subcostal incisions.

3. Use of **nitrous oxide** may cause bowel distention because its solubility is higher than that of nitrogen. Intraluminal gas volume doubles in approximately 10

minutes when high concentrations of nitrous oxide are inspired. Such distention can make closure difficult, and increased intraluminal pressures may cause impaired perfusion of obstructed bowel. For these reasons, nitrous oxide is relatively contraindicated in closed loop obstructions or when anastomoses are being constructed in unprepared bowel.

4. **Nasogastric (NG) tubes** are frequently placed in the preoperative period.

   a. **Preoperative placement** is indicated for decompression of the stomach in patients who have bowel obstruction or who have suffered trauma. A large-bore NG tube can reduce air and the volume of gastric contents but does not eliminate them. Large-particulate material in the stomach may not be removed by an NG tube. NG tubes left in place during induction should be suctioned. However, the NG tube may compromise mask fit and provides a route for reflux of gastric contents past the lower esophageal sphincter. It should be allowed to drain during induction. Cricoid pressure can be applied to prevent reflux when an NG tube is present.

   b. **Intraoperative NG tube placement** is required to drain gastric fluid and air. NG and orogastric tubes should never be placed with excessive force. Lubrication and head flexion may facilitate tube insertion, and they can also be directed into the esophagus using a finger in the oropharynx or by direct visualization using a laryngoscope and Magill forceps. If these methods fail, a large split endotracheal tube (No. 34 or 36) can be used as an introducer for the NG tube. The split tube is introduced orally into the esophagus, and the NG tube is then passed through the lubricated split tube into the stomach. The split tube is then removed while stabilizing the NG tube. A large-bore Ewald tube is best used to lavage upper gastrointestinal tract hemorrhage.

   c. **Confirmation of NG tube placement** can be done by auscultation over the epigastrium while injecting 20–30 cc of air through the tube or by aspiration of gastric fluid.

   d. **Complications.** NG tube insertion can be complicated by bleeding, submucosal dissection in the retropharynx, or placement in the trachea. Intracranial placement has been described in patients with basilar skull fracture. The NG tube should be secured, carefully avoiding excessive pressure on the nasal septum or nostril, which may lead to ischemic necrosis.

5. **Pulmonary compromise may** be seen during retraction of the abdominal viscera with soft packs or rigid retractors, insufflation of gas, or Trendelenburg positioning, often done to improve surgical exposure. These maneuvers may elevate the diaphragm, resulting in diminished FRC and potential hypoxemia. Addition of

positive end-expiratory pressure (PEEP) and ventilation with large tidal volumes (10–15 ml/kg) may counter these effects.

6. **Temperature control.** Heat loss in open abdominal procedures is a common problem. Potential sources and treatment are discussed in Chap. 18.

7. **Bowel or mesenteric manipulation** can lead acutely to facial flushing, hypotension, and tachycardia. Studies have implicated prostaglandin $F_{1\alpha}$, a prostanoid that is found in vascular endothelial cells and luminal cells of the bowel.

8. **Biliary tract spasm** may be caused by narcotics. Clinically, this effect is relatively uncommon, and narcotics are used judiciously in patients with biliary tract disease. Both narcotic premedication and epidural narcotic can produce painful biliary spasm. This response can be specifically reversed with naloxone, and both nitroglycerin and glucagon relieve spasm by nonspecific smooth muscle relaxation. Intraoperative spasm can complicate surgical repair or interpretation of a cholangiogram. Mixed agonist-antagonists such as butorphanol or nalbuphine may provide analgesia without the increase in biliary tone.

9. **Fecal contamination** may occur with perforation of the gastrointestinal tract. Infection and sepsis can progress rapidly.

10. **Hiccoughs** are episodic diaphragmatic spasms that may occur spontaneously or in response to stimulation of the diaphragm or abdominal viscera. Potential therapies include
    a. Increasing the depth of anesthesia, especially if the hiccoughs are due to reaction to the endotracheal tube or reflect diaphragmatic or other visceral stimulation.
    b. Removing the source of diaphragmatic irritation, such as gastric distention, retractors, packs, and suprahepatic hematomas or abscesses.
    c. Increasing the degree of neuromuscular blockade, which may decrease the strength of spasms. Complete diaphragmatic paralysis is difficult to achieve and may be possible only with doses in excess of those required for relaxation of the abdominal muscles.
    d. Chlorpromazine is rarely used intraoperatively. It can be slowly titrated in 5-mg increments IV.

D. **Emergence from anesthesia**
   1. **Reversal of neuromuscular blockade** with an acetylcholinesterase inhibitor should be accomplished at an appropriate time, as discussed in Chap. 12.
   2. **Analgesia for postoperative pain** is essential for a smooth transition upon emergence, as pain can lead to hemodynamic and cardiovascular instability, splinting, and hypoventilation.
      a. **Narcotics** should be titrated to preserve ventilatory drive, and dosage is guided by vital signs including respiratory rate.

        b. Epidural analgesia. Administration of a single dose of preservative-free morphine (Duramorph, 4 mg) has been shown to provide adequate postoperative analgesia for longer than 24 hours. The use of this technique is limited by potential delayed respiratory depression. Fentanyl (50–100 μg in 5–10 ml of preservative-free normal saline) provides 4–6 hours of analgesia with less risk of significant respiratory depression. Combinations of local anesthetic agents and narcotics can be administered by continuous infusion. The standard mix for infusion contains fentanyl, 10 μg/ml, in bupivacaine 0.1% (see Chap. 37).

        c. Other techniques used to provide analgesia include intrapleural anesthesia, intercostal nerve blockade, and field blocks.

IV. Anesthetic considerations for specific abdominal procedures

    A. Splenectomy may be an emergency procedure following blunt or penetrating trauma or may be performed electively for treatment of idiopathic thrombocytopenic purpura or for staging of Hodgkin's lymphoma. Large-bore IV access is required, as it is possible to encounter major blood loss requiring transfusion. General or combined anesthesia and muscle relaxation are required. Occasionally, a transthoracic approach to gain control of the hilar vessels of a very large spleen may be necessary.

    B. Cholecystectomy is a common operation done either as an open laparotomy or by a laparoscopic technique. For either technique, general anesthesia is required, and narcotics should be used judiciously to minimize spasm in the biliary tract and sphincter of Oddi. During laparoscopic cholecystectomy, the patient is placed in the reverse Trendelenburg position, and the gallbladder is dissected from the liver bed using either cautery or laser. Muscle relaxants are required. The amount of hemorrhage is difficult to assess because of the limited field of vision and the high magnification of the scope. Bleeding from the cystic or hepatic artery may be large and difficult to observe. After laparoscopic cholecystectomy, the decline in pulmonary function is greatly reduced, and postoperative pain is minimized. Most patients are discharged on the first postoperative day. The complications of laparoscopy are discussed in Chap. 29.

    C. Partial hepatectomy is used to treat hepatoma, unilobar metastasis of a gastrointestinal carcinoma, arteriovenous malformation, or echinococcal cysts. Major hemorrhage should be anticipated. For this reason, standard monitors are supplemented with arterial and central venous catheters and large-bore IV access. Epidural catheters are placed in patients who have normal coagulation studies. The liver has considerable reserve, and extensive resection must be performed before drug metabolism is clinically impaired. The effects of liver disease on anesthetic management are discussed in Chap. 5.

    D. Orthotopic liver transplantation is performed for patients who have end-stage liver disease. Common etiologies include hepatoma, sclerosing cholangitis, Wilson's disease, alpha$_1$-antitrypsin deficiency, primary biliary cirrhosis, and alcoholic cirrhosis. Such patients typically present for anesthesia with metabolic, hemodynamic, and multiorgan dysfunction.

1. **Preanesthetic considerations**
    a. **Coagulopathy.** Decreased hepatic synthetic function and thrombocytopenia are common.
    b. **Encephalopathy.** Decreased hepatic metabolism may present in any form including coma or increased intracranial pressure. Premedications are omitted for encephalopathic patients.
    c. **Intravascular volume** is usually reduced due to portal hypertension, hypoalbuminemia, and ascites. Many patients may be volume depleted from diuretic therapy prior to transplantation.
    d. **Electrolyte status.** Severe derangements may be seen due to sodium retention, diuretics, and renal insufficiency (hepatorenal syndrome). In some cases, hypoglycemia may be severe.
    e. **Pulmonary function.** Pulmonary shunting and massive ascites frequently lead to hypoxemia.
    f. **Portal hypertension.** Esophageal and gastric varices may be a source of blood loss. Previous portacaval shunting, other abdominal surgical procedures, and prior intraabdominal infections can significantly increase intraoperative bleeding.
    g. **Cardiac function.** Hepatic failure commonly causes shunting in the portal and pulmonary circulations. Development of the collateral circulation causes formation of arteriovenous malformations, leading to a high cardiac output. Although the cardiac output is often notably elevated, these patients may suffer from hypoperfusion at the end-organ level.

2. **Surgery for hepatic transplantation** proceeds in three distinct stages.
    a. **Recipient hepatectomy** includes resection of the gallbladder, hepatic veins, and a section of the inferior vena cava (IVC).
    b. The **anhepatic phase** is marked by decreased venous return when the IVC is cross clamped. Venovenous bypass (typically left femoral and portal to left axillary vein) can often improve venous return.
    c. The **postanhepatic phase** is marked by reperfusion of the donor liver, which delivers a hyperkalemic, hypothermic, and acidic solution (see Chap. 26) to the central circulation. After the vascular anastomoses are completed, the patient's condition usually stabilizes. The biliary anastomoses are performed, followed by donor cholecystectomy, choledochojejunostomy, and placement of a choledochal T tube.

3. **Anesthetic considerations**

a. **Hemorrhage and coagulopathy** are concurrent processes that can produce dramatic blood loss (multiple blood volumes). The period of greatest hemorrhage is usually during recipient hepatectomy. Preexisting coagulopathy may worsen during the anhepatic phase due to fibrinolysis. Both aminocaproic acid (Amicar) and aprotinin have been used (see Chap. 33).

b. **Hypothermia** can occur if preventive measures are not performed from the time of induction (see Chap. 18).

c. **Metabolic derangements** are common.

   (1) Oliguria secondary to hypovolemia and hypoperfusion may lead to renal failure and hyperkalemia. Therapy with diuretics, dopamine, and mannitol is started early in an attempt to prevent these problems.

   (2) Large-volume transfusion of citrated blood products leads to hypocalcemia and increased potassium levels.

   (3) During the anhepatic phase there is a theoretic risk of hypoglycemia, although typically hyperglycemia from dextrose-containing solutions prevails. This phase of the operation will also produce a progressive metabolic acidosis as hepatic metabolism of citrate and lactate is absent and peripheral circulation is compromised.

d. **Hypoxia** can occur from intrapulmonary shunting and thoracic restriction from surgical retraction and the Trendelenburg position. This can be improved by the application of PEEP and high FIO_2.

e. **Hypotension** due to hypovolemia or cardiac dysfunction is anticipated. Vasopressors and inotropes are required until the underlying problem can be corrected.

4. **Anesthetic management**

   a. In addition to the standard monitors, a urinary catheter and right radial arterial catheter are essential. Most patients also receive a pulmonary artery catheter placed through the right internal jugular vein. Venous access is obtained through a large-bore (12-gauge) catheter placed in the right arm and an 8.5 Fr catheter placed in the left internal jugular vein. A rapid transfusion system, capable of delivering 1.0–1.5 L/min at 38°C, supplies the left internal jugular catheter. This system of venous access can be modified as the patient's condition demands.

   b. **Induction of anesthesia** usually includes a rapid sequence technique, as patients may have a full stomach or ascites or be obtunded. Ketamine may be used as an induction agent in unstable patients.

   c. **Maintenance of anesthesia** is usually accomplished with a balanced technique of oxygen, moderate- to high-dose narcotics, and isoflurane. Halothane is avoided because of its ability to decrease hepatic blood flow. Nitrous oxide is avoided because of the possibility of air embolism during venovenous bypass and because it may cause bowel distention.

d. **Laboratory surveillance.** Arterial blood gases, electrolytes, hematocrit, platelet, and coagulation profiles are checked as needed.

e. **Transfusion therapy** relies on autologous transfusion of salvaged blood as well as banked products. Laboratory and clinical assessment of coagulation will determine the need for packed red blood cells, fresh frozen plasma, and other blood products. If possible, transfusion of platelets is delayed until after venovenous bypass is completed. Cryoprecipitate and epsilon-aminocaproic acid (Amicar) are adjuncts that may be required.

f. **Resuscitation** from cardiac collapse may be required at the time of reperfusion. The hyperkalemic, acidemic solution washed out from the donor liver, hypoperfused gut, and lower extremities may cause malignant dysrhythmias or cardiac arrest. Therapy to normalize potassium levels and acid-base status prior to reperfusion includes administration of volume, sodium bicarbonate, diuretics, insulin, dextrose, and small doses of epinephrine (50–100 μg). Hyperventilation is also useful. If necessary, cardiopulmonary resuscitation, calcium chloride, lidocaine, and catecholamine therapy may be required.

g. **Conclusion of the operation** requires that the patient be stable for transport to an intensive care unit. As the donor liver resumes function, coagulopathy generally improves, and ongoing fluid requirements diminish. Patients require additional narcotics for analgesia as well as sedatives.

E. **Operations for patients with portal hypertension.** These patients present with the stigmata of liver failure, and some may await liver transplantation. Operations are performed for palliation of variceal bleeding and ascites.

1. **Portacaval shunts** relieve portal hypertension by shunting blood to the IVC through a surgically created shunt. Complete diversion of portal venous flow to the IVC by an end-to-side anastomosis hastens hepatic failure and has an extremely high postoperative morbidity and mortality. Incomplete "H"-type shunts are usually constructed to permit partial decompression of the portal venous system. Shunting can significantly increase ventricular preload and precipitate heart failure.

2. **Splenorenal shunting** between the splenic and renal veins decompresses esophageal variceal collaterals and thus decreases the incidence of bleeding. Endoscopic sclerotherapy has largely supplanted this surgical technique, but it is still performed in refractory cases. The operation requires complete dissection of the

splenic vein as it crosses the pancreatic bed. Bleeding may be extensive and difficult to control due to coagulopathy.

3. **Peritoneovenous shunting** is performed for treatment of intractable ascites. The operation involves the placement of a valved conduit between the peritoneum and the central venous circulation. Conduits, such as the LeVeen and Denver shunts, allow ascitic fluid to enter the venous system. These operations can usually be conducted with local anesthetic infiltration. Disseminated intravascular coagulopathy precipitated by a shunt is a rare complication and requires prompt removal of the device. Postoperative care is aimed at preventing circulatory overload and requires aggressive diuretic management.

F. **Heterotopic pancreatic transplantation** is usually performed in conjunction with heterotopic renal transplantation. Although recipients may undergo a nephrectomy, their native pancreas is left intact. Anesthetic considerations are primarily related to renal transplantation and management of diabetes and are discussed in Chap. 26. The donor pancreas is most often anastomosed to the recipient's bladder through a portion of duodenum. The exocrine pancreatic secretions then drain into the bladder. Blood glucose should be determined frequently, since it rapidly falls to normal with perfusion of the pancreas. Since there is no pepsin present, trypsinogen and chymotrypsinogen are not activated. Gram-negative urinary tract infection can activate these enzymes, leading to bladder damage and requiring emergency removal of the transplanted pancreas. The pancreas secretes bicarbonate which is lost in the urine, and if kidney function fails, severe metabolic acidosis can result. Pancreatic islet cell transplantation remains an experimental procedure that holds promise for the treatment of diabetes. The procedure consists of purifying islets from cadaveric donors and then injecting them into the liver via the portal vein. The transplantation can be performed percutaneously using local anesthesia. At this time, there have been no long-term successes from islet cell transplantation.

G. **Pancreatectomy for hemorrhagic pancreatitis or pseudocyst** is a surgical procedure resulting in significant bleeding and third-space fluid loss. The inflammatory nature of these diseases may also cause severe peritonitis, ileus, and edema. Release of pancreatic lipases can cause saponification of omental fat, release of fatty acids that sequester calcium, and hypocalcemia.

H. **Whipple procedure** (pancreatojejunostomy with gastrojejunostomy and choledochojejunostomy) is done for resection of adenocarcinoma of the pancreas or for refractory, disabling pancreatitis. These are long and surgically difficult procedures with potential extensive fluid loss.

I. **Intraoperative radiation therapy** for pancreatic or colonic adenocarcinoma usually involves exploratory laparotomy and either a primary resection or a debulking procedure. Before wound closure, the anesthetized patient is moved from the operating room to the radiation therapy suite. Medication and equipment for resuscitation must accompany the patient. The patient is monitored continuously during transportation and ventilated with 100% oxygen. Anesthesia can be maintained with infusion of narcotic or hypnotic (e.g., propofol) until the radiation therapy suite is reached. A fully stocked and checked anesthesia machine must be available in the radiation therapy suite. In the radiation therapy suite, the safety of both the patient and the anesthesiologist must be ensured. Patients are positioned so that monitors and ventilation can be observed on remote television monitors. When the sterile cone of the cyclotron is lowered into the abdominal wound, the patient is checked for signs of aortic or IVC compression. Ventilation should be switched to 100% oxygen to maximize the sensitivity of the tumor to radiation therapy. Treatments usually last 5–20 minutes but may be interrupted if ventilatory or cardiovascular instability develops. Wound closure may be performed in the radiation therapy suite or after transport back to the operating room.

J. Gastrectomy or hemigastrectomy with gastroduodenostomy (Billroth I) or **gastrojejunostomy** (Billroth II) is usually done for gastric adenocarcinoma or for intractable bleeding from gastric or duodenal ulcers. A rapid sequence or awake intubation is usually performed.

K. Gastrostomy can be performed through a small upper abdominal incision or percutaneously with an endoscope. Local anesthesia may be sufficient, particularly in debilitated, elderly patients, but general anesthesia is frequently necessary.

L. Operations for obesity. Patients who are **morbidly obese** are those who weigh more than 100 pounds (45 kg) above their ideal body weight.

    1. Preoperative considerations

        a. Cardiovascular function can be compromised by an increased circulating volume and a tendency toward hypertension. Hypertension may result in ventricular hypertrophy, which combined with a high incidence of coronary artery disease, may severely limit a patient's cardiovascular reverse. Pulmonary artery hypertension may also develop and lead to isolated right ventricular failure.

        b. Obese patients develop a **restrictive ventilatory pattern** with a decrease in FRC. The supine position further compromises ventilation and may lead to significant ventilation-perfusion mismatching and atelectasis.

        c. Decreased gastric emptying time and **increased intragastric pressures and volumes** are seen in obese patients. These result in a higher incidence of symptomatic gastroesophageal reflux.

        d. Insulin resistance develops, and many obese patients require large supplemental doses of insulin for glucose control. Since perfusion of adipose tissue is variable, IV insulin administration is preferred.

2. Anesthetic considerations

a. **Operating tables** may be unable to accommodate the size and weight of the obese patient. It may be possible to modify standard operating tables, but it is preferable to use tables that are designed for obese patients. Extra padding and skin protection are required for even the shortest procedures.

b. Surgery for morbid obesity is often technically difficult, with the possibility of **significant blood loss.** Since venous access may be difficult, the anesthesiologist should anticipate the need for large-bore peripheral or central venous access. A large blood pressure cuff is usually required. Placement of a radial arterial catheter facilitates blood pressure measurement and allows determination of the hematocrit and arterial blood gases. Evaporative and edematous fluid losses are amplified in the obese patient, and central venous pressure measurements may be needed to guide fluid replacement. When cardiovascular function is seriously compromised, a pulmonary artery catheter is required.

c. Obese patients are at **increased risk for aspiration.** Careful airway valuation should be performed (see Chap. 13). The morbidly obese patient requires either a rapid sequence induction or awake intubation. Controlled ventilation by mask may prove impossible because of decreased ventilatory compliance and soft-tissue distortion of airway anatomy.

3. Surgical procedures

to treat morbid obesity have a high rate of complications and failures. Patients who have failed one operation may undergo reoperation with a different procedure. The most successful operation is the Roux-en-Y; however, this procedure has a higher rate of complications. Gastrogastrostomy or vertical banded gastroplasty may be the operation of choice. In each of these procedures the surgeon must mobilize the stomach, and significant blood loss may occur when the short gastric vessels are divided. The surgeon creates a small proximal gastric "pouch," and the anesthesiologist assists in the measurement of pouch volume by inserting an NG tube and instilling a measured volume of saline until the pouch is full.

M. Small-bowel resection is done for penetrating trauma, Crohn's disease, obstructing adhesions, Meckel's diverticulum, carcinoma, or infarction (from volvulus, intussusception, or thromboemboli). Patients are usually hypovolemic from vomiting, diarrhea, ileus, third spacing, or bleeding. Most are considered to have a "full stomach," and muscle relaxation is usually required.

N. Appendectomy is a procedure performed through a small lower abdominal incision. Patients with appendicitis may be dehydrated from fever, poor oral intake, and vomiting, and generous IV hydration is usually indicated prior to induction of anesthesia. In cases where sepsis is absent and hydration is adequate, a spinal or epidural anesthetic may be used. Otherwise, general anesthesia with rapid sequence or awake intubation is necessary.

O. **Colectomy or hemicolectomy** is used to treat adenocarcinoma, diverticulosis, angiodysplasia, abscess, ulcerative colitis, penetrating trauma, and infarction. Emergency colectomy on an unprepared bowel has a high risk of fecal contamination with peritonitis. Many colonic emergencies are treated with an initial diverting colostomy followed later by bowel preparation and elective colectomy. Patients for colectomy must be evaluated for hypovolemia, anemia, and sepsis. All emergency colectomies and colostomies are treated as a "full stomach." Combined anesthetics are commonly performed.

P. **Perirectal abscess drainage, hemorrhoidectomy,** and **pilonidal cystectomy** are relatively noninvasive and brief procedures. Pilonidal cysts are usually excised with the patient in the prone position, while the other procedures may be done in either the prone or lithotomy position. If general anesthesia is employed, deep planes of anesthesia or use of muscle relaxants may be required to achieve adequate sphincter relaxation. Intubation is necessary if general anesthesia is conducted in the prone position. Hyperbaric spinal or caudal anesthesia can be used for procedures in the lithotomy position, while a hypobaric spinal or caudal technique is used for the flexed prone (jackknife) or knee-chest position.

Q. **Inguinal, femoral,** or **ventral herniorrhaphies** can be done under local anesthesia, regional anesthesia (spinal, epidural, caudal or nerve block), or general anesthesia. Maximal stimulation may come at the time of spermatic cord or peritoneal traction, causing a profound vagal response. If general anesthesia is selected, then either a mask technique (e.g., laryngeal mask airway) or deep extubation should be considered to decrease coughing on emergence, which can strain the hernia repair.

SUGGESTED READING

Aitkenhead, A. R. Anaesthesia and bowel surgery. *Br. J. Anaesth.* 56:95, 1984.

Barash, P. G., Cullen, B. F., and Stoelting R. K. *Clinical Anesthesia.* Philadelphia: Lippincott, 1989.

Bigler, D., Hjorts, N.-C., and Kehlet, H. Disruption of colonic anastomosis during continuous epidural analgesia. *Anesthesia* 40:278, 1985.

Busuttil, R. W., et al. Liver transplantation today. *Ann. Intern. Med.* 104:377, 1986.

Chapin, J. W., Newland, M. C., and Hurlbert, B. J. Anesthesia for liver transplantation. *Semin. Liver Dis.* 9(3):195, 1989.

Cousins, M. J., and Bridenbaugh, P. O. *Neural Blockade In Clinical Anesthesia And Management of Pain.* Philadelphia: Lippincott, 1988. P. 1171.

Craig, D. B. Postoperative recovery of pulmonary function. *Anesth. Analg.* 60(1):46, 1981.

Hudson, J. C., et al. Ibuprofen pretreatment inhibits prostacyclin release during abdominal exploration in aortic surgery. *Anesthesiology* 72:443, 1990.

Hurley, R., and Lambert, D. Continuous spinal anesthesia. *Int. Anesthesiol. Clin.* 27(1):46, 1988.

Latimer, R. G., et al. Ventilatory patterns and pulmonary complications after upper abdominal surgery determined by preoperative and postoperative computerized spirometry and blood gas analysis. *Am. J. Surg.* 122:622, 1971.

Manolio, T. A., Christopherson, R., and Pearson, T. A. Regional vs. general anesthesia in high-risk surgical patients. *J. Clin. Anesth.* 1:414, 1989.

Marco, A. P., Yeo, C. J., and Rock, P. Anesthesia for a patient undergoing laparoscopic cholecystectomy. *Anesthesiology* 73:1268, 1990.

Miller, R. D. *Anesthesia.* New York: Churchill Livingstone, 1990.

Scott, N. B., and Kehlet, H. Regional anaesthesia and surgical morbidity. *Br. J. Surg.* 75:299, 1988.

Skolnick, A. Advances in islet cell transplantation: Is science closer to a diabetes cure? *J.A.M.A.* 264:427, 1990.

Sorensen, M. B., et al. Haemodynamics in patients undergoing porto-caval shunt operations. *Acta Anesth. Scand.* 26:425, 1982.

21

Anesthesia for Thoracic Surgery

Richard P. Dutton

I. **Preoperative evaluation**
  A. Patients for thoracic surgery should undergo the usual **preoperative assessment** as detailed in Chap. 1.
    1. Any patient undergoing **elective thoracic surgery** should be carefully screened for underlying bronchitis or pneumonia. Where possible, infections should be treated before surgery.
    2. In patients with **tracheal stenosis,** the history should focus on symptoms or signs of positional dyspnea, static versus dynamic airway collapse, and evidence of hypoxemia.
  B. **Arterial blood gases** (ABGs) will help to clarify the severity of any underlying pulmonary disease.
  C. **Pulmonary function tests** are routinely obtained in all patients scheduled for possible lung resection or where there is underlying severe pulmonary dysfunction (see Chap. 3).
  D. **Differential ventilation-perfusion scans of the chest,** in combination with pulmonary function tests, can be used to estimate the amount of residual lung capacity a patient will have following a major resection such as pneumonectomy. Differential scans should be obtained preoperatively in any patient where they may play a part in determining the surgical plan.
  E. **Computed tomography (CT) scans** are often used to assess the extent of thoracic lesions. The anesthesiologist can use them to examine specific anatomic relationships, including the caliber of affected airways.
  F. **Angiography is performed infrequently** but may provide valuable information regarding the vascularity of some tumors.
  G. **Tracheal tomography** is used to assess the caliber of stenotic airways and can be used to predict the size and length of the endotracheal tube that will be appropriate for the patient. Severe airway stenosis observed preoperatively may change the anesthesiologist's plans for induction and intubation.
  H. **Magnetic resonance imaging (MRI) scans are rarely obtained.**

II. **Preoperative preparation**
  A. **Preoperative sedation** should be given as needed to allay patient anxiety. A small dose of diazepam (5 mg PO) may be supplemented with IV midazolam once the patient is under the direct observation of the anesthesiologist.
    1. In patients with **stenotic airways or severely impaired pulmonary function,** sedation should be used with caution. Small amounts of benzodiazepines may lead to clinically significant hypoventilation, but successful anxiolysis may make breathing easier and facilitate induction of anesthesia.
    2. **Narcotics and larger doses of benzodiazepines**

and spontaneous deep breathing, coughing, and sighing postoperatively, particularly in combination with epidural narcotics.

B. Aspiration prophylaxis, with an oral H_2 antagonist and metoclopramide, should be considered in patients undergoing major thoracic surgery.

C. Glycopyrrolate (0.2 mg IM or IV) may be given to decrease oral secretions.

III. Monitoring

A. Standard monitoring should be used as described in Chap. 10.

B. A radial arterial line should be placed in any patient undergoing major thoracic surgery.

1. **For surgeries in the lateral decubitus position,** placement of the arterial line in the dependent arm will also provide an indicator of intraoperative vascular compromise brought about by positioning or surgical maneuvers.

2. **For tracheal surgery,** placement of the arterial line in the left arm will avoid interference caused by surgical manipulation of the innominate artery.

C. Central venous catheterization is seldom necessary.

D. A pulmonary artery catheter may be placed preoperatively in patients with severe cardiac disease.

1. **Absolute numeric values** may be affected by lateral positioning and opening the chest, although trends in central venous pressure, pulmonary artery pressure, pulmonary artery occlusion pressure, and cardiac output can be followed.

2. **The pulmonary artery catheter** is customarily placed from the nondependent side of the neck, incorporating an extra-long sterile sheath. This facilitates repositioning of the catheter into the dependent pulmonary artery intraoperatively if it does not naturally migrate there. Hypoxic pulmonary vasoconstriction will typically ensure that the catheter migrates to the correct side once the surgical lung is collapsed, but the catheter can always be retracted into the sheath and refloated. Alternatively, the pulmonary artery catheter can be placed preoperatively under fluoroscopic guidance to ensure that the tip is in the correct pulmonary artery.

IV. Endoscopy includes direct or indirect visualization of the pharynx, larynx, esophagus, trachea, and bronchi. Endoscopy may be undertaken to obtain biopsy samples, delineate upper airway anatomy, remove obstructing foreign bodies, assess hemoptysis, or perform laser surgery.

A. Flexible bronchoscopy under local anesthesia. Flexible bronchoscopy may be performed under local anesthesia in the awake, fasting patient. An anesthesiologist may be asked to provide monitored care (MAC) if the patient's medical condition is sufficiently compromised to warrant close monitoring or if assistance with IV sedation or topicalization is required.

1. Most commonly, anesthesia for flexible bronchoscopy is achieved by **topicalization** of the oro- or nasopharynx, larynx, vocal cords, and trachea with a spray of 4%

lidocaine. If this is done patiently, no further anesthesia is required. Premedication with a drying agent such as atropine or glycopyrrolate will limit salivary dilution of the anesthetic, providing quicker and more predictable anesthesia.

2. **Nerve blocks** may be used to supplement airway anesthesia (see Chap. 13).

B. **Flexible bronchoscopy under general anesthesia**

1. **Anesthetic technique** should provide an adequate depth of anesthesia to avoid coughing. The largest possible endotracheal tube should be used, as this will more easily permit ventilation during the procedure.

2. **Multiport adult operating bronchoscopes** require at least a 7.5-mm tube, although pediatric bronchoscopes may pass through tubes as small as 4.5 mm. The fit of the bronchoscope in the endotracheal tube should be checked preoperatively if there is any question of incompatibility.

C. **Rigid bronchoscopy** permits superior visualization and control of the airway compared to fiberoptic bronchoscopy. Adequate operating conditions require general anesthesia.

1. **General considerations**

a. **Hypercarbia secondary to inadequate ventilation** is the most common complication during bronchoscopy and frequently results in ventricular arrhythmias. This mandates that lidocaine be available for immediate use. Most arrhythmias, however, are best treated by increasing ventilation.

b. **Hypoxemia** secondary to intermittent and uneven ventilation may be minimized by using controlled ventilation with 100% oxygen.

c. **Anesthesia machines capable of delivering high flow rates of oxygen** (at least 20 L/min) are necessary to compensate for air leaks occurring around the bronchoscope or during suctioning.

d. **Air leaks around the bronchoscope** may be minimized by compressing the trachea externally.

2. A **rigid bronchoscope with a side arm permitting positive-pressure ventilation** is most commonly used.

a. This type of bronchoscope permits controlled positive-pressure ventilation and the use of inhalation anesthetics.

b. **Manual ventilation** is necessary, since ventilation must be interrupted when the surgeon removes the eyepiece of the bronchoscope to suction or perform a biopsy. In addition, manual ventilation can instantly compensate for changes in effective compliance that may occur when the bronchoscope enters a bronchus.

c. **If difficulty in oxygenating or ventilating the patient occurs during bronchoscopy,** the surgeon should be instructed to withdraw the bronchoscope back into the trachea. Once adequate conditions are reestablished, endoscopy may continue.

3. **Sanders bronchoscopes** use a manually or machine-triggered jet of oxygen with the bronchoscope to entrain air through the proximal end of the tube by the Venturi effect.

   a. An **intravenous anesthetic technique** (see Chap. 14) must be used, since the high fresh gas flow rates may result in unpredictable volatile anesthetic concentrations. Also, the inspired oxygen concentration is uncertain, since the amount of room air entrained cannot be controlled. Muscle relaxation is required for the jet to inflate the lungs adequately.

   b. **Monitoring.** The anesthesiologist should directly observe the effect of each triggered breath, looking at the rise of the chest and listening for adequate breath sounds. Observation of exhalation is equally important, since "ball-valve" obstruction of ventilation will rapidly lead to barotrauma.

   c. End-tidal capnometry is impossible with a jet ventilation system, so **ABGs** should be obtained periodically or at any time the adequacy of ventilation is in question.

   d. The **advantage** of this bronchoscope is that ventilation is not interrupted by suctioning or surgical manipulations, since the proximal end of the bronchoscope is always open. This makes the Sanders bronchoscope suitable for use during laser surgery of the larynx, vocal cords, or proximal trachea.

4. **Anesthetic technique**

   a. **A variety of techniques** may be used in the patient without preexisting airway compromise. Traditionally, volatile agents in oxygen have been used to maintain anesthesia following induction with pentothal or propofol. Short-acting muscle relaxants may be used to lower anesthetic requirements, and controlled ventilation can be applied throughout.

   b. **Total intravenous anesthesia** with combinations of alfentanil, a short-acting muscle relaxant, and a hypnotic agent such as propofol, methohexital, or ketamine, offers the advantage of a constant anesthetic level even during periods of apnea.

   c. **If thoracotomy is to follow the bronchoscopy,** the patient is intubated with a double-lumen endotracheal tube immediately after the bronchoscope is withdrawn.

5. **Complications** of bronchoscopy include dental and laryngeal damage from intubation, injuries to the eyes or lips, airway rupture, pneumothorax, and hemorrhage. Airway obstruction may occur due to excessive bleeding or obstruction from a foreign body or dislodged mass. Inadequate ventilation may lead to hypoxemia, hypercarbia, and ventricular arrhythmias.

D. **Flexible esophagoscopy** may be performed under local anesthesia as described for flexible bronchoscopy (see sec. **A**) or following the induction of general anesthesia and intubation. Use of a smaller-caliber endotracheal tube will allow the surgeon more room to work in the pharynx and proximal esophagus.

E. **Rigid esophagoscopy** is commonly performed under general anesthesia with muscle relaxation to prevent patient movement during the procedure. As with flexible esophagoscopy, a smaller endotracheal tube is used.

V. Mediastinal operations

A. **Mediastinoscopy** is indicated to determine the extrapulmonary spread of pulmonary tumors and to diagnose mediastinal masses. Mediastinoscopy is performed through an incision just superior to the manubrium. A rigid endoscope is then introduced below the sternum, and the anterior surfaces of the trachea, and the hilum are examined.

1. Any **general anesthetic technique** may be used, provided the patient remains immobile. While the procedure is not very painful, intermittent stimulation of the trachea, carina, and main stem bronchi occurs.

2. **Complications** can include pneumothorax, rupture of the great vessels, and damage to the airways. Blood pressures monitored from the right arm may demonstrate intermittent occlusion if the innominate artery is compressed between the mediastinoscope and the posterior surface of the sternum.

B. A **Chamberlain procedure** employs an anterior parasternal incision to obtain lung tissue for biopsy or to drain abscesses.

1. The procedure is performed in the supine position following induction of general anesthesia. If no ribs are resected, the procedure is not usually very painful. Postoperative intercostal blocks spanning the level of the incision will provide adequate analgesia.

2. One-lung ventilation is not required for lung biopsy, but manual ventilation in cooperation with the surgeon(s) can facilitate the procedure.

3. If the **pleural space** is evacuated as it is closed, a chest tube is not generally required postoperatively, although the patient should be carefully monitored for any signs of pneumothorax.

C. **Mediastinal surgery**

1. **Median sternotomy** is performed for resection of a mediastinal tumor or for bilateral pulmonary resections. In descending order of frequency, mediastinal masses include neurogenic tumors, cysts, teratodermoids, lymphomas, thymomas, parathyroid tumors, and retrosternal thyroids.

2. **Thymectomy,** via a median sternotomy, is now considered the treatment of choice for myasthenia gravis, with a 75% positive response rate. Anesthetic considerations for the patient with myasthenia gravis are detailed in Chap. 12.

3. **General anesthesia** may be induced and maintained with any technique.

a. Muscle relaxants are not required to maintain surgical exposure but may be a useful adjunct to general anesthesia. Relaxants should be used with great caution or avoided altogether in the myasthenic patient.

b. During the actual sternotomy, the patient's lungs should be deflated and motionless. Even so, **complications** of sternotomy can include laceration of the right ventricle, atrium, or great vessels (particularly the innominate artery) and unrecognized pneumothorax in either side of the chest.

c. Postoperative pain from a median sternotomy is significantly less than from a thoracotomy and may be managed with epidural or parenteral narcotics.

VI. Pulmonary resection

A. Lateral or posterolateral thoracotomy is the incision most commonly performed for the resection of pulmonary neoplasms or abscesses. Thoracotomy will often be preceded by bronchoscopy, mediastinoscopy, or both. Any lung resection involving a lobe or larger segment will be greatly facilitated by providing a quiet surgical field, produced by selectively ventilating a single lung.

B. Lung isolation

1. Endobronchial tubes. Double-lumen tubes range in size from 28–41 Fr and are designed to conform to either the right or left main stem bronchus, providing separate channels for ventilation of the distal bronchus and the trachea. The right-sided tube has a separate opening for ventilation of the right upper lobe.

a. Insertion

(1) The endobronchial tube, including both cuffs and all necessary connectors, should be carefully checked before placement. The tube should be well lubricated, and a stylet should be placed in the bronchial lumen.

(2) Even though most surgical procedures can be performed with a left-sided double-lumen tube, it is our practice to selectively intubate the dependent (nonoperative) bronchus. This ensures that the endobronchial tube will not interfere with resection of the main stem bronchus, should this be necessary. If the nondependent lung is intubated, ventilation of the dependent lung through the tracheal lumen may be compromised by mediastinal pressure pushing the tube against the tracheal wall and creating a "ball-valve" obstruction.

(3) Following laryngoscopy, the endobronchial tube should be inserted initially with the distal curve facing anteriorly. Once into the trachea, the stylet should be removed and the tube rotated so that the bronchial lumen is toward the appropriate side. The tube is then advanced until resistance is met. If the tube size is appropriate for the patient (39–41 Fr for a man, 35–37 Fr for a woman), the distal end should be seated in the appropriate main stem bronchus.

(4) Alternatively, a fiberoptic bronchoscope can be passed down the bronchial lumen as soon as the

Table 21-1. Results of auscultation with both cuffs inflated and one lumen clamped

Bronchial side ventilated	Tracheal side ventilated	Problem
Clear, unilateral breath sounds, high pressures	Clear breath sounds or no breath sounds	Tube in too far
Bilateral breath sounds	No breath sounds	Tube not in far enough
Unilateral breath sounds on wrong side	No breath sounds or breath sounds on wrong side	Tube in wrong lung

tube is in the trachea and then used to guide the tube into the correct main stem bronchus.

(5) Once the tube has been inserted and connected to the anesthesia circuit, the tracheal cuff is inflated, and manual ventilation is begun. Both lungs should expand evenly with bilateral breath sounds and no detectable air leak. The tracheal side of the adapter is then clamped and the distal tracheal lumen opened to room air via the access port. The bronchial cuff is inflated to a point just sufficient to eliminate air leak from the tracheal lumen, and the chest is auscultated. Breath sounds should now be limited to the nonoperative side of the chest. Moving the clamp to the bronchial side of the adapter and closing the tracheal access port should cause only the operative lung to be ventilated.

(6) Once adequate lung isolation is achieved, the fiberoptic bronchoscope can be used to confirm position. When passed down the tracheal lumen, the bronchoscope should reveal the carina with the top edge of the blue bronchial cuff just visible in the main stem bronchus. Passing the bronchoscope down the bronchial lumen should reveal either the left main stem bronchus or the bronchus intermedius depending on whether a left- or right-sided tube is being placed. The orifice of the right upper lobe should be visible through the side lumen of a right-sided tube. A bronchoscope should be kept available throughout the case.

(7) Both lumens are ventilated, and the patient is positioned for surgery.

b. Table 21-1 illustrates **common errors with endobronchial tube placement.** The most common one with a disposable double-lumen tube is positioning too far into the bronchus so that the distal lumen is only ventilating one lobe.

c. The procedure for **passing an endobronchial tube through an existing tracheal stoma** is virtually identical. Bronchoscopy will help to determine how far the tube should be advanced once it is in the trachea.

2. **Univent tubes** are large-caliber endotracheal tubes encompassing a small integrated channel for a built-in bronchial blocker.

   a. **Insertion.** The Univent tube is inserted into the trachea in the usual fashion and rotated toward the operative lung. Following inflation of the tracheal cuff, the bronchial blocker is advanced into the ipsilateral main stem bronchus under fiberoptic guidance, and the cuff is inflated. Because the Univent tube is made of Silastic rather than PVC, thorough lubrication of the bronchoscope will be required.

   b. **Collapse of the operative lung** occurs through both the small distal opening in the blocker and absorption of oxygen from the lung. This is a slow process but may be hastened by letting the blocker down and disconnecting the anesthesia circuit while observing the lung. Once collapse has occurred, the blocker can be reinflated and the circuit reconnected.

3. **Bronchial blockers** may be used in situations where it is not possible to place an endobronchial tube, typically in pediatric patients, in those with difficult airway anatomy, or in those with prior tracheostomy, or where satisfactory lung isolation cannot be achieved by other means.

   a. **Insertion.** An appropriately sized Fogarty embolectomy catheter is selected and placed in the trachea prior to endotracheal intubation. Following intubation, the balloon tip is positioned with a fiberoptic bronchoscope in the appropriate main stem bronchus and inflated. Lung collapse occurs slowly, via absorption of gases.

   b. While it is occasionally desirable **to place a blocker after endotracheal intubation,** it is often very difficult to pass one around a previously placed tube. Placing the blocker via the bronchoscope adapter through the tube is easy, provided the lumen will accommodate both blocker and bronchoscope.

   c. With either Univent tubes or bronchial blockers, frequent **repositioning** of the blocker may be required.

4. **Complications** of lung isolation techniques include collapse of obstructed segments of the lung, airway trauma, bleeding, and aspiration during prolonged efforts at intubation. Hypoxia and hypoventilation may occur both during placement efforts and as a result of malpositioning.

5. **Positioning.** Thoracotomies for lung resection are most commonly performed in the lateral decubitus position with the bed sharply flexed and the surgical field parallel to the floor.

   a. The **arms** are usually extended in front of the

patient and must be carefully padded to avoid compression on the radial and ulnar nerves or obstruction of arterial and venous cannulas. The dependent brachial plexus must be checked for excessive tension. Various devices exist for supporting the upper arm securely above the lower, leaving the anesthesiologist with good access to the lower arm. Neither arm should be abducted more than 90 degrees.

b. **Head and neck.** The neck should remain in a neutral position, and the dependent eye and ear should be carefully checked to ensure that they are not under any direct pressure.

c. The **lower extremities** should be padded appropriately to avoid compression injuries. In male patients, the scrotum should also be carefully positioned.

d. During the positioning process, the **vital signs** should be closely observed, as pooling of blood in dependent extremities may cause sudden hypotension.

e. **Changes in position** may move the endobronchial tube or blocker and change ventilation-perfusion relationships. Lung compliance, lung isolation, and patient oxygenation should be reassessed after any change in position.

C. **One-lung ventilation.** General anesthesia, the lateral position, an open chest, surgical manipulations, and one-lung ventilation all alter ventilation and perfusion.

1. **Oxygenation**

   a. The **amount of pulmonary blood flow** passing through the unventilated lung (pulmonary shunt) is the most important factor determining arterial oxygenation during one-lung ventilation.

   b. **Diseased lungs** often have reduced perfusion secondary to vascular occlusion or vasoconstriction. This may limit shunting of blood through the non-ventilated operative lung during one-lung ventilation.

   c. **Perfusion of the unventilated lung** is also reduced by hypoxic pulmonary vasoconstriction.

   d. The **lateral position** tends to reduce pulmonary shunting, since gravity will decrease blood flowing to the nondependent lung.

   e. **Monitoring.** Oxygenation needs to be closely monitored, either by clear, constant signal from the pulse oximeter or by frequent ABG assessments.

2. **Ventilation**

   a. **Carbon dioxide tension** should be maintained on one-lung ventilation at the same level as on two lungs.

   b. **Controlled ventilation** is mandatory during open-chest operations.

   c. **Minute ventilation** while on one-lung ventilation is maintained with tidal volume at 10–15 ml/kg and increasing respiratory rate as necessary.

d. Peak airway pressure may increase during one-lung ventilation primarily due to increased elastic recoil from the (relatively) hyperinflated single lung.

e. When switching from two-lung to one-lung ventilation, initial manual ventilation allows instantaneous adaptation to the expected changes in compliance and facilitates assessment of lung isolation. Once tidal volume and compliance have been assessed by hand and lung collapse confirmed visually, mechanical ventilation is reinstituted.

3. Management of one-lung ventilation

a. Anesthetic management. During one-lung ventilation, nitrous oxide is decreased or discontinued if there is any evidence of a significant fall in PaO_2 (i.e., decreases in oxygen saturation).

b. Difficulties with oxygenation during one-lung ventilation may be treated with a variety of maneuvers, all directed at decreasing blood flow to the nonventilated lung (decreasing shunt fraction) or minimizing atelectasis in the ventilated lung.

(1) **Tube position** should be reassessed, ideally by fiberoptic bronchoscopy, and repositioned if necessary.

(2) The tube should be **suctioned.**

(3) **Positive end-expiratory pressure** may be added to the ventilated lung to treat atelectasis but may lower arterial oxygen saturation if more blood flow is forced into the unventilated lung as a result.

(4) **Continuous positive airway pressure** can be applied to the nonventilated lung using a separate Mapleson circuit or any of several commercially available devices. Under direct visualization, the collapsed lung is slowly pressurized to a point just short of when lung expansion is interfering with surgical exposure and then maintained at that level.

(5) **Oxygen insufflation** can be provided to the nonventilated lung at a rate just short of causing any reinflation. This is done by connecting oxygen tubing from a flowmeter to a small suction catheter and then passing the distal tip down the open tracheal lumen.

(6) The nonventilated lung may be briefly inflated with **100% oxygen** and the exhalation port to the operative lung capped. In this way, a motionless, partially collapsed lung is maintained. Reinflation of the lung with oxygen will be necessary every 10–20 minutes.

(7) In the event of **persistent hypoxemia** uncorrectable by combinations of the above therapies or a sudden precipitous desaturation, the surgeon must be notified and the surgical lung reinflated with 100% oxygen. Two-lung ventilation is maintained until the situation has stabilized, and the surgical lung can again be allowed

to collapse. Some patients may require periodic reinflation or even manual two-lung ventilation throughout the procedure to maintain adequate arterial oxygen saturation.

(8) **If hypoxemia persists,** the surgeon can improve ventilation-perfusion matching by clamping the pulmonary artery of the surgical lung or any of its available lobes.

(9) In the **extreme setting,** cardiopulmonary bypass can be instituted to provide oxygenation (see Chap. 23).

c. **When switching from one-lung back to two-lung ventilation,** a few manual breaths with pronounced inspiratory hold will help to reexpand collapsed alveoli. Observation of the lung as it reexpands is useful.

D. **Anesthetic technique.** General anesthesia, in combination with epidural analgesia or anesthesia, is the preferred technique. Thoracic epidural catheters are usually placed (see Chap. 16 for technique).

1. **General anesthesia** is typically induced with thiopental or propofol and a relaxant and maintained with a volatile agent in oxygen.

a. **Nitrous oxide** may be used during the procedure to reduce the requirement for volatile agents.

(1) During one-lung ventilation, shunting and hypoxemia may limit the use of nitrous oxide, although some patients will remain well saturated.

(2) At the conclusion of the procedure with both lungs ventilated, nitrous oxide, in concentrations up to 70%, will provide a smoother emergence than a volatile agent alone. It is essential that the chest tubes are functioning.

b. **Modest doses of fentanyl or alfentanil** given during the induction of anesthesia will diminish the hemodynamic response to intubation, positioning, and incision, while maintaining cardiovascular stability.

c. **Muscle relaxants** are useful adjuncts to general anesthesia. Short-acting agents may be used initially if the thoracotomy is contingent on the results of bronchoscopy or mediastinoscopy.

2. **Epidural analgesia**

a. Bolus injections of **fentanyl** (100 μg in 10 ml normal saline) or a **mixture of bupivacaine and fentanyl** (0.1% and 0.001%, respectively) will reduce the requirement for general anesthesia without producing dense sympathetic blockade. Bupivacaine 0.1% and fentanyl 0.001% may also be used as a continuous infusion at a rate of 4–8 ml/hr.

b. Bolus injections of more concentrated local anesthetics may be associated with dense sympathetic blockade.

(1) The continuous infusion of an **alpha-adrenergic agent** or increased infusion of IV

fluids may be required to maintain adequate blood pressure.

(2) The use of **volatile anesthetics** may exacerbate hypotension from sympathetic blockade but may be necessary for amnesia in the absence of nitrous oxide.

E. **Emergence and extubation.** The goal of the anesthetic technique selected is to have an awake, comfortable, and extubated patient at the end of the procedure.

1. **Prior to closing the chest,** the lungs are inflated to 30 cm H_2O pressure to reinflate atelectatic areas and check for significant air leaks.

2. **Chest tubes are inserted** to drain the pleural cavity and promote lung expansion. Chest tubes usually are placed under water seal and 20 cm H_2O suction, except after a pneumonectomy. Following pneumonectomy, a chest tube, if used, should be placed under water seal only. Applying suction could shift the mediastinum to the draining side and reduce venous return.

3. **Prompt extubation** avoids the potential disruptive effects of endotracheal intubation and positive-pressure ventilation on fresh suture lines. If postoperative ventilation is required, the double-lumen tube should be exchanged for a conventional endotracheal tube with a high-volume, low-pressure cuff. Peak inspiratory pressures should be kept as low as possible.

F. **Postoperative analgesia.** Lateral thoracotomy is a painful incision, involving multiple muscle layers, rib resection, and continuous motion as the patient breathes. Pain treatment should begin before the patient emerges from general anesthesia.

1. **Epidural analgesia** has become the preferred approach for post-thoracotomy pain management (see sec. **D.2** and Chap. 37).

2. **Intercostal nerve blocks**

a. Intercostal nerve blocks may be used in situations where epidural analgesia is impractical or ineffective.

b. **Five interspaces** are usually blocked: two above, two below, and one at the site of the incision.

c. **Technique.** Under sterile conditions, a 23-gauge needle is inserted perpendicular to the skin in the posterior axillary line over the lower edge of the rib. The needle then is "walked" off the rib inferiorly until it just slips off the rib. After a negative aspiration for blood, 2–5 ml of 0.5% bupivacaine with 1:200,000 epinephrine is injected. The procedure is repeated at each interspace to be blocked. In addition, subcutaneous infiltration with bupivacaine is performed in a V-shaped pattern around each chest tube site to reduce the discomfort of chest tube movement. Analgesia lasts from 6–12 hours.

d. If a chest tube is not in place, the **risk of pneumothorax** from the block needs to be considered.

3. **Parenteral narcotics.** If parenteral narcotics are required, they should be administered judiciously.

4. Nonsteroidal anti-inflammatory agents. Ketorolac has proved effective as a supplemental analgesic.

VII. Tracheal resection and reconstruction

A. General considerations.
Surgery of the trachea and major airways involves significant anesthetic risks, including interruption of airway continuity and the potential for total obstruction of an already stenotic airway.

1. The **surgical approach** depends on the location and extent of the lesion. Lesions of the cervical trachea are approached through a transverse neck incision. Lower lesions necessitate a manubrial split. Lesions of the distal trachea and carina may require a median sternotomy and/or single or bilateral thoracotomy.

2. **Extubation** at the conclusion of the surgical procedure is the goal of the anesthetic, as it will put less strain on the fresh tracheal anastomosis.

B. Induction

1. The **anesthetic technique** must include a plan for preserving airway patency throughout induction and intubation, as well as emergency plans and equipment for dealing with any sudden loss of airway control.

2. **Preoperatively,** the patient may be given a nebulized lidocaine treatment (4 ml of 4% solution) to partially anesthetize the upper airway. This will make it easier for the patient to tolerate pungent volatile anesthetics.

3. **If the airway is critically stenotic,** spontaneous ventilation should be maintained throughout the induction, as it may not be possible to ventilate the patient with a mask if apnea occurs. A volatile agent in oxygen is the preferred anesthetic, beginning at low concentrations and slowly increasing. A deep plane of anesthesia must be achieved prior to instrumentation, and this often requires 15–20 minutes in the patient with small tidal volumes and a large functional residual capacity. Hemodynamic support with phenylephrine may be required for the elderly or debilitated patient to tolerate the necessary high concentration of volatile agent.

4. **Muscle relaxants are contraindicated** during induction, since ventilation often depends on the patient's spontaneous efforts alone.

5. **Patients with preexisting mature tracheostomies** may be induced with IV agents, allowing cannulation of the tracheostomy with a cuffed, flexible, armored (Tovell) endotracheal tube. The surgical field around the tube is prepared, and the tube is removed and replaced with a sterile one by the surgeon.

C. Intraoperative management
is complicated by periodic interruption of airway continuity by the surgical procedure.

1. **Rigid bronchoscopy** is commonly performed prior to the surgical incision to delineate tracheal anatomy and caliber.

   a. If the surgeon determines that an endotracheal tube can be placed through the stenotic segment, this should be done as soon as the bronchoscope is withdrawn. Controlled ventilation can then be used safely.

b. If the stenotic segment is too narrow or friable to allow intubation, spontaneous ventilation and anesthesia must continue through the bronchoscope until surgical access to the distal trachea is achieved. Alternatives include having the surgeon "core out" the trachea with the rigid bronchoscope, placing a tracheostomy distal to the stenotic segment, intubating above the lesion, and allowing spontaneous ventilation to continue or using a jet ventilation system to ventilate the patient from above the lesion.

2. **Whenever the airway is in jeopardy or ventilation is intermittent,** 100% oxygen should be used.

3. **For lower tracheal or carinal resections,** a long endotracheal tube with a flexible armored wall can be used. This allows the surgeon to position the tip in the trachea or either main stem bronchus and to operate around it without interrupting ventilation. These "Wilson" tubes are not commercially available but may be constructed by attaching a Tovell tube to the proximal half of a standard red rubber endotracheal tube. They can be inserted using the long stylet from a double-lumen tube.

4. **When the trachea is surgically divided,** the surgeon will ask for the endotracheal tube to be retracted above the division and will then place a sterile Tovell tube in the distal trachea. A suture may be placed in the endotracheal tube before pulling it back into the pharynx to facilitate replacing it in the trachea at the end of the procedure.

a. The **Tovell tube** may be frequently removed and reinserted by the surgeons as they work around it. Manual ventilation during this portion of the procedure will help avoid leakage of gas from the circuit.

b. Once the stenotic segment has been removed and the posterior tracheal reanastomosis completed, the Tovell tube is removed, and the endotracheal tube is readvanced from above. The distal trachea should be suctioned to remove accumulated blood and secretions. The patient's head is then flexed forward, reducing tension on the trachea, and the anterior portion of the anastomosis is completed.

5. **Jet ventilation** through a catheter held by one of the surgeons may be required during carinal resection for airways too small to accommodate an endotracheal tube.

a. It is difficult to administer volatile agents by a jet ventilator, so intravenous agents will be needed during this portion of the surgery.

b. Jet ventilation rate and pressure should be carefully titrated by direct observation of the surgical field. Obstruction of exhalation will lead to "stacking" of breaths, increased airway pressure, and barotrauma.

6. **At the conclusion of the procedure,** a single large suture is placed from chin to anterior chest to preserve neck flexion and thereby minimize tension on the tracheal suture line. This single suture will not support the weight of the patient's head, however, and several blankets under the head to provide flexion will still be required postoperatively. Close attention during emergence, extubation, and transfer to the bed is essential.

D. **Emergence and extubation**
   1. **Spontaneous ventilation** should be resumed as soon as possible after the procedure to minimize trauma to the tracheal suture line. Most patients may be safely extubated, but in those where difficult anatomy or copious secretions make this undesirable, a small tracheostomy may be placed below the tracheal repair.
      a. The patient should be awake enough to maintain spontaneous ventilation and avoid aspiration but should be extubated before head movement damages the surgical repair.
      b. If tracheal collapse, swelling, or secretions cause respiratory distress after extubation, the patient should be reintubated fiberoptically with a small, uncuffed endotracheal tube, preferably with the head maintained in forward flexion.
   2. **Frequent bronchoscopies** may be required in the postoperative period to remove secretions from the lungs. These are performed at the bedside under local anesthesia.
   3. **Pain medications** are often withheld until the patient is wide awake and responsive. Only small amounts of IV morphine are needed to treat the relatively mild pain from neck incisions. Pain from thoracotomies should be managed with epidural analgesia.

E. **Traumatic tracheal disruption** may be caused by airway instrumentation or thoracic trauma and may be signaled by hypoxia, dyspnea, subcutaneous emphysema, pneumomediastinum, or pneumothorax.
   1. The posterior portion of the trachea is most commonly involved. High external pressure to the chest in the setting of a closed glottis, as can occur in motor vehicle accidents, may overpressurize the trachea and "blow out" the membranous wall.
   2. Positive-pressure ventilation will exacerbate the air leak and rapidly worsen symptoms from pneumothorax or pneumomediastinum. If possible, the patient should be allowed to breathe spontaneously, following the protocol for the patient with critical tracheal stenosis.
   3. **Tracheal damage** in the already anesthetized patient may be treated initially by advancement of a small endotracheal tube past the point of injury. If this cannot be accomplished, as in the case of a difficult airway where the tube itself causes the injury, an immediate surgical tracheostomy must be performed and access to the distal trachea secured.
   4. Once a tube has been placed across or distal to the site

of tracheal disruption, controlled positive-pressure ventilation can begin. Further management is as for the patient undergoing elective airway surgery.

VIII. Intrapulmonary hemorrhage. Massive hemoptysis may be caused by thoracic trauma, pulmonary artery rupture secondary to catheterization, or erosion into a vessel by a tracheostomy, abscess, or airway tumor.

   A. The patient must be immediately intubated and ventilated with **100% oxygen.**

   B. An attempt should be made to **suction the airway clear,** ideally with a rigid bronchoscope.

   C. If a unilateral source is identified, **lung isolation** may be undertaken to protect the uninvolved lung and facilitate corrective surgery. Techniques for lung isolation are described in sec. **VI.B.** Obstruction of the endotracheal tube is an ever present danger, and frequent suctioning may be necessary.

   1. Placement of a double lumen endobronchial tube will provide the best isolation but may be technically difficult.

   2. In an emergency, the existing endotracheal tube can simply be advanced into the bronchus of the uninvolved lung and the cuff inflated.

   3. Fiberoptic bronchoscopy is essential for suctioning blood and confirming isolation.

   D. Definitive treatment may require a thoracotomy and surgical repair.

IX. Esophageal surgery includes procedures for resection of esophageal neoplasms, antireflux procedures, and repair of traumatic or congenital lesions.

   A. General considerations

   1. Patients may be **chronically malnourished,** both from systemic illness (carcinoma) and anatomic interference with swallowing.

   2. Both esophageal carcinoma and traumatic disruption of the distal esophagus are associated with **ethanol abuse;** patients may have impaired liver function, elevated portal pressures, anemia, cardiomyopathy, and bleeding disorders.

   3. Patients who have **difficulty swallowing** may be significantly hypovolemic. Cardiovascular instability may be further exacerbated by preoperative chemotherapy with cardiotoxins such as adriamycin.

   4. Most patients presenting for esophageal procedures will be at risk for **aspiration.** Appropriate preoperative prophylaxis should be given, and rapid sequence induction or awake intubation should be planned.

   5. Monitors should include an arterial line and central venous pressure and Foley catheters.

   6. Temperature conservation measures should be aggressively pursued.

   B. Operative approach and anesthesia

   1. Upper esophageal diverticuli are approached through a lateral cervical incision, similar to that for carotid surgery. This incision may also be used for upper esophageal myotomies for swallowing disorders.

      a. Positioning. The patient is positioned supine with the neck extended and the head turned to the contralateral side.

      b. General anesthesia may be induced and maintained with any technique. Postoperative pain and fluid shifts are usually minimal with a cervical incision, and patients may be safely extubated at the conclusion of the procedure. The surgeons may or may not elect to leave a nasogastric tube in place.

2. Carcinoma

      a. Lesions of the upper esophagus are approached through a transverse cervical incision, allowing for a proximal anastomosis in the neck. A right-sided thoracic incision and a midline abdominal incision may also be required to complete the resection and reattach the proximal and distal ends.

      b. Lesions of the middle esophagus are commonly approached through a right-sided thoracotomy, which allows for a proximal anastomosis above the level of the aortic arch. Mobilization of the stomach or jejunum is accomplished through a midline abdominal incision. This combination is known as an **Ivor-Lewis** procedure.

      c. Lower esophageal lesions are approached through an extended left thoracoabdominal incision. Following resection, the surgeon will either primarily reanastomose the esophagus, or the esophagus and stomach, or bring up a roux-en-Y loop of jejunum.

      d. Almost all patients will remain intubated to protect the airway from aspiration, which is a significant postoperative risk.

      e. Virtually any technique may be used. Epidural analgesia is commonly used in the postoperative period.

      f. It is often necessary to change from a double-lumen to a conventional endotracheal tube at the conclusion of an esophageal resection. Dependent tissue edema may significantly narrow the airway, rendering reintubation difficult.

3. Traumatic damage to the entire esophagus (as with lye ingestion) or **extensive cancers** may necessitate a total esophagectomy with subsequent interposition of a segment of colon or jejunum to serve as a conduit between the pharynx and stomach.

      a. Surgical exposure may require two or three incisions. In some cases, the esophagus can be dissected bluntly from the posterior mediastinum through the cervical and abdominal incisions, and no thoracotomy is necessary.

      b. These patients may have a **prolonged postoperative course** with significant fluid shifts, nutritional depletion, and repeated aspirations. They should remain intubated at the conclusion of the surgical procedure.

4. Fundoplication (Belsey Mark IV, Hill, and Nissen) is

performed for relief of gastroesophageal reflux, depending on the preference of the surgeon and the specific anatomy of the patient.

a. **The surgical approach** is transabdominal for the Hill and Nissen procedures and transthoracic for the Belsey. Collapse of the left lung is required for the latter procedure.

b. **Fluid shifts** are usually less than following other esophageal surgeries, and these patients may be safely extubated at the conclusion of the procedure. Postoperative analgesic requirements will be determined by the specific incision made; most patients will benefit from epidural medications.

X. **Lung transplantation** is performed for end-stage respiratory failure (e.g., due to alpha$_1$-antitrypsin deficiency, idiopathic pulmonary hypertension, or cystic fibrosis [necessitating a double-lung transplant]).

A. **General considerations**

1. Most lung transplants occur as **unscheduled procedures.** The patient may have a full stomach and will be extremely anxious. All patients should receive aspiration prophylaxis.

2. In addition to the usual monitoring for pulmonary resection, **a pulmonary artery catheter should be placed,** incorporating a long sterile sheath to facilitate intraoperative repositioning.

3. An **epidural catheter** should be placed for postoperative pain management, unless there is a strong possibility that the patient will need cardiopulmonary bypass and full heparinization.

4. **Antibiotics and immunosuppressants** will be recommended by the surgical team.

B. **Anesthetic technique.** High-dose narcotic and 100% oxygen provide cardiovascular stability. Muscle relaxants are used throughout, and small doses of benzodiazepines or volatile anesthetics are used to provide amnesia.

1. **The surgical approach** is via a standard posterolateral incision or a bilateral subcostal thoracotomy, extended toward the side of the transplant. A separate abdominal incision may be made to provide an omental flap to cover the tracheobronchial anastomosis. For the transverse incision, the patient is maintained in the supine position, with the arms extended. For a lateral thoracotomy, the patient is usually rolled 45 degrees to the operative side, allowing access to both the chest and the abdomen.

2. **Lung isolation** is best achieved with a contralateral endobronchial tube. In the event of a double-lung transplant, a left-sided tube is used with the left-sided bronchial anastomosis performed distal to the tip.

3. **Equipment** should be available for peripheral arteriovenous or venovenous bypass through an oxygenator if hypoxemia becomes a significant problem.

4. **Full cardiopulmonary bypass** may be necessary for the safe transplantation of the patient with pulmonary hypertension, who would not otherwise tolerate unilat-

eral pulmonary artery clamping. Indications for bypass include arterial oxygen saturation less than 90% following clamping of the pulmonary artery, cardiac index less than 3.0 despite therapy with dopamine and nitroglycerin, or systolic blood pressure less than 90 mm Hg. Management of the patient on bypass is discussed in Chap. 23.

C. **Postoperatively,** the patient remains intubated, ventilated, and sedated until the transplanted lung begins to function well and symptoms of acute rejection are controlled. The patient is extubated only when breathing well, comfortable, and hemodynamically stable.

   1. **Serial ABGs** are followed to document the function of the transplanted lung. Acute rejection may manifest as decreasing compliance with worsening arterial oxygenation.

   2. The patient must also be observed for **signs of toxicity from the immunosuppressive regimen,** including acute renal failure.

   3. **Epidural analgesia** will greatly facilitate emergence and extubation.

D. **Repeated bronchoscopies and biopsies of the transplanted lung** will be necessary in the days, weeks, and months following surgery. These can generally be managed under local anesthesia with IV sedation.

SUGGESTED READING

Cicala, R. S., et al. Initial evaluation and management of upper airway injuries in trauma patients. *J. Clin. Anesth.* 3:91, 1991.

Eisenkraft, J. B., Cohen, E., and Kaplan, J. A. Anesthesia for Thoracic Surgery. In P. G. Barash (ed.), *Clinical Anesthesia.* Philadelphia: Lippincott, 1989.

Geffin, B., Bland, J., and Grillo, H. Anesthetic management of tracheal resection and reconstruction. *Anesth. Analg.* 48:884, 1969.

Kaplan, J. A. *Thoracic Anesthesia* (3rd ed.). New York: Churchill Livingstone, 1991.

Lee, B. S., Sarnquist, F. H., and Sarner, V. A. Anesthesia for bilateral single-lung transplantation. *J. Cardiothorac. Vasc. Anesth.* 6:201, 1992.

Sabiston, D. C., and Spencer, F. C. (eds.) *Surgery of the Chest* (5th ed.). Philadelphia: Saunders, 1990.

Scheller, M. S., et al. Airway management during anesthesia for double-lung transplantation using a single-lumen endotracheal tube with an enclosed bronchial blocker. *J. Cardiothorac. Vasc. Anesth.* 6:204, 1992.

Young-Beyer, P. and Wilson, R. S. Anesthetic management for tracheal resection and reconstruction. *J. Cardiothorac. Anesth.* 2(6):821, 1988.

22

Anesthesia for Vascular Surgery

David Clement

I. **Preoperative assessment and management** should be aimed at identifying coexisting disease, optimizing specific therapies, and anticipating intra- and postoperative problems.

A. **Cardiovascular system.** Coronary artery disease is present in 40–80% of vascular surgery patients and is their major source of morbidity and mortality. Myocardial infarction (MI) accounts for about one-half of the early postoperative deaths. Cardiac risk factors including congestive heart failure, MI, hypertension, valvular heart disease, angina, and arrhythmias should be identified and evaluated as described in Chap. 2.

1. **Coexisting medical conditions** such as claudication, disability from a prior stroke, and emphysema limit the history as a tool to assess cardiac function.

2. **Specialized cardiac testing** such as ambulatory Holter monitoring, exercise stress testing, dipyridamole-thallium stress testing, echocardiography, and cardiac catheterization help to stratify cardiac risk, as discussed in Chap. 2.

3. Due to the widespread nature of atherosclerosis, the presence of major differences in **blood pressure readings** between arms is not uncommon and should be determined preoperatively.

4. Risk stratification may help with decisions regarding perioperative management, and **high-risk patients** may profit from

a. Optimizing medical therapy (with beta blockers, nitrates, and diuretics).

b. Coronary revascularization (percutaneous transluminal coronary angioplasty and coronary artery bypass grafting).

c. Modifying surgical procedures (using axillobifemoral rather than aortofemoral bypass grafting).

B. **Respiratory system.** Many vascular patients have a significant smoking history, compromising their pulmonary function. This must be assessed as detailed in Chap. 3.

C. **Renal system.** Renal insufficiency is common, secondary to atherosclerosis, hypertension, diabetes, inadequate perfusion, overzealous diuresis, and angiographic dye-related acute tubular necrosis.

D. **Central nervous system.** Patients should be examined for carotid bruits. Their presence warrants further evaluation prior to major vascular surgery.

E. **Endocrine system.** Diabetics may manifest diffuse, accelerated atherosclerosis, as well as distal small-vessel disease. Long-standing diabetics may have autonomic neuropathy, giving rise to silent ischemia, diabetic nephropathy, and reduced resistance to infection. Preoperative insulin orders and related management are discussed in Chap. 6.

F. **Hematologic system.** Vascular surgical patients are often treated with anticoagulants (heparin, warfarin, dipyridamole, or aspirin). A history of easy bruising, petechiae, or ecchymosis should be sought and evaluated with a prothrombin time, partial thromboplastin time, platelet count, and bleeding time where appropriate. This may impact on choice of regional anesthetic technique and intraoperative blood loss.

G. **Infection.** There is a high mortality associated with infection in patients with vascular grafts. Patients with any evidence of infection should receive appropriate antibiotics preoperatively, and consideration should be given to postponing cases where heterologous graft materials will be used.

II. Preoperative medication

A. Specific **cardiac medications** are continued as discussed in Chap. 2.

B. **Anticoagulation.** Heparin is generally withheld 4 hours prior to surgery in consultation with the surgical staff if regional anesthesia is planned.

C. **Sedatives.** The goals and regimens for sedative premedicants are generally the same as for elderly patients undergoing other major procedures (see Chap. 1).

III. Carotid endarterectomy

A. **General considerations.** Carotid endarterectomy is performed in patients with stenotic or ulcerative lesions of the common carotid artery and its internal and external branches. These lesions lead to carotid bruits, which may be clinically symptomatic. The asymptomatic carotid bruit may have significant hemodynamic alterations as measured by noninvasive studies.

1. As with other vascular surgical patients, **atherosclerotic disease** in other arteries (e.g., the coronary vessels) is often present.

2. The normal range of **blood pressure** and **heart rate** should be ascertained.

3. Patients will frequently give a history of **transient ischemic attacks.**

4. **Preexisting neurologic deficits** should be documented so that new deficits can be determined postoperatively. Patients may exhibit neurologic symptoms with extreme neck motion as would occur during positioning for surgery. This should be noted preoperatively.

B. **Monitoring**

1. **Standard, plus arterial line.** Central venous pressure (CVP) line or pulmonary artery (PA) catheter may be placed where needed, as detailed in Chap. 10.

2. The **electroencephalogram** (EEG) is used to ensure adequate perfusion during carotid cross-clamping and to identify patients who may require shunting to preserve cerebral blood flow (see Chap. 24).

C. **Anesthetic technique**

1. Minimal sedation is employed to facilitate early post-

operative neurologic examination. Cardiac medications are continued, and a baseline EEG is obtained in the preinduction period.

2. Regional anesthesia

  a. Regional anesthesia may be performed with a superficial and deep cervical plexus block (see Chap. 17).

  b. This technique requires an alert, cooperative patient who is able to tolerate lateral head position under the surgical drapes.

  c. Continuous neurologic assessment is facilitated with an awake patient.

3. General anesthesia

  a. General anesthesia provides control of ventilation, oxygenation, and reduced cerebral metabolic demand.

  b. Blood pressure should be maintained at the patient's high-normal range and may require a vasopressor such as phenylephrine.

  c. Induction requires the slow titration of anesthetic drugs to preserve cerebral perfusion while minimizing hemodynamic alterations detrimental to the patient with coronary artery disease. Ventilation should be adjusted to maintain normocarbia, to avoid hypocapnic cerebral vasoconstriction. Hypercarbia has no clinical benefit.

  d. A steady state of **"light" anesthesia** (e.g., nitrous oxide–narcotic–relaxant) is commonly used, as this will facilitate interpretation of EEG changes with carotid cross-clamping.

  e. Surgical traction on the carotid sinus may cause an intense vagal stimulus, leading to hypotension and bradycardia. Infiltration with local anesthetic may abolish the response. Withdrawal of stimulus and IV atropine may be required.

  f. Carotid cross-clamping

   (1) Heparinization (heparin, 5000 units IV) is used prior to cross-clamping.

   (2) EEG changes indicate the need for shunt placement. Blood pressure may be temporarily increased during this time to increase cerebral perfusion.

  g. Unclamping. During unclamping, reflex vasodilation and bradycardia may be seen. Vasopressors may be required during this adaptation of baroreceptors and may extend into the postoperative period.

  h. Emergence. The goals during this transition include hemodynamic stability, smooth extubation, and immediate neurologic examination.

D. Postoperative neurologic deficits may occur from hypoperfusion or emboli (shunts, ulcerated plaques). Minor neurologic changes usually resolve, but sudden major changes require immediate reexploration.

E. Postoperative management. Patients are monitored during transport to the postanesthesia care unit, where they remain overnight for observation. Major concerns include frequent neurologic assessment, hemodynamic stability, and evidence of postoperative hemorrhage, which may lead to edema and airway obstruction.

IV. Peripheral vascular surgery

A. **General considerations.** Peripheral vascular surgery is performed to bypass occlusive disease or aneurysms, remove emboli, and repair pseudoaneurysms and catheter injuries. Though peripheral vascular surgery is less of a physiologic insult than aortic surgery, their risks are comparable.

B. **Femoral-popliteal and distal lower extremity bypass grafting.** Lower extremity occlusive arterial disease is most often bypassed with a saphenous vein graft. The preparation of the vein and subsequent anastomoses to the arterial circulation may be time-consuming but rarely place significant hemodynamic stress on the patient. The use of synthetic Gortex grafts in selected patients and limited disease in others may shorten these procedures. Though blood loss is usually minimal, revision of previous peripheral vascular procedures and surgically difficult cases may result in significant blood loss.

1. **Monitoring.** In relatively healthy patients undergoing limited surgery, routine monitoring, as outlined in Chap. 10, is sufficient. As a case proceeds, hemodynamic lability, excessive blood loss, poor urine output, or cardiac ischemia may dictate placement of invasive monitors (arterial, CVP, and PA lines). For compromised or unstable patients, invasive monitoring is used. A Foley catheter is placed routinely.

2. **Regional anesthesia.** A continuous lumbar epidural catheter is commonly used. It provides excellent anesthesia and a route to administer postoperative analgesia. Spinal anesthesia is appropriate if the length of the procedure can be predicted with some assurance. A catheter spinal technique is useful during prolonged procedures for patients in whom epidural anesthesia proves technically difficult or unsatisfactory.

   a. An alpha-adrenergic agent (phenylephrine) should always be available to treat the **hypotension associated with sympathetic blockade.**

   b. **Anticoagulation**

      (1) There is no evidence that heparinization after atraumatic epidural catheter placement increases the risk of epidural hematoma formation.

      (2) The anticoagulated patient must either have his clotting abnormality corrected (with fresh-frozen plasma, vitamin K, or protamine) prior to catheter insertion or receive a general anesthetic.

      (3) During these procedures, heparin is given prior to arterial occlusion. The heparin is not usually reversed with protamine, and occasionally a dextran solution is started at the end of the operation.

   c. **Monitoring during regional anesthesia** may be facilitated by the conscious patient who may be able to relate any chest pain.

   d. Attention to **patient comfort** is particularly important when using regional techniques during long procedures. Appropriate back and shoulder padding and freedom of the neck and arms should be provided. Sedation is aimed at reducing patient anxiety without producing confusion, respiratory depression, or unresponsiveness. Blankets and other warming measures are important, as heat loss from vasodilated extremities is significant. Shivering is not only unpleasant but may also be detrimental.

   3. General anesthesia. Any of the techniques of general anesthesia is appropriate provided hemodynamic stability is maintained.

C. Iliofemoral and iliodistal bypass grafting can usually be performed with spinal or epidural anesthesia. A higher anesthetic level is needed (i.e., T8) due to proximal extension of the incision and peritoneal retraction for exposure of the iliac artery. Monitoring needs and anesthetic considerations are the same as for femoral-popliteal surgery (see sec. **B**).

D. Peripheral embolectomy and femoral pseudoaneurysm repair frequently involve patients with unstable cardiovascular status (e.g., recent myocardial infarction). Many of these patients are anticoagulated or have received thrombolytic agents, thus precluding regional anesthesia. Field blocks with local anesthesia provided by the surgeon are appropriate in these situations. Surgical embolectomy and flushing of the thrombi from an obstructed artery may be associated with significant blood loss and hypotension.

E. Femoral-femoral bypass grafting is used to treat symptomatic unilateral iliac occlusive disease. Monitoring and anesthesia are the same as for femoral-popliteal bypass grafting (see sec. **B**).

F. Peripheral aneurysms, such as popliteal aneurysms, rarely rupture but are associated with a high rate of thrombosis and embolism. Bypass grafting and ligation of the aneurysm are performed using monitoring and anesthesia as for femoral-popliteal surgery (see sec. **B**).

G. Axillofemoral bypass grafting provides arterial blood flow to the lower extremities. This approach is chosen when there is an active abdominal infection or an infected aortic bypass graft or when a patient is medically unfit for abdominal aortic surgery. Routine monitoring is supplemented by an arterial catheter, which should be placed in the arm opposite the surgery. CVP and PA lines are used as necessary. Most patients undergo a combined epidural and general anesthetic technique.

H. Vascular surgery of the upper extremity usually includes distal embolectomy and repair of traumatic injuries. The surgical technique is localized, but there may be a need to harvest a vein graft elsewhere. Monitoring is similar to that for femoral-popliteal surgery (see sec. **B**). Anesthetic technique may include field block, regional, or general anesthesia. More proximal vascular surgical procedures (e.g., vertebral stenosis and thoracic outlet syndrome) may require an intrathoracic approach and/or temporary interruption of carotid blood flow.

I. **Postoperative care.** These patients should have careful hemodynamic control (heart rate, blood pressure) and adequate analgesia. Intravascular volume and oxygenation should be optimized. Graft occlusion in the immediate postoperative period may occur, requiring reexploration. Epidural catheters are left in place for the postoperative period.

V. Abdominal aortic surgery

A. Infrarenal aortic surgery

1. Abdominal aortic surgery may be required for **atherosclerotic occlusive disease** or **aneurysmal dilatation.** These processes involve the aorta and any of its major branches, leading to ischemia, rupture, and exsanguination. Ninety-five percent of all abdominal aortic aneurysms occur below the renal arteries. Patients with abdominal aortic aneurysms over 5 cm in diameter, especially those shown to be expanding, have a better prognosis if they undergo elective resection. The annual risk of rupture of an expanding 5-cm aneurysm is about 4%. The operative mortality for elective abdominal aortic aneurysm resection is less than 2%, while the overall mortality of aneurysm rupture is 70–80%.

2. The **surgical technique** includes a transabdominal or retroperitoneal approach.

3. **Monitoring.** A large peripheral IV (14-gauge), ECG (II and V5 leads), a central venous catheter, arterial line, and Foley catheter, in addition to the usual monitoring, are required. PA catheters are employed where indicated, as outlined in Chap. 10. All monitoring catheters (except the Foley) are inserted prior to induction, and initial baseline values are obtained to guide anesthetic management. Transesophageal echocardiography may be used to assess regional wall motion abnormalities and ventricular function. Vasoactive agents (nitroglycerin and phenylephrine) must be available for every case.

4. **Anesthetic technique**
   a. **General considerations.** Most patients receive combined general and epidural anesthesia with the epidural catheter placed at about the T8 level. While general anesthesia alone is acceptable, a combined technique reduces anesthetic requirement, facilitates early extubation, and provides a method for postoperative analgesia.
   b. **Induction.** The epidural catheter is injected with lidocaine 2% and a sensory level confirmed prior to administration of general anesthesia. Reduction in blood pressure associated with the onset of epidural anesthesia is treated with phenylephrine. General anesthesia is induced in a slow and controlled fashion, titrating drugs to hemodynamic and anesthetic effect. Many drugs are appropriate, but if extubation is contemplated at the end of the proce-

dure, a high-dose narcotic technique is not appropriate.

c. **Maintenance**

(1) **Anesthesia** is primarily provided by epidural blockade. This is supplemented by nitrous oxide, muscle relaxants, and occasionally an inhalation agent. A continuous infusion of dilute bupivacaine 0.1% and fentanyl, 10 μg/ml, is begun early in the anesthetic.

(2) **Heat conservation.** Heat loss during aortic procedures may be considerable. Strategies for heat conservation are discussed in Chap. 14.

(3) **Bowel manipulation** is usually necessary to gain access to the aorta and may be accompanied by skin flushing, a fall in systemic vascular resistance, and hypotension, which is exaggerated in the setting of sympathetic blockade. These changes are due to release of prostaglandins and possibly other vasodilators from the bowel and last for approximately 20–30 minutes. Treatment consists of phenylephrine, reducing anesthetic depth, and infusing additional volume.

(4) **Fluid management.** Intravascular volume is depleted by hemorrhage, third spacing into the bowel and peritoneal cavity, and insensible losses associated with large abdominal incisions.

(a) **Crystalloid** is used for volume replacement at an approximate rate of 10–15 ml/kg/hr.

(b) **Colloids** are reserved for patients with severe ongoing blood loss and patients who cannot tolerate large amounts of crystalloid (renal failure, severe pulmonary disease).

(c) **Hematocrit** should be maintained above the 30% range. With blood losses greater than 2000 ml, coagulation profiles and appropriate replacement of platelets, clotting factors, and calcium should be considered.

(d) **Autotransfusion devices** should be employed whenever possible. This processed blood is composed of washed packed red blood cells deficient in plasma, clotting factors, and platelets.

(5) **Aortic cross-clamping**

(a) **Heparin** (5000 units IV) is given several minutes prior to applying an aortic cross clamp. Increased afterload following aortic cross-clamping is well tolerated by patients with normal hearts. Those with compromised left ventricular function may exhibit a rise in pulmonary capillary wedge pressure, a decrease in cardiac output, and/or ischemic changes on the electrocardiogram (ECG). The use of nitroglycerin and occasionally afterload reduction with nitroprusside improve myocardial oxygen supply-demand balance. When a combined technique is used, this is infrequently encountered.

(b) Prolonged aortic occlusion produces peripheral ischemia and accumulation of anaerobic metabolites, with subsequent profound distal vasodilatation. Intravascular volume must be maintained in the normal to high range, anticipating a fall in systemic vascular resistance following release of the aortic cross clamp.

(6) **Renal preservation.** The incidence of renal failure is 1–2% for infrarenal surgery. Preoperative angiographic dye studies and preexisting renal artery atherosclerosis augment this risk. Renal cortical blood flow and urine output decrease with infrarenal aortic cross-clamping. The mechanism may include microcirculatory derangement, effects on the renin-angiotensin system, and microembolization. Adequate hydration and maintenance of urine flow seem to reduce the incidence of acute renal failure. Mannitol (0.25–0.5 gm/kg IV) and possibly furosemide should be given prior to aortic occlusion if urine output is inadequate (< 1 ml/kg/hr). If the diuresis is inadequate during the cross-clamp period, additional mannitol, furosemide, or low-dose dopamine infusion (1–5 µg/kg/min) may be given. Patients with chronically elevated creatinine levels (> 2 mg/dl) have substantially higher morbidity and mortality after vascular surgery.

(7) **Aortic unclamping.** Cross-clamp release leads to both venous and arterial dilatation, resulting in hypotension. The washout of anaerobic metabolites also may contribute a negative inotropic effect. Volume loading, decreasing anesthetic depth, discontinuing vasodilators, infusing a vasopressor, and a slow, controlled release of the aortic cross clamp will minimize hypotension. Reperfusion of the lower extremities results in hyperemia with washout of anaerobic products and possibly systemic acidosis. This is directly related to duration of cross-clamp time and degree of collateral flow. Sodium bicarbonate administration is rarely necessary. Protamine is usually given to reverse the effect of heparin once distal perfusion has been ensured.

(8) **Emergence.** Most patients are extubated at the end of the procedure. Patients with unstable cardiac or pulmonary function, ongoing bleeding, or severe hypothermia (temperature < 33° C) are left intubated. Hypertension, tachycardia, pain, and shivering should be anticipated and treated.

(9) **Transport.** All patients should receive supplemental oxygen. Blood pressure and ECG monitoring are mandatory.

B. **Suprarenal abdominal aortic surgery.** Surgical repair may require cross-clamping the aorta at various levels above the renal arteries. Anesthetic considerations are similar to those for infrarenal aortic surgery (see sec. **A**), with the following caveats:

1. PA lines are routinely used.
2. There is a potential for greater blood loss.
3. Renal perfusion is further compromised. This is related to cross-clamp time and potential cholesterol emboli.
4. Cross-clamping above the celiac and superior mesenteric artery leads to visceral ischemia and further acidosis.

C. **Renal artery surgery.** Renal artery stenoses or aneurysms are repaired with a variety of techniques. Aortorenal bypass and transaortic endarterectomy require aortic cross-clamping, while hepatorenal (right) and splenorenal (left) bypass procedures avoid cross-clamping. The anesthetic considerations are the same as for abdominal aortic surgery (see sec. **A**). The postoperative concerns include ongoing hypertension and deterioration in renal function.

D. **Emergency abdominal aortic surgery.** Patients present with a wide spectrum of signs and symptoms and can be divided into two groups:

1. The **hemodynamically stable patient** (with an expanding, tender, contained rupture) has the same anesthetic considerations as previously described (see sec. **V.A**), but the preoperative preparation must proceed expeditiously. In addition, some patients come to the operating room stabilized in Military Anti-Shock Trousers (MAST) or a G suit. This suit should be kept inflated until the surgeon is scrubbed and anesthesia is ready to proceed.

   a. **Foley catheter and nasogastric tube insertion** should be delayed until after induction, to avoid Valsalva maneuvers (or hypertension) that may aggravate bleeding or cause frank rupture.

   b. **Induction proceeds after preoxygenation** using placement of cricoid pressure and careful titration of hypnotic agents, narcotics, and muscle relaxant. Hypertension must be avoided and anesthesia can be supplemented with esmolol, nitroprusside, or both.

2. The **hemodynamically unstable patient** (rupture) requires resuscitative measures. Mortality can be limited by restoration of intravascular volume, judicious use of vasoconstrictors, and rapid surgical control. Under the best of situations, there is a 40–50% mortality, usually resulting from the physiologic consequences of hypotension and massive blood transfusion. The incidence of MI, acute renal failure, respiratory failure, and coagulopathy is high. Survival depends on coordination between the emergency room, operating room, and surgical, anesthesia, and intensive care unit staffs.

   a. **General considerations**
      (1) Several large-bore IVs are necessary.
      (2) Blood samples should be sent immediately for

cross-matching and any other pertinent laboratory studies. Blood components should be ordered immediately, but universal donor-type blood (type O-negative) should be obtained if type-specific blood is unavailable. Colloid should be available. The autotransfusion team should be notified and equipment set up.

b. Surgical technique. The immediate surgical priority will be to control bleeding by cross-clamping the aorta in the chest or abdomen.

c. Monitoring. Although time is of the essence in a dire emergency, the minimum monitoring standards (see Chap. 10) should still be applied. Placement of arterial and PA catheters must await volume resuscitation.

d. Anesthetic technique

(1) Induction

(a) In the moribund patient, intubation should be performed immediately.

(b) In the hypotensive patient, a rapid sequence induction is indicated. Oxygen, scopolamine, ketamine, and/or a benzodiazepine and a relaxant may be all that are tolerated.

(2) Maintenance

(a) Once the aorta has been clamped to control bleeding, resuscitative efforts should continue until hemodynamic stability is achieved. Incremental doses of narcotic and supplemental anesthetics are given as tolerated.

(b) Blood products (including fresh-frozen plasma and platelets) are administered when available. Serial laboratory studies may guide further management.

(c) Hypothermia is common and contributes to the acidosis, coagulopathy, and myocardial dysfunction that commonly complicate aortic aneurysm repair. Warming the operating room and other means outlined in Chap. 14 should be utilized.

(d) To prevent renal failure, aggressive efforts should be made to preserve urine output with volume replacement, mannitol, furosemide, and low-dose dopamine. Mortality in patients developing renal failure following ruptured abdominal aortic aneurysm approaches 100%.

(3) Emergence. The fluid shifts, hypothermia, acid-base, electrolyte, and coagulation abnormalities make the immediate postoperative period complex. Most patients remain intubated, relaxed, and heavily sedated at the end of the procedure.

VI. Thoracic aortic surgery. Diseases of the thoracic aorta may result from atherosclerosis, degenerative disorders of connective tissue (Marfan's and Ehlers-Danlos syndromes, cystic medical necrosis), infection (syphilis), congenital defects (coarctation or congenital aneurysms of the sinus of Valsalva), trauma (penetrating and deceleration injuries), and inflammatory processes (Takayasu's aortitis).

The most common problem affecting the thoracic aorta is **atherosclerotic aneurysm of the descending portion,** accounting for some 20% of all aortic aneurysms. When these dissect proximally, they may involve the aortic valve or coronary ostia. Distal dissection may involve the abdominal aorta, renal, or mesenteric branches. The next most frequent problem is **traumatic disruption of the thoracic aorta.** Adventitial false aneurysms may form distal to the left subclavian artery at the insertion of the ligamentum arteriosum as a result of penetrating or deceleration injuries. These false aneurysms may dissect anterograde, involving the arch and its major branches.

A. **Ascending aortic aneurysms** are approached by median sternotomy and require cardiopulmonary bypass with arterial cannulation through the femoral artery, the distal ascending aorta, or the aortic arch.

B. **Transverse aortic arch repair** requires median sternotomy, cardiopulmonary bypass, and hypothermic total circulatory arrest to ensure central nervous system protection.

C. **Descending aortic aneurysms** are often approached by left lateral thoracotomy with cross-clamp placement distal to the left subclavian artery.

D. **Thoracoabdominal aneurysms** are approached by a combined left thoracotomy and abdominal incision.
   1. **Classification** (Crawford)
      a. **Type I.** Aneurysm of the descending thoracic aorta distal to the subclavian artery, ending above the visceral vessel take off.
      b. **Type II.** Aneurysm from the subclavian artery take off to the distal abdominal aorta including the visceral and renal arteries.
      c. **Type III.** Aneurysm from the mid-descending thoracic aorta down to include the visceral and renal arteries.
      d. **Type IV.** Aneurysm from the diaphragm down to the distal aorta below the renal arteries.
   2. **Associated findings**
      a. **Airway deviation or compression,** particularly of the left main stem bronchus, leading to atelectasis.
      b. **Tracheal displacement or disruption,** leading to difficulties with intubation and ventilation. Longstanding aneurysms may damage the recurrent laryngeal nerves, resulting in vocal cord paralysis and hoarseness.
      c. **Hemoptysis** secondary to erosion of the aneurysm into an adjacent bronchus.
      d. **Esophageal compression** with dysphagia and an increased risk of aspiration.
      e. **Distortion and compression of central venous and arterial anatomy,** leading to markedly asymmetric pulses and difficult internal jugular cannu-

lation. A right radial artery catheter is placed because cross-clamping of the aorta may occlude flow through the left subclavian artery.

   f. **Hemothorax and mediastinal shift** from rupture or leakage, with resultant respiratory and circulatory embarrassment.

   g. **Reduced distal perfusion** secondary to aortic branch vessel occlusion, leading to renal, mesenteric, spinal cord, or extremity ischemia.

3. **Surgical technique.** During repair of the aneurysm, the affected aortic segment is isolated, and an interposition graft is inserted. Proximal blood flow to collaterals provides the only distal perfusion. Some institutions provide distal perfusion through a heparin-bonded Gott shunt or pump-assisted bypass. The **inclusion technique** involves using the native aorta containing the celiac, superior mesenteric, and renal ostia as a component of the bypass graft.

4. **Monitoring.** Routine monitoring is supplemented with
   a. A right radial arterial line.
   b. A VIP PA catheter. An extra-long sheath facilitates manipulation of the catheter.
   c. A 7.5 Fr introducer is used for a volume line.
   d. **Spinal cord monitoring**
      (1) The **anterior spinal artery** branches from the vertebral arteries at the base of the skull and anastomoses with **aortic radicular arteries.** The latter arise segmentally (a few in the lumbar and lower thoracic regions, but none or one in the upper thoracic region).
      (2) The dominant vessel is the **artery of Adamkiewicz** (usually found between T9 and T12); cross-clamping may compromise flow, depriving the anterior spinal artery of flow and producing spinal cord ischemia.
      (3) Manifestations of the **anterior spinal artery syndrome** are paraplegia, rectal and urinary incontinence, and loss of pain and temperature sensation, but sparing of vibratory and proprioceptive sensation. The incidence of paraplegia resulting from the anterior spinal artery syndrome is 1% (type IV) to 41% (type II with dissection), with an overall rate of 11%. Risk factors include the duration of the cross clamp, the location of proximal and distal cross clamps, increased body temperature, the degree of collateralization of the spinal cord circulation, and reperfusion with cross-clamp removal.
         (a) Steroids, hypothermia, barbiturates, free radical scavengers, cerebrospinal fluid (CSF) drainage, intrathecal papaverine, magnesium, naloxone, thiopental, and reanastomosis of intercostal vessels have all been tried without convincing evidence that any technique reduces the incidence of paraplegia.
         (b) Mild hypothermia is permitted, and glucose-

containing solutions are avoided, since experimental evidence indicates that hyperglycemia is detrimental during ischemia and may worsen neurologic outcome.

e. As the spinal fluid pressure is the downstream pressure of the spinal cord arterial bed, lowering CSF pressure may increase spinal cord perfusion. Therefore, a lumbar CSF catheter (19-gauge) is inserted to monitor and control CSF pressure.

f. It may be possible to detect spinal cord ischemia by monitoring somatosensory evoked potentials (SSEPs) (see Chap. 24), but this is not done at the Massachusetts General Hospital.

g. The use of vasopressors such as phenylephrine or norepinephrine and of vasodilators such as nitroglycerin, nitroprusside, and mannitol/furosemide/dopamine is required, and these drugs should be available prior to induction.

h. Foley catheter.

5. Anesthetic technique

a. Prior to induction of general anesthesia, a **thoracic epidural catheter** is inserted, and a sensory level is achieved with 2% lidocaine.

b. **General anesthesia** is induced as detailed in sec. **V.A.4.b.**

c. **A double-lumen endobronchial tube** is placed to facilitate surgical access and protect the left lung from trauma during left thoracotomy (see Chap. 21).

d. **Muscle relaxation** is usually provided with an infusion of atracurium. This facilitates neurologic examination at the end of the procedure.

6. Positioning. The patient is turned to the right lateral decubitus position and prepared for incision.

7. Maintenance

a. **Anesthesia** is continued as in sec. **V.A.4.c,** and one-lung ventilation is begun as described in Chap. 21.

b. **Fluid management** includes colloids, fresh-frozen plasma, red blood cells, and platelets almost exclusively after induction, in an attempt to limit the development of a coagulopathy and excessive edema. Autotransfusion and a Level One D300 blood warmer are always used.

8. Aortic cross-clamping

a. Prior to cross-clamping, **CSF pressure is lowered** by withdrawal of 20 ml of CSF. Thereafter, further CSF withdrawal is done to maintain CSF pressure at or below baseline values.

b. **Marked hypertension is universal** with a proximal aortic cross clamp and is treated with IV narcotics, epidural anesthesia, nitroglycerin, and nitroprusside.

c. **Renal function** is preserved by infusion of iced Lactated Ringer's solution into the orifices of the renal arteries through a catheter placed by the surgical team.

9. **Aortic unclamping** produces hypotension by the mechanism discussed in sec. **V.A.4.c.(7).** Volume loading prior to and during unclamping, slow release of the cross clamp, and use of vasopressors are continued until myocardial function and vascular tone have normalized.

10. **Systemic acidosis is universal** following release of the aortic cross clamp. An infusion of bicarbonate during the cross-clamping period will prevent severe acidosis with reperfusion.

11. **Emergence.** The double-lumen tube is replaced with a standard endotracheal tube. Dependent tissue edema may significantly narrow the airway, rendering reintubation difficult.

12. **Transport.** The patient remains intubated and sedated for transport to the intensive care unit. Both ECG and blood pressure are monitored.

VII. **Postoperative considerations.** Intensive care is required following most vascular surgical procedures. Attention to urine output, cardiac output, distal extremity perfusion, respiratory adequacy, hematocrit, and hemostasis is required. The most frequent complications include MI, renal failure, bowel ischemia or infarction, pancreatitis, sepsis, disseminated intravascular coagulation, peripheral embolization, respiratory insufficiency, and paraplegia.

SUGGESTED READING

Baron, J. F., et al. Combined epidural and general anesthesia versus general anesthesia for abdominal aortic surgery. *Anesthesiology* 75:611, 1991.

Boucher, C. A., et al. Determination of cardiac risk by dipyridamole-thallium imaging before peripheral vascular surgery. *N. Engl. J. Med.* 312:389, 1985.

Crawford, E. S., et al. Thoracoabdominal aortic aneurysms: Preoperative and intraoperative factors determining immediate and long-term results of operations in 605 patients. *J. Vasc. Surg.* 3:389, 1986.

Diehl, J. T., et al. Complications of abdominal aortic reconstruction. *Ann. Surg.* 197:49, 1983.

Eagle, K. A., et al. Combining clinical and thallium data optimizes preoperative assessment of cardiac risk before major vascular surgery. *Ann. Intern. Med.* 110(11):859, 1989.

Goldman, L. Cardiac risks and complications of noncardiac surgery. *Ann. Intern. Med.* 98:504, 1981.

Isaacson, I. J., et al. The value of pulmonary artery and central venous monitoring in patients undergoing abdominal aortic reconstructive surgery. *J. Vasc. Surg.* 12:754, 1990.

Mangano, D. T. Perioperative cardiac morbidity. *Anesthesiology* 72:153, 1990.

Miller, D. C., and Myers, B. D. Pathophysiology and prevention of acute renal failure associated with thoracoabdominal or abdominal aortic surgery. *J. Vasc. Surg.* 5:518, 1987.

Odoom, J. A., and Sih, I. L. Epidural analgesia and anticoagulant therapy. *Anaesthesia* 38:254, 1983.

Raby, K. E., et al. Correlation between preoperative ischemia and major cardiac events after peripheral vascular surgery. *N. Engl. J. Med.* 321:1296, 1989.

Rao, T. L. K., and El-Etr, A. A. Anticoagulation following placement of epidural and subarachnoid catheters: An evaluation of neurologic sequelae. *Anesthesiology* 55:618, 1981.

Shah, K. B., et al. Reevaluation of perioperative myocardial infarction in patients with prior myocardial infarction undergoing noncardiac operations. *Anesth. Analg.* 71:231, 1990.

Tuman, K. J., et al. Effects of epidural anesthesia and analgesia on coagulation and outcome after major vascular surgery. *Anesth. Analg.* 73:696, 1991.

Yeager, M. P., et al. Epidural anesthesia and analgesia in high risk surgical patients. *Anesthesiology* 66:729, 1986.

Steven Thorup and Mansoor Husain

I. Preanesthetic assessment

A. **A complete history and physical examination** are required as described in Chaps. 1 and 2. Particular issues pertinent to cardiac surgical procedures and the physiologic impact of extracorporeal bypass and elective arrest include the following:

1. **Prior surgery** on the thorax, heart, great vessels, or lungs technically complicates cardiac surgery.

2. **Prior admissions** for peripheral vascular disease, including transient ischemic attacks or cerebral vascular accidents, and results of noninvasive and invasive vascular studies should be noted. Symptomatic or documented carotid arterial disease may warrant endarterectomy prior to or simultaneous with cardiac operations requiring cardiopulmonary bypass (CPB).

3. **A history of bleeding tendency** may reveal a condition responsive to pre- or intraoperative therapy.

4. **Renal insufficiency** may indicate the need for various intraoperative renal protective measures.

5. **Post-CPB pulmonary dysfunction** can be life-threatening, and patients with pulmonary disease may benefit from preoperative bronchodilators, corticosteroids, or chest physiotherapy.

B. **Cardiac evaluation** should determine the major anatomic and physiologic characteristics of the cardiovascular system, the likelihood of intraoperative ischemia, and the functional reserve of the heart, which in turn will reflect the ability to tolerate elective arrest and separation from CPB.

1. **Radionuclide imaging** may demonstrate the regions and extent of myocardium at risk for ischemia.

2. **Radionuclide ventriculography** delineates cardiac chamber volume, ejection fraction, and right-to-left stroke volume ratios.

3. **Echocardiography** can assess global ventricular function, valvular dysfunction, intracardiac defects, thrombus, myxoma, aortic dissection, pericardial effusions, and tamponade. Regional wall motion abnormalities may reflect ischemia or a prior myocardial infarction.

4. **Cardiac catheterization** provides anatomic and functional data often not available from noninvasive studies.

   a. **Anatomic data.** Coronary angiography reveals the location and extent of coronary stenoses, distal runoff, collateral flow, and coronary dominance. **Significant stenosis** implies a greater than 70% reduction in luminal diameter. The dominant coronary system supplies the atrioventricular node and the posterior descending coronary artery.

   b. **Functional data.** Ventriculography may demonstrate wall motion abnormalities, mitral regurgita-

Table 23-1. Normal intracardiac pressure and oxygen saturation

	Pressure (mm Hg)	O_2 saturation (%)
Superior vena cava		71
Inferior vena cava		77
Right atrium (mean)	1–8	75
Right ventricle (systolic/diastolic)	15–30/0–8	75
Pulmonary artery (systolic/diastolic)	15–30/4–12	75
Pulmonary capillary wedge pressure (mean)	2–12	
Left atrium (mean)	2–12	98
Left ventricle (systolic/ diastolic/end-diastolic)	100–140/0–8/2–12	98
Aorta (systolic/diastolic)	100–140/60–90	98

tion, left ventricular (LV) outflow obstruction, and
intracardiac shunts; LV ejection fraction is normally greater than 0.6. Impaired ventricular performance, as assessed by abnormally elevated filling
pressures and decreased ejection fraction, is a useful
predictor of increased surgical risk.

c. **Hemodynamic data** are compiled from both right
and left heart catheterization. Intracardiac and pulmonary vascular pressures reflect volume status,
cardiac valve function, and the presence of pulmonary vascular disease (normal values are presented
in Table 23-1). An elevated left ventricular end-
diastolic pressure (LVEDP) (measured at the down
slope of the a wave) may be due to ventricular
failure and dilation, volume overload (mitral or
aortic regurgitation), poor compliance from ischemia or hypertrophy, or a constrictive process.
The LVEDP may rise substantially in patients with
coronary artery disease after dye injection for ventriculography or coronary angiography, despite otherwise normal hemodynamic values.

d. **Left-to-right intracardiac shunts** are demonstrated by an arterial oxygen saturation (SaO_2)
"step up" in the right heart. Systemic and pulmonary flow and flow ratios can be calculated by Fick
principles (see section **IV. C. 1.c** for equations).

e. **Cardiac output** is determined by thermodilution,
and hemodynamic indices can be derived (Table
23-2).

C. **Laboratory studies.** At a minimum, routine studies for
patients undergoing CPB include a complete blood count,
prothrombin time, partial thromboplastin time, platelet
count, electrolytes, blood urea nitrogen, creatinine, glucose, aspartate aminotransferase, lactate dehydrogenase,
creatine kinase, urinalysis, chest x-ray, and a 12-lead
electrocardiogram (ECG) with a rhythm strip.

Table 23-2. Ventricular function indices

Formula	Units	Normal value
$SV = \dfrac{CO}{HR} \times 1000$	ml/beat	60–90
$SI = \dfrac{SV}{BSA}$	ml/beat/m^2	40–60
$LVSWI = \dfrac{1.36(MAP - \overline{PCWP})}{100} \times SI$	$\dfrac{gram\text{-}meters/m^2}{beat}$	45–60
$RVSWI = \dfrac{1.36(\overline{PAP} - \overline{CVP})}{100} \times SI$	$\dfrac{gram\text{-}meters/m^2}{beat}$	5–10
$SVR = \dfrac{MAP - \overline{CVP}}{CO} \times 80$	dynes-sec/cm^5	900–1500
$PVR = \dfrac{\overline{PAP} - \overline{PCWP}}{CO} \times 80$	dynes-sec/cm^5	50–150

Key: BSA = body surface area; CO = cardiac output; $\overline{CVP}$ = mean central venous pressure; HR = heart rate; LVSWI = left ventricular stroke work index; MAP = mean systemic arterial pressure; $\overline{PAP}$ = mean pulmonary artery pressure; $\overline{PCWP}$ = mean pulmonary capillary wedge pressure; PVR = pulmonary vascular resistance; RVSWI = right ventricular stroke work index; SI = stroke index; SV = stroke volume; SVR = systemic vascular resistance.

II. Anesthetic management
A. Patient education.
Anxieties are often allayed by an explanation of what is to be expected, both immediately before and after surgery. Preoperative teaching by cardiac nurse educators, intensive care unit (ICU) staff, and respiratory therapy personnel improves continuity of care, increases patient confidence in the health care team, and may improve patient cooperation postoperatively in the ICU.
B. Premedication
1. Cardiac medications
a. Beta agonists, calcium channel blockers, and nitrates, including IV nitroglycerin, are routinely continued on schedule until arrival in the operating room. Shorter-acting beta blockers (e.g., metoprolol, propranolol) may be substituted for longer-acting drugs (e.g., atenolol, nadolol). Long-acting preparations of calcium channel blockers may be changed to standard formulations preoperatively.
b. Digitalis preparations are commonly held for 24 hours preoperatively due to inherent toxicity (especially in the presence of hypokalemia) and a long elimination half-life. When rate control is critical, as in mitral stenosis, digitalis should be continued preoperatively.
c. Antihypertensives, including vasodilators and diuretics, are continued when blood pressure is labile. Otherwise, they are withheld for at least 12 hours. Long-acting ACE inhibitors may produce refractory hypotension in the perioperative period.

d. Antidysrhythmics are generally continued to the time of surgery. Type I agents (quinidine, procainamide, disopyramide, and oral lidocaine derivatives) may suppress automaticity and conduction, especially when patients are hyperkalemic. Disopyramide is a particularly potent myocardial depressant and is often discontinued earlier. Amiodarone has a long half-life of 30 days; hence preoperative discontinuation within a few days of surgery will have a minimal effect on serum levels. Therapy is associated with pulmonary toxicity, decreased atrioventricular nodal conduction, atropine-resistant bradycardia, and myocardial depression.

e. Aspirin and dipyridamole (Persantine) inhibit platelet function and are routinely discontinued 10–14 days preoperatively. In patients undergoing coronary revascularization, however, 1 or 2 doses of dipyridamole are frequently given on the day before surgery, as long-term graft patency may be improved by antiplatelet therapy.

f. Warfarin (Coumadin) is held 10–14 days preoperatively.

g. Heparin infusions, initiated for unstable angina or for patients with left main coronary disease, are routinely continued until the patient is fully heparinized prior to CPB.

2. Sedation and analgesia are warranted in almost all cardiac surgical patients. Combinations of benzodiazepines, morphine, and scopolamine will provide excellent amnesia and analgesia for preinduction catheter insertion, with an acceptable degree of cardiorespiratory depression in all but the most debilitated patients.

a. For full-size adults with good LV function, lorazepam, 1–2 mg PO, is given the night before and again 2 hours prior to arrival in the operating room, and morphine, 0.1–0.15 mg/kg IM (SQ if patient is anticoagulated), combined with scopolamine, 0.3–0.4 mg IM or SQ, is given at least 1.5 hours prior to induction. A higher incidence of perioperative delirium is seen in debilitated and elderly patients (> 70 years of age) undergoing CPB, and scopolamine may best be avoided in this population.

b. Alternative sedative regimens may include midazolam, 0.07–0.1 mg/kg IM. The hypertensive patient may benefit from co-premedication with clonidine, 0.1 mg PO.

c. Patients with mitral valve disease may develop life-threatening pulmonary hypertension with sedation-induced hypoventilation and hypoxemia. These patients may also be extremely sensitive to the central effects of sedation, and these premedications should be reduced by 50%.

d. In patients requiring anesthesia transport to the operating room, premedication can be titrated IV.

3. Supplemental oxygen therapy should be given to all

cardiac surgical patients following sedative premedication.

4. **Other medications.** Patients with active pulmonary disease may benefit from preoperative steroid administration.

C. **Monitoring**

1. **Standard monitors** (see Chap. 10)

    a. **Electrocardiogram.** Continuous display of both leads II and V_5 will facilitate the diagnosis of ischemia and rhythm disturbance. Other leads to monitor regions of myocardium known to be at risk (e.g., V_{4R} for right ventricular ischemia) may be indicated.

    b. **Temperature monitoring** includes measurement of the "core" temperature, measured in the nasopharynx and reflective of brain and other highly perfused tissues, the "blood" temperature, measured by the pulmonary artery catheter, and the "shell" temperature, measured in the rectum and reflective of less perfused regions.

2. **Central venous and pulmonary artery pressures.**

    a. Patients with normal ventricular function undergoing cardiac surgery can be effectively managed with central venous pressure (CVP) monitoring. However, cardiac output and reliable filling pressure data readily obtained from a pulmonary artery (PA) catheter greatly facilitate rational drug and volume therapy throughout the perioperative period.

    b. **Pacing PA and Paceport catheters** provide pacing capability for the management of a variety of valvular lesions (aortic insufficiency and mitral regurgitation) and conduction disorders and for "redo" operations during which rapid access for epicardial pacing may not be possible. Right ventricular (RV) ejection fraction can be estimated with PA catheters equipped with a fast response thermistor and may be helpful in the management of patients with pulmonary hypertension and RV failure. Mixed venous oxygen saturation ($S\bar{v}O_2$) monitoring is available continuously with PA catheters specially equipped with a fiberoptic linked oximeter. A decrease in $S\bar{v}O_2$ is the result of either decreased cardiac output, decreased hemoglobin, increased oxygen consumption, or decreased SaO_2.

3. **Transesophageal echocardiography** is of clear value in the assessment of intraoperative valvular function, especially for mitral valve reconstruction. It is useful for imaging aortic dissection and the adequacy of repair of intracardiac shunts and may become an efficient intraoperative monitor of ischemia through the detection of regional wall motion abnormalities.

D. **Preinduction.** Upon the patient's arrival in the operating room, vital signs are checked, an adequate SaO_2 is ensured, and additional premedication, if indicated, is titrated.

1. **Peripheral venous access** is established. In adults, one large-bore (14-gauge) peripheral IV is usually

sufficient. If excessive bleeding is expected (e.g., a redo operation or a patient with a preexisting coagulopathy), a second peripheral line will facilitate blood product administration.

2. **Arterial cannulation** is performed with either an 18- or 20-gauge catheter.

   a. When possible, in patients undergoing **left internal mammary dissection,** the right radial artery is cannulated so that the left arm may be safely tucked.

   b. Right radial artery pressure is monitored whenever **aortic arch** surgery is planned or whenever the left subclavian artery may be obstructed.

   c. Cannulation distal to a previous brachial artery cutdown site should be avoided. Pressure gradients may occur across arteriotomies, especially during and after CPB.

   d. If blood pressure measurements are asymmetric, the arterial catheter should be placed on the side with the higher value.

   e. Femoral artery cannulation is a safe and reliable alternative to radial artery cannulation.

   f. **Intraaortic balloon lumen pressure (IABP)** can be transduced as a temporary monitor of central arterial pressure.

3. **Central venous access** may be established pre- or postinduction, depending on the clinical situation.

4. A **defibrillator** and **external pacemaker generator** must be available, as should a **pacemaker magnet,** if applicable.

5. **Typed and cross-matched blood** must be present and checked. If excessive post-CPB bleeding is deemed likely, appropriate blood products should be requested.

6. **Baseline hemodynamics,** including cardiac output, and a 7-lead ECG are recorded prior to induction.

7. **Medications** available should include heparin, protamine, calcium chloride, lidocaine, inotropes, vasopressors, and nitroglycerin.

E. **Induction** is one of the most critical times in the anesthetic management of the cardiac surgical patient. A surgeon should be available, and the CPB pump should be primed in the event that a hemodynamic emergency occurs. The choice of agents and sequence of events are dependent on the specific cardiac lesions, the patient's underlying condition, and the surgical plan. A systematic, gradual induction with frequent assessment of the degree of cardiovascular depression and depth of anesthesia (as determined by hemodynamic response to graded stimuli including oral airway insertion and Foley catheterization) will minimize hemodynamic instability.

1. **Agents** useful in the induction and maintenance of anesthesia in the coronary artery bypass graft patient include the following:

   a. **Intravenous narcotics** produce varying degrees of vasodilation and bradycardia without significant myocardial depression. A high-dose technique utilizes fentanyl (50–100 µg/kg) or sufentanil (10–20 mg/kg) as both the induction and primary maintenance agent. Alternatively, a lower induction bolus may be supplemented with a continuous narcotic infusion, or lower doses (fentanyl, 10–25 µg/kg, or sufentanil, 1–5µg/kg) may be used in conjunction with other central nervous system depressants as part of a "balanced technique." An extremely gradual hydromorphone (Dilaudid, 0.25 mg/kg) or morphine (1–3 mg/kg) induction is often useful in the management of severely debilitated patients with poor ventricular function, who are frequently dependent on maximal endogenous sympathetic tone.

b. **Sedative hypnotics and amnestics,** including thiopental, propofol, ketamine, and etomidate, though myocardial depressants, may be useful as coinduction agents in particular situations.

c. **Potent inhalation anesthetics** are useful supplementary agents, especially in the treatment of hypertension.

d. **Nitrous oxide,** if used in the prebypass period, should be discontinued prior to initiation of CPB and should not be used post-CPB due to the enhanced potential for gas emboli.

e. **Muscle relaxants** with minimal cardiovascular effects are commonly chosen (e.g., vecuronium, doxacurium). Pretreatment with a "priming dose" and early relaxant administration help to counteract chest wall rigidity often encountered during narcotic inductions. Succinylcholine may cause bradycardia, particularly when used after fentanyl or sufentanil. Gallamine or pancuronium can be used to produce a graded increase in heart rate.

2. **Valvular heart disease**

a. **Aortic stenosis.** Hemodynamic goals include adequate intravenous volume, slow sinus heart rate and rhythm, and maintenance of contractility and systemic vascular tone. Anesthetic agents that reduce vascular tone should be used with particular caution, and vasopressors should be available for induction.

b. **Aortic regurgitation.** Patients are often highly dependent on endogenous sympathetic tone. Hemodynamic goals include adequate intravascular volume, maintenance of an increased heart rate and contractile state, and decreased systemic vascular tone to facilitate forward flow. Atrial fibrillation is common, but sinus rhythm is maintained when possible.

c. **Mitral stenosis.** Hemodynamic goals mandate maintenance of a slow sinus rhythm and adequate intravascular volume, contractility, and systemic resistance. Elevated pulmonary vascular resistance (PVR), often secondary to hypoventilation, should be avoided.

d. **Mitral regurgitation.** Hemodynamic goals include

maintenance of volume status, contractility, a normal to elevated heart rate, and a reduction of systemic vascular tone. Elevated PVR should be avoided.

e. In patients with **mixed valvular lesions,** the most hemodynamically significant lesion will predominate the management goals.

F. The **prebypass period** is characterized by variable levels of stimulation during preparation for the initiation of CPB. Particularly stimulating periods include sternal splitting and retraction, pericardial incision, and aortic root dissection and cannulation. Spontaneous cooling should occur.

1. Baseline laboratory data, including an arterial blood gas (ABG), control activated clotting time (ACT), and hematocrit, are obtained. Phlebotomy and hemodilution may be considered in otherwise healthy patients with a starting hematocrit of 40% or greater, thus providing fresh autologous whole blood for transfusion following CPB and heparin reversal.

2. Lungs are deflated during sternal splitting. Anatomic changes in chest wall configuration will produce ECG changes, especially T-wave changes, which should be noted to avoid confusion with ischemia-induced changes.

3. **Left internal mammary artery dissection** may account for significant occult blood loss into the left chest.

4. **Anticoagulation for cannulation**
   a. Prior to induction of anesthesia, 300 IU/kg of heparin should be preprared in case emergency initiation of CPB is necessary. Administration is through a centrally placed catheter; blood is aspirated both before and after injection. Alternatively, in emergencies or in pediatric cases, the surgeon may inject heparin directly into the right atrium.
   b. Vasodilation often follows a heparin bolus.
   c. The ACT, determined approximately 5 minutes after heparin administration, is used to monitor the degree of anticoagulation. Control values are 80–150 seconds, while heparinization sufficient to prevent microthrombus formation during CPB correlates with an ACT of longer than 400 seconds (at > 35°C). Patients on continuous IV heparin preoperatively may become relatively "heparin resistant" and often require a 400–500 IU/kg bolus to achieve an ACT longer than 400 seconds. If an ACT longer than 400 seconds is not achieved with standard heparin dose regimens, an additional 100 IU/kg is administered. Fresh-frozen plasma may be necessary to correct an unrecognized antithrombin III deficiency.

5. **Aortic root dissection and cannulation** may produce hypertension and tachycardia, which should be aggressively treated with short-acting IV agents to minimize the risk of aortic tear or dissection.

6. An improperly placed side-biting clamp or arterial

cannula may occlude more than 50% of the aortic lumen and markedly increase afterload, causing myocardial decompensation. The early signs are hypotension, elevation of PA pressures, and ST-segment or T-wave changes on the ECG.

7. The right atrium (or superior and inferior vena cavae individually) is then cannulated. Maintenance of normal CVP may help prevent atrial fibrillation during cannulation.

8. **Proximal saphenous vein graft** to aorta anastomosis may precede CPB, thus shortening CPB time.

G. **Cardiopulmonary bypass (CPB)**

1. **CPB circuit.** The fundamental components of a CPB circuit are a series of pumps, a reservoir, an oxygenating device, and a heat exchanger. The primary circuit supplies oxygenated blood to the aortic perfuser and will incorporate either a centrifugal or roller pump. Centrifugal pumps require a separate flow-measuring device, whereas roller pumps are calibrated with fixed-volume Silastic tubing fitted into an appropriately occluded pump head. The venous limb of the circuit draws blood by gravity from either a single two-stage right atrial cannula or two separate caval cannulae. Venous blood is oxygenated in either a **bubble oxygenator,** which requires defoaming, or a **membrane oxygenator,** which physically separates gas from blood with a semipermeable membrane, thereby reducing red cell trauma and eliminating the formation of foam. A reservoir accommodates excess volume and provides a safety mechanism against pumping air. Prior to perfusion into the patient, blood is filtered and temperature is regulated by passage through a fluid-filled heat exchanger. A 2-liter lactated Ringer's pump prime accounts for the roughly 12 percentage point hematocrit drop seen following initiation of CPB in the average adult patient. Blood may be required in the prime, most often for small or anemic patients, to ensure a hematocrit greater than 20% during CPB. Smaller roller pumps are used to create suction for the left ventricle returning heparinized blood from the surgical field back into the pump reservoir. A fourth roller system is commonly used for delivery of cardioplegic solution.

2. **Initiation of CPB.** Adequate heparinization must be ensured prior to initiation of CPB. The inferior vena cava line is unclamped first, and adequate venous drainage is confirmed. The superior vena cava (SVC) line is subsequently opened, and volume permitting (i.e., if venous drainage is adequate), pump speed is progressively increased to a flow of 2.0–2.4 L/min/m^2 or roughly 50 ml/min/kg for adults. A mean arterial pressure (MAP) of 40–140 mm Hg may be achieved by such flow, depending on vascular resistance, intravascular volume, and blood viscosity changes. Once adequate flows and venous drainage are established, volatile anesthetics from the anesthesia machine, IV fluids, and positive-pressure ventilation are discontin-

ued, and oxygen flows are reduced to 200 ml/min. Muscle relaxants are supplemented to prevent shivering, which increases oxygen consumption, and may produce acidosis during cooling. Anesthesia is maintained by IV agents or by inhalation agents administered through a vaporizer in the oxygen line of the oxygenator. It is advisable to pull the PA catheter back 1–5 cm to prevent migration of the catheter tip into wedge position during CPB. CVP should be monitored from the side port of the PA catheter introducer during CPB, thus ensuring measurement of SVC pressure, rather than from the right atrial port, which may be below the SVC tourniquet. As cerebral perfusion pressure is equal to MAP minus the SVC pressure, obstruction of the SVC cannula and consequent rising SVC pressures must be detected to avoid potentially disastrous neurologic injury. Following fibrillation or arrest, mean PA pressures are displayed. A vent cannula may be inserted into the left ventricle to prevent distention.

3. **Maintenance of CPB**

   a. **Myocardial protection during CPB** is primarily achieved by reducing myocardial oxygen consumption through either hypothermia, arrest, or both. Intermittent cold cardioplegia is currently the most commonly used technique. Cold fibrillation and warm continuous blood cardioplegia techniques both maintain coronary flow.

      (1) **Cardioplegia solutions,** given after application of the aortic cross clamp, produce electromechanical arrest of the heart. All solutions contain K^+. Other components include buffers, Ca^{2+}, Mg^{2+}, nitroglycerin, mannitol, lidocaine, blood, and metabolic substrate (e.g., glucose, insulin, glutamate); some solutions are oxygenated. Anaerobic metabolism continues during arrest, and by-products should be washed out by reinfusion. Cold cardioplegia (4–6°C) is often given intermittently (q20–30min), whereas warm blood cardioplegia is given continuously, thus maintaining arrest while providing continuous metabolic support and waste washout. Solutions may be delivered antegrade through the aortic root, coronary ostia, or vein graft or retrograde through the coronary sinus.

      (2) **Topical cooling** is an important consideration in cold protection techniques.

      (3) **Cold fibrillating techniques** (no aortic cross clamp) require elevated systemic pressure (MAP > 80 mm Hg) for adequate myocardial perfusion.

   b. **Hypothermia** (20–34°C) is commonly employed during CPB. Oxygen consumption, and thereby flow requirements, are reduced while blood viscosity increases, thus counteracting prime-induced hypoviscosity. Adverse effects of hypothermia include impaired autoregulatory, enzymatic, and cellular membrane function, decreased oxygen delivery (leftward shift of the hemoglobin oxygen dissociation curve), and potentiation of coagulopathy.

c. **Hemodynamic monitoring** during CPB is the shared responsibility of the perfusionist, anesthesiologist, and surgeon.

(1) **Hypotension** during initiation of CPB is usually due to hemodilution and hypoviscosity. Other important causes include inadequate pump flow, vasodilation, acute aortic dissection, or incorrect placement of the aortic cannula (e.g., directing flow toward the innominate artery not supplying the cannulated radial artery). The PA pressure and LV vent flow rate should be inspected to ensure that aortic incompetence has not compromised forward pump flow. A phenylephrine drip may be required to treat transient hypotension. In the presence of carotid stenosis, MAP should be maintained at a higher level than usual (e.g., 80–90 mm Hg), and hypocarbia should be avoided.

(2) **Hypertension** (MAP > 90 mm Hg) may be treated with vasodilators or anesthetics. Elevated PA pressures indicate left heart distention, which may be due to inadequate venting, aortic regurgitation, or inadequate isolation of venous return. Severe distention may result in irreversible myocardial damage.

d. **Metabolic acidosis and oliguria** suggest inadequate systemic perfusion. Additional volume (blood or crystalloid dependent on hematocrit) may be required to achieve increased flow. Brisk urine output should be established within the first 10 minutes of CPB.

(1) **Oliguria** (< 1 ml/kg/hr) should be treated with a trial of increased perfusion pressure and/or flow, mannitol (0.25–0.5 gm/kg), or dopamine (1–5 μg/kg/min). Patients on chronic furosemide therapy may require their usual dose during CPB to sustain diuresis.

(2) **Hemolysis** during CPB is usually due to physical trauma to red blood cells by the pump suction; released pigments may cause acute renal failure postoperatively. For hemoglobinuria, diuresis is maintained with mannitol or furosemide, and when severe, the urine is alkalinized by administering 0.5–1.0 mEq/kg of sodium bicarbonate.

e. **Additional heparin** may be needed for prolonged CPB. A 100 IU/kg hourly reinforcement dose is given starting 2 hours after the initial dose. An artificially elevated ACT is seen during aprotinin therapy and when blood temperature is lower than 35°C. The duration of heparin anticoagulation may be shorter in patients on chronic heparin therapy or during cases in which systemic hypothermia is not employed.

H. Discontinuing CPB implies transferring cardiopulmonary function from the bypass system back to the patient. In preparation for this transition, the anesthesiologist must critically examine and optimize the patient's metabolic, anesthetic, and cardiorespiratory status.

1. **Preparation** for discontinuing CPB begins during rewarming. The arterial perfusate is warmed. The core temperature should reach 37°C, and the shell (rectal) temperature, reflective of less highly perfused tissues, should reach 33–35°C prior to discontinuation from CPB.

2. **Laboratory data** to acquire during rewarming include an ABG, K^+, Ca^{2+}, glucose, hematocrit, and ACT (> 35°C).

   a. Adequate **anticoagulation** during rewarming and separation from CPB is ensured with additional heparin if necessary.

   b. **Metabolic acidosis** should be treated with sodium bicarbonate, and appropriate ventilatory changes, as determined by the ABG, should be instituted by the perfusionist.

   c. **Hyperkalemia,** commonly seen following the use of cardioplegia, is allowed to correct spontaneously by redistribution and diuresis; however, serum K^+, if trending to less than 4 mEq/L at the time of separation from CPB, should be supplemented.

   d. **Severe hyperglycemia** (blood glucose > 400–500 mg/dL), most commonly seen in diabetic patients following a warm cardioplegia technique, may require insulin by infusion for correction.

   e. A **hematocrit** over 21% should be achieved prior to separation, either by transfusion or hemoconcentration, as indicated by the CPB reservoir volume status. A higher or lower hematocrit may be appropriate, depending on the patient's age and underlying condition.

3. **Anesthetic considerations** during rewarming include maintenance of adequate neuromuscular blockade, analgesia, and amnesia. Supplementary relaxants and narcotics are routinely given at this time, as are benzodiazepines (midazolam, lorazepam), which will decrease the likelihood of recall during this period. The anesthetic system, including breathing circuit and machine, is briefly rechecked. Pressure transducers are recalibrated and zeroed. Volatile anesthetics in use on the CPB system are discontinued. If MAP is elevated, sodium nitroprusside may be used for blood pressure control, as well as to facilitate rewarming. The temperature in the operating room is raised.

4. **Separation from CPB**

   a. Following procedures where the heart has been opened (e.g., valve replacements), **"de-airing maneuvers"** are necessary to prevent air embolism to the cerebral or coronary circulations. Sustained positive-pressure ventilation will move air forward from the pulmonary veins. Air in the ventricular trabeculae can be liberated by shifting the operating room table from side-to-side and lifting the apex of the heart; it can then be evacuated by needle aspiration of the apex. Deliberately obstructing carotid flow for the first few heartbeats following removal of the aortic cross clamp also may prevent air embolization to the brain. Direct aspiration of air bubbles visible within coronary artery vein grafts will help prevent ischemia in the relevant zone of myocardium.

b. **Aortic cross-clamp removal** reestablishes coronary perfusion. A lidocaine bolus (1 mg/kg) is administered, and an infusion (1 mg/min) is begun. Extensive distal vascular disease (common in diabetics) may predispose to persistent ischemia following revascularization and may warrant reinstitution of IV nitroglycerin.

c. **Defibrillation** may be spontaneous; ventricular fibrillation is treated with directly applied 10–30 joule DC countershock. Other treatments for ventricular arrhythmias include epicardial or endocardial (through the PA line) pacing, correction of hypokalemia or ischemia, or additional antiarrhythmics (e.g., procainamide, bretylium).

d. **Rhythm** is assessed. With slow rhythms, atrial pacing is established through epicardial wires, but if the PR interval is prolonged or there is complete heart block, ventricular pacing is added. Hypothermia, hypocalcemia, hyperkalemia, and magnesium from cardioplegia solutions may contribute to a high incidence of reversible heart block immediately following CPB. Atrial tachydysrhythmias may be treated with fentanyl, overdrive pacing, cardioversion, and then, if necessary, antidysrhythmics (esmolol, propanolol, or verapamil if there is minimal LV dysfunction; otherwise digitalis may be indicated).

e. The **ECG** should be inspected for evidence of ischemia (possibly related to intracoronary air), heart block, and pacemaker capture.

f. **LV filling** may be guided during separation from CPB by mean PA, PA occlusion pressure, or a surgically placed left atrial line. Comparison is made between central (aortic) and peripheral (radial) arterial pressures to ensure that no significant gradient exists.

g. **Compliance of the lungs** is tested with a few trial breaths (ventilation should be reestablished when LV ejection, even on bypass, occurs). To facilitate expansion of the lungs, the stomach is suctioned, and if previously opened, the pleural cavities are drained. If the lungs are noncompliant after reinflation, suctioning or bronchodilators may be indicated (e.g., metaproterenol [Alupent] or albuterol [Ventolin] by inhaler, epinephrine [0.5–2.0 μg/min], or prostaglandin E_1 PGE_1, [.05–.3 μg/kg/min]).

h. Visual inspection of the heart confirms atrioventricular synchrony; contractility is assessed both by gross appearance and by systolic performance, as estimated by peak systolic and pulse pressure, taking into account pump flow and left atrial and PA pressure. If poor myocardial performance is demonstrated or anticipated (impaired preoperative function, intraoperative ischemia), initiation of inotropic support prior to separation from CPB may be indicated. Pump flow rate is checked and compared with the patient's preoperative cardiac output. Significantly higher flows indicate the need to increase vascular tone (norepinephrine, phenylephrine).

i. Ionized Ca^{2+} may be corrected slowly. Rapid Ca^{2+} administration, especially in the presence of myocardial ischemia, is associated with Ca^{2+}-induced myocardial injury (Ca^{2+} paradox). Calcium chloride will increase both contractility and systemic vascular resistance (SVR).

j. At the time of **actual separation from CPB,** venous lines are slowly clamped, allowing the heart to gradually fill, ejection occurring with each contraction. Prolonged partial venous line occlusion allows for "partial bypass," during which time cardiopulmonary function is shared and hemodynamics are optimized. Following complete venous line occlusion, once adequate filling pressures are achieved, perfusion through the aortic cannula is stopped, and the heart alone provides systemic perfusion. Manual ventilation with full tidal volumes and short inspiratory times facilitates ventricular performance.

(1) Pressure maintenance. Transfusion from the CPB reservoir maintains the left atrial pressure or PA occlusion pressure at an optimal level. Guides to determine optimal filling include blood pressure, cardiac output, and direct observation of the heart. Care is taken not to overdistend the heart; however, should this occur, the surgeon may "empty" the heart by transiently unclamping a venous line.

(2) If cardiac output is low despite adequate cardiac filling and rhythm, a positive inotrope may be indicated. Dopamine started at 200 μg/min and titrated as necessary is a common first-line agent. Dobutamine and amrinone are alternatives. Myocardial ischemia is commonly the cause of low cardiac output post-CPB and may result from inadequate myocardial protection, air or thromboembolism, coronary dissection, or acute coronary graft occlusion or kinking. Although it is important to identify and treat the cause of myocardial ischemia, it is critical to maintain coronary perfusion pressure. If inotropes are ineffective, other options include returning to CPB, inserting an IABP, or utilizing an LV assist device.

(3) **If cardiac output is high but blood pressure is low,** a vasoconstrictor is needed. If pulmonary hypertension is present, pressors can be administered through a left atrial line.

(4) **Hypertension** with adequate cardiac output should be treated to prevent bleeding at suture lines and cannulation sites. Either vasodilators, (e.g., nitroprusside) narcotics, or volatile anesthetics may be appropriate.

(5) **RV dysfunction** is heralded by a CVP rising out of proportion to left atrial pressure or PA occlusion pressure or by the appearance of RV distention on the surgical field. (The CVP/left atrial pressure ratio is normally < 1.) RV failure may precipitate LV failure, either by diminished preload or by changes in intracardiac geometry (i.e., septal shift). Predictors of RV failure include mitral valvular disease and pulmonary hypertension. Management includes the following:

(a) Treatment of known causes of elevated PVR: light anesthesia, hypercarbia, hypoxemia, and acidemia. Vasopressors and calcium chloride should be administered through a left atrial line if available.

(b) Vasodilator therapy, including nitroglycerin, sodium nitroprusside, or PGE_1 (begin 0.05 µg/kg/min, titrate as necessary) through a right-sided line. Systemic vasodilatation often necessitates compensatory vasopressor support through a left atrial line.

(c) Inotropic support is maintained with either dobutamine, dopamine, or with isoproterenol for maximal pulmonary vasodilatation, as well as for maintenance of coronary perfusion pressure. Mechanical support (IABP or RV assist devices [see secs. **V.A** and **B**]) may be necessary.

(6) **Failure to separate from CPB** may be due to LV or RV failure or both. If a return to CPB is necessary, adequate anticoagulation must be ensured, and a full heparinizing dose is indicated if any protamine has been given. Surgically correctable causes of ventricular dysfunction are treated, physiologic parameters are optimized, and more aggressive pharmacologic or mechanical support for subsequent weaning attempts as determined by the clinical situation are planned.

I. **Post-bypass period**

1. **Hemodynamic stability** is the primary goal, as myocardial function is impaired and physiologic reserve is often minimal. Maintenance of adequate volume status, perfusion pressure, and appropriate rate and rhythm is critical, and continuous reassessment facilitates prompt treatment of any cardiovascular disorders.

2. **Hemostasis.** Once cardiovascular stability has been achieved, **protamine administration** begins. Initially

25–50 mg is given over 5 minutes, and hemodynamic response is observed. Protamine often causes systemic vasodilatation and varying degrees of pulmonary hypertension, both dependent on the rate of administration; hence, slow infusions are prudent. Rarely, an **anaphylactic or anaphylactoid reaction** or catastrophic pulmonary hypertension is encountered. Upon severe reaction, the drug is immediately discontinued, appropriate resuscitative measures are employed, and if necessary, the patient is reheparinized and CPB is reinitiated.

  a. Insulin-dependent diabetics previously treated with protamine zinc insulin preparations and patients previously exposed to protamine (e.g., "redo" operations) are particularly prone to developing adverse hemodynamic responses.

  b. It is advisable to **monitor PA pressures** while administering protamine (even if left atrial pressure is available).

  c. In general, 1 mg of protamine is administered for each mg (100 IU) of heparin administered throughout the procedure.

  d. After protamine, the ACT is measured and compared to baseline. Further protamine is given to return the ACT toward control.

  e. During transfusion of heparinized "pump blood," additional protamine (25–50 mg) is also given.

  f. Desmopressin, aminocaproic acid (Amicar), aprotinin, and various blood products may each be of value in the treatment of post-CPB coagulopathy. Strategies for the diagnosis and management of intraoperative bleeding diatheses are discussed in Chap. 33.

3. Pulmonary dysfunction may follow CPB. Aggressive treatment of bronchospasm prior to sternal closure is imperative.

4. Pulmonary hypertension may arise during the post-CPB period. See sec. **I.H.4.j.(5)** for approaches to management.

5. Sternal closure may precipitate acute cardiovascular decompensation. Cardiac tamponade may develop from compression of the heart and great vessels in the mediastinum.

  a. Volatile anesthetics and other negative inotropes are avoided in anticipation of sternal closure. Intravascular volume should be optimized.

  b. Immediately after sternal closure, the left atrial pressure, or PWCP, and cardiac output are compared to preclosure values, and appropriate adjustments in volume or drug infusions are made.

  c. Mediastinal and chest tubes are placed on suction to prevent tamponade and quantitatively evaluate blood loss.

  d. The left atrial waveform and the ability of pacemakers to capture are rechecked to verify that displacement has not occurred during sternal closure.

J. Transfer to the ICU

1. Patients should always be hemodynamically stable **prior to transport.** The patient's bed should be equipped with a full cylinder of oxygen, an Ambu bag, and essential monitoring equipment. Drugs and equipment for resuscitation should accompany the patient during transport and include calcium chloride, lidocaine, a vasopressor, and a mask, as well as spare intubation equipment, a defibrillator, and extra crystalloid or colloid.

2. **During transfer,** the ECG and arterial and PA pressures are monitored. Portable oximetry is useful.

3. **Mediastinal and pleural drainage** tubes are attached to suction. The ECG and pressure transducers are attached and calibrated to the ICU monitors. The patient is placed on the ICU ventilator, and ventilation is ensured. An **anteroposterior chest x-ray** and a 12-lead ECG are obtained, and blood samples are sent for ABG, electrolytes, hematocrit, platelet count, prothrombin time, and partial thromboplastin time. A **thorough report** is provided to the ICU team, including pertinent hemodynamics, vasoactive drips and dosages, and the problems that are anticipated. Prior to leaving the ICU, the anesthesiologist should review the ECG and ABG and should check the chest x-ray for the presence of abnormal findings (e.g., atelectasis, pneumothorax, malpositioned tubes and catheters, or a widened mediastinum or pleural effusion, suggestive of bleeding).

III. Postoperative care

A. Warming. Most cardiac surgical patients will arrive in the ICU hypothermic, and their initial course is notable for warming and vasodilation. A temperature overshoot phenomenon is common, and patients will, on average, reach a maximal temperature at 6–12 hours into their ICU stay. Pressor and volume requirements should be anticipated. Adequate sedation (narcotics, benzodiazepines), either by periodic bolus or continuous infusion, will prevent early waking and shivering during this period.

B. Extubation. Coincident with emergence from anesthesia, ventilatory support is withdrawn, and most patients are extubated 12–18 hours after arrival in the ICU. Intracardiac cannulae and chest tubes are removed, and hemodynamic support is then gradually withdrawn.

C. Complications

1. **Dysrhythmias and myocardial ischemia** are common in the immediate postoperative period. Diagnosis and management are discussed in Chap. 18.

2. **Unexplained profound hypotension,** unresponsive to volume and pharmacologic resuscitation, is an indication for immediate reopening of the chest in the ICU. The operating room should be notified and blood products requisitioned.

3. **Cardiac tamponade** may occur insidiously and may be difficult to diagnose. Most often an accumulation of blood in the mediastinum and inadequate chest tube

drainage secondary to clot are responsible. Placing mediastinal tubes on suction as soon as the sternum is closed and frequent tube "stripping" will help to prevent the development of tamponade. Reopening the sternum may be lifesaving. The diagnosis is considered with hypotension or low output syndrome. Equilibration of mean CVP, PA pressure, and PA occlusion pressure, accompanied by compensatory tachycardia, hypotension, and venous congestion are pathognomonic.

IV. Pediatric cardiac anesthesia

A. Transition from fetal to adult circulation.

The transition from fetal to adult circulation is a transformation from two parallel to two serial circulations. After birth, as the lungs are expanded, PVR decreases. Initially there is right-to-left shunting of blood across the ductus arteriosus; this eventually becomes left-to-right shunting as PVR falls below SVR. There is an increase in pulmonary blood flow, an improvement in RV compliance, a decrease in right-sided filling pressures, and eventual closure of the foramen ovale associated with this fall in PVR. The ductus arteriosus normally closes by the second to third day of life, and the circulation is then assumed to be in an adult pattern. The persistence of a transitional circulation is common in many cases of congenital heart disease (CHD) and can occasionally be lifesaving.

B. Difference between neonatal and adult cardiac physiology

1. In infants there is parasympathetic nervous system dominance that reflects the relative immaturity of the sympathetic nervous system at birth. Infant hearts are stimulated more by circulating catecholamines than by sympathetic nervous system innervation.

2. Neonatal hearts have more inelastic membrane mass than elastic contractile mass. Consequently, infant hearts have less myocardial reserve, a greater sensitivity to drugs causing myocardial depression, and a greater tendency for volume overload. The relatively noncompliant ventricles make stroke volume less variable and cardiac output more heart rate dependent.

3. The right and left ventricles are equal in muscle mass at birth. A left to right muscle mass ratio of 2 : 1 is not achieved until the age of 4–5 months.

C. Congenital heart disease.

In CHD the clinical presentation is dependent on the anatomy and the physiologic changes secondary to intracardiac shunts and obstructive lesions.

1. **Shunt classification.** A shunt is an abnormal communication between the systemic and pulmonary circulations.

   a. **Simple shunts** are not associated with an obstruction to blood flow. Pulmonary and systemic blood flow is determined solely by the relative ratios of PVR and SVR.

   b. **Complex shunts** are lesions where a shunt is accompanied by an obstruction to blood flow. The direction and magnitude of blood flow are largely fixed by the obstructive lesion. Blood flow depends less on the PVR/SVR ratio and more on the size of the obstruction.

c. **Shunt flow calculation.** The amount of systemic arterial desaturation due to CHD is determined by the relative amount of pulmonary-to-systemic blood shunting ($\dot{Q}p/\dot{Q}s$) and the saturation of the venous blood.

$$\dot{Q}p/\dot{Q}s = (SaO_2 - S\bar{v}O_2)/(S_{pv}O_2 - S_{pa}O_2)$$

$\dot{Q}p/\dot{Q}s > 1$ left-to-right shunt

$\dot{Q}p/\dot{Q}s < 1$ right-to-left shunt

$\dot{Q}p$ = pulmonary blood flow; $S\bar{v}O_2$ = mixed venous oxygen saturation; $\dot{Q}s$ = systemic blood flow; $S_{pv}O_2$ = pulmonary venous oxygen saturation; SaO_2 = systemic arterial oxygen saturation; $S_{pa}O_2$ = pulmonary artery oxygen saturation.

Since we are calculating the ratio of flows, oxygen saturations can be used instead of oxygen contents. To simplify calculation, if systemic blood is fully saturated, one can approximate that there is no significant right-to-left shunting and that pulmonary venous oxygen saturation is equal to systemic oxygen saturation ($S_{pv}O_2 = SaO_2$).

2. The **effects of shunts** on the cardiovascular and pulmonary systems include volume overload (from left-to-right shunt), increased PA pressures, increased PVR, and ventricular dysfunction.

3. **Clinical presentation**

   a. **Cyanosis** due to CHD is caused by either inadequate pulmonary blood flow (e.g., pulmonary or tricuspid atresia) or intracardiac right-to-left shunts (tetralogy of Fallot); the presence of a common mixing chamber (single ventricle, common atrioventricular canal); or transposition of the great arteries.

   b. **Congestive heart failure (CHF)** may be due to either left-to-right shunt and excessive pulmonary blood flow (atrial septal defect, ventricular septal defect, or patent ductus arteriosus) or left ventricular outflow obstruction and pressure overload (congenital subvalvular, valvular, or great-vessel obstruction). Mixed lesions can give rise to both cyanosis and CHF.

D. **Anesthetic management**

   1. **Preoperative workup**

      a. The **history** should provide an assessment of the extent of cardiopulmonary impairment (presence of cyanosis or CHF, exercise tolerance, cyanotic "spells," activity level, feeding and growth patterns, associated syndromes, and anatomic abnormalities).

      b. **Physical examination** should make note of skin color, activity level, respiratory pattern and frequency, and appropriateness of development for given age. The heart and lungs should be auscultated and close attention given to the patient's airway and IV access. Peripheral pulses should be palpated and blood pressure obtained in both arms and the lower extremities if coarctation is suspected.

c. The **chest x-ray** is examined for evidence of increased heart size, presence of CHF, decreased pulmonary blood flow, abnormalities in heart position, and the presence of any thoracic cage abnormalities.

d. The **ECG** may be normal even in the presence of CHD. However, abnormalities can be important clues to underlying cardiac lesions (refer to a pediatric cardiology text for a comprehensive discussion).

e. **Echocardiography** will show anatomic abnormalities and, with Doppler, provide information about flow patterns and pressure gradients.

f. **Cardiac catheterization** is, at present, the best window into the patient's central circulatory system. Anatomy can be defined, pulmonary and systemic shunt flows and vascular resistances quantified, and intracardiac chamber pressures obtained.

2. **Premedication.** Infants younger than 6 months of age, cyanotic or dyspneic children, and patients who are critically ill generally receive no premedication. Older or more vigorous children may be given atropine (0.02 mg/kg IM) and morphine (0.15 mg/kg IM). An alternate intramuscular regimen is ketamine (3–5 mg/kg) in combination with midazolam (0.5–1.0 mg) and glycopyrrolate (0.1–0.2 mg) given in the preanesthetic holding area. Dosages are reduced in cases where lowering SVR would increase right-to-left shunting. Fasting guidelines must be adjusted based on the patient's age and cardiac condition. Cyanotic infants are usually polycythemic and may be prone to vital organ thrombi if not hydrated with IV fluids preoperatively.

3. **Monitoring and equipment** (Table 23-3). In addition to the standard monitoring required for all patients, a precordial or esophageal stethoscope, three temperature probes (tympanic membrane, esophageal, and rectal), and a Doppler flow probe to use with cuff pressure measurements should be available. Intraarterial pressure monitoring is usually necessary (note that previous surgical procedures [e.g., classic Blalock-Taussig shunt and coarctation repair] may influence the site of radial artery cannulation). Central venous catheters are regularly inserted for infusion of vasoactive drugs, CVP measurement, and volume administration. Our practice is to use a 4 Fr double-lumen catheter for infants weighing 10 kg or less and a 5 Fr double-lumen catheter for larger children. A warming/cooling blanket, radiant heating lamps, and a heated humidifier are useful perioperatively.

Table 23-3. Checklist for a pediatric cardiopulmonary pump procedure

Equipment

Mapleson D circuit if patient is under 10 kg
500-ml and 1-liter breathing bags
Bain circuit adapter for machine
Humidifier and appropriate tubing
Pediatric anesthesia machine with air tank (full) and extra air
    tanks
Halothane, isoflurane, and enflurane vaporizers
Noninvasive automatic blood pressure machine
Pediatric and neonatal cuffs
Pulse oximeter probes (infant and pediatric)
Appropriate size masks, airways, laryngoscope blades, endotracheal
    tubes (ETTs), stylet, Magill forceps
Lidocaine/phenylephrine solution for nose (nasal ETT and nasogas-
    tric tube)
Nasogastric tubes
Tympanic/esophageal temperature monitor
Tympanic temperature probe
Esophageal stethoscope with built-in temperature probe
Hat
End-tidal carbon dioxide connector
Precordial stethoscope and stickers
Suction catheters
Rectal temperature probe

Drugs

Pancuronium
Fentanyl (100 μg/kg)
Atropine (0.02 mg/kg)
Succinylcholine (4 mg/kg for IM use)
Ketamine (10, 50, or 100 mg/ml for IV or IM use)
Calcium gluconate (100 mg/ml)
Thiopental
Midazolam
Dopamine, dobutamine, epinephrine, isoproterenol, amrinone, and
    prostaglandin E_1 drips as needed (see Chap. 19 for guide to prep-
    aration and dosing)
Phenylephrine (10 μg/ml, 100 μg/ml syringes)
Epinephrine (10 μg/ml, 100 μg/ml syringes)
Sodium bicarbonate

4. **Resuscitation drugs** and infusions of inotropic medications for appropriate pediatric dosages must be
   available. **Air bubbles must be meticulously removed from all IV lines, IV line junctions, and
   syringes.** Air filters should be used whenever possible.
   Even in the absence of shunts, paradoxical air emboli
   may, under some conditions, traverse a probe-patent
   foramen ovale.

5. **Induction.** The choice between an inhalation and
   intravenous induction is based primarily on ventricular function and the need for postoperative ventilation.
   A slow, carefully titrated induction by either technique

usually provides for a safe and stable anesthetic. Theoretically, patients with right-to-left shunts should have a delayed induction with inhalation agents, since blood is shunted past the lungs. Similarly, patients with a significant right-to-left shunt should see blood concentrations of IV anesthetic rise much faster and consequently have a faster onset of induction. An alternative anesthetic induction is intramuscular ketamine (3–5 mg/kg) along with an antisialogogue such as atropine (0.02 mg/kg) or glycopyrrolate (0.01 mg/kg). This alternative is especially suited for the uncooperative child or a child surviving primarily on sympathetic stimulation. Nasal intubation is preferred, since this provides the greatest comfort, stability, and ease of management postoperatively.

E. **Cardiopulmonary bypass**
1. **Pump prime volume** ranges between 700 and 1200 ml depending on the weight of the infant. Packed red blood cells are frequently added to yield a final hematocrit of 25%. Typical constituents of pump prime include sodium bicarbonate (to counteract acidosis), mannitol (to promote diuresis), and calcium (to offset the effects of the citrate in citrate-dextrose-phosphate preserved blood).
2. Infants and children generally lack vasoocclusive disease. Consequently, blood flow during CPB is more important than arterial pressure. Flows as high as 150 ml/kg/min may be used (in infants < 5 kg), while MAP as low as 30 mm Hg is well tolerated provided that SVC pressure is low (indicating that venous drainage is adequate).
3. **Deep hypothermic circulatory arrest (DHCA)** is used extensively for infants weighing less than 10 kg. Up to 1 hour of circulatory arrest is tolerated at a core and brain temperature of 15–20°C without neurologic injury. Phentolamine (Regitine, 0.2 mg/kg) and furosemide (Lasix, 0.25 mg/kg) are frequently administered to encourage even cooling and renal tubule protection in preparation for DHCA. Key management points include
   a. Adequate brain hypothermia (e.g., packing the head with ice packs).
   b. Hemodilution.
   c. Acid-base balance.
   d. Muscle relaxation.
   e. Avoidance of increased blood glucose.

F. **Procedures not requiring CPB**
1. **Closed heart cases** without the use of CPB include patent ductus arteriosus ligation, coarctation of the aorta repair, PA banding, and most shunts designed to increase pulmonary blood flow (e.g., modified Blalock-Taussig shunt).
2. **Open heart cases** without CPB include those that can be accomplished through normothermic caval inflow obstruction, such as pulmonary valvulotomy, aortic valvulotomy, and creation of atrial septal defects.

G. **Management of specific CHD lesions** (Table 23-4)
  1. **Cyanotic lesions**
     a. **Right-to-left shunting** includes lesions such as tetralogy of Fallot, tricuspid atresia, pulmonary atresia, and acute pulmonary hypertension.
        (1) **Goal** is to decrease PVR, increase pulmonary blood flow, maintain SVR, and maintain central volume.
        (2) **Anesthetic maneuvers** include hypocarbia, 100% oxygen, maintaining normal FRC, and avoiding acidosis. For tetralogy of Fallot, a negative inotrope (e.g., propranolol) to relax infundibular spasm may help increase pulmonary blood flow. PGE_1 (0.1 µg/kg/min IV) helps support ductus arteriosus patency, decreases PVR, and increases pulmonary blood flow. A peripheral vasoconstrictor should be readily available.
     b. **Mixing lesions** include hypoplastic left heart syndrome (plus right-to-left shunt), truncus arteriosus, total anomalous pulmonary venous return, double-outlet right ventricle with pulmonary stenosis, double-inlet left ventricle, single atrium or ventricle, and transposition of the great arteries.
        (1) **Goal** is to decrease pulmonary blood flow and maintain adequate systemic perfusion.
        (2) **Anesthetic maneuvers** include normocarbia and limiting inspired oxygen concentration.
  2. **Lesions with CHF**
     a. **Left-to-right shunting** includes lesions such as atrial septal defect, ventricular septal defect, patent ductus arteriosus (amenable to the addition of regional [caudal, lumbar, or thoracic epidural] anesthesia), and atrioventricular canal.
        (1) **Goal** is to avoid myocardial depressants and excessive pulmonary blood flow.
        (2) **Anesthetic maneuvers** include IV induction (opiates, ketamine), avoiding negative inotropes (inhalation agents, pentothal), normocarbia, limiting inspired oxygen concentration, and positive end-expiratory pressure.
     b. **Left ventricular outflow obstruction** includes coarctation of the aorta (see sec. **a** regarding patent ductus arteriosus), aortic stenosis, and hypoplastic left heart syndrome.
        (1) **Goal** is to decrease SVR and to maintain ductal patency to allow for right-to-left flow.
        (2) **Anesthetic maneuvers** are the same as in sec. **a.(2)**. PGE_1 infusion may help maintain ductal patency.
H. **Anesthesia for cardiac catheterization.** The goal is to provide sufficient sedation to allow the procedure to be completed without excessive movement while avoiding sedative-induced hemodynamic changes and hypoventilation.
  1. An **anesthesia machine** (fitted with compressed air as well as oxygen) and all standard monitoring equip-

Table 23-4. Specific congenital heart disease lesions

Lesion (incidence)	Anatomy	Pathophysiology	Surgical correction	Anesthetic considerations
Atrial septal defect (ASD) (9.8%)	Three varieties: 1. Ostium secundum; defect in septum primum (most common). 2. Ostium primum (endocardial cushion defect). 3. Caval-atrial (sinus venosus).	L→R shunt. RV volume overload. Minimal symptoms until late age, when CHF may develop.	Suture or patch closure. Percutaneous catheterization baffle/umbrella closure.	Inhalation or intravenous induction. Potential extubation at end of procedure. Avoid air bubbles.
Ventricular septal defect (VSD) (30.5%)	Membranous versus muscular.	L→R shunt. ↑ Pulmonary blood flow. Pulmonary hypertension as late effect (Eisenmenger's syndrome).	Dacron patch closure. Usually difficult to locate muscular defect.	Hypocarbia to ↓ pulmonary blood flow. Avoid myocardial depressants. Potential need for pacing (second-degree heart block not uncommon) and inotropic support for correction. Avoid air bubbles.
Coarctation (6.8%)	Narrowing usually distal to origin of left subclavian artery; usually preductal in neonates and postductal in older children.	Increased blood flow to upper extremities and head. Systemic hypoperfusion. Pressure overload of LV.	L. thoracotomy. Subclavian artery flap angioplasty or resection and end-to-end anastomosis.	PGE₁ in neonates with LV failure to maintain R→L. Non-CPB case. Arterial line on right. Suitable for regional anesthesia supplementation.

	Anatomy	Physiology	Surgical treatment	Anesthetic management
Patent ductus arteriosus (PDA) (9.7%)	Patent ductus arteriosus.	R→L shunt when PVR high. L→R shunt as PVR decreases. Necessary for survival with certain CHD lesions.	L thoracotomy. Ligation and division of PDA. Cardiac catheterization laboratory closure.	Usually premature infants with concomitant hyaline membrane disease. Avoid high FiO_2 (risk of retrolental fibroplasia). Risk of recurrent laryngeal nerve damage.
Tetralogy of Fallot (5.8%)	1. VSD. 2. Pulmonary outflow obstruction. 3. RV hypertrophy. 4. Overriding aorta.	R→L shunt through VSD into overriding aorta. Systemic desaturation.	Closure of VSD. RV outflow. Tract reconstruction and excision of infundibular muscle band.	Management of "Tet spell": 100% O_2, MSO_4i Valsalva/knee-chest position, ↑ SVR (phenylephrine), ↓ PVR, augment intravascular volume ⇒ ↑ pulmonary blood flow.
Transposition of the great arteries (4.2%)	Isolation of pulmonary and systemic circulations due to transpositions of aorta to RV; PA to LV.	ASD, VSD, or PDA required for survival.	1. Atrial baffle (Mustard, Senning). 2. Arterial switch (Jatene procedure). 3. If associated with VSD, a Rastelli procedure (RV→PA conduit) may be considered.	Duct/mixing lesion dependent CHD lesion. Balloon atrial septostomy (Rashkind) if insufficient mixing. PGE_1 to maintain ductus arteriosus patency.
Truncus arteriosus (2.2%)	Single great artery that gives rise to aorta, PA, coronary arteries. Associated VSD.	Mixing of R + L blood. Increased pulmonary blood flow. Mild hypoxemia.	VSD closure. RV to PA valved conduit. Valvuloplasty of truncal valve.	Decrease pulmonary blood flow, increase PVR precorrection. Inotropes, ↓ PVR postcorrection.

Table 23-4. (continued)

Lesion (incidence)	Anatomy	Pathophysiology	Surgical correction	Anesthetic considerations
Atrioventricular (AV) canal (< 1%)	Common AV valve. Deficiency of atrial and ventricular septae.	Mixing of blood between all 4 chambers; increased pulmonary blood flow.	Closure of ASDs and VSDs. Mitral valvuloplasty and repair of mitral cleft.	Increased or decreased pulmonary blood flow. Associated with Down's syndrome (expect airway difficulty). Need for inotropes postoperatively.
Hypoplastic left heart syndrome (< 1%)	Atretic/hypoplastic mitral valve, LV, ascending aorta.	L→R shunt (obligatory) at atrial level with complete mixing. Ductus arteriosus dependent for R→L and systemic perfusion.	Fontan procedure: ASD closure, anastomosis of right atrium to right or main PA. 1st stage = Norwood procedure (atrial septectomy, reconstruction of aortic arch, and pulmonary artery).	Avoid myocardial depressants; usually critically ill neonates. Manipulate PVR and SVR to provide adequate systemic perfusion without decreasing pulmonary blood flow critically.

L = left; R = right ventricle/ventricular; LV = left ventricle/ventricular; CHF = congestive heart failure; PGE₁ = prostaglandin E₁; CPB = cardiopulmonary bypass; PVR = pulmonary vascular resistance; CHD = congenital heart disease; SVR = systemic vascular resistance; PA = pulmonary artery.

ment, resuscitation drugs, airway management equipment, and a defibrillator (with appropriately sized paddles) must be present.

2. **Premedication** is similar to that mentioned in sec. **D.2.** Patients are generally well sedated and maintain a good airway with a continuous combined ketamine (2 mg/kg/hr) and midazolam (0.1 mg/kg/hr) infusion (500 mg of ketamine + 5 mg of midazolam in 50 ml; ketamine = 10 mg/ml, midazolam = 0.1 mg/ml) with supplemental boluses as needed.

3. **General endotracheal anesthesia** may be utilized in children prone to airway obstruction (Down's syndrome, nasopharyngeal defects) and in children with suprasystemic RV pressures where cyanosis from pulmonary hypertension may improve after anesthesia reduces sympathetic tone. General endotracheal anesthesia should be readily available in cases of premedication and drug bolus overdose.

V. **Mechanical support devices**

A. **The intraaortic balloon pump (IABP)** is indicated in patients with **cardiogenic shock** who are known to have surgically correctable lesions, with unstable angina that cannot be stabilized with any medical regimen including high-dose nitroglycerin and heparin, or following CPB where myocardial failure is expected to be relatively transient.

   1. The IABP **improves myocardial performance** by augmenting aortic diastolic pressure while reducing the impedance to LV ejection. The left ventricle is allowed to eject at a pressure lower than that at which the coronary arteries are perfused.

   2. The IABP is **inserted** through a femoral artery and advanced until the tip is just distal to the left subclavian artery in the descending thoracic aorta. It may occasionally be placed transthoracically if iliofemoral occlusive disease precludes use of a femoral artery.

   3. **Inflation** of the IABP is synchronized with either the patient's ECG, a pacemaker potential, or the arterial blood pressure trace. Balloon inflation occurs early in diastole, augmenting aortic pressure by driving blood both proximally (toward the coronary bed) and distally (toward the systemic circulation). Deflation occurs just prior to systole, reducing LV stroke work and hence myocardial oxygen consumption. Intraoperative triggering directly from a pacemaker generator will eliminate interference otherwise caused by electrocautery or blood sampling.

   4. **Complications** of IABPs include distal embolization (to extremities, kidneys, brain, and the gastrointestinal tract), femoral arterial spasm with lower extremity ischemia, bleeding from heparinization, and consumptive coagulopathies.

B. **Ventricular assist devices** provide temporary circulatory support by assuming varying degrees of pump function. The specific pumping device may be pulsatile or nonpulsatile. The left ventricular assist devices (LVAD) may perfuse the ascending aorta with blood drawn from a variety of sites, most commonly the left atrium. Right ventricular support (RVAD), biventricular support, and the total artificial heart (TAH), though less commonly encountered, are all options for the hemodynamic support of patients in extremis, for whom some form of corrective therapy will soon become available.

VI. **Other cardiac procedures**
  A. **"Redo" cardiac surgery**
    1. **Multiple previous indwelling catheters** may make percutaneous arterial and jugular cannulation difficult.
    2. The **heart, major vessels, vascular grafts,** or **lungs** may be adherent to the underside of the sternum; sternotomy can be complicated by catastrophic lacerations and hemorrhage. In emergency situations, venous return may be supplied from the pump suction line on the field, thus "sucker bypass" is initiated. Manipulation of atheromatous grafts may send emboli to the coronary circulation. Femoral vessels may be isolated prior to sternotomy, since partial bypass may be lifesaving.
    3. **Diffuse bleeding** (from extensive dissection of scar tissue) may occur following CPB, so these patients are more likely to require transfusion.
    4. **Epicardial pacing** may be difficult from scarring on the surface of the heart; Paceport or pacing PA catheters are frequently useful in this setting.
  B. **Cardiac tamponade.** Ketamine, though itself a myocardial depressant, may be a useful induction agent for patients presenting with cardiac tamponade. Volume resuscitation is often required to maintain cardiac output despite elevated filling pressures.
  C. **Cardiac transplantation**
    1. **Management of the donor.** See Chap. 20.
    2. **Anesthetic management of the recipient**
      a. These patients have extremely low ejection fractions and poor organ perfusion.
      b. **Full stomachs** are the rule, as cases are done on an emergency basis.
      c. **Anticoagulation** with warfarin (Coumadin) is common and may require corrective measures including vitamin K and fresh-frozen plasma.
      d. **Cyclosporine,** an immunosuppressant, may be administered orally or by nasogastric tube prior to induction (10–12 mg/kg); the nasogastric tube should not be aspirated once cyclosporine has been given.
      e. **Invasive monitoring** consists of arterial and CVP catheters.
      f. **Inotropes** may be required prior to CPB.
      g. **Weaning from CPB** may be complicated by right heart failure secondary to recipient pulmonary hypertension. Dopamine and nitroglycerin may be necessary. Isoproterenol may be particularly useful, not only as an inotrope and pulmonary vasodilator, but also as a positive chronotrope for the denervated heart.

h. **After weaning** from CPB, the immunosuppressants azathioprine (Imuran, 5 mg/kg IV) and methylprednisolone (Solu-Medrol, 500 mg IV) are administered.

D. **Antiarrhythmia surgery** may involve aneurysmectomy (with or without electrophysiologic mapping), cryoablation of accessory bundles responsible for Wolff-Parkinson-White syndrome, endocardial resection, or implantation of an AICD system.

1. **Aneurysmectomy.** It is crucial to prevent hyperdynamic responses; stress on the ventricular suture line is life-threatening. Large resections may compromise ventricular stroke volume. Thus, patients may be rendered highly rate dependent to achieve adequate cardiac output.

2. **AICD surgery.** Patients presenting for AICD procedures often have profound ventricular dysfunction, frequent malignant dysrhythmias, and a high incidence of coexisting disease. Therapeutic electrical discharge from the device may be delivered through transvenous lead systems, patch electrodes, or a combination of the two. Patch electrodes may be either subcutaneous, pericardial (thoracotomy or subxyphoid approach), or epicardial (thoracotomy or median sternotomy). Subcutaneous tunneling is required to connect lead systems with the pulse generator, most commonly placed in an abdominal subcutaneous pouch. The specific surgical procedure will, to a large extent, determine appropriate anesthetic techniques.

   a. **Standard monitoring and access** include an arterial line and central venous catheter.

   b. **Anesthetic techniques** may include combined epidural/general anesthesia and occasionally double-lumen endobronchial intubation. Postoperative epidural analgesia provides superior postthoracotomy pain relief.

   c. **Ventricular fibrillation** is routinely induced. Backup defibrillator systems must be immediately available, as should antidysrhythmics including lidocaine, procainamide, and bretylium. Adequate oxygenation must be ensured prior to periods of arrest.

   d. **Defibrillation thresholds** may be affected by anesthetic agents.

   e. Report to the postoperative care team must include information on device status (i.e., ON or OFF), as well as rate-sensing parameters.

VII. **Anesthesia for cardioversion and electrophysiology procedures.** In addition to providing anesthesia for elective and emergent cardioversions, anesthesia services may also be requested for a variety of electrophysiology procedures including pediatric radiofrequency ablation, as well as the AICD-related testing procedures IPS (invasive programmed stimulation) and NIPS (noninvasive programmed stimulation). During these latter procedures, malignant dysrhythmias (ventricular tachycardia, ventricular fibrillation) are deliberately induced for brief periods of time, to be treated by either internal or external pacing, cardioversion, or defibrillation.

A. Intubating equipment drugs, a source of oxygen and positive-pressure ventilation, suction, an IV, blood pressure cuff, and oximeter, as well as a defibrillator, pacing equipment, and resuscitating drugs must be immediately available.

B. After preoxygenation, methohexital (0.5–1.0 mg/kg IV), thiopental (1.0–1.5 mg/kg IV), or propofol (0.5–1.0 mg/kg IV) may be used for brief periods of anesthesia. Onset of action may be delayed because of relatively low cardiac output due to the arrhythmia. As soon as consciousness is lost, the appropriate charge may be delivered. The airway is maintained and ventilation supported until consciousness is regained.

C. Following emergence, a short period in the postanesthesia care unit (where monitoring cardiac rhythm continues) is usually necessary.

SUGGESTED READING

Becker, R. C., and Alpert, J. S. The impact of medical therapy on hemorrhagic complications following coronary artery bypass grafting. *Arch. Intern. Med.* 150:2016, 1990.

Bristow, M. R. The surgically denervated transplanted human heart (editorial). *Circulation* 82:658, 1990.

deBruijn, N. P., and Clements, F. Intraoperative Use of Echocardiography. *Society of Cardiovascular Anesthesiologists Monograph.* Philadelphia: Lippincott, 1991.

Hensely, F. A., Jr., and Martin, D. E. (eds.). *The Practice of Cardiac Anesthesia.* Boston: Little, Brown, 1990.

Hickey, P. R., and Wessel, D. L. Anesthesia for Treatment of Congenital Heart Disease. In J. A. Kaplan (ed.), *Cardiac Anesthesia* (2nd ed.). New York: Grune & Stratton, 1987.

Hoffman, J. I., and Spaan, J. A. Pressure-flow relations in coronary circulation. *Physiol. Rev.* 70:331, 1990.

Jacobs, M. L., and Norwood, W. I. *Pediatric Cardiac Surgery.* Boston: Butterworth-Heinemann, 1992.

Kaplan, J. A. *Cardiac Anesthesia* (2nd ed.). New York: Grune & Stratton, 1987.

Kennedy, J. W., et al. Multivariate discriminant analysis of the clinical and angiographic predictors of operative mortality from the collaborative study in coronary artery surgery (CASS). *J. Thorac. Cardiovasc. Surg.* 80:876, 1980.

Lake, C. L. (ed.). *Pediatric Cardiac Anesthesia.* Norwalk, CT: Appleton and Lange, 1988.

Lichtenstein, S. V., Salerno, T. A., and Slutsky, A. S. Warm continuous cardioplegia versus intermittent hypothermic protection during cardiopulmonary bypass. Pro: Warm continuous cardioplegia is preferable to intermittent hypothermic cardioplegia for myocardial protection during cardiopulmonary bypass. *J. Cardiothorac. Anesth.* 2:279, 1990.

Lowenstein, E., et al. Catastrophic pulmonary vasoconstriction associated with protamine reversal of heparin. *Anesthesiology* 59:470, 1983.

Miller, D. C., et al. Discriminant analysis of the changing risks of coronary artery operations: 1971–1979. *J. Thorac. Cardiovasc. Surg.* 85:197, 1983.

Royston, D. High-dose aprotinin therapy: A review of the first five years' experience. *J. Cardiothorac. Vasc. Anesth.* 6:76, 1992.

Rung, G. W., et. al. Anesthetic Management for Patients with Congenital Heart Disease. In F. A. Hensley, and D. E. Martin (eds.), *The Practice of Cardiac Anesthesia.* Boston: Little, Brown, 1990.

Slogoff, S., et al. Rise of perfusion pressure and flow in major organ dysfunction after cardiopulmonary bypass. *Ann. Thorac. Surg.* 50:911, 1990.

24

Anesthesia for Neurosurgery

Takahisa Goto and David Kliewer

I. Physiology

A. **Cerebral blood flow** (CBF) is equal to cerebral perfusion pressure (defined as the difference between mean arterial pressure [MAP] and intracranial pressure [ICP] or central venous pressure, whichever is higher) divided by the cerebral vascular resistance. CBF averages approximately 50 ml/100 gm of whole brain tissue/min in the normal brain and is affected by blood pressure, $PaCO_2$, and PaO_2. It is also regulated regionally to meet the metabolic needs of the tissue.

1. **Blood pressure.** CBF is maintained at a constant level between 50 and 150 mm Hg MAP by constriction and dilation of resistant arterioles (**autoregulation**) in the normal person (Fig. 24-1). CBF varies directly with MAP beyond these limits. Chronic hypertension shifts the autoregulatory curve to the right, rendering patients susceptible to cerebral ischemia at blood pressures considered normal in healthy individuals. Chronic antihypertensive therapy may bring the autoregulatory range back toward normal. Cerebral ischemia, trauma, hypoxia, hypercarbia, edema, mass effect, and volatile anesthetics attenuate or abolish autoregulation and make blood flow to the affected brain dependent on MAP.

2. **$PaCO_2$** has profound effects on CBF by its effect on the pH of brain extracellular fluid. CBF increases linearly with increasing $PaCO_2$ in the range from 20–80 mm Hg, with an absolute change of 1–2 ml/100 gm/min for each mm Hg change in $PaCO_2$. However, the effect of $PaCO_2$ on CBF diminishes over 12–24 hours, because of slow adaptive changes in brain ECF bicarbonate concentration. With sustained hyperventilation, CSF HCO_3 production decreases, allowing CSF pH to gradually decrease as well. Rapid normalization of $PaCO_2$ after a period of hyperventilation raises the pH of brain ECF, with resulting vasodilation and increased intracranial hypertension.

3. **PaO_2.** Hypoxia is a potent cerebral vasodilator; CBF increases markedly below a PaO_2 of 60 mm Hg.

B. **Cerebral metabolic rate** ($CMRO_2$) and CBF are coupled, as the brain requires a constant supply of substrate to meet its relatively high metabolic demands. Regional or global increases in $CMRO_2$ elicit a corresponding increase in CBF, possibly mediated by metabolic by-products. Factors that affect $CMRO_2$ (and CBF through this mechanism) include

1. **Anesthetics** (see secs. II.A and B).

2. **Temperature.** Hypothermia decreases $CMRO_2$ 7% per 1°C, and hyperthermia increases it.

3. **Seizures** increase $CMRO_2$.

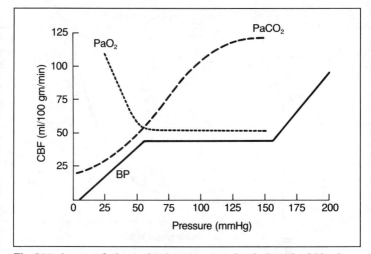

Fig. 24-1. Autoregulation maintains a constant level of cerebral blood flow (CBF) over a wide range of carotid artery mean blood pressure (BP). Independent of this effect, CBF is elevated by hypercarbia ($PaCO_2$) and hypoxemia (PaO_2); hypocarbia diminishes CBF.

   C. **Intracranial pressure** reflects the relationship between the volume of the intracranial contents (brain, blood, and cerebrospinal fluid [CSF]) and the volume of the cranial vault.
      1. Since the **cranial vault** is rigid, its capacity to accommodate increases in intracranial volume is limited. A developing intracranial mass (e.g., tumor, edema, hematoma, hydrocephalus) initially displaces one or more of the intracranial components and ICP remains relatively normal (Fig. 24-2A). As intracranial volume increases further, however, intracranial compliance decreases, and ICP rises rapidly (Fig. 24-2B). Thus, patients with decreased compliance may develop marked increases in ICP even with small increases in intracranial volume (i.e., cerebral vasodilation due to anesthesia, hypertension, or carbon dioxide retention) (Fig. 24-2B).
      2. Methods commonly used to **measure ICP**:
         a. The **subarachnoid bolt** is a hollow screw easily placed through a burr hole and connected to a pressure transducer through nonheparinized, saline-filled tubing. The bolt is used for both measurement and treatment of ICP. CSF cannot be withdrawn through it.
         b. A **ventriculostomy catheter** can be inserted through a burr hole into a lateral ventricle. This may be more accurate than a subarachnoid bolt and is also useful for draining CSF. However, its placement requires passage through brain tissue and may be difficult in patients with compressed or

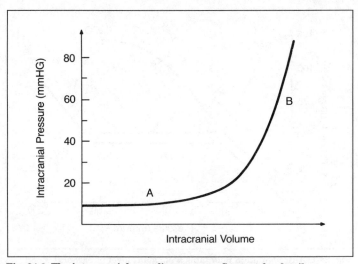

Fig. 24-2. The intracranial compliance curve. See text for details.

distorted ventricles. Complications include infection and hemorrhage.

c. A **Camino catheter** can be inserted intracerebrally for a continuous numerical display of ICP.

3. **Clinical features of elevated ICP.** Normal ICP is 5–15 mm Hg. Intracranial hypertension is defined as sustained ICP greater than 15–20 mm Hg. ICP elevation decreases cerebral perfusion pressure and may cause ischemia in regions of the brain where autoregulation is defective and CBF is dependent on cerebral perfusion pressure. The signs and symptoms of increased ICP include headache, nausea, vomiting, and decreased levels of consciousness. As ICP rises higher, distortion and ischemia of the brainstem and/or brain herniation may ensue and result in hypertension with brady- or tachycardia, irregular respiration, oculomotor (third cranial) nerve palsy leading to ipsilateral pupillary dilation with no light reflex, abducens (sixth cranial) nerve palsy, contralateral hemiparesis or hemiplegia, and finally coma and respiratory arrest.

4. **Treatment of elevated ICP** involves strategies aimed at decreasing the volume of one of the intracranial components.

a. **Reduction of cerebral blood volume**

(1) Both hypoxia and hypercarbia cause cerebral vasodilation and therefore should be avoided. **Meticulous airway management** is crucial.

(2) **Hyperventilation** to a $PaCO_2$ of 25–30 mm Hg produces cerebral vasoconstriction and is useful in acute management of increased ICP. Since there is little additional decrease in CBF below 20–25 mm Hg $PaCO_2$ and biochemical evidence

of cerebral ischemia may develop, excessive hyperventilation should be avoided.

   (3) Venous drainage should be promoted by elevating the head 30 degrees, avoiding excessive flexion or rotation of the neck, and preventing increases in intrathoracic pressure (e.g., coughing and straining and elevated airway pressures). Positive end-expiratory pressure should also be kept to the lowest level that provides adequate oxygenation.

   (4) Malignant hypertension should be treated. Pain and anxiety should be reduced.

   (5) Potent pharmacologic vasoconstrictors such as **barbiturates** may be used in patients resistant to other modes of therapy.

   b. Reduction of brain tissue volume

   (1) Maintaining **high serum osmolality** (305–320 mOsm/L) removes water from the brain and thereby effectively decreases brain volume. Fluid management is designed to achieve this goal (see sec. **IV.A.5**). Mannitol (0.5–2.0 gm/kg IV) produces a hyperosmolar state and is effective in acute reduction of brain volume. Mannitol initially increases intravascular volume and may precipitate congestive heart failure in susceptible patients; it may also cause hypokalemia from renal excretion of potassium.

   (2) Furosemide in combination with **mannitol** provides greater reduction in ICP and brain edema than either alone. Furosemide reduces CSF production and leads to dehydration. It is slower in onset and less reliable than mannitol when used alone.

   (3) Steroids reduce edema associated with tumors but appear to be ineffective in treating edema secondary to trauma or hypoxia. Because their effects occur slowly (over 12 hours), steroids are not useful for acute treatment of elevated ICP.

   c. Reduction of CSF volume can be achieved by draining CSF through a lumbar subarachnoid or ventriculostomy catheter.

II. Pharmacology

   A. Inhalation anesthetics

   1. The effect of **nitrous oxide** is controversial, but it probably is a cerebral vasodilator. This effect can be greatly attenuated or abolished by hyperventilation or IV anesthetics. Nitrous oxide slightly increases $CMRO_2$.

   2. Halothane, enflurane, and **isoflurane** are direct cerebral vasodilators causing increases in CBF. Autoregulation can be attenuated or abolished by increasing concentration of these drugs, but responsiveness to carbon dioxide seems to be preserved. Institution of hyperventilation prior to administration of the agent may attenuate the rise in ICP. Enflurane at concentrations greater than 1.5 minimum alveolar concentration (MAC) when combined with hypocarbia ($PaCO_2 < 30$

mm Hg) has been shown to induce seizure activity on the electroencephalogram (EEG), although the clinical significance has not been established.

3. **Volatile anesthetics** produce dose-dependent reduction in metabolism ($CMRO_2$), probably by depressing neuronal electrical activity. Isoflurane is the most potent in this respect and is the only volatile agent that induces an isoelectric EEG at clinically relevant concentrations (2 MAC).

B. **Intravenous anesthetics** (barbiturates, benzodiazepines, narcotics, etomidate, propofol) cause coupled reduction in CBF and $CMRO_2$ in a dose-dependent manner. This is also due to depression of neuronal electrical activity with minimal or no effect on cellular function. Barbiturates and etomidate are potent depressants of CBF and $CMRO_2$, while narcotics cause only modest or insignificant changes. Benzodiazepines seem to have intermediate effects. Ketamine increases CBF up to 60% or more of normal and increases $CMRO_2$ and for this reason is used infrequently in neuroanesthesia. Autoregulation and carbon dioxide responsiveness appear to be preserved with these IV agents.

C. **Muscle relaxants** have no direct effect on CBF and $CMRO_2$ because they do not cross the blood-brain barrier. However, they may indirectly alter cerebral hemodynamics through their effects on blood pressure (e.g., curare, atracurium) and heart rate (pancuronium) (see Chap. 12). **Succinylcholine** alone causes an increase in CBF and $CMRO_2$, probably secondary to increased cerebral afferent input from muscle spindles stimulated by fasciculation. Its clinical significance is controversial but is probably minimal if administered after induction of adequate anesthesia or defasciculating dose of nondepolarizing muscle relaxant.

D. **Vasoactive drugs**
1. **Vasopressors.** Phenylephrine, epinephrine, and norepinephrine may increase CBF indirectly by increasing cerebral perfusion pressure but have little direct effect on cerebral vasculature because they do not cross the blood-brain barrier.
2. **Vasodilators.** Sodium nitroprusside, nitroglycerin, and hydralazine can increase CBF and ICP by direct cerebral vasodilation if arterial blood pressure is maintained. Trimethaphan, a ganglionic blocking agent, does not increase CBF and ICP as much as the direct vasodilators. However, trimethaphan causes cycloplegia and mydriasis, which may confuse the postoperative neurologic assessment. Beta-blocking agents probably have minimal effects if cerebral perfusion pressure is maintained. Despite these profiles, all of these agents have been used safely in neuroanesthesia.

E. **Cerebral protection**
1. **Cerebral ischemia** can be classified into three types:
   a. **Focal,** characterized by the presence of surrounding nonischemic brain and possible collateral blood flow

to the ischemic region (e.g., stroke, arterial occlusion, embolization).

b. **Incomplete global,** some but insufficient blood supply to the whole brain (e.g., hypotension, increased ICP).

c. **Complete global,** no CBF (e.g., cardiac arrest).

2. **Agents**

a. **Barbiturates** may improve the neurologic recovery from focal or incomplete global ischemia, probably by decreasing metabolic rate. Maximum beneficial effects are achieved when the EEG is made isoelectric because metabolic depression by barbiturates is caused by suppression of neuronal electrical activity. In contrast, barbiturates have been shown to be of no benefit following cardiac arrest. This is probably because cardiac arrest abolishes the electrical activity of brain neurons almost instantly, and therefore, administration of barbiturates cannot produce further metabolic depression.

b. **Isoflurane** also has no beneficial effect in global ischemia. In contrast to barbiturates, the effects of isoflurane in focal or incomplete global ischemia seem to be less consistent even when an isoelectric EEG is produced.

c. **Hypothermia** can reduce metabolism for both neuronal and cellular functions, but the associated risks of marked cardiovascular and respiratory depression, arrhythmias, tissue hypoperfusion, and coagulopathy limit its use largely to cardiac surgery.

d. **Hyperglycemia** may worsen neurologic outcome following ischemic insult, probably because anaerobic metabolism of glucose produces excessive lactate, leading to cellular acidosis.

e. The calcium channel antagonist, **nimodipine**, has been shown in some studies to improve outcome after stroke and attenuate cerebral hypoperfusion following global ischemia, although with inconsistent neurologic recovery. Nimodipine's beneficial effects on vasospasm after subarachnoid hemorrhage are well established.

f. **Steroids** have not been found to be beneficial after stroke or severe head injury in the majority of studies. High-dose methylprednisolone has been shown to produce modest improvement in neurologic recovery following acute spinal cord injury if the treatment is started within 8 hours of injury.

III. **Electrophysiologic monitoring**

A. **Electroencephalography** (EEG) measures electrical activity of the neurons of the cerebral cortex and is thus a threshold marker that is able to detect ischemia from inadequate CBF. It is used frequently during procedures that jeopardize cerebral perfusion such as carotid endarterectomy and cardiopulmonary bypass.

1. The **EEG waveforms** are classified by their frequencies.

   a. **Alpha** activity (8–13 Hz) predominates in awake patients with closed eyes and is most evident over the occipital region.
   b. **Beta** activity (14–30 Hz) is predominant anteriorly in the normal awake patient.
   c. Slower frequencies (**delta** [1–3 Hz] and **theta** [4–7 Hz]) appear during stages of natural sleep and in pathologic states.
   d. **EEG waveform changes** that may reflect inadequate CBF during surgery include loss of fast activity (alpha and beta), loss of amplitude, and increased slow-wave activity (delta and theta).

2. **Reduction of CBF.** When CBF decreases below 20–25 ml/100 gm/min under nitrous oxide–oxygen–halothane anesthesia, EEG slowing occurs; in the vicinity of 18 ml/100 gm/min, the EEG becomes isoelectric ("flat"). Sustained reduction of CBF to 8–10 ml/100 gm/min results in tissue infarction. Thus, EEG changes can warn of ischemia before CBF becomes insufficient to maintain tissue viability. The critical level of cerebral blood flow is defined as that degree of cerebral blood flow below which signs of ischemia are seen on EEG, and it is roughly correlated with the extent to which each anesthetic depresses $CMRO_2$. The level of critical cerebral blood flow varies from 20 ml/100 gm/min for halothane, to 18 ml/100 gm/min for enflurane, and 10 ml/100 gm/min for isoflurane.

3. The EEG may exhibit **changes intraoperatively with no demonstrable neurologic deficit** during postoperative examination. Cerebral ischemia can produce electrical dysfunction without causing actual neuronal cell damage because the blood flow threshold for electrical failure is higher than that for metabolic failure.

4. **Factors other than anesthetics that may affect the EEG** include hypothermia (which may limit its usefulness during cardiopulmonary bypass), hypotension, hypoxia, tumors, vascular abnormalities, and epilepsy. Hypocarbia has few effects. The abnormal EEG in patients with preexisting neurologic deficits, strokes in evolution, and recent reversible ischemic neurologic deficits can also make it difficult to interpret new changes.

5. **Anesthetic effects on the EEG.** Anesthetic effects are generally global, which often helps distinguish them from the focal changes of ischemia. All anesthetics cause a combination of slow frequencies and superimposed fast activity. As the anesthetic depth increases from "light" to "deep," a progression in activity to a predominance of slow activity is seen. "Deep" anesthesia may cause marked EEG slowing, making detection of superimposed ischemic changes during carotid clamping more difficult to interpret. Maintaining a constant level of anesthesia during critical periods (i.e., carotid clamping) facilitates EEG interpretation.

B. **Evoked potential monitoring**

1. **Sensory evoked potentials** (EPs) are electrical potentials generated within the neuraxis in response to stimulation of a peripheral or cranial nerve. These potentials are recorded as they travel from the periphery to the brain by electrodes placed over the scalp as well as along the transmission pathway. EPs are of lower voltage compared to background EEG activity, but summation of hundreds of signals using computerized devices makes it possible to extract them by averaging out the random background EEG. A normal response implies that the conduction pathway is intact. Damage to the pathway generally manifests as a decrease in amplitude or a prolongation in latency (i.e., time from peripheral stimulus to arrival of potentials at the recording site) of the peaks of a waveform. EPs are classified according to the nerve tract being evaluated.

   a. **Somatosensory evoked potentials** (SSEPs) are obtained by stimulating a peripheral nerve (e.g., median nerve at the wrist, posterior tibial nerve at the ankle or in the popliteal fossa) and recording the elicited signals over the spinal cord (spinal SSEPs) or cerebral cortex (cortical SSEPs). SSEPs are used most commonly to monitor spinal cord function during spinal cord or vertebral column surgery (e.g., Harrington rod instrumentation) and may also be used during peripheral nerve, brachial plexus, or thoracic aortic surgery (to detect spinal ischemia during aortic cross-clamping). Since SSEPs are conducted primarily by the posterior column in the spinal cord, there are concerns about the reliability of SSEP monitoring for detecting threatened motor function (anterior spinal cord). For this reason, the **wake-up test** is used by some (see sec. **V.B.1**), and **motor evoked potential** monitoring has been developed recently.

   b. **Brainstem auditory evoked potentials** (BAEPs) are recorded by delivering a "clicking" sound to one ear through an ear-insert headphone. BAEPs reflect the transmission of electrical impulses along the auditory pathway and are monitored during posterior fossa surgery in an attempt to avoid brainstem or auditory (eighth cranial) nerve damage.

   c. **Visual evoked potentials** are generated by light flashes to the eyes and have been used during surgery around the optic nerve and tracts (e.g., pituitary surgery). Because of the inability to deliver patterned stimuli in anesthetized patients, they are rarely used.

2. **Motor evoked potentials,** although still investigational, may be more reliable than SSEPs in detecting threatened motor function of the spinal cord. The motor cortex is stimulated by a pulsed magnetic field or directed electrical stimulation generated by a coil placed over the scalp. Electrical activity resulting from the discharge of cortical motor neurons is detected with

electrodes placed over the spinal cord or peripheral nerves or by observing the electromyograph or muscle movement. A significant limitation is that even small doses of anesthetics depress the responses profoundly and make interpretation difficult.

3. **Confounding factors.** Interpretation of EP changes are confounded by factors similar to those that affect the EEG (i.e., anesthetics, temperature, hypotension, hypoxia, anemia, preexisting neurologic lesions).

4. **Anesthetic effects**

   a. **Volatile anesthetics** can depress EPs significantly by reducing the amplitude or prolonging the latency. IV anesthetics have diminished effect; barbiturates and fentanyl (up to 50 μg/kg) are compatible with effective monitoring of cortical SSEPs and BAEPs.

   b. **Spinal SSEPs and BAEPs** appear to be more resistant to the depressive effects of anesthetics than cortical SSEPs.

5. **False positives.** Like the EEG, changes in EPs occur frequently and are often not associated with postoperative neurologic complications. Further work is required to establish the nature, magnitude, and duration of EP changes associated with irreversible damage.

IV. Specific neurosurgical procedures

A. Supratentorial mass lesions

1. **Preoperative considerations**

   a. **Intracranial compliance** may be decreased by intracranial mass lesions (e.g., tumor, hematoma, abscess). In addition, there may be compression of surrounding normal brain tissue leading to brain edema and loss of autoregulation of cerebral vessels in that area. Signs and symptoms that suggest elevated ICP are discussed in sec. **I.C.3.**

   b. **A computed tomography (CT) scan** should be reviewed as midline shift, and compressed ventricles or cisterns may suggest the presence of diminished intracranial compliance. The degree of brain edema surrounding the mass and the site of the lesion in relation to major intracranial vessels and structures should be noted. Lesions near the dural venous sinuses may require exposure of the sinuses to the atmosphere and may be associated with higher risk of venous air embolism (see sec. **IV.D.3**).

   c. The **pathology of the mass** is also important in anticipating possible perioperative problems. Vascular lesions (e.g., meningiomas, some metastatic brain tumors) may cause massive intraoperative bleeding. Infiltrating malignant tumors may render the patient particularly prone to postoperative brain swelling and may justify more strict fluid restriction than usual.

   d. **Fluid and electrolyte imbalance** and **glucose intolerance** are common due to fluid restriction, diuretics, poor oral intake, steroids, and centrally-mediated endocrine abnormalities.

    e. Patients may require **anticonvulsants** for seizure control and **steroids** for treatment of edema. These drugs should be continued preoperatively.

2. **Premedication** should be prescribed cautiously, since patients with intracranial disease may be extremely sensitive to the effects of central nervous system (CNS) depressants. Frequently no premedication is given, and if sedation is needed, diazepam (0.1–0.2 mg/kg PO) is often used. Additional sedation in the form of IV midazolam can be given once the patient arrives in the operating room. Narcotics should be avoided.

3. Besides standard **monitoring** (see Chap. 10), **arterial catheters** are used in most patients undergoing craniotomy. Capnography is particularly useful when controlling ICP by hyperventilation. An indwelling urinary catheter is placed for fluid management and forced diuresis. Invasive monitoring (e.g., pulmonary artery catheter) may be indicated for patients with severe cardiac, renal, or pulmonary disease in the face of marked diuretic-induced fluid shifts. Since access to the neck is limited during neurosurgery, placing central lines by the brachial or subclavian approaches should be considered. A second IV catheter for drug administration is often useful.

4. **Intraoperative management.** Anesthetic goals for intracranial procedures include amnesia, immobility, control of ICP and cerebral perfusion pressure, and a "relaxed brain" (i.e., optimal surgical conditions). The anesthetic plan should provide an awake, extubated patient who can be evaluated neurologically at the end of the procedure when possible.

    a. **Induction** of anesthesia must be accomplished smoothly without increasing ICP or compromising CBF. Hypertension, hypotension, hypoxia, hypercarbia, and coughing should be avoided.

        (1) While **thiopental** (3–7 mg/kg), **propofol** (2.0–2.5 mg/kg), **midazolam** (0.2–0.4 mg/kg), and **etomidate** (0.3–0.4 mg/kg) are all reasonable choices, the hemodynamic effects caused by these agents must be anticipated.

        (2) A patent mask airway is essential. Following induction, hyperventilation by mask is started with either a **nitrous oxide–oxygen mixture or 100% oxygen.**

        (3) An intubating dose of **muscle relaxant** is given. A nondepolarizing agent such as vecuronium or pancuronium is commonly chosen. Adequate relaxation should be obtained to avoid coughing and straining on intubation.

        (4) **Narcotics** cause minimal change in cerebral hemodynamics and are useful in blunting responses to intubation and craniotomy. Since intubation, placement of head pins, and craniotomy (skin incision, manipulation of the periosteum) represent the most stimulating periods during intracranial procedures, generous doses

of narcotics are given prior to these manipulations. Fentanyl (5–10 µg/kg) and sufentanil (0.5–1.0 µg/kg) are most commonly used, as both have rapid onset and high potency. Lidocaine (1.5 mg/kg IV) has also been shown to attenuate the cardiovascular and ICP response to intubation.

(5) **Low concentrations of a potent inhalation agent** are frequently added to prevent hypertension during the initial surgical stimulation.

(6) **Following intubation,** the eyes are covered with watertight patches to prevent irritation from surgical preparation solutions, the head is carefully checked to ensure good venous return, and close attention is paid to the airway, since access to the airway is limited during neurosurgical procedures. Breath sounds and adequate ventilation should be checked after final positioning to ensure proper placement of the endotracheal tube, and all connections in the breathing circuit should be secured tightly.

b. **Maintenance**

(1) Adequate brain relaxation is necessary **prior to opening the dura.** This is achieved by ensuring adequate oxygenation, muscle relaxation, depth of anesthesia, good venous return, hyperventilation to a $PaCO_2$ of 25–30 mm Hg, and administration of furosemide (10–20 mg IV) and mannitol (0.5–1.5 gm/kg IV) before the craniotomy is completed. A need for further brain relaxation, as assessed by the surgeon checking the tension of the dura, may be met by IV thiopental or drainage of CSF through a lumbar subarachnoid catheter.

(2) **After craniotomy and dural opening,** anesthetic requirement is substantially lower, since brain parenchyma is devoid of sensation. If supplemental narcotics are needed, small doses of morphine, fentanyl, or sufentanil can be given. Long-acting narcotics and sedatives are usually avoided during the last 1–2 hours of the procedure to facilitate neurologic examination at the end of surgery and prevent prolonged postoperative obtundation. A volatile anesthetic (isoflurane) may be used to decrease the incidence of awareness and to control hypertension. Hypertension may also be treated with a vasodilator.

(3) **Muscle relaxants** are frequently continued throughout the procedure to prevent movement. In patients with upper motor nerve lesions and a flaccid limb, placement of the twitch monitor on the flaccid limb may lead to overdose. Patients on anticonvulsants (e.g., phenytoin) may require more frequent administration of muscle relaxants.

(4) **Hyperventilation** is continued.

    c. Emergence should occur promptly without straining or coughing. Muscle relaxation is usually maintained until the head dressing is completed and then reversal agents may be given. IV lidocaine may be given to suppress the cough reflex. $PaCO_2$ is normalized gradually toward the end of the procedure. Hypertension must be controlled to minimize bleeding; rapidly-acting IV agents such as labetalol, esmolol, sodium nitroprusside, or nitroglycerin are often used. Before leaving the operating room, the patient should be awake so that a brief neurologic examination can be performed. The presence of new, unexpected deficits may necessitate further evaluation, CT scan, or immediate reexploration.

5. Perioperative fluid management is designed to decrease brain water content and thereby reduce ICP and provide adequate brain relaxation while maintaining hemodynamic stability and cerebral perfusion pressure.

    a. The **blood-brain barrier** is selectively permeable. Gradients for osmotically active substances ultimately determine the distribution of fluids between the brain and intravascular spaces.

      (1) Water freely passes through the blood-brain barrier. Intravascular infusion of free water will thus increase brain water content and may elevate ICP. Isosmotic glucose solutions (e.g., 5% dextrose in water) have the same effect, since the glucose is metabolized and free water remains.

      (2) The blood-brain barrier is impermeable to most **ions** including Na^+. Therefore, unlike in peripheral vasculature, total osmolality rather than colloid oncotic pressure determines the osmotic pressure gradient across the blood-brain barrier. Consequently, maintenance of high-normal serum osmolality can decrease brain water content, while administration of a large amount of hyposmolar crystalloid solution may increase it.

      (3) Large, polar substances cross the blood-brain barrier poorly. Albumin has little effect on brain extracellular fluid, since the colloid oncotic pressure contributes to only a small portion of total plasma osmolality (approximately 1 mOsm/L).

      (4) If the blood-brain barrier is disrupted (e.g., by hypoxia, head trauma, or tumor), permeability to mannitol, albumin, and saline increases such that these molecules have equal access to brain extracellular fluid. Under such circumstances, administration of isosmolar colloid and crystalloid seems to have similar effects on edema formation and ICP.

    b. Severe fluid restriction can result in marked hypovolemia, leading to hypotension, a fall in CBF, and ischemia of the brain and other organs while producing only a modest decrease in brain water content. Excessive hypervolemia may cause hypertension and cerebral edema.

c. **Specific treatment recommendations.** The overall goal is to maintain normal intravascular volume and to produce a hyperosmolar state.

(1) **Fluid loss.** The fluid deficit incurred by an overnight fast is usually not replaced. Physiologic maintenance fluids are given. Third-spacing of fluids during intracranial surgery is minimal and usually ignored. Two-thirds of intraoperative urine output is replaced with crystalloid. If signs of hypovolemia develop, additional fluid is administered.

(2) **Blood loss** may be replaced with 3 ml of crystalloid to every 1 ml of blood. Transfusion is guided by hematocrit using criteria identical to those for other types of surgery. Assessment of blood loss may be difficult during intracranial procedures because significant amounts can be hidden under the drapes, and irrigating solutions are used generously by the neurosurgeon.

(3) The **serum osmolality** is increased to 305–320 mOsm/L. Isosmolar crystalloid such as 0.9% normal saline (309 mOsm/L) may be preferable to hyposmolar solutions such as lactated Ringer's (272 mOsm/L). Mannitol (0.25–2.0 gm/kg IV) and/or furosemide (5–20 mg IV) is also administered (see sec. **I.C.4.b**). The large diuresis produced by these agents demands close monitoring of intravascular volume and electrolytes.

(a) **Hypokalemia** may develop from the use of steroids or potassium-wasting diuretics and is exacerbated by hyperventilation. Administration of potassium is rarely necessary, however.

(b) **Hyponatremia** may be seen secondary to diuretic usage or syndrome of inappropriate antidiuretic hormone secretion (SIADH).

(c) **Hyperglycemia** may worsen neurologic outcome after ischemia (see sec. **II.E.2.d**). Glucose-containing solutions are avoided in patients at risk for CNS ischemia.

(d) **Marked hyperosmolarity** may produce obtundation, seizures, and renal dysfunction.

6. **Immediate postoperative care.** Patients are observed closely in an intensive care setting. The report to the intensive care or postanesthesia care unit staff includes the patient's preoperative neurologic condition as well as anticipated postoperative neurologic deficits and other pertinent history as described in Chap. 34.

a. **The head of the bed** should be elevated 30 degrees to promote venous drainage.

b. **Neurologic function** including the level of consciousness, orientation, pupillary size, and motor strength should be assessed frequently. Deterioration of any of these may indicate development of brain edema, hematoma, hydrocephalus, or herniation.

c. **Adequate ventilation and oxygenation** are particularly important in patients with reduced level of consciousness.

d. **Continuous monitoring of ICP** may be indicated if intracranial hypertension exists at the time of dural closure or is anticipated in the postoperative period.

e. **Serum electrolytes and osmolarity** should be checked.

f. **SIADH** can be diagnosed by hyponatremia and serum hyposmolality with high urine osmolality. Treatment is centered on free water restriction.

g. **Diabetes insipidus** may occur after any intracranial procedure but is most common after pituitary surgery. Polyuria is associated with hypernatremia, serum hyperosmolality, and urine hyposmolality. Conscious patients can compensate by increasing their fluid intake; otherwise, adequate IV replacement is mandatory. Aqueous vasopressin (5–10 USP units SQ or 3 units/hr by IV infusion) may be given. Larger doses may cause hypertension from its vasopressor action. Alternatively, desmopressin (DDAVP) (1–2 µg IV or SQ q6–12h) can be used and is associated with a lower incidence of hypertension.

h. **Seizures** may indicate the presence of an expanding intracranial hematoma. If a seizure occurs, airway control, oxygenation, and ventilation must be ensured. For acute control, thiopental (50–100 mg IV), midazolam (2–4 mg IV), or diazepam (5–20 mg IV for adults) may be used. Phenytoin (15 mg/kg IV over 20 minutes as a loading dose followed by 300–500 mg/day PO or IV for adults) can be started to prevent recurrence.

i. **Tension pneumocephalus** may occur and should be suspected after failure to awaken from anesthesia. Skull x-rays confirm the diagnosis; treatment consists of opening the dura to release the air.

B. **Intracranial aneurysm.** Patients may present for surgery either electively or acutely following subarachnoid hemorrhage.

1. The optimal **timing** of surgery after subarachnoid hemorrhage is controversial. Early surgery (within 48 hours of hemorrhage) can be associated with suboptimal surgical conditions but may reduce the incidence of major complications such as rebleeding and vasospasm, which are most common 1–4 and 5–9 days after hemorrhage, respectively. Delaying surgery provides time for brain swelling to subside and the aneurysm to "firm" but increases the incidence of hydrocephalus, rebleeding, and vasospasm.

2. The **presurgical treatment of aneurysm patients** is designed to reduce the risk of rebleeding and to prevent

Table 24-1. Classification of patients with intracranial aneurysms according to surgical risk (Hunt and Hess)

GRADE I	Asymptomatic or minimal headache and slight nuchal rigidity
GRADE II	Moderate to severe headache, nuchal rigidity, no neurologic deficit other than cranial nerve palsy
GRADE III	Drowsiness, confusion, or mild focal deficit
GRADE IV	Stupor, moderate to severe hemiparesis, possibly early decerebrate rigidity, and vegetative disturbances
GRADE V	Deep coma, decerebrate rigidity, moribund appearance

vasospasm. Current regimens include sedatives, bed rest, antifibrinolytics (epsilon-aminocaproic acid), calcium channel antagonists (nimodipine), and volume expansion.

3. **Preoperative evaluation** should include the neurologic grade classification by Hunt and Hess (Table 24-1) and determination of the degree of vasospasm. Hydrocephalus may also be present due to impairment of CSF circulation by blood in the subarachnoid space. ICP is likely to be elevated in patients with poor Hunt and Hess grade (Grades III–V), hydrocephalus, or intracranial hematoma. Electrocardiographic changes are common following subarachnoid hemorrhage, including ST-segment and T-wave changes due to autonomic hyperactivity induced by subarachnoid hemorrhage. Patients with preexisting ischemic heart disease or evidence of myocardial dysfunction require further workup.

4. **Specific anesthetic goals**
   a. **Avoidance of hypertension** is essential to prevent bleeding or rebleeding, which is associated with a very high morbidity and mortality.
   b. **Hypotension** is of concern if vasospasm or elevated ICP is present.
   c. **Adequate brain relaxation** is necessary to optimize surgical conditions. However, lowering ICP may also reduce the tamponade effect of the hematoma and precipitate hemorrhage and should be done cautiously prior to dural opening.

5. **Controlled hypotension** during surgical dissection will decrease transmural pressure across the aneurysm and reduce the risk of rupture. An MAP of 50–60 mm Hg is acceptable in healthy patients but may not be tolerated by patients with other cerebral or cardiovascular diseases. The cerebral arteries feeding the aneurysm are sometimes clipped temporarily to isolate the aneurysm from the arterial pressure and reduce the risk of rupture by surgical manipulation. Moderate hypertension can then be induced to improve the collateral flow to the brain regions that were perfused by the clipped arteries.

6. **Intraoperative aneurysm rupture** can produce rapid and massive blood loss. Induced hypotension or, occasionally, manual pressure on the ipsilateral carotid artery in the neck may be helpful. These patients may be extremely sensitive to hypotensive agents. Accurate estimation of blood loss is essential to guide volume repletion.

7. Once all the permanent clips are placed on the aneurysm, **prevention of postoperative vasospasm** becomes important. Blood pressure is increased moderately, and fluid is increased to achieve a mildly positive fluid balance.

C. **Arteriovenous malformation** (AVM) is a direct communication between cerebral arteries and veins without an intervening capillary bed. Since AVMs are a high-flow, low-resistance system, surrounding brain regions may be hypoperfused by diversion of the blood to the AVM (steal). These may manifest as subarachnoid hemorrhage, seizures, mass effect, or focal cerebral ischemia.

1. The **anesthetic management** of AVMs is similar to that of aneurysms, with the primary focus on tight blood pressure control.

2. **Complications**
   a. **Hypotension** can be potentially deleterious to the normal brain regions surrounding the AVM because the vessels in these regions are maximally vasodilated and unable to autoregulate due to chronic hypoperfusion. After excision of the AVM, these vessels regain autoregulation only slowly.
   b. **Reperfusion** of these areas may lead to severe edema, increased ICP, and hemorrhage aggravated by hypertension.

D. **Posterior fossa surgery**
1. **Tumors of the posterior fossa** may cause cranial nerve palsies, cerebellar dysfunction, and hydrocephalus due to obstruction of the fourth ventricle. Tumors or surgery around the glossopharyngeal and vagus nerves may impair the gag reflex and increase the risk of aspiration. Resection of tumors in the floor of the fourth ventricle may damage respiratory centers and necessitate mechanical ventilation postoperatively.

2. **Cardiovascular instability resulting from surgical manipulation** is common. Sudden severe bradycardia and hypertension occur if the trigeminal nerve is stimulated, while bradycardia and hypotension may follow stimulation of the glossopharyngeal or vagus nerve. The surgeon should be notified immediately. Cessation of the stimulus usually improves the instability, and further treatment is rarely necessary.

3. The **sitting position** is sometimes used for posterior fossa surgery. Its advantages include better surgical exposure, diminished bleeding due to improved venous drainage, and better access to the airway and chest for the anesthesiologist. However, it is associated with a higher incidence of venous air embolism and cardiovascular instability. Modified supine or prone position-

ing may be substituted for the sitting position because of these concerns (see Chap. 18 for detection and management of venous air embolism).

4. **At the end of surgery,** the ability to protect the airway and the adequacy of respiration should be checked before extubation. Surgical manipulation may have caused damage to the cranial nerves or respiratory center in the brainstem, with resulting pharyngeal or respiratory dysfunction. Postoperative infarction, edema, or hematoma formation in the posterior fossa can cause rapid clinical deterioration. Close observation and prompt support including intubation, mechanical ventilation, and circulatory management may be lifesaving.

E. **Transsphenoidal resection of the pituitary gland** is performed through either a nasal or labial incision.

1. Although nonfunctioning **pituitary adenomas** are the most common tumor type, some patients have endocrine deficiencies due to hypothalamopituitary compression. Various hyperpituitarism syndromes may accompany a functioning adenoma, including Cushing's disease, acromegaly, and amenorrhea-galactorrhea (see Chap. 6).

2. **ICP** is not a concern in most cases because tumors are small and unlikely to compromise intracranial compliance. Uncontrollable bleeding is rare but can be massive and catastrophic. Frontal craniotomy may ultimately be required to achieve hemostasis. It is prudent to have at least one large-bore IV in place.

3. **Monitoring.** Access to the patient's head is obstructed by the operating microscope, so the endotracheal tube must be firmly secured. Continuous monitoring of ventilation is essential, while arterial line monitoring is rarely necessary.

4. **Insertion of a throat pack** will prevent blood from accumulating in the stomach and may reduce postoperative vomiting. The throat pack must be removed prior to extubation.

5. **At the conclusion of surgery,** nasal breathing will be obstructed by packs. Therefore the patient must be conscious and the oropharynx suctioned prior to extubation.

6. **Diabetes insipidus** may occur after transsphenoidal hypophysectomy. Treatment with IV fluids or vasopressin may be necessary (see sec. **IV.A.6.g** and Chap. 6).

F. **Stereotactic surgery** is performed through a burr hole, using a three-dimensional reference grid attached to the head with pins placed in the outer table of the skull. This approach allows localization of a discrete area of brain for biopsy or ablation (by cryoprobe, proton beam, or radiofrequency). In most cases, the procedure can be performed under local anesthesia with IV sedation. Since the stereotactic apparatus precludes full access to the airway, sedation must be given with extreme caution. If endotracheal intubation and general anesthesia are needed after the frame is placed, the technique of securing the airway is selected based on the urgency of airway management and whether the stereotactic frame interferes with the mask airway. The frame may also prevent optimal head positioning for mask ventilation and direct laryngoscopy. Awake intubation, preferably with a fiberoptic scope, may be indicated. The stereotactic frame may need to be removed in an emergency.

G. **Epilepsy surgery** is performed in patients with epilepsy of focal origin who are refractory to medical therapy or intolerant of side effects from anticonvulsants. The procedures include cortical excision of an area of epileptiform activity and temporal lobectomy for temporal lobe epilepsy. Electrophysiologic mapping of the epileptic focus and other cortical areas serving important functions (e.g., language, memory, sensorimotor) is often performed to maximize the resection of the epileptogenic lesion while minimizing the neurologic deficits. Awake craniotomy with local anesthesia of the scalp and IV sedation allows efficient conduction of the mapping procedure, which requires patient cooperation. General anesthesia offers the advantages of patient comfort, immobility, a secure airway, and ability to control $PaCO_2$ and other variables to provide optimum operating conditions but may interfere with electrophysiologic monitoring. A nitrous oxide–narcotic–relaxant technique is often used. EEG signals can be augmented with methohexital, etomidate, or ketamine during the mapping period. Since there is often an initial increase in seizure activity postoperatively, anticonvulsant agents should be resumed as soon as possible.

H. **Head trauma.** Anesthetic management of the patient with head trauma is complicated by the challenging combination of a "tight" head, full stomach, and potentially unstable cervical spine. While following the "ABCs" of resuscitation, the anesthesiologist should ascertain the mechanism and extent of injury. Cervical spinal cord injury must be suspected and the neck stabilized until cervical vertebral fracture is ruled out.

1. **Patients who are responsive and ventilating adequately** should receive supplemental oxygen and be observed closely for evidence of neurologic deterioration while being prepared for surgery (e.g., monitors applied, IVs inserted).

2. **Comatose patients** require immediate endotracheal intubation for airway protection. In addition, hypercarbia and hypoxia must be corrected, since they can exacerbate increases in ICP and contribute to secondary brain injury.

3. **Endotracheal intubation** should be accomplished rapidly, with minimal blood pressure lability, and without coughing or straining.

   a. A **rapid sequence induction** is most commonly performed. If a cervical spine fracture has not been ruled out, the assistant (preferably the neurosurgeon) should immobilize the neck with manual in-line stabilization. The anterior part of the cervical collar may need to be removed to apply cricoid pressure and obtain sufficient mouth opening. A short-acting induction agent such as methohexital, thiopental, or etomidate is given to induce anesthesia, which is immediately followed by an intubating dose of muscle relaxant. Hyperventilation via mask is started until sufficient muscle relaxation is obtained if its benefits (i.e., ICP reduction, maintenance of adequate PaO_2) are considered to outweigh the risk of aspiration. A muscle relaxant should have rapid onset of action and short duration; succinylcholine satisfies both of these conditions and can be used safely unless contraindicated by other reasons (e.g., associated burns, severe muscle trauma, or motor deficits from brain or spinal cord injury more than 24–48 hours old). ICP effects of succinylcholine are discussed in sec. **II.C.** Vecuronium may also be used.

  b. Awake intubation (e.g., blind nasal, fiberoptic) is sometimes advocated because of full-stomach considerations, the potential for worsening neck injuries during manipulation of the airway, and anticipation of a difficult airway due to associated facial injuries. However, this approach is often impractical in head-injured patients due to lack of cooperation, and may increase ICP further by inducing hypertension, coughing, and straining.

  c. Nasal intubation and nasogastric tube placement are contraindicated in the presence of basilar skull fracture (e.g., CSF rhinorrhea, otorrhea, Le Fort III facial fracture), since the tube could further traumatize the intracranial vault.

4. Hypertension in head-injured patients may be the body's compensatory effort to maintain cerebral perfusion pressure in the face of elevated ICP. **Hypotension**, on the other hand, can be detrimental in patients with already elevated ICP. Hypotension combined with tachycardia should lead one to suspect bleeding from associated injuries (intrathoracic, intraabdominal, retroperitoneal, or orthopedic) until proved otherwise. Interventions to stop bleeding and restore intravascular volume should precede surgical treatment of head injury.

5. If severely or progressively elevated ICP is suspected, **ICP monitoring** can be performed.

6. Seizures may accompany direct cerebral injury or signal the expansion of an intracranial hematoma.

7. Although diffuse brain contusion is the most common type of injury, **surgery** may be indicated for the following situations:

  a. Acute epidural hematoma most commonly results from a skull fracture and laceration of a branch of the middle meningeal artery. Ligation of the vessel and early evacuation of hematoma are performed to improve outcome.

  b. Acute subdural hematoma is usually the result of

blunt trauma and is caused by arterial or venous bleeding from bridging veins or contused brain. Subdural hematomas, although much more common than epidural hematomas, carry a worse prognosis. Intracranial hypertension is frequently seen even after evacuation of hematomas because of severe brain swelling.

    c. Penetrating brain injury requires early debridement of injured tissue and removal of bone fragments and hematoma.

    d. Skull fractures may require cranioplasty and repair of dural lacerations after thorough neurologic evaluation for associated intracranial lesions. Compound skull fractures require early debridement.

  8. Anesthetic management follows the general rules of maintaining cerebral perfusion pressure and reducing ICP and cerebral edema. Postoperative intubation and ventilatory support are frequently required for ICP control and airway protection in patients with prolonged loss of consciousness or an inadequate gag reflex. Preoperative alteration in the level of consciousness is not likely to be improved immediately by the surgery and is helpful in predicting the need for postoperative intubation.

V. Surgery on the spine and spinal cord is undertaken for a variety of conditions, including intervertebral disk diseases, spondylosis, stenosis, neoplasm, scoliosis, and trauma. The spinal cord is controlled by the same physiologic principles as the brain even though absolute rates of blood flow and metabolism are lower. Maintaining spinal cord perfusion pressure (which equals MAP minus extrinsic pressure on the cord) and reducing cord compression are clinical management objectives.

  A. The prone position is frequently used. Most patients can be anesthetized on a stretcher and "logrolled" onto the operating room table after endotracheal intubation. Awake intubation should be considered for patients with tenuous neurologic conditions that may be worsened by the transfer (e.g., patients with unstable cervical or thoracic spine injuries). Awake intubation may also be prudent in patients with symptomatic cervical spine disease, a "tight" cervical spinal canal, or morbid obesity. An abbreviated neurologic examination should be performed after intubation and transfer to ensure that injury has not occurred. The anesthesiologist should ensure that all pressure points are well padded, neck and extremities are not in excessive flexion or extension, there is no pressure on the eyes, nose, or elsewhere, and that all monitors and lines are secured in place and functioning satisfactorily. Special attention should be paid to the endotracheal tube because it can move significantly or even kink in the oropharynx with the patient prone.

  B. Correction of scoliosis can be accompanied by significant blood loss. Various techniques are often employed to reduce blood loss, including hypotension to an MAP of approximately 60 mm Hg, hemodilution, autologous blood transfusion, and use of a cell saver. This procedure is accompanied by a 1–4% incidence of serious postoperative neurologic complications including paraplegia secondary to spinal cord ischemia caused by spinal instrumentation and distraction. Intraoperative monitoring of spinal cord function (i.e., the wake-up test and/or SSEP monitoring) is widely accepted.

1. **The wake-up test.** During the procedure when spinal instrumentation and distraction are complete, patients are instructed to move their legs (which may require reversal of muscle relaxant or narcotic). If there is no movement, the spine distraction is released gradually until leg movement is observed.

2. **SSEP monitoring** provides a continuous evaluation of posterior spinal cord function (see sec. **III.B**).

3. **Nitrous oxide–narcotic–relaxant anesthesia** is commonly selected because it usually provides a faster, smoother, and pain-free wake-up test and is less likely to interfere with SSEP monitoring than a pure inhalation technique. Inhalation agents may be added to a nitrous oxide–narcotic anesthetic to help lower blood pressure but should be maintained at a constant level during the crucial periods of surgery.

C. Surgery is occasionally performed after **acute spinal cord injury** for decompression and stabilization of the spinal cord. The primary goal in the initial management of acute spinal cord injury is to prevent secondary damage to the injured spinal cord. This is accomplished by stabilizing the spine and correcting circulatory and ventilatory abnormalities that can exacerbate the primary injury. The presence of cervical cord injury should lead one to suspect associated head, face, or tracheal trauma; thoracic and lumbar spine injuries are often associated with chest or intraabdominal trauma.

1. **Spinal shock** may persist for days to weeks after the initial insult.

    a. Vasodilation, hypotension, and, if the lesion involves the cardiac accelerator nerves (T1–T4), bradycardia, bradyarrhythmias, atrioventricular block, and cardiac arrest may occur due to functional transection of sympathetic innervation below the lesion with unopposed vagal activity. Bradycardia can be treated by atropine. Hypotension can be treated by fluid, vasopressors, or both. A pulmonary artery catheter may be helpful when associated injuries are present or surgery is planned. Patients with high spinal cord injury may be unusually sensitive to the cardiovascular depressant effects of anesthetics because of an inability to increase sympathetic tone.

    b. Lesions above C3–C4 necessitate intubation and mechanical ventilatory support because of loss of innervation to the diaphragm (C3–C5). Lesions below C5–C6 may still cause as much as a 70% reduction in vital capacity and FEV_1 and impair ventilation and oxygenation.

      c. Atony of the gastrointestinal tract and urinary bladder necessitates a nasogastric tube and indwelling urinary catheter, respectively. These patients are also prone to heat loss because of inability to vasoconstrict.

    2. Chronic spinal cord injuries are discussed in Chap. 26.

    3. Airway management of patients with cervical spine injury is discussed in sec. **IV.H.**

SUGGESTED READING

Crosby, E., and Liu, A. The adult cervical spine: Implications for airway management. *Can. J. Anaesth.* 37:77, 1990.

Cucchiara, R. F., and Michenfelder, J. D. (eds.), *Clinical Neuroanesthesia.* New York: Churchill Livingstone, 1990.

Cucchiara, R. F., et al. Anesthesia for Intracranial Procedures. In P. G. Barash, B. F. Cullen, and R. K. Stoelting (eds.), *Clinical Anesthesia.* Philadelphia: Lippincott, 1989.

Domino, K. B. Fluid Management for the Neurosurgical Patient. In *ASA Refresher Course Lectures.* Park Ridge, IL: American Society of Anesthesiologists, 1989.

Drummond, J. C., and Shapiro, H. M. Cerebral Physiology. In R. D. Miller (ed.), *Anesthesia.* New York: Churchill Livingstone, 1990.

Goto, T., and Crosby, G. Anesthesia and the spinal cord. *Anesth. Clin. North Am.* 10:493, 1992.

Hall, R., and Murdoch, J. Brain protection: Physiological and pharmacological considerations. Part II: The pharmacology of brain protection. *Can. J. Anaesth.* 37:762, 1990.

Hastings, R. H., and Marks, J. D. Airway management for trauma patients with potential cervical spine injuries. *Anesth. Analg.* 73:471, 1991.

Herrick, I. A., and Gelb, A. W. Anesthesia for intracranial aneurysm surgery. *J. Clin. Anesth.* 4:73, 1992.

Hoffman, W. E., and Grundy, B. L. Neuroanatomy and Neurophysiology. In P. G. Barash, B. F. Cullen, and R. K. Stoelting (eds.), *Clinical Anesthesia.* Philadelphia: Lippincott, 1989.

Lam, A. M. Monitoring Neurologic Evoked Responses. In *ASA Peer-Reviewed Refresher Courses in Anesthesiology.* Park Ridge, IL: American Society of Anesthesiologists, 1989. Vol. 17, p. 13.

Messick, J. M., et al. Principles of neuroanesthesia for the nonneurosurgical patient with CNS pathology. *Anesth. Analg.* 64:143, 1985.

Michenfelder, J. D. (ed.), *Anesthesia and the Brain.* New York: Churchill Livingstone, 1988.

Murdoch, J., and Hall, R. Brain protection: Physiologic and pharmacologic considerations. Part I: The physiology of brain surgery. *Can. J. Anaesth.* 37:663, 1990.

Shapiro, H. M., and Drummond, J. C. Neurosurgical anesthesia and intracranial hypertension. In R. D. Miller (ed.), *Anesthesia.* New York: Churchill Livingstone, 1990.

25

Anesthesia for Head and Neck Surgery

Martin Acquadro

I. **Anesthesia for eye surgery**
  A. **General considerations.** Anesthetic management requires an understanding of the physiology of intraocular pressure and the oculocardiac reflex, in addition to the specific surgical needs for each procedure.
    1. **Intraocular pressure (IOP)** is determined by the rate of production of aqueous humor in relation to its rate of drainage (normal = 10–22 mm Hg; abnormal $\geq$ 25 mm Hg).
      a. **Factors increasing IOP.** Patient movement, coughing, straining, vomiting, venous congestion, hypercarbia, increased muscle tone, and hypertension.
      b. **Factors decreasing IOP.** Drugs (e.g., central nervous system depressants, ganglionic blockers, mannitol, acetazolamide), hyperventilation, and hypothermia.
    2. **Glaucoma** is characterized by increased IOP that eventually leads to damage of the optic nerve and loss of vision. It is the second leading cause of blindness in the United States.
      a. **Open-angle glaucoma** usually arises from chronic obstruction of aqueous humor drainage and is characterized by a progressive, insidious course, which may not be associated with pain.
      b. **Closed-angle glaucoma.** Aqueous outflow is obstructed by a narrowing of the anterior chamber of the eye and usually presents with acute eye pain from pupillary dilation.
    3. **Oculocardiac reflex**
      a. The oculocardiac reflex is most often triggered by increased pressure on the globe or by traction on the extrinsic eye muscles causing bradycardia. Performance of a retrobulbar block may also elicit this response.
      b. The afferent arc of this reflex is mediated by the trigeminal (fifth cranial) nerve and efferent arc by the vagus (tenth cranial) nerve. The oculocardiac reflex should be promptly treated by cessation of the stimulus. Occasionally atropine (0.007 mg/kg IV) and even local infiltration of lidocaine near the extrinsic eye muscles may be necessary. The reflex fatigues quickly with repeated stimulation.
    4. **Commonly used drugs**
      a. **Topical.** Most ophthalmic medications are highly concentrated solutions that are administered topically, which can produce systemic effects when absorbed.
        (1) **Mydriatics**
          (a) **Phenylephrine** eye drops may cause hyper-

tension, especially when administered as a
10% solution. For this reason, they are most
commonly given as a 2.5% solution.

   (b) **Cyclopentolate** may produce CNS toxicity
(confusion, seizures).

  (2) **Miotics. Acetylcholine** may lead to bradycardia, salivation, bronchorrhea, and perspiration.

  (3) **Agents that decrease IOP**

    (a) **Beta-adrenergic antagonists**

      (i) **Timolol** has been reported to cause
bradycardia and bronchospasm.

      (ii) **Betaxolol** is beta-1 specific and may be
less likely to cause bronchospasm in asthmatic patients.

    (b) **Anticholinesterases** such as echothiophate
(Phospholine) depress plasma cholinesterase
activity for 2–4 weeks, resulting in a prolonged response to succinylcholine.

  (4) **Cocaine** may potentiate sympathomimetics.

 b. Systemic. Acetazolamide (Diamox), a carbonic
anhydrase inhibitor, is administered systemically
to control aqueous humor secretion. Chronic use
may lead to hyponatremia, hypokalemia, or metabolic acidosis.

B. Anesthetic management

 1. Preoperative evaluation. Patients undergoing eye
surgery are often elderly with significant concomitant
diseases, which require careful evaluation (see Chaps.
2–7).

 2. Premedication

  a. Visually impaired patients may be very apprehensive about surgery and require constant verbal
orientation about identities, surroundings, and procedures. In addition, they may be susceptible to
changes in IOP and postoperative nausea and vomiting. Therefore, the ideal premedication for these
patients should control anxiety and postoperative
nausea without altering IOP or cooperation.

  b. Ophthalmic procedures performed under local anesthesia require that the patient be sedated and calm
yet awake and cooperative.

  c. Premedication regimens will not increase IOP. There
is no evidence that premedication with IM atropine
causes increased IOP, even in glaucoma patients.

  d. Benzodiazepines such as midazolam and diazepam are effective anxiolytics with good amnestic
properties. In very large doses, they may cause
mydriasis, which is to be avoided in patients with
acute narrow-angle glaucoma. Midazolam, 2–4 mg
IM 30 minutes preoperatively or 1–2 mg IV immediately before a retrobulbar block, is very effective.
Alternatively, diazepam, 5–10 mg PO 1 hour preoperatively, is used.

  e. Narcotics, if used, should be given in combination
with some antiemetic such as promethazine (Phenergan), hydroxyzine (Vistaril), or droperidol.

      f. Barbiturates produce variable degrees of sedation of long duration but do not provide analgesia, amnesia, or control of anxiety.

3. **Unexpected patient or eye movements** during delicate microscopic intraocular surgery can lead to increased IOP, choroidal hemorrhage, expulsion of vitreous material, and loss of vision. Therefore, the avoidance of coughing, sudden movement, or straining is a major priority during anesthesia for ophthalmic procedures.

4. **Anesthetic technique.** Ophthalmic procedures can be performed under either local or general anesthesia. The choice of technique reflects patient safety, cooperation, and surgical difficulty. While current studies are inconclusive, it seems that a well-conducted regional anesthetic for ophthalmic procedures probably has the least morbidity.

    a. Local (retro- or peribulbar block)

        (1) Ophthalmic procedures such as cataract extraction, corneal transplant, and anterior chamber irrigation among others can be done following a retrobulbar block and light intravenous sedation.

        (2) Technique. The **retrobulbar block** is achieved in a fully monitored patient by injecting 5–7 ml of a 50 : 50 mixture of 2% lidocaine and 0.75% bupivacaine (both with 1 : 200,000 epinephrine) into the muscle conus behind the globe near the ciliary nerve and ganglion through an inferior approach. The facial nerve's motor branch to the orbicularis oculi muscle is blocked separately to prevent active squeezing.

        (3) Patient cooperation and lack of head motion are important for the success of this technique. Patients who are unable to understand due to deafness, senility, psychosis, or language barrier or are unable to hold still due to a chronic cough, involuntary tremor, or arthritis may not be good candidates for delicate eye procedures under local anesthesia.

        (4) During the procedure, **fresh air** at 10–15 L/min flow is provided for the patient under the drapes using a large face mask. This helps remove exhaled carbon dioxide. Oxygen may be used for patients with a history of coronary artery disease, but the surgeon should be notified not to use cautery while the oxygen is flowing.

        (5) Intravenous sedation may be used just prior to the retrobulbar block injection. Titration of midazolam (0.015 mg/kg), diazepam (0.03 mg/kg), or propofol (0.3 mg/kg) will aid in patient comfort during the procedure. During supplementation, the patient should not become unresponsive. Standard monitoring should be supplemented with a precordial stethoscope and observation of ventilation. Undue restlessness may be a sign of hypoxia or oversedation in the elderly.

(6) The **advantages** of a retrobulbar block include a lower incidence of coughing, straining, and emesis upon emergence. This technique is also useful for ambulatory patients and provides adequate postoperative analgesia.

(7) **Complications** of retrobulbar block are infrequent but include direct optic nerve trauma, retrobulbar hemorrhage, and transient globe compression with increased IOP. The oculocardiac reflex may be stimulated during injection or by eye compression (see sec. **I.A.3**). Intravascular injection may cause seizures or myocardial depression. Rarely, the local anesthetic may dissect along the neural sheath affecting the central nervous system and cause temporary (15 minutes) loss of consciousness without seizures. The patient may become apneic briefly but usually maintains a strong pulse and blood pressure.

b. **General anesthesia**

(1) The eye is a very sensitive, highly innervated organ. Eye surgery requires a proper **depth of general anesthesia** to prevent eye motion, coughing, straining, or hypertension. General endotracheal anesthesia using a potent inhalation agent is usually satisfactory. This may be supplemented by a short-acting nondepolarizing muscle relaxant.

(2) The lack of access to the airway during the procedure requires **endotracheal intubation.** Intravenous lidocaine (1.0–1.5 mg/kg) or 4% lidocaine spray to the larynx and trachea may help prevent straining. The endotracheal tube should be firmly supported and taped in place to prevent disconnection and stimulation of a cough reflex by motion.

(3) Ketamine causes blepharospasm, nystagmus, increased arterial pressure, and vomiting and may increase IOP. For these reasons, **ketamine is usually a poor choice for most ophthalmic surgery.**

(4) Smooth **emergence** and **extubation** are particularly desirable following ophthalmic surgery. This may be facilitated by thorough posterior pharyngeal suctioning while the patient is deeply anesthetized, IV lidocaine (1.0–1.5 mg/kg) 5 minutes before planned extubation, and administration of IV narcotic to reduce the cough reflex. The patient may then be extubated awake with intact airway reflexes. Deep extubation also is an option but does not guarantee a smooth emergence.

C. **Specific procedures**

1. **Open-eye injury.** Penetrating eye trauma is a surgical emergency, frequently occurring in patients who

have recently eaten. It requires a carefully conducted anesthetic designed to prevent not only aspiration but also those factors that increase IOP (see sec. **I.A.1**). A sudden increase in IOP can result in extrusion of ocular contents and permanent loss of vision.

a. **Succinylcholine** administered during a rapid sequence induction will slightly increase IOP, but this response may be attenuated by a prior defasciculating dose of a nondepolarizing relaxant.

b. Alternatively, a "modified" rapid sequence induction using high-dose **vecuronium** (0.2–0.3 mg/kg) while maintaining cricoid pressure may be employed, bearing in mind that satisfactory intubating conditions may not be available for up to 90 seconds.

c. In either technique, **an adequate depth of anesthesia and degree of neuromuscular blockade must be ensured** prior to laryngoscopy and intubation to prevent increases in IOP associated with coughing and straining.

d. In **children,** an inhalation induction with cricoid pressure may be necessary, since IV placement in a crying, struggling child could result in an acute increase in IOP.

2. **Strabismus repair** is a common pediatric ophthalmic procedure with the following anesthetic considerations:

a. **Succinylcholine** administration may interfere with interpretation of the forced duction test through its increase in IOP. Typically, nondepolarizing **muscle relaxants** are used to facilitate endotracheal intubation and ensure patient immobility.

b. **Surgical manipulation** may elicit the oculocardiac reflex (see sec. **I.A.3**).

c. **Postoperative nausea and vomiting** are common. Metoclopramide (0.1–0.15 mg/kg IV) or droperidol (25–30 µg/kg IV) is often administered intraoperatively to reduce postoperative emesis. Droperidol in higher doses (70 µg/kg) may be a more effective antiemetic but can lead to delayed emergence and dysphoria. The use of propofol and the avoidance of nitrous oxide may be of benefit as well.

d. The incidence of **malignant hyperthermia** appears to be higher in patients with strabismus. Body temperature, heart rate, and end-tidal carbon dioxide should be carefully monitored and blood gas analysis performed if there is any question of the diagnosis.

3. **Retinal surgery** for detachment is often performed on diabetics with the full range of associated medical problems (see Chap. 6).

a. **Unexpected patient movement** during the delicate (sometimes intraocular) retinal repair may result in loss of vision. Therefore, deep inhalation anesthesia, supplemented with an intermediate-acting muscle relaxant during the intraocular part of the procedure, is recommended. Postoperatively, excessive coughing, straining, or vomiting should be prevented.

b. An **intravitreal gas bubble,** containing an inert, high-molecular-weight, low-diffusivity gas such as SF_6 or C_3F_8 may be injected at the conclusion of surgery to reduce intravitreal bleeding. Nitrous oxide will result in rapid expansion of the bubble and possibly increase IOP. Subsequent cessation of nitrous oxide at the end of the procedure will result in rapid shrinkage of this bubble and loss of its mechanical advantage. Thus, if the surgeon intends to use an intravitreal bubble, the anesthesiologist should be aware and discontinue nitrous oxide prior to bubble injection. This intravitreal gas bubble will remain for about 5 days, and nitrous oxide should be avoided if subsequent surgery is required during this time.

II. Anesthesia for ear, nose, and throat surgery
A. General considerations
1. **Airway.** During ear, nose, and throat (ENT) surgery, the anesthesiologist must frequently share the patient's airway with the surgeon. The airway may be compromised by bleeding, pathology, or surgical manipulation and may not always be accessible. Preoperative evaluation, intraoperative planning, and surgical cooperation are essential to avert management problems.
2. Besides standard **monitoring,** major head and neck procedures also mandate monitoring of urinary output and intraarterial blood pressure.
3. **Extubation** following any upper airway surgery must be carefully planned. Posterior pharyngeal packs are removed, the pharynx is suctioned and inspected for blood, the patient is fully oxygenated, and extubation is performed when full protective laryngeal reflexes return. Excessive upper airway bleeding, edema, or pathology may preclude extubation.

B. Ear surgery
1. **Preoperative considerations**
   a. Ear surgery often involves dissecting and preserving the **facial** (seventh cranial) **nerve.**
   b. The **middle ear** normally communicates with the nasopharynx via the eustachian tube. If eustachian tube function is compromised by trauma, edema, inflammation, or congenital deformity, normal venting of middle ear pressure cannot occur. When used in high concentration, nitrous oxide diffuses into the middle ear faster than nitrogen escapes (approximately 34 : 1), and in the presence of a blocked eustachian tube, the middle ear can attain pressures of 300–400 mm Hg after 30 minutes. Positive-pressure ventilation can further increase the rate of rise. Acute cessation of nitrous oxide can result in rapid resorption and a net negative pressure in the middle ear. These changes may result in altered middle ear

anatomy, tympanic membrane rupture, disarticulation of artificial stapes, disruption of surgical grafts, and postoperative nausea and vomiting.
- c. **Positioning.** During surgery, the patient's head is often turned to the side. Extremes of head position should be assessed preoperatively so that limits in range of motion can be determined.

2. **Anesthetic technique.** After induction with a hypnotic and a short-acting muscle relaxant, anesthesia is usually maintained with an inhalation technique.
   - a. This technique obviates the need for muscle relaxants, allowing the surgeon to locate the facial nerve with direct nerve stimulation.
   - b. It allows for discontinuation of **nitrous oxide** if necessary. The use of nitrous oxide should be discussed with the surgeon, as it may need to be limited to 50% or even discontinued altogether for surgical convenience.
   - c. **Delicate microsurgery** of the ear requires diminished bleeding for accurate surgery. Volatile agents administered with controlled ventilation (often supplemented with labetalol IV in 5- to 10-mg increments) work well to lower blood pressure. In addition, a 15-degree head-up tilt to decrease venous congestion and application of topical epinephrine in small amounts will provide satisfactory operating conditions.
   - d. **Antiemetics** should be administered, since postoperative emesis is very common.

C. **Nasal surgery**
1. **Anesthetic technique.** Nasal surgery may be performed under either local or general anesthesia. Even during general anesthesia, ENT surgeons will inject 2% lidocaine with epinephrine and place 4% cocaine nasal packs for vasoconstrictive effects. These agents may cause tachycardia, hypertension, and arrhythmias, especially when used in the presence of halothane. They do, however, attenuate the painful stimuli of surgery. Hence, general anesthesia is needed mainly for amnesia, patient immobility, and toleration of the endotracheal tube.
2. Following nasal cosmetic surgery, the nose is unstable, and face mask application is not desirable. Smooth **emergence** and **extubation** are important to decrease postoperative bleeding and avoid laryngospasm and use of the face mask.
3. **Blood loss** during nasal surgery may be substantial and difficult to estimate. A posterior pharyngeal pack may decrease postoperative vomiting by preventing the passage of blood into the stomach. This pack must always be removed prior to extubation. An orogastric tube placed at the completion of surgery may aid in evacuating any swallowed blood.
4. Patients with **severe epistaxis** presenting for internal maxillary artery ligation are often anxious, tired, and hypertensive and may be hypovolemic and anemic. A

posterior nasal pack may cause edema and hypoventilation. These patients need reassurance, rehydration, and careful sedation. They are assumed to have a full stomach (blood) and should be induced and intubated accordingly. Since the extent of preoperative blood loss is deceptive, patients should have adequate intravenous access (14–16 gauge IV) and blood available. Removal of a posterior pack may be followed by substantial bleeding.

D. Upper airway surgery

1. Tonsillectomy and adenoidectomy

a. Preoperative evaluation should seek a history of airway obstruction, bleeding disorders, and loose teeth while confirming that coagulation studies are normal. Many of these patients have recurrent upper respiratory infections, which should be evaluated preoperatively.

b. Anesthetic technique

(1) An inhalation induction, followed by a balanced anesthetic consisting of a short-acting nondepolarizing muscle relaxant (e.g., atracurium or vecuronium), narcotic (e.g., morphine, 0.1 mg/kg IV), and volatile agent, is usually preferred. Glycopyrrolate (5–10 µg/kg IV) is sometimes administered on induction to decrease secretions.

(2) **At the end of surgery,** an orogastric tube should be passed to empty the stomach of blood and the posterior pharynx carefully suctioned. Extubation is undertaken when the patient is awake with intact airway reflexes. Coughing on the endotracheal tube may be reduced with lidocaine (1.0–1.5 mg/kg IV). Deep extubation may be attempted in an effort to decrease coughing but may lead to airway problems in the PACU.

(3) After extubation, patients are placed in the **"tonsillar" position** (on their side, head lower than hips), administered 100% oxygen, and observed for unobstructed breathing. In the PACU, patients are given humidified oxygen by mask, observed for at least 90 minutes, and checked for a dry pharynx before discharge.

c. Specific considerations

(1) **Arrhythmias** are common and may be due to hypoventilation or light anesthesia.

(2) Inadvertent **endotracheal tube displacement** can occur during head and mouth gag manipulations.

(3) **Fluid replacement.** Even though these procedures are short, full replacement of the fluid deficit should be attempted through a well-functioning IV line due to the potential for large blood losses.

2. Bleeding tonsil

a. Rebleeding following a pediatric tonsillectomy requiring surgery is an emergency with an incidence of approximately 1%. It most frequently occurs within 24 hours after operation but may be delayed (5–10 days postoperatively). Hematemesis, tachycardia, hypotension, frequent swallowing, pallor, or airway obstruction may be seen. The extent of blood loss is often underestimated until the patient vomits a large amount of swallowed blood.

b. A large IV cannula must be inserted if not already present, and the patient should be adequately **hydrated** before reoperation. Hematocrit and coagulation studies should be rechecked, and transfusion may be necessary. Inducing general anesthesia in a bleeding, hypovolemic child can result in severe hypotension and even cardiac arrest.

c. Rapid sequence induction should be performed with two suctions set up, a styletted endotracheal tube one size smaller than predicted for the patient's age, and the surgeon(s) at the bedside.

3. Tonsillar abscess may present with painful trismus, dysphagia, and a distorted, compromised airway. Before induction, the surgeon may be able to reduce the abscess size by needle aspiration. This will decrease the risk of rupture and aspiration during intubation. Careful instrumentation is required, since an abscess may be friable and partially block the upper airway. Anesthetic management and extubation procedures are similar to those discussed for tonsillectomies (see sec. 1).

4. Direct laryngoscopy is indicated for therapeutic (vocal cord polyp removal) or diagnostic (tumor biopsy) purposes and may involve potentially compromised airways. Successful anesthetic management requires a careful history, physical examination, and discussion with the surgeon. Evaluation of previous studies (computed tomography scan, magnetic resonance imaging, and pulmonary function tests) may help identify airway abnormalities and potential intraoperative problems. Many patients are former smokers with resultant severe pulmonary pathology.

a. Anesthetic management is the same as described in Chap. 21, sec. IV.

b. Postoperative airway edema may develop. If anticipated intraoperatively, dexamethasone (Decadron), 8 mg IV, may be given prior to extubation. Once in the PACU, treatment options include elevating the head of the bed, administering humidified oxygen by mask, and inhalation therapy (beta agonists or racemic epinephrine).

5. Laser is light amplification by stimulated emission of radiation. A laser produces a high-energy density beam of coherent light that generates a focused thermal effect on contact with tissue. The emission media used to produce the monochromatic coherent light determines the wavelength.

a. Short-wavelength (1 μm) **lasers** (argon gas, ruby, yttrium aluminum garnet [YAG]) in the red-green visible part of the electromagnetic spectrum are poorly absorbed by water but well absorbed by pigmented tissues such as retina and blood vessels.

b. The **infrared** (10 μm) **carbon dioxide laser** is well absorbed by water and superficial surface cells. The carbon dioxide laser is commonly used for laryngeal lesions. It cannot be transmitted through fiberoptics.

c. **Eyes** must be protected from the laser beam. Operating room personnel must wear appropriate safety goggles (green-tinted for argon lasers, amber for YAG lasers, and clear for carbon dioxide lasers), and the patient's eyes should be taped closed and covered with wet gauze.

d. The most serious complication of laser surgery of the upper airway is **airway fire.** The likelihood of fire depends on the gas environment in the airway, the laser energy level, the manner in which the laser is used, the presence of moisture, and the type of endotracheal tube. Nitrous oxide supports combustion as well as oxygen. A safe gas mixture during laser upper airway surgery is 25–30% oxygen in nitrogen. Helium (60–70%) is a fire quencher but is only protective at laser energy less than 12.5 watts.

e. **Safe laser use.** Lasers should be used intermittently, in the noncontinuous mode, at moderate power (10–15 watts). Surgeons should not use the laser as a cautery and should share responsibility for fire prevention by limiting the energy input, allowing time for heat dispersal, packing aside nontarget tissue and endotracheal tube cuffs with moist gauze, and maintaining moisture (as a heat sink) in the field.

f. **Airway options during laser surgery.** Red rubber tubes are more flame resistant than PVC tubes and, when properly wrapped with metallic tape, are safe in a 25% oxygen-nitrogen environment at moderate beam energy levels. Metal endotracheal tubes and/or special impregnated, disposable, fire-resistant endotracheal tubes (Xomed-Treace Laser-Shield II endotracheal tube) are often selected for lesions involving the anterior commissure. The use of a jet-Venturi technique eliminates the need for an endotracheal tube, but dry tissue can still spark and inflame, causing a blowtorch effect with jet oxygen. Endotracheal tube cuffs can be filled with saline as a precaution against an inadvertent hit by the laser beam.

g. **If an airway fire occurs,** stop ventilation, pour saline into the pharynx to absorb the heat, extubate, and reintubate with a new endotracheal tube. Follow-up should include a chest x-ray, bronchoscopy, steroids, and arterial blood gases. Late complications include tracheal and/or laryngeal granulation tissue formation or stenosis.

h. The **anesthetic technique** for laser surgery is similar to that described for endoscopy (see Chap. 21). Goals include adequate surgical visualization, fire prevention, decreased laryngeal reflexes, absence of vocal cord motion, and rapid return of airway reflexes prior to extubation. Any of the techniques to control the airway described in sec. **f** may be used, usually in an environment of 30% oxygen-nitrogen. Since airway edema may occur, the patient is given humidified oxygen postoperatively and observed closely in the PACU. Steroids or racemic epinephrine may be necessary.

III. Anesthesia for head and neck procedures

A. The primary anesthetic concern during head and neck surgery is establishing and maintaining a **secure airway.**

1. An **armored** (Tovell) **endotracheal tube** may be necessary to prevent kinking.

2. **Inhalation anesthesia** with carefully titrated doses of narcotic without muscle relaxants is commonly employed to facilitate the intraoperative identification of nerves during complicated dissection.

3. **Vocal cord paralysis.** Injury to one recurrent laryngeal nerve causes unilateral vocal cord paralysis, a benign condition limited to hoarseness and a weak voice. Bilateral vocal cord paralysis, however, is more serious and causes increasing upper airway obstruction and stridor. Obstruction may be temporarily relieved by positive-pressure face mask ventilation while preparations are being made for immediate reintubation. Partial obstruction caused by vocal cord edema may be treated by humidified oxygen, nebulized racemic epinephrine (0.5 ml in 1.5 ml of saline), and the head-up position.

4. **Bleeding.** Following thyroid or parathyroid surgery, operative site bleeding may compress the trachea, causing difficulty in breathing. Placing a sterile hemostat through the incision to open the wound allows egress of trapped blood. Emergency endotracheal intubation may be difficult due to tracheal displacement.

5. **Teflon injection** of the vocal cords must be done during awake laryngoscopy so that the patient can cooperate and phonate while the quality of the voice is assessed. Therefore, these procedures should be done with an adequate laryngeal block and light sedation.

B. Radical neck dissection

1. **Patient condition.** Radical neck dissections, in previously irradiated patients, may be associated with large blood loss. These patients are often elderly, chronically debilitated, with a history of heavy alcohol and tobacco use. Preoperative evaluation and choice of monitoring should take this into account.

2. **Anesthetic technique.** Controlled hypotensive anesthesia (see Chap. 19) may be considered, but this is not usually needed if a 15-degree head-up tilt and positive-pressure ventilation with a potent volatile agent are

used to keep systolic blood pressures at 90–100 mm Hg.

3. During dissection, traction or pressure on the carotid sinus may cause **arrhythmias** such as a bradycardia or cardiac arrest. Treatment includes immediate cessation of the surgical stimulus. If necessary, the surgeon may use lidocaine to block the carotid sinus, or atropine (0.07 mg/kg IV) may be used as a vagolytic.

4. **Air embolism** through large open veins during neck surgery is possible but infrequent.

5. If the surgical dissection places the patient at risk for **pneumothorax,** bilateral precordial stethoscopes can be placed for early detection of unequal breath sounds.

6. An **elective tracheostomy** may be performed at the end of the procedure if soft-tissue edema or neck bleeding is expected to cause airway compromise during the first 48–72 hours postoperatively. Alternatively, a nasotracheal tube may be left in place during this period.

SUGGESTED READING

Donlon, J. V. Anesthetic management of patients with compromised airways. *Anesth. Rev.* 7:22, 1980.

Donlon, J. V. Anesthesia for Eye, Ear, Nose, and Throat. In R. D. Miller (ed.), *Anesthesia.* New York: Churchill Livingstone, 1985. Pp. 1837–1894.

Hermens, J. M., Bennett, M. J., and Hirshman, C. A. Anesthesia for laser surgery. *Anesth. Analog.* 62:218, 1983.

Latto, I. P., and Rosen, M. *Difficulties in Tracheal Intubation.* Philadelphia: Saunders, 1985.

Libonati, M. M., Leahy, J. J., and Ellison, N. The use of succinylcholine in open eye surgery. *Anesthesiology* 62:637, 1985.

Lopez, N. R. Mechanical problems of the airway. *Clin. Anesth.* 3:8, 1978.

McGoldrick, K., Bruce, R. A., and Oppenheimer, P. *Anesthesia for Ophthalmology.* Birmingham, AL: Aesculapius, 1982.

Moreno, R. J., Kloess, P., and Carlson, D. W. Effect of succinylcholine on intraocular contents of open globes. *Ophthalmology* 98:636, 1991.

Morrison, J. D., Mirakhur, R. K., and Craig, H. J. *Anesthesia for Eye, Ear, Nose and Throat Surgery.* New York: Churchill Livingstone, 1985.

Murphy, D. T. Anesthesia and intraocular pressure. *Anesth. Analg.* 64:520, 1985.

Murphy, T. Somatic Blockade for Head and Neck. In M. J. Cousins and P. O. Bridenbaugh (eds.), *Neural Blockade.* Philadelphia: Lippincott, 1980. Pp. 420–432.

Patil, V., Stehling, L., and Zauder, H. (eds.). *Fiberoptic Endoscopy in Anesthesia.* Chicago: Year Book, 1983.

Symposium on anesthesia for eye surgery. *Br. J. Anaesth.* 52:641–703, 1980.

Zahl, K., and Meltzer, M. A. Preoperative evaluation and choice of anesthesia for ophthalmic surgery. *Ophthal. Clin. North Am.* 3(1), 1–11, 1990.

26

Anesthesia for Urologic Surgery

Thomas Hill

I. Preoperative evaluation

A. Patients presenting for surgery of the urogenital tract comprise a diverse population both in age and extent of underlying disease. Elderly patients constitute a large percentage of the urology population.

B. **Physiologic changes with aging**

1. **Cardiovascular.** About 50–60% of elderly patients have cardiovascular disease.

a. Myocardial fibrosis and increased ventricular wall thickness occur, leading to decreased myocardial compliance and cardiac output.

b. Heart rates are slower at rest and with moderate and maximal exercise. Valvular calcification is common.

c. Increased large artery stiffness causes elevated systolic pressure.

d. Patients are slow to compensate for changes in position, intravascular volume, and depth of anesthesia due to diminished autonomic nervous system function. This may also cause a decreased maximal response to inotropic and chronotropic agents.

2. **Pulmonary**

a. Chest wall calcification causes decreased chest wall compliance.

b. Decreased pulmonary elasticity leads to increased lung compliance. These changes lead to an increased functional residual capacity, decreased FEV_1, decreased total lung capacity, and a significant reduction in vital capacity.

c. Increased alveolar and anatomic dead space leads to atelectasis and ventilation-perfusion mismatching with an increased A-a gradient.

d. The ventilatory response to hypoxia and hypercarbia is depressed.

3. **Central nervous system.** Cerebral blood flow and cerebral metabolic rate are both decreased with age, but coupling is maintained. Cerebral autoregulation is maintained with aging.

4. **Renal**

a. Progressive loss of glomeruli and renal function occurs, leading to decreased renal blood flow and glomerular filtration rate.

b. There is a decreased ability to conserve sodium and concentrate urine.

c. Despite loss of renal function, serum creatinine is often maintained due to diminished muscle mass.

5. **Hepatic** blood flow is decreased, and there is diminished hepatic elimination of drugs.

6. **Endocrine.** Elderly patients are glucose intolerant.

C. **Pharmacokinetics and pharmacodynamics in the elderly**

1. As discussed, **decreased hepatic and renal function** will affect the metabolism and excretion of drugs in the elderly.
2. Qualitative and quantitative changes in **protein binding** lead to exaggerated pharmacologic effects due to higher free drug levels.
3. Skeletal muscle mass, blood volume, and lean body mass are decreased, leading to altered drug effects.

D. **Anesthetic considerations in the elderly**
1. Elderly patients have an increased incidence of **concurrent medical problems,** management of which will impact their perioperative course.
2. Patients with osteoporosis, arthritis, poor skin, or soft-tissue perfusion will require care when moving or positioning for surgery.
3. Elderly patients are very susceptible to both intraoperative hypothermia and the cardiopulmonary consequences of shivering in the postoperative period.
4. **Anesthetics**
    a. The minimum alveolar concentration for inhalation anesthetics is **decreased** by up to 30%.
    b. Elderly patients have a **diminished** requirement for narcotics, barbiturates, benzodiazepines, and local anesthetics. Muscle relaxants may have prolonged duration due to altered pharmacokinetics.

II. **Anesthesia for specific urologic procedures**
A. **Endoscopy** is performed to visualize and evaluate the **upper** (ureter, kidney) and **lower** (bladder, prostate, urethra) **urinary tracts.** These procedures are performed for diagnosis and treatment of a variety of conditions such as hematuria, pyuria, calculi, trauma, and cancer.
1. These operations are performed in the **lithotomy** position, which presents certain problems.
    a. **Nerve injuries**
        (1) The **common peroneal nerve** may be injured due to compression of the leg brace against the nerve at the fibular head.
        (2) The **saphenous nerve** may be compressed at the medial tibial condyle.
        (3) The **sciatic nerve** may be injured due to excessive external rotation of the legs or extension of the knees.
        (4) The **obturator and femoral nerve** may be stretched with excessive flexion of the thigh to the groin.
    b. **Altered vascular capacitance** (venous pooling) occurs when elevating and lowering the legs.
2. **Cystoscopy** involves the passage of a rigid scope through the urethra into the bladder.
    a. Minor procedures may be done with **2% lidocaine jelly** to anesthetize the urethra, particularly in females.
    b. **Urethral stimulation** (especially if dilatation is required) and bladder distention may be quite painful, requiring general anesthesia or regional anesthesia.

    c. If a regional anesthetic is selected, a **T10 sensory level** is required to eliminate the pain of bladder distention.

3. Cystoscopy with retrograde ureteral catheterization is performed to visualize the ureter and renal calyces with dye, to place stents, to drain obstructions, and to remove renal calculi.

    a. Cystoscopy is described in sec **A.2.**

    b. Instrumentation of the ureters requires a sensory level to T6. Rigid ureteroscopy stretches the bladder trigone and is extremely stimulating. These procedures may be prolonged depending on the surgical difficulties encountered.

    c. General or **regional anesthesia** is required.

4. Transurethral resection of the bladder. Endoscopic resection and electrodesiccation are used in the treatment of superficial bladder tumors.

    a. General anesthesia satisfies the surgical requirements; however, coughing and straining must be avoided to prevent bladder perforation.

    b. With **regional anesthesia,** the bladder becomes atonic and may become thinner when distended, increasing the risk of perforation. Tumors of the anterior bladder may be more difficult to visualize with distention.

    c. Blood loss, hypothermia, and **bacteremia** may occur.

    d. If the **peritoneal cavity** is entered, shoulder discomfort, nausea, and vomiting may be seen in the awake patient.

    e. Perforation in the presence of high-grade malignancy risks **seeding** of the peritoneum.

5. Transurethral resection of the prostate (TURP) is usually undertaken for prostatic enlargement up to 60 gm. Neoplastic or obstructive prostatic tissue is removed by electrosurgical resection under direct endoscopic vision. This is performed by application of a high-frequency current to a wire loop. Hemostasis is affected by sealing the vessels with the coagulation current. An optically clear, nonconductive, nonhemolytic, nontoxic solution is required to distend the bladder. Glycine 1.5% or cytal 3.2% (a mixture of mannitol and sorbitol) meet these requirements.

    a. Anesthetic considerations

        (1) General anesthesia can be employed, although coughing and straining must be avoided, as they increase the risk of bleeding.

        (2) Benefits of spinal anesthesia

            (a) The bladder will be atonic with a large capacity; thus glycine infusion pressure can be low, and emptying is less frequent, facilitating resection.

            (b) Postoperative bladder spasm is prevented, allowing for a period of quiescence during which hemostasis occurs.

(c) An awake patient may facilitate early detection of complications.

b. **Complications of TURP**

(1) **Blood loss** is variable and difficult to quantify. In appropriate patients, invasive monitoring with an arterial line and a central venous pressure (CVP) line may be used but is rarely necessary.

(2) **Venous absorption of irrigating fluid** may occur during resection of the prostatic bed; open venous sinuses provide direct communication with the circulation. Principal determinants of fluid absorption are irrigation pressure (height of the irrigation container) and duration of exposure of the open sinuses. Absorption ranges from none to more than 4 liters but is less of a problem with newer resectoscopes. Increased intravascular volume and dilutional hyponatremia may occur.

(a) **Clinical features.** Early signs include hypertension and tachycardia; CVP may rise as cardiac decompensation begins to occur. Pulmonary artery pressure monitoring may be necessary in patients with impaired cardiac function. The awake patient may complain of dyspnea or nausea. Hypoxia and/or hyponatremia may result in apprehension, disorientation, convulsions, and coma. This is commonly referred to as the **TURP syndrome.** Symptoms of early glycine toxicity include nausea and vomiting, progressing to altered mental status and eventual coma.

(b) **Management.** When significant venous absorption of irrigation fluid is suspected, the surgeon should be asked to control bleeding and quickly terminate the resection. A blood sample should be sent for serum electrolytes; an acute decrease in serum sodium (Na^+) to less than 120 mEq/L is serious. This hypervolemic **hyponatremia** can usually be corrected by fluid restriction and diuretics (furosemide, 10–20 mg IV). If hyponatremia is severe, hypertonic (3%) saline solutions should be given. The correction is calculated as follows: Na^+ deficit (mEq) = (140 − serum Na^+) × 0.6 × body weight (kg). Hyponatremia must be cautiously corrected to avoid precipitating the syndrome of central pontine myelinolysis (see Chap. 4).

(c) **Normal saline** or **Ringer's lactate** is the IV fluid of choice. Procedures should be postponed, if possible, when serum Na^+ is low ($\leq$ 125 mEq/L).

(3) **Perforation with extravasation of irrigation fluid** may occur during deep dissection in the

prostatic bed. If perforation into the periprostatic space occurs, the awake patient will experience suprapubic fullness, abdominal spasm, and pain. Hypertension and tachycardia are usually seen early after perforation and may be followed by sudden and severe hypotension. Intraperitoneal perforation is manifested by abdominal pain, distention, and cardiovascular collapse.

(4) **Bacteremia** may occur.

(5) **Hypothermia.** Cool irrigation solutions intended to cause local vasoconstriction may produce systemic cooling; solutions warmed to body temperature will decrease this risk. A temperature drop of 1.5°C/hr has been reported.

(6) **Coagulopathy.** Severe postoperative hemorrhage following TURP may be due to disseminated intravascular coagulation triggered by release of prostatic thrombogenic substances, particularly with carcinoma of the prostate. Pronounced hematuria may occur due to release of urokinase. If present, renal insufficiency is associated with platelet dysfunction, and the risk of postoperative hemorrhage may be increased.

If **hemolysis** occurs, the circulation should be supported, urine output maintained at 1 ml/kg/hr or greater, and blood products transfused as needed. The current treatment of TURP-induced fibrinolysis involves administration of packed red cells, fresh-frozen plasma, platelets, cryoprecipitate, and, rarely, epsilon-aminocaproic acid (Amicar).

(7) The possibility of an **open surgical procedure** necessitated by bladder perforation or other complications should be anticipated.

B. **Open prostatic procedures** are performed for resection of large prostatic masses (> 60 gm). Surgical approaches include transvesicular, perineal, and suprapubic. For the transvesicular and suprapubic approach, the patient is supine with the table slightly flexed and placed in the Trendelenburg position. The perineal approach requires an extreme lithotomy position.

1. **Anesthetic considerations**

a. These procedures can be performed with **regional and/or general anesthesia.** Large-bore IV access is required.

b. **Diagnostic dyes** may be used during these procedures.

(1) **Methylene blue** 1% (1 ml IV) is administered to color the urine to facilitate identification of the ureters into the bladder. IV bolus administration may be associated with hypotension.

(2) **Indigo carmine dye** 0.8% (5 ml) has an alpha-sympathomimetic effect that can increase blood pressure.

(3) Both methylene blue and indigo carmine have

been found artificially to reduce oxygen saturation measured by pulse oximetry. Oxygen saturation measurements of approximately 65% for
1–2 minutes have been recorded. Methylene
blue has the greatest effect on SaO_2 measurement.

2. **Complications** are usually related to blood loss and
include hypothermia, anemia, and coagulopathy. Subsequent obstruction or malposition of a Foley catheter
may require surgical replacement.

C. **Nephrectomy.** Indications for nephrectomy include
chronic infection, trauma, cystic or calculous disease, and
neoplasm.

1. A simple nephrectomy can be performed through a
lateral retroperitoneal or anterior abdominal incision.
The lateral approach is performed with maximal flexion and use of the kidney bar to elevate the kidney.
This may cause vena caval compression and hypotension. Radical nephrectomy may require a thoracoabdominal incision in the lateral position. Either a general or combined anesthesia technique is used.
Adequate hydration of the donor and attention to
preserving renal blood flow are goals.

2. **Cadaver donor.** See Chap. 20.

3. **Kidney preservation.** Cold-storage solutions have
been developed to preserve cadaveric kidney grafts and
prolong graft survival with minimal tissue necrosis
and edema. The goal of cold storage (4°C) is to **reduce
metabolic demands** and provide nutrients to maintain **metabolic activity.** To reduce tissue edema,
continuous perfusion of the kidney is performed using
pulsatile flow of cold preservation solution pumped at
40–60 mm Hg. Two solutions are currently used:

a. **Belzer (University of Wisconsin [UW])** cold-
storage solution is composed of glucose polymers
with a potassium concentration of 140 mEq/L, magnesium, allopurinol, adenosine, glutathione, and
sodium hydroxide adjusted to a pH of 7.4. Calculated
osmolarity is 320 mOsm. Additional additives may
include glucocorticoids, regular (recombinant) insulin, and antibiotics.

b. **Euro-Collins solution.** Similar in composition to
the UW solution, a 3.57% glucose solution is used
along with potassium, sodium bicarbonate, and
heparin.

c. Several **additives** in the cold-storage solutions may
trigger a hypersensitivity reaction in the recipient,
including allopurinol, mannitol, heparin, and antibiotics. With continuous renal perfusion, grafts may
be stored for up to 72 hours. For cold-stored grafts,
48 hours is the maximum allowed before ischemic
necrosis jeopardizes graft survival.

4. **Transplant recipient.** The medical condition of the
patient should be optimized whenever possible prior to
transplantation. Serum potassium should be normalized and metabolic acidosis corrected. Anemia is com-

mon and usually well tolerated. Hypertension, cardiac dysfunction, and pleural effusions may be present. Patients are placed supine with a roll under the hip. The kidney is most frequently anastomosed to the external iliac arteries in the pelvis, although recipient nephrectomy occasionally permits an end-to-end vascular and ureteral anastomosis.

a. **Anesthetic considerations**

(1) **IV access** may be difficult and catheters should not be placed in an extremity containing a fistula or functional shunt.

(2) **General anesthesia** is usually provided using nitrous oxide, isoflurane, and narcotic. Full-stomach considerations apply to patients who are uremic, diabetic, or presenting for urgent surgery. Since succinylcholine may raise serum potassium by 0.5–1.0 mEq/L, it should be avoided in hyperkalemic patients. An intubating dose of atracurium is commonly used.

(3) **Regional anesthesia** may be relatively contraindicated by preexisting coagulopathy and concern regarding immunosuppression.

(4) **Normal saline solution** is preferred to lactated Ringer's solution to avoid infusing potassium.

(5) **Adequate hydration with crystalloid, colloid, and blood** is critical for revascularization of the kidney. Methylprednisolone and diuretics (mannitol and/or furosemide) are also given at this time. Low-dose dopamine may be added if oliguria persists.

(6) **Extubation** at the end of the procedure is routine.

b. **Complications.** Hyperkalemia and delayed renal function or graft failure may occur.

D. **Radical cystectomy and ileal/colonic conduit.** Patients with invasive bladder tumors may require cystectomy. Other patients with pelvic malignancies, neurogenic bladder, chronic lower urinary tract obstruction, or postradiation bladder dysfunction may require an ileal or colonic diverting procedure. The procedure can be performed in one operation so that radical cystectomy with lymph node dissection occurs first, followed by preparation of the ureter and bowel segment and creation of the ureteroileal anastomosis and ileostomy. These operations are done in a supine position.

1. **Anesthetic considerations.** General or combined anesthesia is used. Standard monitoring is usually supplemented with arterial and CVP lines.

a. **Large-bore IV access** is required.

b. **Fluid shifts** can be extensive during long procedures. Urine output is difficult to evaluate once the ureters are disconnected. Since judging the adequacy of volume replacement may be more difficult, a CVP catheter is useful. If thought necessary, diuretics may be used to stimulate urine output.

c. The use of **dyes** such as indigo carmine and methylene blue may be necessary to identify the ureteral orifices (see sec. **B.1.b**).

2. **Complications.** Hypothermia, inadequate volume replacement, and need for postoperative ventilation may occur.

E. **Laser surgery.** The use of **l**ight **a**mplification by **s**timulated **e**mission of **r**adiation (laser) has been extended to the ablation of perineal lesions, bladder tumors, and the fragmentation of ureteral calculi (see Chap. 25 for a discussion of laser surgery).

F. **Orchidopexy, orchiectomy, and urogenital plastic procedures** are performed to treat congenital deformities, neoplasms, and impotence. Patients with torsion of the testicle may require emergency reduction and orchidopexy to prevent ischemia. These operations are done with the patient in either the supine or lithotomy position. **General or regional anesthesia** can be used.

1. A **T9 sensory level** is required (due to innervation of the testicle from its embryologic origin).

2. Some procedures may be performed under **local anesthesia** with sedation.

3. **Regional nerve blocks** may be useful.

   a. **Ilioinguinal** nerve block for scrotal and testicular surgery should include blockade of the external pudendal nerve.

   b. For circumcision, **penile** block provides postoperative analgesia.

G. **Shunts/fistulas.** Arteriovenous fistulas or shunts are placed as access for hemodialysis. These are performed with the patient supine with the arm extended.

1. **General anesthesia, regional anesthesia** (brachial plexus blockade), and **local infiltration** are all appropriate.

2. This **patient population** includes those debilitated from renal dysfunction (with medical problems such as anemia, coronary artery disease, and diabetes).

III. **Extracorporeal shock wave lithotripsy (ESWL)**

A. ESWL breaks upper urinary tract stones with external shock waves by creating vibration at tissue-stone interfaces. ESWL devices utilize a cushion to interface with skin or require submersion of the patient in a water tank. The lithotriptor delivers a shock wave triggered by the QRS complex of the electrocardiogram (ECG).

B. **Positioning.** The patient may initially be placed in lithotomy for cystoscopy and placement of ureteral stents, then transferred to a suspension frame (most often in a beach chair position) prior to immersion in the tank. Appropriate padding is required in the suspension frame. All catheters must have occlusive dressings.

C. **Monitoring.** Standard monitoring is used. Interference is encountered when ECG leads become wet and is minimized by covering the electrode with a transparent occlusive dressing. Noninvasive blood pressure cuffs are fastened with clips and tape, and pulse oximetry probes must be kept above the water level.

D. Anesthetic techniques include regional or general anesthesia.

1. **General anesthesia.** Tracheal intubation is required. A decreased tidal volume is often employed to minimize stone movement with ventilation. Heart rate should be maintained between 70 and 115 beats/min, as bradycardia prolongs the procedure and tachycardia may create discoordination between the ESWL device and the cardiac cycle. Emergence and extubation should be performed when the patient is removed from the tank and on the postanesthesia care unit stretcher.

2. **Epidural anesthesia** with a catheter should provide a T4 sensory level. Catheter placement after loss of resistance to saline is performed to minimize air entry into the epidural space. Epidural sites should be sealed with occlusive dressings.

E. Adequate IV hydration with occasional diuretic supplementation may aid passage of stone fragments.

F. A **stretcher** should always be available in the event that emergency removal from the tank is required.

G. Temperature monitoring of both the patient and the water bath is essential. Hyperthermia ($> 40°C$) could occur if the inflow water temperature is high.

H. Complications

1. **Hypotension** may occur from sympathetic blockade accompanying epidural anesthesia or simply from immersion in the warm tank, leading to a reduction in systemic vascular resistance.

2. **Hypothermia** may occur from cold immersion temperature or following immersion from evaporation.

3. **Ureteral colic** soon after the procedure may manifest as nausea, vomiting, or bradycardia.

4. **Hematuria** is commonly seen and treated with volume expansion and diuretics.

IV. Patients with spinal cord pathology. Patients with paraplegia or quadriplegia require repeated urologic evaluation, as they are susceptible to infection, urinary tract obstruction, and renal calculi. In addition to other medical problems, neurologically compromised patients may have suffered from trauma, neoplasm, vascular pathology, or congenital anomalies such as meningomyelocele. Patients with spinal cord lesions or meningomyelocele require care in positioning, as some may have restrictive bony defects or large decubitus ulcers. Repeat urinary catheterization may cause latex allergy. Following neurologic trauma, two physiologic responses occur: spinal shock and autonomic hyperreflexia.

A. Spinal shock. Total absence of neurologic activity may last for 4–28 days. It is characterized by complete loss of visceral and somatic sensation and absence of sweating below the level of the lesion, hypesthesia above the level of the lesion, absent deep tendon reflexes, a positive Babinski response, paralytic ileus, urinary and fecal retention, and postural hypotension.

B. Reflex autonomism. With the loss of supraspinal inhibitory influence, sensory input from the dermatomes below

the spinal lesion becomes unrestrained. Spinal cord responses are now characterized by
1. Motor hyperreflexia (rigidity and spasticity).
2. Flexor responses initiated by pain, bladder distention, and surgical stimulus.
3. Late return of extensor reflexes.
4. Autonomic hyperreflexia.

C. **Autonomic hyperreflexia.** Transverse spinal cord lesions leave the sympathetic outflow functionally disconnected from the brainstem and hypothalamus. Uncontrolled sympathetic discharge may occur with distention of the bowel or bladder. However, lesions below T7 are rarely associated with autonomic hyperreflexia. **Clinical features** include
1. Nausea and apprehension.
2. Skin flushing cephalad to the lesion.
3. Severe hypertension, which may progress to headache, convulsions, or cerebral hemorrhage.
4. Bradycardia, ventricular arrhythmias, or cardiac arrest.

D. **Repeat operative intervention** may be required, so anesthesia and hospital records should be reviewed for evidence of autonomic lability.
1. **Procedures below the level of spinal cord damage** may not require anesthesia to prevent pain but rather to prevent autonomic hyperreflexia. An arterial line may be used in conjunction with standard monitoring.
2. **General anesthesia**
   a. Any general anesthetic **technique** is appropriate provided that a deep anesthetic level is maintained.
   b. **Antihypertensives** may be available, and options include nitroprusside, trimethaphan, labetalol, and hydralazine.
   c. **Muscle spasms** may be eliminated by administration of nondepolarizing neuromuscular blockers, but succinylcholine must **not** be used because of excessive potassium release from denervated muscle.
   d. **Absence of autonomic hyperreflexia** during a prior surgical procedure does not guarantee that it will not occur during a subsequent procedure.
3. **Regional anesthesia** prevents autonomic hyperreflexia by blocking afferent and efferent pathways. Spinal or epidural anesthesia will prevent reflex muscle spasm and autonomic hyperreflexia. Saddle block to a T10 level is sufficient to block afferents from the bladder; however, testing the level may be difficult.

SUGGESTED READING

Abrams, P. H., et al. Blood loss during transurethral resection of the prostate. *Anesthesia* 37:71, 1982.

Bardoczky, G. I., Rausin, I., and Hennart D. Bronchospasm following revascularization of cadaver kidney graft. *Anesthesiology* 74:200, 1991.

Cassady, F. F. Regional anesthesia for urologic procedures. *Urol. Clin. North Am.* 14(1):43, 1987.

Duvall, O., and Griffith, D. P. Epidural anesthesia for extracorporeal shock wave lithotripsy. *Anesth. Analg.* 54:544, 1985.

Gelb, A. W., et al. Isoflurane alters the kinetics of oral cyclosporine. *Anesth. Analg.* 72:801, 1991.

Harper, K. W., et al. Age and nature of operations influence the pharmacokinetics of midazolam. *Br. J. Anaesth.* 57:866, 1985.

Kraus, J. W., et al. Effects of aging and liver disease on disposition of lorazepam. *Clin. Pharmacol. Ther.* 24:411, 1985.

Krechel, S. W. *Anesthesia and the Geriatric Patient.* Orlando: Grune & Stratton, 1984.

Lambert, D. H., Deane, R. S., and Mazuzan, J. E. Anesthesia and the control of blood pressure in patients with spinal cord injury. *Anesth. Analg.* 61:344, 1982.

Levin, K., Nyren, O., and Pompeius, R. Blood loss, tissue weight and operating time in transurethral prostatectomy. *Scan. Urol. Nephrol.* 15:197, 1982.

Linde, H. W., et al. Cardiovascular effects of isoflurane and halothane during controlled ventilation in older patients. *Anesth. Analg.* 54:701, 1975.

Manning, J. K. Surgical management of renal cell carcinoma. *Monogr. Urol.* 5:98, 1984.

Ovassapian, A., Oshi, C. W., and Brunner, E. A. Visual disturbance: An unusual symptom of transurethral prostatic resection reaction. *Anesthesiology* 57:332, 1982.

Peterson, G. N., Krieger, J. N., and Glauber, D. T. Anesthetic experience with percutaneous lithotripsy. *Anaesthesia* 40:460, 1985.

Salter, J. E. Rubber anaphylaxis. *N. Engl. J. Med.* 320:1126, 1989.

Theiss, M., Wirth, M. P., and Frohmuller, H. G. Extracorporeal shock wave lithotripsy in patients with cardiac pacemakers. *J. Urol.* 143:479, 1990.

Vacanti, C. A., and Kanchan, L. L. Fatal massive air embolism during transurethral resection of the prostate. *Anesthesiology* 74:186, 1991.

Wetchler, B. V. Outpatient general and spinal anesthesia. *Urol. Clin. North Am.* 14(1):31, 1987.

Wickstrom, I. Enflurane anesthesia in living donor renal transplantation. *Acta Anaesth. Scand.* 25:263, 1981.

27

Anesthesia for Neonatal Surgery

Maria Markakis

I. **Developmental physiology**
   A. **Organogenesis** is virtually complete after the twelfth gestational week, and further cellular growth occurs until delivery.
   B. **Respiratory development**
      1. **Anatomic.** The lungs begin as a bud on the embryonic gut in the fourth week of gestation. Failure of separation of the lung bud from the gut can result in the formation of a tracheoesophageal fistula. The diaphragm forms during the tenth week of gestation, dividing the abdominal and thoracic cavities. If the diaphragm is not completely formed when the midgut reenters from the umbilical pouch (tenth week of gestation), the abdominal contents can enter the thorax. The posterior part of the diaphragm is the last part to close, the left side closing after the right; this is the most common location for a diaphragmatic hernia. The presence of abdominal contents occupies space within the thorax and appears to arrest lung growth on this side. The distribution and total number of pulmonary arterioles in the involved side are inadequate for the size of the infant, and the smooth muscle in the pulmonary vasculature of both lungs is abnormally thick and reactive, resulting in a marked increase in pulmonary vascular resistance.
      2. **Physiologic development of the lung** is insufficient for survival until the twenty-third week of gestation. Secretion of surfactant, which reduces alveolar wall surface tension and promotes alveolar aeration, is inadequate until the last month of gestation. Following birth, the first breath and the onset of postnatal breathing are stimulated by hypoxemia, hypercarbia, tactile stimulation, and a decrease in plasma prostaglandin E_2. Following aeration and oxygenation of the lung, pulmonary arteriolar smooth muscle relaxes, pulmonary vascular resistance falls, and pulmonary blood flow increases.
   C. **Cardiovascular development**
      1. **Anatomic**
         a. The **primitive cardiac tube** forms during the first month of gestation and consists of the sinoatrium, the primitive ventricle, the bulbus cordis (primitive right ventricle), and the truncus (primitive main artery). During the second month of gestation, a heart with two parallel pumping systems develops out of this initial tubular system. During this process, various structures divide and migrate, at which time numerous abnormalities can occur:
            (1) **Division of the sinoatrium into the two atria.** Failure of division results in a single atrium.

Improper closure results in an atrial septal defect.

   (2) **Migration of the ventricular septum and atrioventricular valve between the primitive ventricle and the bulbus cordis.** Failure of migration can result in a double-outlet left ventricle (single ventricle). Minor migrational defects can result in a ventriculoseptal defect.

   (3) **Division of the truncus into the pulmonary artery and the aorta.** Failure of division results in truncus arteriosus.

   b. **The aortic arch system** initially consists of six pairs of arches, of which only the third, fourth, and sixth develop further.

   (1) The **third arches** form the connections between the external and internal carotid arteries.

   (2) The **sixth arches** produce the pulmonary arteries. The ductus arteriosus develops from the distal portion of the right sixth arch; the left proximal sixth arch usually degenerates but can persist to form an aberrant left ductus arteriosus.

   (3) The left **fourth arch** becomes the segment of aorta between the left carotid and the subclavian arteries. The right fourth arch becomes the proximal subclavian artery.

   (4) **Failure of regression of various portions of the aorta and arch system** can result in aberrant vessels and even a double aortic arch. Regression of the left but not the right side can result in a right-sided aortic arch.

2. **Physiologic.** After the twelfth week, the circulatory system is in its final form. Blood supplying oxygen to the fetal organs passes through the umbilical vessels, through the ductus venosus, returning to the heart. There the majority of the blood bypasses the pulmonary circulation by passing through the foramen ovale and the ductus arteriosus into the left-sided circulation. At birth, umbilical placental circulation ceases, thus reducing flow through the ductus venosus, which then passively closes in 3–7 days. The fall in venous return results in decreased right atrial pressure and functional closure of the foramen ovale. At the same time, gas exchange is transferred from the placenta to the lungs, and pulmonary resistance falls as adequate pulmonary circulation is established. With increasing PaO_2, constriction of the ductus arteriosus occurs, with functional closure within several hours.

D. **Body composition**

1. **Extracellular fluid** (ECF) accounts for a smaller fraction of total body water as the fetus grows. Thus, ECF represents 90% of total body weight at 30 weeks, 85% at 36 weeks, and 75% at term.

2. After birth, a **physiologic diuresis** occurs, with the infant losing about 5–10% of ECF in the first few days of life.

Table 27-1. Normal vital signs in the neonate

Vital sign	Term	Preterm
Pulse (beats/min)	110–120	140–180
Respirations (breaths/min)	35–40	50–70
Blood pressure (mm Hg)	60–90/40–60	40–60/20–40
Temperature (°C)	37.5 (rectal)	37.5

3. Before 32 weeks of gestation, the **neonatal kidney** is immature and less able to concentrate urine or handle solute loads. This improves with advancing gestational and postnatal age.

II. General assessment

A. History

1. **Prenatal.** The history of the neonate begins in utero. Fetal growth and development are affected by maternal disorders, including hypertension, diabetes, and drug, cigarette, or alcohol use. Polyhydramnios, abnormal alpha-fetoprotein, maternal infections, and premature labor may be associated with neonatal problems.

2. **Perinatal** history should include gestational age, time of onset of labor and rupture of membranes, use of tocolytics and fetal monitors, signs of fetal distress, type of anesthesia, mode of delivery (spontaneous, forceps assisted, or cesarean), condition of the infant at delivery, APGAR scores, and immediate resuscitation steps required. Ensure that vitamin K and eye antibiotic ointment were given.

B. Physical examination

1. **General inspection.** A careful, complete, systematic evaluation is needed. No assumptions concerning the development, location, or function of organ systems should be made. An abnormality in one system may be associated with abnormalities in another.

2. **Vital signs** provide a useful physiologic screen of organ function; if cardiac disease is suspected, upper and lower extremity blood pressure measurement is required. Normal vital signs are summarized in Table 27-1.

3. **APGAR score** (Table 27-2) reflects the degree of intrapartum stress as well as the effectiveness of initial resuscitation. Different points are awarded for each of the five criteria, with the maximum score being 10.

4. **Gestational age** influences care, management, and survival potential of the neonate. An infant is considered term if gestational age is 37–42 weeks, preterm if less than 37 weeks, and post-term if greater than 42 weeks. Although date of conception and ultrasound can be used to predict gestational age, a physical examination and Dubowitz scoring to determine gestational age should be performed. The Dubowitz scoring system involves evaluation of physical characteristics of the skin, external genitalia, ears, breasts, and neuromuscular behavior to assess gestational age.

Table 27-2. APGAR score

Sign	Score		
	0	1	2
Heart rate	Absent	<100/min	>100/min
Respiratory effort	Absent	Irregular	Good, Crying
Muscle tone	Limp	Some flexion	Active motion
Reflex irritability	Absent	Grimace	Cough/sneeze
Color	Blue	Acrocyanosis	Completely pink

5. **Weight determination,** as a function of gestational age, is an important part of the evaluation of the neonate. Infants who are small for gestational age often have had intrauterine growth retardation. This may be the result of chromosomal defects, maternal hypertension, maternal cigarette or drug use, chronic placental insufficiency, or congenital infection. These infants have a high incidence of hypoglycemia, hypocalcemia, and polycythemia. Infants who are large for gestational age may be products of maternal diabetes and should be evaluated for potential hypoglycemia.

6. **Respiratory.** Signs of respiratory distress include grunting, nasal flaring, intercostal retractions, rales, rhonchi, asymmetry of breath sounds, and apneic periods. Pulse oximetry has become a standard noninvasive screen of respiratory function in neonates.

7. **Cardiovascular.** Central cyanosis and capillary refill should be assessed. Distal pulses should be palpated, noting whether they are bounding or whether a delay between brachial and femoral pulses exists. Note the character and location of murmurs and splitting of the second heart sound. Murmurs may appear or disappear during the first 48 hours as intracardiac pressure gradients change and the ductus arteriosus closes.

8. **Gastrointestinal.** Signs of gastrointestinal anomalies include a scaphoid abdomen, an abnormal number of vessels in the umbilical cord (usually two arteries, one vein), and the size of the liver, spleen, and kidneys. Note the location and patency of the anus, as well as the presence of hernias or abdominal masses.

9. **Neurologic.** A thorough examination includes evaluation of motor activity, strength, symmetry, tone, and newborn reflexes (Moro, tonic neck, grasp, suck, and stepping reflexes). Full-term newborns should have an upgoing Babinski reflex and brisk deep tendon reflexes.

10. **Genitourinary.** The gonads may be differentiated or ambiguous, and the testes should be palpable. The location of the urethra should be determined, remembering that hypospadias precludes a circumcision.

11. **Musculoskeletal.** Any deformities, unusual posturing, or asymmetric limb movement should be noted, and the hips should be examined for possible dislocation. Clavicles may be fractured during a difficult delivery.

12. **Craniofacial.** One should determine head circumference, the location and size of the fontanelles, and the presence of hematoma or caput. The patency of both nares can be assessed by alternately occluding each naris and assessing any effect on respiration.

C. **Laboratory studies.** There are no "routine" laboratory studies aside from an initial hematocrit and serum glucose. Additional studies should be guided by the individual problem; some suggested tests are as follows:

1. **Fluids.** Insensible water loss increases with lower birth weight, phototherapy, or radiant warmer use. These losses must be replaced, as well as those from pathologic causes (e.g., omphalocele). Infants who are mechanically ventilated absorb free water from their respiratory system. Fluid replacement guidelines include the following:

   a. Volume varies from 50–150 ml/kg/day.

   b. An isosmolar solution using 5–10% dextrose is initially started.

   c. Attempt to maintain urine output at 0.5 ml/kg/hr.

2. **Electrolytes.** In the initial postpartum period, the neonate does not require electrolyte infusions. Usual requirements thereafter include

   a. Na^+, 2–4 mEq/kg/day.

   b. K^+, 1–3 mEq/kg/day.

   c. Ca^{+2}, 150–220 mEq/kg/day.

D. **Nutrition.** The physiologic needs of the infant may be met enterally or parenterally. The gastrointestinal tract is functional after 28 weeks' gestation but is of limited capacity. Requirements vary with each neonate.

1. **Calories.** Requirements are 100–130 kcal/kg/day.

2. **Protein.** Requirements are 2–4 gm/kg/day.

3. **Fat.** Requirements begin at 1 gm/kg/day. Fat should provide 40% of calories.

4. **Vitamins.** A, B, D, E, C, and K should be replaced.

5. **Iron.** Requirements are 2 mg/kg/day.

6. **Minerals.** Calcium, phosphate, magnesium, zinc, copper, manganese, and iron need to be replaced.

7. **Enteral feedings.** A formula that simulates human milk with a high whey-casein ratio is preferred. Preterm infants often have lactose intolerance, for which numerous nonlactose formulas are available. Infants under 32 weeks' gestation often have poor suck and swallow reflexes and require gavage feedings. With all premature infants or ill neonates, small feedings with a slowly advancing schedule should be used.

8. **Parenteral feeding.** When needed, parenteral nutrition should be started as soon as possible to promote positive nitrogen balance and growth. Up to a 12.5% dextrose solution can be administered peripherally. The infant should be followed closely to adjust the solutions to the infant's needs and to identify signs of toxicity from hyperalimentation. Usual studies include serum glucose, electrolytes, osmolality, liver function tests, blood urea nitrogen (BUN), creatinine, lipid levels, and platelet count.

III. Common neonatal problems
  A. **Respiratory disorders**
  1. **Differential diagnosis.** Many diseases share the same signs and symptoms as pulmonary parenchymal disease and should be considered when evaluating an infant with respiratory distress.
     a. **Airway obstruction.** Choanal atresia, vocal cord palsy, laryngomalacia, tracheal stenosis, and obstruction of the trachea by external masses (e.g., cystic hygroma, hemangioma, and vascular ring).
     b. **Developmental anomalies.** Tracheoesophageal fistula, congenital diaphragmatic hernia, congenital emphysema, and lung cysts.
     c. **Nonpulmonary.** Cyanotic heart disease, persistent pulmonary hypertension of the newborn (PPHN), congestive heart failure, and metabolic disturbances (e.g., acidosis).
  2. **Laboratory studies** for an infant in respiratory distress should include an arterial blood gas, pre- and postductal oxygen saturation by pulse oximetry, hematocrit, 12-lead electrocardiogram (ECG), and chest x-ray.
  3. **Apnea**
     a. **Etiologies.** Apnea is differentiated in terms of its etiology.
        (1) **Central apnea** is due to immaturity or depression of the respiratory center (e.g., narcotics).
        (2) **Obstructive apnea** is due to the inability to consistently maintain a patent airway.
        (3) **Mixed apnea** represents a combination of both central and obstructive apnea.
     b. **Central apnea** is related to the degree of prematurity and is exacerbated by metabolic disturbances such as hypoglycemia, hypocalcemia, hypothermia, hyperthermia, and sepsis. Central apnea due to immaturity of the respiratory center is often treated with methylxanthines such as theophylline and caffeine.
     c. **Apnea of an obstructive or mixed origin** is responsible for the majority of apneic episodes in preterm infants and may be due to incomplete maturation and poor coordination of upper airway musculature. These forms of apnea may respond to changes in head position, insertion of an oral or nasal airway, or placing the infant in a prone position. Occasionally, administration of continuous positive airway pressure (CPAP) may be beneficial.
  4. **Respiratory distress syndrome (RDS)**
     a. **Pathophysiology.** RDS (formerly referred to as hyaline membrane disease) results from physiologic surfactant deficiency. This leads to decreased lung compliance, alveolar instability, and progressive atelectasis. The resultant ventilation-perfusion mismatch results in intrapulmonary shunting. All of these events produce cyanosis, hypoxemia, respiratory distress, and failure.

b. **Infants at risk for RDS** include premature infants, infants of diabetic mothers, and infants born by cesarean delivery. Infants at risk may be identified prenatally by amniocentesis and evaluation of the amniotic fluid for lung maturity using the lecithin-sphingomyelin ratio (L : S > 2 : 1), saturated phosphatidylcholine level (SPC > 500 μg/dl), or presence of phosphatidylglycerol in the specimen.

c. **Glucocorticoids** given at least 2 days before delivery greatly attenuate the severity of RDS and may help prevent the syndrome.

d. **Clinical features** include tachypnea, nasal flaring, grunting, retractions, hypoxemia, and cyanosis that appears shortly after birth.

e. The **chest x-ray** will show a "ground-glass" pattern, air bronchograms, and low lung volumes.

f. **Treatment** is guided by the degree of respiratory failure. With mild distress, warmed, humidified oxygen is administered by hood, and arterial pH, PaO_2, and PCO_2 are followed. The FIO_2 should be adjusted to maintain the PaO_2 between 50 and 80 mm Hg (SaO_2 < 96%) and thus avoid hyperoxia or hypoxemia. If deterioration occurs requiring FIO_2 greater than 60%, CPAP can be attempted at 5 cm H_2O. With more severe disease, intubation and ventilation with positive end-expiratory pressure may be required. Endotracheally administered exogenous surfactant may be utilized to decrease the severity, morbidity, and mortality of the disease.

g. Since RDS is indistinguishable from pneumonia, **broad-spectrum antibiotics** are begun after appropriate cultures.

h. RDS may be **self-limited**; clinical improvement after 2–3 days may be associated with a spontaneous diuresis.

i. **Prognosis** is quite good with over 80% survival, and most patients have normal lungs by 1 month of age. Morbidity and mortality are directly related to the degree of prematurity, the perinatal resuscitation, and the coexistence of other problems (e.g., patent ductus arteriosus). Pneumothoraces and pulmonary interstitial emphysema may complicate the recovery and may be associated with the evolution to chronic lung disease.

5. **Bronchopulmonary dysplasia (BPD)**

a. **Etiology.** BPD is defined as the continued need for respiratory support with oxygen therapy or mechanical ventilation beyond 1 month of age. BPD usually follows severe RDS, and even though the primary cause is unclear, oxygen toxicity, chronic inflammation, mechanical injury, and excessive intake of fluid and salt all contribute to this condition. BPD can be worsened by the presence of a patent ductus arteriosus and resultant pulmonary edema.

b. **Clinical features** include retractions, rales, lung hyperinflation, and lung hyperresonance.

c. **Treatment** consists of supportive respiratory care, adequate nutrition, and diuretic therapy to offset pulmonary edema and improve lung compliance. Bronchodilator therapy is used to treat bronchospasm as needed.

d. **Prognosis** varies with the severity of the disease. Of severely affected infants, 25% die within the first year. Most infants are asymptomatic by 2 years of age, and only the rare infant has signs and symptoms of BPD after 5 years of age.

6. **Pneumothorax**

a. **Etiology.** Pneumothorax is a frequent complication in mechanically ventilated infants and may occur spontaneously in otherwise normal full-term infants. Although the cause is unknown, uneven ventilation with overdistention of airways and alveoli may be associated. The incidence is 2% in cesarean deliveries, 10% with meconium staining, and 5–10% in RDS.

b. **Clinical features.** The diagnosis should be considered in any neonate with respiratory distress or in the ventilated infant with an acute deterioration in condition (e.g., bronchospasm, sudden cyanosis, hypotension, or agitation). Although difficult to appreciate, one may observe asymmetric chest movement with ventilation and asymmetric breath sounds. An endobronchial intubation should be ruled out.

c. **Laboratory studies.** Transillumination of the chest with a strong light usually will show a hyperlucent hemithorax. A chest x-ray will confirm the diagnosis.

d. **Treatment**

(1) In an otherwise **healthy infant with minimal respiratory distress,** close observation and nitrogen washout by breathing a high concentration of oxygen may be the only therapy required.

(2) In the **unstable infant,** immediate aspiration of the pleural space with an intravenous catheter should be performed even before obtaining a chest x-ray. Reaccumulation of air after aspiration warrants immediate placement of a chest tube.

7. **Meconium aspiration syndrome**

a. **Meconium staining of amniotic fluid** occurs in 10% of all births and may be associated with fetal distress and asphyxia.

b. **Infants delivered through meconium-stained fluid** should be intubated and have their airways suctioned, preferably before they take their first breath.

c. **Meconium aspiration** may produce complete obstruction of the airways, resulting in distal atelectasis. Alternatively, meconium may produce partial obstruction of the airway and overinflation of distal air spaces by a ball-valve effect, leading to pneumothorax. The bile may contribute a chemical component of meconium pneumonitis and airway edema. Meconium aspiration syndrome has also been associated with PPHN (see sec. **B.5**).

d. **Treatment** includes respiratory support as indicated and broad-spectrum antibiotic coverage.

8. Congenital diaphragmatic hernia

a. Congenital diaphragmatic hernia occurs in 1:4000 live births. It has a high mortality, with 50% stillborn or dying within the newborn period. Seventy percent of the defects occur on the left. The embryology and pathophysiology are discussed in sec. **I.B.**

b. **Clinical features.** The defect can often be seen on prenatal ultrasound. At birth, a scaphoid abdomen is often noted, and breath sounds are absent on the involved side. Rarely, bowel sounds are heard in the affected hemithorax. Early and often severe respiratory distress is seen.

c. The **diagnosis** is best confirmed by chest x-ray which shows intestine, stomach, and often liver in the thorax.

d. **Treatment** consists of cardiovascular and respiratory support as indicated. Hypotension and shock are often seen secondary to large gastrointestinal fluid losses. The main causes of mortality are respiratory insufficiency and PPHN. Pneumothorax in the unaffected lung is common and is often the cause of death during resuscitation.

e. **Surgical repair** involves replacing the abdominal contents and repairing the diaphragm. In the past this was performed urgently in the critically ill infant. With the advent of extracorporeal membrane oxygenation (ECMO) (see sec. **B.6**), many infants are now stabilized on ECMO, with surgical repair performed while still on bypass. Survival even after repair depends on the degree of lung hypoplasia and PPHN seen.

B. Cardiovascular disorders

1. Laboratory studies. In the infant with signs and symptoms of cardiovascular disease, relevant studies include an arterial blood gas, pre- and postductal oxygen saturations, determination of arterial blood gas tension during inhalation of pure oxygen ("hyperoxia test"), hematocrit, chest x-ray, and ECG. Two-dimensional echocardiography is frequently performed.

2. Patent ductus arteriosus

a. **Clinical features.** Patent ductus arteriosus is commonly seen in the premature infant and is characterized by a murmur at the left sternal border radiating to the back, bounding pulses, widened pulse pressure, evidence of increased pulmonary blood flow, and excessive weight gain.

b. **Treatment** consists of fluid restriction and diuretic therapy. If the degree of shunt through the ductus arteriosus becomes clinically significant, pharmacologic closure with indomethacin may be attempted.

Surgical closure is reserved for the infant who has failed therapy, who does not tolerate indomethacin, or whose growth and respiratory weaning are hindered by the open ductus.

3. **Cyanosis**
   a. **Etiology.** There are many causes of cyanosis, including respiratory diseases and polycythemia. These need to be considered when evaluating an infant with cyanosis.
   b. **Arterial desaturation** is characteristic of cardiac lesions that cause right-to-left shunting. Blood entering the right heart may be shunted to the left (usually through the foramen ovale) because of structural obstruction or rearrangement of the outflow tracts. Deoxygenated blood bypasses the lungs, resulting in cyanosis.
   c. **Ductal-dependent lesions** include transposition of the great vessels, pulmonic stenosis or atresia, tetralogy of Fallot, and Ebstein's anomaly. These lesions depend on the patency of the ductus to provide flow to the lungs. Most of these infants become symptomatic as the ductus arteriosus closes at 2–3 days of life.
   d. **The diagnosis of increased shunt** can be confirmed by a hyperoxic challenge. The infant breathes 100% oxygen, and arterial oxygen tension is measured. A significant shunt will produce a PaO_2 below 150 mm Hg when breathing 100% oxygen.
   e. **Initial management** consists of respiratory and cardiovascular support. If a fixed shunt exists, the infant should be placed in an atmosphere of 40% oxygen or less, as a higher inspired oxygen concentration will not improve arterial saturation but may contribute to pulmonary toxicity.
   f. If a **ductal-dependent lesion** exists, prevention of ductal closure is critical to maintain pulmonary blood flow. This may be accomplished with a prostaglandin E1 infusion. Side effects include apnea, hypotension, and seizure activity.

4. **Arrhythmias**
   a. The most frequent arrhythmia seen in neonates is **paroxysmal atrial tachycardia.** This may be self-limited and well tolerated, but if hypotension or desaturation occurs, treatment may be required.
   b. **Treatment** consists of vagal maneuvers such as nasopharyngeal stimulation. Massage of the eye should be avoided, as this may lead to disruption of the lens in neonates. Esophageal pacing has also been used successfully.
   c. **Digitalization** will usually convert paroxysmal atrial tachycardia to sinus rhythm; maintenance therapy for 1 year is subsequently indicated. Propranolol and quinidine are second-line medications. Adenosine has also been helpful.
   d. If the patient is hemodynamically unstable, **DC conversion** is indicated.

5. **Persistent pulmonary hypertension of the newborn (PPHN)**
   a. **Pathophysiology.** PPHN, previously referred to as persistent fetal circulation, is manifested by an increase in pulmonary vascular resistance (PVR) with resulting pulmonary arterial hypertension, right-to-left shunting across the foramen ovale and the ductus arteriosus, and profound cyanosis. Alveolar hypoxia may be the initial event that triggers an increase in PVR.
   b. **Etiology.** There are many predisposing conditions including asphyxia, meconium aspiration, bacterial pneumonia, sepsis, and congenital diaphragmatic hernia.
   c. **Clinical features.** Markedly cyanotic infants may present after a stormy delivery with severe respiratory distress, cyanosis, and decreased pulmonary markings on chest x-ray. Patients often have marked hypoxemia with PaO_2 less than 60 mm Hg despite breathing 100% oxygen. Echocardiography is needed to rule out congenital heart disease.
   d. **Treatment**
      (1) **Intubation and mechanical ventilation** with high respiratory rates to maintain $PaCO_2$ in the 25–30 mm Hg range and high FiO_2 to help diminish PVR.
      (2) **Paralysis** may aid ventilation, and **profound analgesia** with narcotics (e.g., fentanyl at 1–3 μg/kg/hr) may ablate PVR elevations from noxious stimuli.
      (3) **Bicarbonate infusion** is used to treat systemic acidosis.
      (4) **Preload** is maintained with crystalloid, colloid, or pressors (e.g., dopamine or isoproterenol).
      (5) A trial of **tolazoline** (1 mg/kg IV over 10 minutes) to dilate the pulmonary arteries is reasonable. Unfortunately, this agent often produces systemic hypotension.
      (6) **Inhaled nitric oxide** has, in our experience, proved efficacious for reversing or stabilizing PPHN. Inhaled nitric oxide in low concentrations appears to be a selective pulmonary vasodilator and bronchodilator without significant toxic effects.
      (7) **ECMO** is performed if the above measures fail and if entry criteria are met.

6. **Extracorporeal membrane oxygenation** (ECMO) is a modality to provide oxygen delivery to an infant with severe respiratory failure or PPHN.
   a. The **circuit** consists of tubing, a reservoir, a pump, the membrane oxygenator, and a heat exchanger.
   b. **Access.** In most cases, the right common carotid artery and the right internal jugular vein are cannulated for access. Occasionally, the femoral artery and vein may be used.
   c. There are many **exclusion criteria** because of the

potential risks associated with ECMO. Infants less than 35 weeks' gestation, less than 2000 gm, or with intraventricular hemorrhage are excluded because of their unacceptable risk of hemorrhage while heparinized. Also excluded are infants with multiple congenital anomalies, severe neurologic impairment, or cyanotic congenital heart disease.

d. **Selection criteria** vary between centers, but most reserve ECMO for the infant with a high mortality risk. These infants are identified as those having a large A-a gradient (> 600 mm Hg) with high mean airway pressures for more than 4 hours.

e. **Morbidity.** Heparinization can cause intracranial hemorrhage and bleeding from other sites. Right-sided cerebral injuries are seen secondary to cannulation and ligation of the right internal carotid artery. These include focal left seizures, left hemiparesis, and progressive right cerebral atrophy after decannulation.

f. **Mortality** has fallen drastically from over 80% to 20% with the advent of ECMO.

C. **Hematologic disorders**

1. **Hemolytic disease of the newborn (erythroblastosis fetalis)**

a. **Isoimmune hemolytic anemia** in the fetus is caused by the passage of maternal antibody against fetal erythrocytes transplacentally into the fetus. Only IgG can cross the placenta.

b. **Rh hemolytic disease** is usually caused by the anti-D antibody but can also be caused by antibodies to minor antigens including Kell, Duff, Kidd, or Ss antigens. The absence of D antigen makes one Rh negative and occurs in 15% of whites and 5% of blacks. A mother can be sensitized to fetal antigens by leakage of fetal blood into the maternal circulation during pregnancy, delivery, abortion, or amniocentesis. To prevent sensitization, an unsensitized Rh-negative mother is given a 300-μg dose of anti-D immune globulin (RhoGAM) during pregnancy and another dose after delivery. Once sensitized, immune prophylaxis is of no value. Even if treated with immune globulin, a mother can still be sensitized during pregnancy if a large fetomaternal transfusion occurs.

c. **ABO hemolytic disease** can occur without maternal sensitization, since a mother with group O blood has naturally occurring anti-A and anti-B antibodies in her circulation. These are usually IgM antibodies, but some may be IgG. This disease tends to be milder than Rh disease, with little or no anemia, mild indirect hyperbilirubinemia, and rarely a need for exchange transfusion.

d. An **indirect Coombs' test** on maternal blood can detect the presence of IgG antibodies in her serum.

e. A **direct Coombs' test** on the infant's blood can

detect cells already coated with antibody, thus indicating a risk for hemolysis.

f. **Hemolysis** occurs when antibody crosses the placenta, attaches to the corresponding antigen on fetal erythrocytes, and causes hemolysis. Hepatosplenomegaly results from increased hematopoiesis triggered by hemolysis.

g. **Clinical features.** Physical examination may reveal hepatosplenomegaly, edema, pallor, or jaundice.

h. **Laboratory studies** often reveal anemia, thrombocytopenia, a positive direct Coombs' test, indirect hyperbilirubinemia, hypoglycemia, hypoalbuminemia, and an elevated reticulocyte count that increases proportionally with the severity of the disease. Serial hematocrit and indirect bilirubin levels should be followed.

i. **Treatment** consists of phototherapy. An exchange transfusion may be required if the rate of rise of bilirubin exceeds 1 mg/dl/hr.

2. **Hydrops fetalis**

a. Hydrops fetalis is defined as the **excessive accumulation of fluid by the fetus** and can range from mild peripheral edema to massive anasarca.

b. **Etiologies.** Hydrops can be seen in hemolytic disease and is thought to be due to increased capillary permeability secondary to anemia. Other etiologies of hydrops include anemias (e.g., fetomaternal hemorrhage, donor twin-twin transfusion), cardiac arrhythmias (e.g., complete heart block, supraventricular tachycardia), congenital heart disease, vascular or lymphatic malformation (e.g., hemangioma of the liver, cystic hygroma), or infection (e.g., viral, toxoplasmosis, syphilis).

c. **Treatment.** The main goals of therapy include prevention of intrauterine or extrauterine death from anemia and hypoxia, restoration of intravascular volume, and avoidance of neurotoxicity from hyperbilirubinemia.

(1) Survival of the **unborn infant** may be improved by in utero transfusion via the umbilical vein.

(2) Care of the **liveborn infant** should include correction of hypovolemia and acidosis, as well as potential exchange transfusion.

(3) **Late complications** include anemia; mild graft vs host reactions; inspissated bile syndrome (characterized by persistent icterus with elevated direct and indirect bilirubin); and portal vein thrombosis (as a complication of umbilical vein catheterization).

D. **Gastrointestinal disorders**

1. **Hyperbilirubinemia**

a. **Pathophysiology.** Bilirubin is formed from the breakdown of heme, then bound to albumin, transported to the liver (where it is conjugated with glucuronide), and delivered to the intestine in bile. In the intestine, it is either deconjugated by intestinal bacteria and reabsorbed or converted to excretory urobilinogen.

b. **Etiology.** Hyperbilirubinemia results from overproduction (e.g., hemolysis, absorption of sequestered blood, polycythemia), underconjugation (e.g., immature or damaged liver), or underexcretion (e.g., biliary atresia). It is often seen in sepsis, asphyxia, and metabolic disorders (e.g., hypothyroidism, hypoglycemia, galactosemia) as well as in healthy newborns and breast-fed infants.

c. **Toxic effects.** Unconjugated (indirect) bilirubin is lipid soluble and is capable of entering the central nervous system. Toxic levels result in bilirubin staining and necrosis of neurons in the basal ganglia, the hippocampus, and the subthalamic nuclei. This process, known as bilirubin encephalopathy or **kernicterus,** may have clinical symptoms ranging from mild lethargy and fever to convulsions. Infants with respiratory distress, sepsis, metabolic acidosis, hypoglycemia, hypoalbuminemia, or severe hemolytic disease are at increased risk for kernicterus. Survivors evaluated in childhood are found to have neurologic sequelae ranging from diminished cognitive function to mental retardation and choreoathetoid cerebral palsy.

d. **Physiologic jaundice** results from increased red cell turnover and an immature hepatic conjugation system. It occurs in 60% of newborns, and peak bilirubin levels occur by day 2–4 of life. Premature infants have an increased incidence (80%) and later bilirubin peak (day 5–7).

e. **Breast milk jaundice** develops gradually, occurring in the second or third week of life, with peak bilirubin levels of 15–25 mg/dl, which may persist for 2–3 months. Other causes should be excluded before making this diagnosis. Interrupting nursing for a few days results in a marked decrease in serum levels, at which time nursing can be restarted. This is a benign type of jaundice without adverse sequelae.

f. **Laboratory studies** include total and direct bilirubin, direct Coombs' test, reticulocyte count, blood smear for red cell morphology, electrolytes, BUN, creatinine, and appropriate cultures if sepsis is suspected.

g. **Treatment**

(1) Management of **physiologic or mild hemolytic jaundice** consists of monitoring serial bilirubin levels and starting early feeding to reduce enterohepatic cycling of bilirubin.

(2) Phototherapy is used if **moderate indirect bilirubin levels** or an accelerated rate of rise is noted (e.g., indirect bilirubin level > 5 in a full-term infant on day 1 of life). Light therapy of

420- to 470-nm wavelength results in photoisomerization of bilirubin, making it water soluble. Eyes must be shielded to prevent retinal damage.

(3) For **severe hyperbilirubinemia,** exchange transfusion is indicated (e.g., indirect bilirubin > 25 mg/dl in a full-term infant).

2. **Esophageal atresia**
   a. **Pathophysiology.** The proximal blind esophageal pouch has a small capacity, resulting in overflow aspiration. This leads to the classic triad of coughing, choking, and cyanosis. Occasionally, only drooling requiring frequent suctioning may be noted.
   b. The **diagnosis** is confirmed by the inability to pass a nasogastric tube into the stomach. Anterior and lateral x-rays with water-soluble contrast agents will confirm this.
   c. The majority of esophageal atresias are of the blind pouch variety with a distal tracheoesophageal fistula. Reflux of gastric contents into the distal airway worsens respiratory symptoms.
   d. **Medical treatment** consists initially of protection from aspiration. A nasogastric tube is placed on continuous low suction and the head of the bed is elevated 40 degrees. With severe respiratory compromise, endotracheal intubation and ventilation may be required.
   e. **Surgical treatment** consists of initial gastrostomy tube placement to decompress the stomach. The definitive repair may be performed concomitantly in very healthy infants or as a staged repair following gastrostomy tube placement.

3. **Duodenal atresia**
   a. **Clinical features.** Duodenal atresia usually presents with bile-stained emesis, upper abdominal distention, and increased volume of gastric aspirates. It is associated with Down's syndrome and may coexist with other intestinal malformations.
   b. An **abdominal x-ray** often reveals a "double bubble," representing air in the stomach and upper duodenum.
   c. **Treatment** consists of nasogastric decompression and surgical correction.

4. **Pyloric stenosis**
   a. Although usually presenting in the second or third week of life, pyloric stenosis may present in the immediate newborn period.
   b. **Clinical features** include persistent nonbilious emesis and a metabolic alkalosis from loss of gastric hydrochloric acid. With significant vomiting, the patient may present with acidosis and shock. An abdominal mass consisting of the hypertrophic pylorus or "olive" is often palpable.
   c. An **abdominal x-ray** usually shows gastric dilatation. The diagnosis is confirmed by abdominal ultrasound or by barium swallow.

d. **Treatment** consists of rehydration, correction of metabolic alkalosis, and nasogastric drainage before surgical repair.

5. **Omphalocele and gastroschisis**

a. An **omphalocele** is caused by migration of intestinal contents out of the umbilicus and failure of the abdominal wall to close completely. The viscera remain outside the abdominal cavity, where they are covered with intact peritoneum. Omphaloceles may be associated with cardiac lesions.

b. **Gastroschisis** occurs later in fetal life from interruption of the omphalomesenteric artery. The resulting abdominal wall defect allows exposure of the bowel to the intrauterine environment without peritoneal coverage; bowel loops are often edematous and covered with an inflammatory exudate.

c. **Medical stabilization** includes nasogastric drainage, IV hydration, and protection of the viscera before imminent surgical repair. If the peritoneal sac is intact, the omphalocele should be covered with sterile, warm, saline-soaked gauze to decrease heat and water loss and the risk of infection. If the sac has ruptured or if the infant has gastroschisis, saline-soaked gauze should be used to wrap the exposed viscera; the infant should then be wrapped in warm sterile towels prior to surgical repair.

6. **Necrotizing enterocolitis**

a. Necrotizing enterocolitis is an **acquired intestinal necrosis** that appears in the absence of functional (e.g., Hirschsprung's) or anatomic (e.g., malrotation) lesions. It occurs predominantly (90%) in premature infants and may be endemic or epidemic in nature. It usually develops during the first few weeks of life, almost always after the institution of enteral feedings. Mortality may be as high as 40%.

b. **Pathogenesis** is unclear but involves critical stress of an immature gut by ischemic, infectious, or immunologic insults. Enteral feedings seem to potentiate mucosal injury.

c. **Clinical features** include abdominal distention, ileus, increase in gastric aspirates, abdominal wall erythema, or bloody stool. The infant may demonstrate systemic signs such as temperature instability, lethargy, respiratory and circulatory instability, oliguria, and bleeding diathesis.

d. **Laboratory studies** should include an abdominal x-ray (which may show pneumatosis intestinalis, fixed loops of bowel, portal air, or free intraperitoneal air), complete blood count (CBC) (revealing leukocytosis, leukopenia, thrombocytopenia), arterial blood gases (demonstrating acidosis), stool guaiac, and stool Clinitest (showing evidence of carbohydrate malabsorption). Since the differential diagnosis includes sepsis, cultures of blood, urine, and stool should also be obtained. If the patient is stable and disseminated intravascular coagulation is not evident, cerebrospinal fluid (CSF) should be obtained by lumbar puncture for gram stain and culture.

    e. **Treatment.** When necrotizing enterocolitis is suspected, enteral feedings are discontinued, and the stomach is decompressed with a nasogastric tube. The child is kept NPO for at least 2 weeks and supported with parenteral feedings. Broad-spectrum antibiotics are begun (ampicillin, an aminoglycoside, and if perforation is suspected, clindamycin).

    f. **Surgical consultation** is indicated, although laparotomy is usually reserved for intestinal perforation.

  7. **Volvulus**

    a. Volvulus may occur as a primary lesion or more commonly as the result of intestinal malrotation. If present in utero, intestinal necrosis may be present at birth, and immediate resection is indicated.

    b. **Clinical features** may include abdominal distention, bilious emesis, and signs of sepsis or shock.

    c. The **diagnosis** of malrotation is made by barium enema, which demonstrates an abnormally positioned ligament of Treitz.

    d. **Treatment** involves volume resuscitation, placement of a nasogastric tube, and surgical repair.

E. Neurologic disorders

  1. **Seizures**

    a. Seizures may be generalized, focal, or subtle. Even jitteriness alone may be a manifestation of a seizure disorder.

    b. **Etiologies** include birth trauma, intracranial hemorrhage, postasphyxial encephalopathy, metabolic disturbances (hypoglycemia or hypocalcemia), drug withdrawal, and infections.

    c. **Laboratory evaluation** should include

      (1) Electrolytes, glucose, calcium, magnesium, serum/urine amino acids.

      (2) Appropriate cultures, including CSF.

      (3) Cranial ultrasound and/or computed tomography (CT) scan.

      (4) Electroencephalogram before and after pyridoxine administration.

    d. **Treatment** includes supportive care and correction of underlying problems (e.g., hypoglycemia, hypocalcemia). Anticonvulsants are started, and if indicated, a test dose of pyridoxine (50 mg IV) is administered.

    e. **Anticonvulsants**

      (1) **Phenobarbital,** 0.15 mg/kg IV load; maintenance dose of 2.5 mg/kg bid to maintain a serum level of 20–40 µg/ml.

      (2) **Phenytoin** (Dilantin), 10 mg/kg IV load over 15 minutes; maintenance dose of 2.5 mg/kg bid to maintain a therapeutic level of 15–30 µg/ml.

(3) **Benzodiazepine** (e.g., diazepam), 0.1–0.3 mg/kg IV.

(4) **Paraldehyde,** 0.2 ml/kg (rectally).

2. **Intracranial hemorrhage**

a. **Intraventricular hemorrhage** occurs in over 40% of infants with birth weights below 1500 gm. Subdural and subarachnoid hemorrhages are much less common.

b. **Clinical features.** Intraventricular hemorrhage is often asymptomatic, although it may present with unexplained acidosis, lethargy, anemia, apnea, or seizures.

c. **Laboratory studies.** Diagnosis is made by cranial ultrasound or CT scan.

d. **Grading of intraventricular hemorrhage**

(1) **Grade I.** Subependymal bleeding only.

(2) **Grade II.** Intraventricular bleeding without dilatation of ventricles.

(3) **Grade III.** Intraventricular bleeding with dilatation of ventricles.

(4) **Grade IV.** Grade III with intraparenchymal blood.

e. The major **complication** of intraventricular hemorrhage is CSF obstruction resulting in hydrocephalus. This is followed by measuring daily head circumferences and by serial ultrasounds. Intraventricular shunting is often required.

f. **Hypertonic agents** (e.g., 25% dextrose in water for treatment of hypoglycemia) have been implicated in the etiology of intraventricular hemorrhage and should be avoided.

3. **Retinopathy of prematurity** (ROP)

a. **Etiologies**

(1) ROP is seen in infants with birth weights less than 1700 gm, with an 80% incidence in infants less than 1000 gm. The risk of ROP is increased in neonates requiring oxygen therapy and depends on the duration and FiO_2. To prevent this, a PaO_2 of 45–60 mm Hg is recommended, and SaO_2 is maintained in the range of 94–96%.

(2) Factors other than hyperoxic exposure and prematurity may produce ROP, as it has been demonstrated in full-term infants, infants with cyanotic heart disease, stillborn infants, and infants with no hyperoxic exposure, as well as in a single eye. Factors that may increase risk include anemia, infection, intracranial hemorrhage, acidosis, and patent ductus arteriosus.

b. **Pathophysiology.** ROP begins in the temporal peripheral retina, which is the last part of the retina to vascularize. An elevated ridge demarcating vascularized and nonvascularized retina is initially seen. Fibrovascular proliferation from this border extends posteriorly, and in 90% of patients, gradual resolution occurs from this stage. These patients may develop strabismus, amblyopia, myopia, or peripheral retinal detachment in later life.

c. In 10% of patients, fibrovascularization extends into the vitreous, resulting in vitreous hemorrhage, peripheral retinal scarring, temporal dragging of the disk and macula, and partial retinal detachment. In severe disease, extensive fibrovascular proliferation can result in a retrolental white mass (leukokoria), complete retinal detachment, and loss of vision.

d. All infants at risk are examined with **indirect ophthalmoscopy** after 1 month of age. If ROP is identified, the infant is reexamined at 2-week intervals until spontaneous resolution occurs. New cases of ROP do not occur after 3 months of age.

e. **Treatment** for severe manifestations of ROP has included photocoagulation, diathermy, cryotherapy, and vitrectomy, though none has proved to be effective.

F. **Infectious diseases**

1. **Environment**

a. **Preterm infants and neonates** are particularly vulnerable to infection. They have decreased cellular and humoral immune defense systems and are at increased risk for colonization and nosocomial infection.

b. **Prevention.** Infectious transmission may be reduced by using separate equipment and isolettes for each infant, by scrupulous hand washing before and after each contact, and by wearing cover gowns.

2. **Risk factors for infection.** Prolonged rupture of membranes is associated with a high incidence of amnionitis and subsequent ascending bacterial and viral infection in the neonate. Maternal fever, maternal leukocytosis, and fetal tachycardia are also associated with neonatal infection.

3. **Laboratory studies** include Gram stain and culture of gastric aspirate, CBC with differential, and blood cultures. A lumbar puncture for culture and analysis of CSF may be indicated. If appropriate, viral cultures are indicated.

4. **Neonatal sepsis**

a. **Organisms** responsible for infections soon after birth are usually acquired in utero or during passage through the birth canal. These can include group B beta-hemolytic streptococcus, *Escherichia coli, Listeria,* and herpes. Later-onset infections may be caused by *Staphylococcus aureus* and *Staphylococcus epidermidis.*

b. The **clinical features** of sepsis include fulminant respiratory failure, seizures, or shock. Often subtle signs, including respiratory distress, apnea, irritability, or poor feeding, are seen first and warrant a high index of suspicion.

c. **Laboratory studies** should include cultures of

blood, urine and CSF, CBC with platelet count, urinalysis, and chest x-ray.

d. **Antibiotic coverage** with ampicillin or oxacillin and an aminoglycoside is begun and continued for 48–72 hours. If culture results are positive, treatment should continue as indicated by the severity and location of infection. Aminoglycoside serum levels should be monitored and dosages adjusted to prevent toxicity.

SUGGESTED READING

Avery, G. B. *Neonatology. Pathophysiology and Management of the Newborn* (3rd ed.). Philadelphia: Lippincott, 1987.

Barry, J. E., and Auldist, A. W. The Vater association: One end of a spectrum of anomalies. *Am. J. Dis. Child.* 128:769, 1974.

Bartlett, R. H., et al. Extracorporeal circulation in neonatal respiratory failure: A prospective randomized study. *Pediatrics* 76:479, 1985.

Drummond, W. H., et al. The independent effects of hyperventilation, tolazoline, and dopamine on infants with persistent pulmonary hypertension. *J. Pediatr.* 98:603, 1982.

Gersony, W., Peckham, G., and Ellison, R. Effects of indomethacin in premature infants with patent ductus arteriosus: Results of a national collaborative study. *J. Pediatr.* 102:895, 1983.

Gregory, G. Life-threatening apnea in the ex-premie. *Anaesthesia* 59:495, 1983.

Hannerman, C., and Aramburo, M. H. Prolonged indomethacin therapy for the prevention of recurrences of patent ductus arteriosus. *J. Pediatr.* 117:771, 1990.

Kurth, C. D. et al. Postoperative apnea in premature infants. *Anesthesiology* 66:483, 1987.

Lang, P., et al. Inhaled nitric oxide: A selective vasodilator for the treatment of pulmonary artery hypertension in congenital heart disease. *Pediatr. Res.* 31:A104, 1992.

Liu, L. M. P., et al. Life threatening apnea in infants recovering from anesthesia. *Anesthesiology* 59:506, 1983.

O'Rourke, P. P., et al. Extracorporeal membrane oxygenation and conventional medical therapy in neonates with persistent pulmonary hypertension of the newborn: A prospective randomized therapy. *Pediatrics* 84:957, 1989.

Peckham, G., and Fox, W. Physiologic factors affecting pulmonary artery pressure in infants with persistent pulmonary hypertension. *J. Pediatr.* 93:1005, 1978.

Roberts, J. D., Jr., Cote, C., and Todres, I. D. Neonatal Emergencies. In C. Cote and J. Ryan (eds.), *A Practice of Anesthesia for Infants and Children* (2nd ed.). Philadelphia: Saunders, 1992.

Roberts, J. D., Jr., et al. Inhaled nitric oxide (NO): A selective pulmonary vasodilator for the treatment of persistent pulmonary hypertension of the newborn (PPHN). *Circulation* 84:A1279, 1991.

Rudolph, A. M., and Yuan, S. Response of the pulmonary vasculature to hypoxia and H^+ ion concentration changes. *J. Clin. Invest.* 45:399, 1966.

Shannon, D. C., et al. Prevention of apnea and bradycardia in low-birthweight infants. *Pediatrics* 55:589, 1975.

Soll, R. F., et al. Multicenter trial of single dose Survanta for prevention of respiratory distress syndrome (RDS). *Pediatrics* 85:1092, 1990.

Steward, D. J. Preterm infants are more prone to complications following minor surgery than are term infants. *Anesthesiology* 56:304, 1982.

I. Anatomy and physiology

A. Upper airway

1. Neonates are **obligate nose breathers.** Their nares are relatively narrow, and a significant fraction of the work of breathing is needed to overcome their resistance. Hence, occlusion of the nares by bilateral choanal atresia or tenacious secretions can cause complete airway obstruction. Placement of an oral airway or an endotracheal tube may be necessary to reestablish airway patency.

2. Infants have a relatively **large tongue,** which makes mask ventilation and laryngoscopy challenging. If excessive submandibular pressure is applied during mask ventilation, the tongue can easily cause total airway obstruction.

3. Infants and children have a more **cephalad glottis** (C3 in premature infants, C4 in infants, C5 in adults) and a narrow, long, angulated epiglottis, which can make visualization of the glottis during laryngoscopy more difficult.

4. In infants and children younger than 7–10 years old, the narrowest part of the airway is at the **cricoid ring** rather than at the glottis (as in adults). An endotracheal tube that passes through the cords may still meet obstruction distally.

5. **Deciduous teeth** erupt within the first year of age and may be shed from 6 years old through adolescence. To avoid dislodging a loose tooth, it is safest to open the mandible without blindly introducing a finger into the oral cavity. In some instances very unstable teeth should be removed prior to laryngoscopy. Parents and patients should be apprised of this possibility in advance.

6. **Airway resistance** in infants and children can be dramatically increased by subtle changes in an already small-caliber system. Poiseuille's law describes airway dynamics, whereby resistance to laminar flow varies inversely with airway radius to the fourth power. Even a small amount of edema can significantly increase airway resistance and cause airway compromise.

B. Pulmonary system

1. Neonates have high metabolic rates, resulting in an elevated **oxygen consumption** (7–9 ml/kg/min) when compared with adults (3 ml/kg/min).

2. Neonatal lungs have **high closing volumes,** which fall within the lower range of their normal tidal volume. Below closing volume, alveolar collapse and shunting occur.

3. Infants have a **higher minute ventilation** and **lower functional residual capacity** (FRC) per kilogram of body weight than adults. Their high minute ventila-

tion/FRC ratio results in the rapid induction of anesthesia with inhalation agents.

4. **Anatomic shunts** including patent **ductus arteriosus** and patent **foramen ovale** may have augmented flow with increases in pulmonary artery pressure (e.g., under conditions of hypoxia, hypoventilation, or excessively high positive airway pressure).

5. All of these characteristics of the infant's pulmonary system contribute to **rapid desaturation** during apnea. Moreover, profound desaturation can occur even with a properly positioned endotracheal tube when the infant coughs or strains, with resultant alveolar collapse. Treatment may require deepening anesthesia with intravenous agents or the use of succinylcholine.

6. The **diaphragm** is the infant's major muscle of ventilation. Compared with the adult diaphragm, the newborn has only half the number of type 1 slow-twitch oxidative muscle fibers essential for sustained increased respiratory effort. Thus, the infant's diaphragm fatigues earlier than the adult's.

7. The **pliable rib cage** of a newborn collapses with increases in negative intrathoracic pressure. This diminishes the efficacy of the infant's attempts to increase ventilation.

8. Anesthetic breathing systems can significantly increase an infant's **dead space,** which under normal circumstances is only about 5 ml (2 ml/kg is the approximate dead space in an infant, as in an adult).

9. Infants' **high minute ventilation,** particularly under conditions of stress, limits their ability to increase their ventilatory effort effectively. Therefore it is recommended that young infants under anesthesia be managed with controlled ventilation.

10. Premature infants weighing less than 1600 gm and gestational age less than 38 weeks are at risk for **retinopathy** and **pulmonary dysplasia** when exposed to conditions of hyperoxia. The routine use of 100% oxygen intraoperatively is discouraged unless these patients are hypoxemic (oxygen saturation < 95%).

11. **Apnea and cardiovascular instability** following general anesthesia occur with increased frequency in infants who are premature and less than 60 weeks' postconceptual age, as well as in infants who have sepsis or other systemic infection, hypothermia, central nervous system (CNS) disease, hypoglycemia, or other metabolic derangement. These patients should have cardiorespiratory monitoring for a minimum of 24 hours postoperatively. It follows that these infants are not candidates for ambulatory day surgery.

C. **Cardiovascular system**

1. **Cardiac output** is 180–240 ml/kg/min in newborns, which is two to three times that in adults. The relatively high cardiac output is necessary to meet high metabolic demands.

2. The ventricles are **noncompliant** and have a rela-

tively smaller muscle mass in newborns and infants; therefore there is minimal compensatory reserve. There is some limited ability to increase contractility, but increases in cardiac output are largely rate dependent. Bradycardia is the most deleterious dysrhythmia in infants, resulting in direct, proportional decreases in cardiac output.

3. **Heart rate** and **blood pressure** vary with age and should be maintained at age-appropriate levels perioperatively (Tables 28-1 and 28-2).

D. **Fluid and electrolyte balance**
1. The **glomerular filtration rate (GFR)** at birth is 15–30% of normal adult values. Adult values are reached by age 1 year. Renal clearance of drugs and their metabolics are correspondingly diminished during the first year.
2. Newborns tolerate water or salt loads poorly because of low GFR and decreased **concentrating ability.**
3. The **total body water (TBW)** in the preterm infant is 90% of body weight. In term infants, it is 80%; at 6–12 months, it is 60%. This increased percentage of the TBW affects drug volumes of distribution, and therefore the dosages of some drugs (e.g., thiopental, succinylcholine, and pancuronium) are 20–30% greater than the equally effective dose for adults.

E. **Hematologic system**
1. The **blood volume** in preterm infants is 90–100 ml/kg; it is 80 ml/kg at term. It reaches the adult value of 70 ml/kg by age 1 year.
2. Normal values for hematocrit are listed in Table 28-1. The nadir of **physiologic anemia** is at 3 months and may reach as low as 28% in an otherwise healthy infant.
3. At birth, **fetal hemoglobin (HbF)** is predominant but is largely replaced with the adult type (HbA) by 3–4 months. Fetal hemoglobin has a higher affinity for oxygen (left shift of oxyhemoglobin dissociation curve), but this does not normally prove clinically significant. By 6 months, the HbA/HbF ratio of adulthood is attained.

F. **Hepatobiliary system**
1. **Liver enzyme systems** important in drug metabolism are immature in the infant, particularly those involved in phase II (conjugation) reactions.
2. **Jaundice,** which is common in neonates, can be physiologic or have pathologic causes.
3. Hyperbilirubinemia and displacement of bilirubin from albumin by drugs can result in **kernicterus.** Premature infants develop kernicterus at lower levels of bilirubin than do those at term.

G. **Endocrine system**
1. Newborns, particularly premature babies and those small for gestational age, have diminished **glycogen stores** and are more susceptible to hypoglycemia. Infants of diabetic mothers, who have high insulin levels following prolonged exposure to elevated maternal serum glucose, are also prone to **hypoglycemia.**

Table 28-1. Age-dependence of typical respiratory parameters

Variable	Newborn	1 Year	3 Years	5 Years	Adult
Respirations (breaths/min)	40–60	20–30	Gradual decrease to 18–25	18–25	12–20
Tidal volume (ml)	15	80	110	250	500
Minute ventilation (L/min)	1	1.8	2.5	5.5	6.5
Hematocrit (%)	47–60	33–42	—	—	40–50
Arterial pH	7.30–7.40	7.35–7.45	—	—	—
$PaCO_2$ (mm Hg)	30–35	30–40	—	—	—
PaO_2 (mm Hg)	60–90	80–100	—	—	—

Table 28-2. Cardiovascular variables

Age	Heart rate (beats/min)	Blood pressure (mm Hg) Systolic	Diastolic
Preterm neonate	120–180	45–60	30
Term neonate	100–180	55–70	40
1 Year	100–140	70–100	60
3 Years	84–115	75–110	70
5 Years	80–100	80–120	70

Infants who fall into these groups may have dextrose requirements as high as 5–15 mg/kg/min.

2. **Hypocalcemia** is common in infants who are preterm, small for gestational age, asphyxiated, or offspring of diabetic mothers or who have received transfusions with citrated blood or fresh-frozen plasma. Serum calcium concentration should be monitored and calcium chloride administered if the ionized calcium is less than 1.0 mmol/L.

H. **Temperature regulation**
   1. Compared to adults, infants and children have a **greater surface to body weight ratio.** This results in greater losses of body heat by radiation, evaporation, convection, and conduction.
   2. Infants less than 3 months old cannot compensate for cold by shivering.
   3. Infants respond to **cold stress** by increasing norepinephrine production, which enhances metabolism of brown fat. While increasing body heat production, norepinephrine also produces pulmonary and peripheral vasoconstriction. If profound, right-to-left shunting, hypoxia, and metabolic acidosis can result. Sick and preterm infants have limited stores of brown fat and therefore are more susceptible to cold. Strategies to prevent cold stress are discussed in sec. **IV. C.**

II. **The preanesthetic visit.** General principles of the preanesthetic visit are discussed in Chap. 1. The preoperative visit is an excellent opportunity to **allay anxiety** on the part of the child and the parent.
   A. **History**
      1. Maternal health during gestation, including alcohol or drug use, smoking, and viral infections.
      2. Gestational age and weight.
      3. Events during labor and delivery, including APGAR scores.
      4. Neonatal hospitalizations.
      5. Congenital anatomic or metabolic anomalies or syndromes.
      6. Recent upper respiratory infections, croup, or asthmatic episodes.
   B. **Physical examination**
      1. **General appearance** includes alertness, color, tone, congenital anomalies, and head size and shape.

2. **Vital signs,** height, and weight in kilograms.
3. The presence of **loose teeth** or craniofacial anomalies that could complicate airway management should be determined.
4. The respiratory system should be examined for evidence of **upper respiratory infection** as well as for signs of reactive airways disease. These conditions may predispose the patient to laryngospasm and bronchospasm during anesthesia and during the postoperative period.
5. The **cardiovascular system** should be examined with particular attention to the presence of murmurs, which may indicate flow through anatomic shunts. Vascular access is also assessed.
6. **Neurologic examination** should reveal any abnormalities in tone, strength, and developmental milestones.

C. **Laboratory data** that are appropriate for the child's illness and proposed surgery should be obtained.

III. **Premedication and NPO guidelines**

A. **Premedication**

1. Children at any given age show a spectrum of social development. Their behavior may be influenced by experiences they have had at home, in day care or school, and during previous hospitalizations. Honesty about procedures and possible pain involved is necessary to maintain the trust of children regardless of their level of development. Reassuring the parents is often the best way to relieve a child's anxiety.
2. **Infants less than 6 months old** generally tolerate short periods of separation from parents well and require no premedication.
3. **Children 6 months to 5 years** cling to their parents and usually require sedation prior to the induction of anesthesia (see sec. **V.B**).
4. **Older children** generally respond well to information and reassurance. Parental and patient anxiety may be reduced by having parents accompany children to the operating room or to an adjacent holding area. A particularly anxious child may benefit from premedication for transport from his or her room to the operating room holding area. Diazepam, 0.2–0.3 mg/kg PO given 2 hours before surgery, is frequently selected; it causes sedation with minimal respiratory depression. Narcotics, on the other hand, do cause respiratory depression and are best avoided except when specifically indicated (e.g., for children with congenital heart disease). Chloral hydrate at a dose of 25–50 mg/kg per rectum may be used for premedication provided the child is monitored for possible respiratory depression.
5. Premedication with IM anticholinergics is not recommended. If vagolytic drugs are indicated, they are usually administered IV at the time of induction.
6. In the presence of a **hiatal hernia** or **gastroesophageal reflux**, cimetidine, 7.5 mg/kg PO, can be used 2 hours prior to surgery to raise gastric pH and reduce gastric volume.

Table 28-3. Fasting guidelines (hours)

Age	Milk/solids	Clear liquids
< 6 MONTHS	4	2
6–36 MONTHS	6	3
> 36 MONTHS	8	3

7. Children on medication for control of **chronic systemic illnesses** such as asthma, seizures, or hypertension should continue to take these medications preoperatively.

B. **NPO guidelines**

1. **Milk, formula**, and **solid foods** should be restricted as outlined in Table 28-3.

2. The **last feeding** should consist of clear fluids or sugar water. Recent studies suggest that there may be no increased risk of aspiration if clear fluids are offered up to 2 hours preoperatively. In addition, offering clear fluids closer to the time of surgery may decrease the chance of **preoperative dehydration** and **hypoglycemia** and contribute to a smoother induction and more stable operative course. We currently suggest that patients receive clear fluids until 3 hours before surgery is scheduled. Infants less than 6 months old and premature infants should have an IV started for maintenance fluid or receive a clear liquid feeding 2 hours before surgery. Patients are then made NPO (see Table 28-3).

3. If **surgical delays** occur, patients may need to have an IV started for hydration.

IV. **Preparation of the operating room**

A. **Anesthetic circuit**

1. The **semi-closed circuit** normally used in adults is not usually used in infants because

a. The mask, metal connectors, and large-bore tubing significantly increase dead space.

b. The inspiratory and expiratory valves increase the work of breathing.

c. The large volume of the absorber system acts as a reservoir for anesthethic agents.

2. In **children 10 kg or less**, the nonrebreathing, open circuit solves these problems. The **Mapleson D circuit**, which we use most often, is described in Chap. 9.

a. **Rebreathing** is prevented by using fresh gas flows 2.0–2.5 times the minute expiratory volume to wash out carbon dioxide. **Capnography** is helpful in recognizing rebreathing ($F_1CO_2 > 0$) and avoiding excessive hyperventilation.

b. It is essential to use a **heated humidifier** in the circuit.

c. **Reservoir bag volume** should be at least as large as the child's vital capacity but small enough so that a comfortable squeeze does not overinflate the chest.

General guidelines are newborns, 500-ml bag; 1–3 years, 1000-ml bag; and over 3 years, 2000 ml bag.

3. In **children 10–12 kg or more**, the semi-closed circuit-absorber system can be utilized with a smaller reservoir bag and a circuit with small-caliber tubing.

B. **Airway equipment**

1. A **mask** with minimum dead space should be chosen. A clear plastic type is preferred, since it allows observation of the lips (for color) and the mouth (for secretions and vomitus).

2. An appropriate size of **oral airway** can be estimated by holding the airway in position next to the child's face. The tip of the oral airway should reach to the angle of the mandible.

3. **Laryngoscopy**

   a. A narrow handle is preferred.

   b. A straight blade (Miller or Wis-Hipple) is recommended for children less than 2 years old. The smaller flange and long tapered tip of the straight blade provide better visualization of the larynx and manipulation of the epiglottis in the confined spaces of a small oral cavity.

   c. Curved blades are generally used for patients over 5 years old.

   d. Guidelines for laryngoscope blade sizes:

Miller 0	Neonate and premature infant
Miller 1	Up to 6–8 months old
Wis-Hipple 1.5	9 months–2 years old
Miller 2	2–5 years old
Macintosh 2	Child over 5 years old

4. **Endotracheal tubes.** Uncuffed tubes are used for children under age 6–7 years (5.5-mm endotracheal tube). The ideal size will have a leak at 15–20 cm H_2O airway pressure. If the leak is present at less than 10 cm, the endotracheal tube should be changed to the next larger size. At the time of intubation, endotracheal tubes that are one size larger and smaller than the estimated size should be available. Special techniques of endotracheal intubation are discussed in sec. **VI.** Guidelines for endotracheal tube sizes are as follows:

Age	Size (mm internal diameter)
Premature newborn	2.5–3.0
Full-term newborn	3.0
6–12 months	3.5
12–20 months	4.0
2 years	4.5
Over 2 years	$\dfrac{16 + \text{age (years)}}{4}$
French size	Age (years) + 18
Tube length at mouth (cm)	$\dfrac{10 + \text{age (years)}}{2}$

C. **Temperature control**
   1. The **operating room should be warmed** to 80–90°F prior to the child's arrival, and a heating blanket placed on the operating room table. Infants should be kept covered with a blanket and a hat.
   2. A **servocontrolled radiant warmer** will keep infants warm while monitoring is being applied. However, skin temperature should not be allowed to exceed 39°C as measured by a skin thermometer. The servocontrol from a core thermistor should never be used.
   3. **Gases** should be heated and humidified; humidifiers can *actively* warm a child weighing less than 10 kg (0.5 m^2) and prevent *passive* losses in larger children.
   4. **Fluids** and **blood** should also be warmed.

D. **Monitoring**
   1. A **precordial** or **esophageal stethoscope** should be used at all times.
   2. **Electrocardiogram.**
   3. **Blood pressure**
      a. A blood pressure cuff should cover at least two-thirds of the upper arm but not encroach on the axilla or antecubital space.
      b. Blood pressure can also be obtained by using a pediatric-model automated blood pressure device. For children less than 2 years old, a Doppler flow probe may provide more reliable blood pressure readings.
   4. **Pulse oximeters** are particularly useful because infants and small children desaturate rapidly; they also aid in avoiding hyperoxic complications in premature infants.
   5. **Capnographs** are helpful when using nonrebreathing circuit to ensure the adequacy of ventilation. It should be realized that the observed reading for end-tidal carbon dioxide usually will be lower than the patient's because of dilution from fresh inspired gases.
   6. **Temperature** should always be monitored. In small infants it is preferable to monitor esophageal or rectal temperature, rather than axillary temperature, as they are more accurate in reflecting core temperature.
   7. **Urine output** is an excellent reflection of volume status in children. In newborns, 0.5 ml/kg/hr is adequate; for infants over 1 month of age, 1.0 ml/kg/hr usually indicates that renal perfusion is not impaired.

E. **Intravenous set-up**
   1. For **children under 20 kg**, a control chamber (burette) should be used to prevent inadvertent overhydration.
   2. For **older children**, a pediatric infusion set is used where 60 drops equal 1 ml.
   3. Extension tubing with a short T-piece connection is used so that injection ports are not draped out of reach, but drugs should be administered as close to the IV insertion site as possible to avoid the use of excess fluids.
   4. Extra care should be taken to purge IV tubing of air, since, in principle, it is possible for infants to shunt

right-to-left through a patent foramen ovale. Neonates
and children known to have intracardiac shunts should
always have air filters in the IV tubing.

V. Induction techniques

A. **Infants less than 6–8 months old** can be transported to
the operating room without sedation; anesthesia can then
be induced by an inhalation technique (see sec. C). The
vessel-rich organs are proportionately larger and the
muscle and fat groups smaller in neonates than in adults.
This will affect uptake and distribution of inhalation
agents (see Chap. 11).

B. Sedation options for **children 6 months to 5 years old**
not already premedicated include

1. **Rectal methohexital (Brevital)**, 25–30 mg/kg dissolved in sterile water in a 10% solution. The dose is
administered with a syringe fitted with soft plastic
tubing into the distal 1 inch of the rectum. (Blood flow
to the proximal third of the rectum is drained into the
portal circulation, where there is a significant first-
pass effect for methohexital.) Peak effect is after 10–15
minutes; if no sedation occurs after 20 minutes, the full
dose is repeated. Resuscitation equipment and an anesthesiologist should be present after administering
the drug, as it can produce respiratory depression.
Parents should be advised that children frequently
become excited or agitated before reaching a state of
sedation.

2. **Midazolam**, 0.5–1.0 mg/kg, in parenteral solution
dissolved in sweet syrup PO, as an alternative to
methohexital. Sedation is usually produced within 20
minutes, though the time to onset of action can be
somewhat unpredictable. Patients often remain awake
but sedated with this dose, but generally they will
have no recall of leaving their parents or of induction
of anesthesia.

C. **Inhalation induction**

1. This is the method of choice for most pediatric patients,
except when rapid sequence induction is required. In
older children, placement of an IV catheter makes IV
induction an option.

2. An "excitement stage" of anesthesia is often encountered during inhalation induction. For this reason,
stimulation from noise and activity in the operating
room should be minimized.

3. **Techniques**

a. Children 6 months to 5 years old may be induced
after profound sedation with rectal methohexital or
midazolam (called a **"steal" induction**). Specifically, the face mask is held near, but not touching,
the child's face, and low flows (1–3 liters) of oxygen
and nitrous oxide are begun. Then, the volatile
agent (halothane is the least irritating to the airways and is best tolerated) is gradually increased
from 0.5–4.0% in 0.5% increments. When the lid
reflex disappears, the mask can be applied to the
child's face and the jaw gently lifted.

    b. A **slow inhalation induction** may also be used for induction of engageable toddlers and older children who have not been premedicated. Children are shown how to breathe through a clear anesthethic mask painted with flavor extract of their choice. The child's attention is then engaged by telling him a story while he begins to breathe through the face mask attached to an anesthesia circuit. Induction begins with oxygen via face mask, followed by addition of nitrous oxide and gradual incremental addition of volatile anesthetic as in **a.**

    c. Children 6 years old to teenager (with/without oral sedating premedication) may be induced from the awake state with a **single-breath induction.**

        (1) The minimum alveolar concentration of halothane necessary to cause loss of consciousness can be achieved with a single vital capacity breath of 4% halothane in 70% nitrous oxide–oxygen.

        (2) The circuit should be prefilled with nitrous oxide–oxygen (3 : 1) and 4–5% halothane. The end of the circuit should be occluded with a plug or another reservoir bag and pop-off valve left open to minimize nonscavenged anesthetic spillage.

        (3) Painting the mask with flavor extracts will increase acceptance by children.

        (4) The child is instructed to take a deep breath (vital capacity) of room air, blow it all out (forced expiration), and then hold his or her breath. At this point, the anesthesiologist gently places the mask on the patient's face. Then the child takes a deep inspiration (vital capacity) and again holds his or her breath.

        (5) Most children will be asleep in 30–60 seconds; a few children will need more than one breath.

    d. Children can become frightened during an inhalation induction, making them uncooperative and even combative. Should this occur, it is imperative to be prepared with a **backup method,** such as an IM induction or the IV induction through a butterfly needle described in sec. **E.**

D. Intramuscular induction. For the uncooperative or retarded child who is not otherwise controllable, anesthesia may be induced with ketamine (4–10 mg/kg IM), which takes effect in 3–5 minutes. Atropine (0.02 mg/kg IM) or glycopyrrolate (0.01 mg/kg IM) should be mixed with the ketamine to prevent excess salivation. Midazolam, 0.2–0.5 mg/kg IM, may also be added to reduce the chance of emergence delirium that may be associated with ketamine.

E. Intravenous induction

    1. For **children over 10 years old,** the option of having an IV placed should be offered and anesthesia induced as it is in adults; children may require up to 6 mg/kg of thiopental.

    2. A **"butterfly" induction** may be performed in smaller children. A small IV or butterfly needle is quickly inserted, and the child is given an IV induction dose of thiopental. IV induction in such a setting is often preferable to struggling through a potentially difficult mask induction.

F. Children with full stomachs
1. **Rapid sequence induction.** In general, the same principles apply to infants and children as for adults. In addition:
   a. Atropine (0.02 mg/kg, minimum dose 0.1 mg) may be given IV prior to administration of succinylcholine to prevent bradycardia.
   b. Children require larger doses of thiopental (4–6 mg/kg) and succinylcholine (1.5–2.0 mg/kg).
   c. Infants with gastric distention should have their stomachs decompressed by orogastric tubes placed prior to induction to minimize the chance of aspiration.
   d. Cimetidine (7.5 mg/kg PO or IV) can be used to decrease gastric volume and raise gastric pH.
2. **Awake intubations** are often preferable for very sick infants. Those with anatomically abnormal airways also should be intubated awake.

VI. Endotracheal intubation
A. Oral approach
1. Older children are placed in the "sniffing" position using a blanket. Infants and small children have large occiputs, and blankets are often not necessary.
2. The larynx is located during laryngoscopy as in adults, but the tip of the blade is used to elevate the epiglottis.
3. The distance from the glottis to the carina is about 4 cm in a term neonate. Pediatric endotracheal tubes have a single black mark located 2 cm from the tip and a double mark at 3 cm; these markings should be observed as the tube is passed beyond the glottis.
4. If resistance is met during intubation, the next smaller (by one-half size) tube should be tried.
5. Following intubation, the chest should be examined for bilateral equal expansion and the lungs auscultated for equal breath sounds. There should be a leak around the uncuffed tube when 15–20 cm H_2O positive-pressure is applied.
6. Extension of the head can result in extubation, while flexion can result in tube advancement into the right main stem bronchus. Therefore, the chest should be auscultated after *every* change in head position to verify equal bilateral breath sounds.
7. Endotracheal tubes should be **securely taped** using benzoin and tape, and the numerical marking on the tube closest to the gingiva noted; migration of the endotracheal tube will be apparent from any change in this relation.

B. Nasal approach
1. This method is generally similar to that for adults (see Chap. 13).
2. The anterior position of the infant larynx makes an

unaided pass difficult; Magill forceps are almost always needed to guide the tip of the tube through the vocal cords.

3. Nasal intubation should be performed only when specially indicated (e.g., oral surgery), due to the risk of epistaxis from swollen adenoids and tonsils.

4. Apneic infants will become hypoxic within 30–45 seconds, even after preoxygenation. If bradycardia, cyanosis, or desaturation occurs, intubation attempts should cease immediately and 100% oxygen administered until recovery is complete.

C. **Muscle relaxants**

1. Depolarizing and nondepolarizing muscle relaxants are often used to facilitate endotracheal intubation. Muscle relaxants may be contraindicated in infants and children with abnormal airway anatomy.

2. The use of a combination of halothane and succinylcholine during induction may be associated with an increased incidence of masseter spasm. Therefore, this combination is rarely used in current practice; instead, nondepolarizing relaxants are generally selected unless rapid sequence induction is specifically indicated.

3. Succinylcholine can lead to bradycardia, which may be exaggerated with repeated doses. If atropine has not been administered prior to the first dose of succinylcholine, it should be given before the second dose.

VII. **Fluid management.** The following calculations may be used to estimate fluid requirements for infants and children. Other reflections of volume status, including blood pressure, heart rate, urine output, central venous pressure, and pulmonary artery pressure may suggest further adjustments.

A. **Maintenance fluid requirements**

1. Administer 4 ml/kg/hr for the first 10 kg of body weight (100 ml/kg/day), 2 ml/kg/hr for the second 10 kg (50 ml/kg/day), and then add 1 ml/kg/day for more than 20 kg (25 ml/kg/day). (For example, maintenance fluids for a 25-kg child would be $[4 \times 10] + [2 \times 10] + [1 \times 5] = 65$ ml/hr.)

2. The "standard" solution for the healthy child for replacement of fluid deficits and ongoing losses is lactated Ringer's solution. Solutions of 5–10% dextrose are frequently used in the perioperative period for premature infants, septic neonates, infants of diabetic mothers, and those on total parenteral nutrition. These patients should have blood sugar levels periodically checked with Dextrostix.

B. **Estimated blood volume (EBV) and blood losses**

1. **EBV** = 90 ml/kg in neonates
   = 80 ml/kg in infants up to 1 year old
   = 70 ml/kg thereafter

2. **Estimated red cell mass** (ERCM) = EBV × hematocrit/100.

3. **Acceptable red cell loss** (ARCL) = ERCM − $ERCM_{30}$, which is the ERCM at a hematocrit of 30%.

4. **Acceptable blood loss** (ABL) = ARCL × 3.

   a. If the amount of the blood loss is less than one-third

of the ABL, it can be replaced with lactated Ringer's solution.

b. If the amount of blood loss is greater than one-third of the total ABL, it should be replaced with colloid, preferably 5% albumin.

c. If the amount of blood loss is greater than ABL, replace with packed red blood cells and an equal amount of colloid.

d. The above calculations are based on 30% as the minimal acceptable hematocrit, below which transfusion of packed cells is indicated. Under some circumstances, it may be desirable to keep the hematocrit somewhat higher, as when a patient is experiencing rapid ongoing operative blood loss with significant further losses anticipated. In other situations, the hematocrit may be allowed to fall below 30% without significantly increasing risk to the patient. Since it is sometimes difficult to measure small-volume blood losses precisely in young children, monitoring of hematocrit will both help avoid unnecessary transfusions and alert the anesthesiologist to the need for homologous blood transfusion.

C. Estimated fluid deficit (EFD) = (maintenance fluid/hr) × hours since the last oral intake. The entire EFD is replaced during all major cases; the first half is given during the first hour, and the remaining deficit is divided over the next 1–2 hours.

D. Third-space losses may require up to an additional 10 ml/kg/hr of lactated Ringer's solution or normal saline if there is extensive exposure of the intestine or a significant ileus.

VIII. Emergence and postanesthesia care

A. Extubation. As infants and children enter stage II (excitement) during emergence from anesthesia, they are at significant risk for **laryngospasm.** It is important to avoid extubation during this critical period. The patient may be extubated "deep" while still in stage III. This is most appropriate in cases such as inguinal hernia repairs where coughing on emergence is undesirable or in patients with reactive airways disease. Obviously a "deep" extubation would not be appropriate where there is an increased risk of aspiration. In the majority of cases, children are extubated after emerging through stage II. Coughing is not a sign that the child is ready for extubation. Rather, patients should demonstrate "purposeful" activity (e.g., reaching for the endotracheal tube, squeezing fingers on command) or eye opening before extubation.

B. During transport to the postanesthesia care unit (PACU) on supplemental oxygen, the child's color, respiratory pattern, and gas exchange should be continuously monitored.

C. In the PACU, the child is maintained on oxygen via face mask or tent and monitored with pulse oximetry until fully awake. Early reunion of children with their parents is desirable.

IX. Specific pediatric anesthesia problems

A. The compromised airway

1. **Etiologies**
   a. Congenital abnormalities (e.g., choanal atresia, Pierre Robin syndrome, tracheal stenosis, laryngeal web).
   b. Inflammation (e.g., croup, epiglottitis, pharyngeal abscess).
   c. Foreign bodies in the trachea or esophagus.
   d. Neoplasms (e.g., congenital hemangioma, cystic hygroma, thoracic lymphadenopathy).
   e. Trauma.
2. **Management**
   a. Administer 100% oxygen by face mask.
   b. Keep the child as calm as possible. Evaluation should be kept to a minimum, since it may increase agitation and cause further airway compromise. Parents are invaluable in their ability to pacify their children and should remain with them as long as feasible.
   c. An anesthesiologist must be present during transport to the operating room. Oxygen, a Hope-type resuscitation bag and mask, laryngoscope, atropine, succinylcholine, and appropriate-size endotracheal tubes must also be available.
   d. **Induction of anesthesia**
      (1) **Minimize manipulation of the patient.** A precordial stethoscope and pulse oximeter are all the monitoring that is necessary during the initial phase of induction.
      (2) **A gradual inhalation induction** in a sitting position with the parents present is begun using 100% oxygen and halothane. Airway obstruction with poor air exchange will prolong induction.
      (3) Parents are then asked to leave when the child becomes unconscious, and an IV is started. **Atropine** may be given at this time.
      (4) **Patients with croup** may benefit from gentle application of continuous positive airway pressure, but any positive pressure can cause acute airway obstruction in patients with epiglottitis or a foreign body.
      (5) The **oral endotracheal tube** chosen should be styletted and at least one size smaller than the one predicted.
      (6) At this point, patients are usually hypercarbic (end-tidal carbon dioxide 50–60 mm Hg), but it is generally well tolerated provided they are not also hypoxic. Bradycardia is an indication of hypoxia and requires immediate establishment of a patent airway.
      (7) Perform **laryngoscopy** only when the patient is deeply anesthetized. Muscle relaxants are contraindicated, except as a true last resort. Orotracheal intubation should be accompanied before any further airway procedures are attempted,

except in cases of large upper airway foreign bodies of friable subglottic tumors (e.g., hemangiomas), when bronchoscopy is indicated prior to intubation.

(8) For **illnesses that require several days of intubation** (e.g., epiglottitis), a nasal tube may be better tolerated. Orotracheal tubes may be changed to nasotracheal tubes at the end of the procedure and carefully secured, provided the oral intubation was easily accomplished.

(9) Children should be sedated for **transport** to an intensive care unit; a combination of a narcotic and a benzodiazepine is particularly effective. Breathing may be spontaneous or assisted during the immediate postoperative period.

B. Intraabdominal malformations

1. These include pyloric stenosis, gastroschisis, omphalocele, atresia of the small intestine, and volvulus.

2. **Management**

   a. Gastrointestinal emergencies frequently lead to marked **dehydration** and **electrolyte abnormalities**. Repair of pyloric stenosis should be delayed as long as necessary to replenish intravascular volume and correct hypochloremic metabolic alkalosis. However, the situation is more urgent with the other lesions, and rehydration may need to be accomplished intraoperatively.

   b. Abdominal distention in infants and young children rapidly causes **respiratory compromise**, so nasogastric drainage is mandatory. Even so, many patients require intubation prior to the induction of anesthesia; awake intubation is often all that is tolerated.

   c. Children with less severe physiologic disturbances and only mild or moderate distention can be managed with **rapid sequence inductions.**

   d. In **toxic children**, arterial and central venous pressure catheters and a Foley catheter may be needed.

   e. **Anesthetics** with minimal cardiac depression and vasodilatation are the safest agents for such cases; oxygen/air mixtures, narcotics, and relaxants are usually better tolerated than the potent inhalation agents. Nitrous oxide should be avoided, since it will add to the abdominal distention.

   f. **Fluid and heat losses.** When the bowel is exposed and manipulated, third-space losses may be excessive, and remarkable fluid volumes may be needed to maintain blood pressure. Even when employing all the possible warming strategies, heat loss is usually unavoidable.

   g. **Postoperative ventilatory support** is often indicated until abdominal distention is diminished, body temperature normalizes, and fluid shifting ceases.

C. Thoracic emergencies

1. **Tracheoesophageal fistula**

   a. Tracheoesophageal fistula and esophageal atresia
   can present in several combinations.
   (1) **Esophageal atresia with a fistula between
   the trachea and the distal segment of the
   esophagus** is the most common of these lesions
   (about 90%). Neonates with this anomaly choke
   and become cyanotic during their first feeding.
   The diagnosis is confirmed by the inability to
   pass a feeding tube into the stomach, and chest
   x-ray demonstrates the feeding tube curled in
   the proximal esophageal pouch. Air in the stomach and bowel confirms the presence of a fistula.
   (2) The H-**type fistula without esophageal
   atresia** is the next most common of these lesions.
   These children usually present somewhat later
   in life with a history of frequent pulmonary
   infections.
   b. The most common **complication** in all forms of
   tracheoesophageal fistula is pneumonitis secondary
   to pulmonary aspiration.
   c. Preoperative management
   (1) Neonates should be kept **NPO** when this diagnosis is suspected.
   (2) Maintaining the **upright position** minimizes
   the chance of gastric reflux and pulmonary aspiration of gastric fluid.
   (3) Saliva in the proximal pouch is frequently aspirated. Thus, a **nasogastric tube** should be
   placed in the pouch and continuously suctioned.
   (4) **Chest x-ray** and **cardiac echocardiogram**
   should be obtained to rule out associated cardiac
   anomalies.
   (5) **Pulmonary complications** are present in
   nearly all patients and should be treated prior to
   surgery. Surgical intervention is urgent, but not
   an emergency. If repair must be delayed, a
   percutaneous gastrostomy tube may be placed in
   the interim under local anesthesia to diminish
   gastric distention.
   d. Intraoperative management
   (1) Usually an **awake or rapid sequence intubation** is done. Narcotics and inhalation agents
   may be used as tolerated; muscle relaxants are
   usually necessary to facilitate access to the abdomen or chest.
   (2) The **endotracheal tube** should be positioned
   below the fistula, which usually enters 1–2 cm
   above the carina. One technique for placement is
   to perform a deliberate endobronchial intubation, then withdraw until bilateral breath
   sounds are first heard. In this position, the
   endotracheal tube will almost always be below
   the fistula.
   (3) Prior to tracheoesophageal fistula repair, a **gastrostomy tube** may be placed to decompress the
   stomach.

       (4) After the fistula is ligated, the **esophagus** is primarily repaired. However, the gastrostomy is left in place, since esophageal motility is usually abnormal. Gastroesophageal reflux is commonly encountered postoperatively, ultimately requiring fundoplication in about 50% of these patients.

  e. The **postoperative** course is usually dominated by the presence of pulmonary complications or associated anomalies.

2. **Congenital diaphragmatic hernia** (see Chap. 27 for pathogenesis and presentation).

  a. **Pathophysiology**

    (1) **Mechanical compression** of lung tissue.

    (2) **Abnormal pulmonary parenchymal development** with diminished numbers of alveoli.

    (3) **Right-to-left shunting.** In neonates, hypoxemia and acidosis inhibit normal closure of the **ductus arteriosus** and at the same time cause pulmonary vasoconstriction (**pulmonary hypertension**). The net result is a return to fetal-type circulation in which most of the cardiac output bypasses the lungs; this is the cause of the intractable hypoxia associated with congenital diaphragmatic hernia. Severe right-to-left shunting may intermittently appear during surgery and is also the most frequent cause of death in the postoperative period.

  b. **Anesthetic considerations**

    (1) A **nasogastric tube** should be placed to relieve distention and minimize respiratory compromise.

    (2) Positive-pressure ventilation by mask should not be applied, since it can cause inflation of the bowel and precipitate decompensation.

    (3) Most of these patients require emergency **intubation** prior to arrival in the operating room. After intubation, ventilation should be controlled using minimal positive pressure to prevent overinflation of the contralateral lung. If there is a sudden deterioration, a pneumothorax of the contralateral side should be suspected.

    (4) Nitrous oxide is contraindicated, since it will cause bowel distention.

    (5) Initially, **100% oxygen** and **muscle relaxation** may be all that are tolerated until the thorax is decompressed. Afterward, judicious doses of **narcotics** are desirable, since adequate anesthesia seems to help prevent episodic right-to-left shunting. Recent experimental evidence suggests that nitric oxide may also act as a potent pulmonary vasodilator.

    (6) **Acidosis** and **hypercarbia** must be corrected with hyperventilation and sodium bicarbonate to avoid elevations in pulmonary vascular resistance.

(7) **Hypothermia** and **light anesthesia** should be vigorously treated, sine they too can precipitate a return to fetal-type circulation.

c. **Postoperative care**

(1) These infants have atelectatic and/or hypoplastic lungs and continue to require **ventilation** postoperatively. When possible, high airway pressures should be avoided.

(2) Due to the frequency of pneumothorax, **bilateral chest tubes** are frequently placed prophylactically.

(3) **Pulmonary artery hypertension** persists in 40% of cases. A "preductal" arterial catheter and often a central venous catheter are needed for optimal postoperative management.

(4) **Prognosis** is poor in patients with severely hypoplastic lungs. Despite aggressive therapy, in the past most patients died of intractable hypoxia and acidosis. In recent years, advances with extracorporeal membrane oxygenation in infants have improved survival among these patients (see Chap. 27).

D. **Congenital heart disease.** For relevant physiologic and anesthetic considerations, see Chap. 23 and references cited therein.

E. **Head and neck procedures**

1. **Strabismus repair** is the most common pediatric ocular surgery performed in the United States. Anesthetic considerations include the oculocardiac reflex, postoperative nausea and vomiting, and an increased risk of masseter spasm in these patients. See Chap. 25 for a full discussion.

2. **Tonsillectomy, adenoidectomy,** and emergency surgery in the child with **bleeding tonsils** are outlined in Chap. 25.

X. **Regional anesthesia.** A better understanding of the pharmacokinetics and pharmacodynamics of local anesthetics in infants and children and the development of regional anesthetic techniques and equipment specifically designed for children have facilitated the use of regional anesthesia for pediatric patients.

A. **Pharmacology of local anesthetics**

1. **Protein binding** of local anesthetics is decreased in neonates due to decreased levels of serum albumin. Resultant increases in free drug concentration may occur, especially for bupivacaine.

2. **Plasma cholinesterase** activity is decreased by approximately 50% in infants under 6 months old, theoretically diminishing clearance of amino esters.

3. **Hepatic microsomal enzyme systems** are immature in the neonate, leading to decreased clearance of amino amides.

4. **Increased volume of distribution** in the infant and child, on the other hand, acts to decrease free local anesthetic concentrations in the blood significantly.

5. Systemic toxicity is the most frequent complication of regional anesthetics, and doses should be carefully calculated on a per kilogram basis. The risk of accumulation of free drug following repeated doses of local anesthetics is increased in infants and children.

B. **Spinal anesthesia**
   1. **Indications**
      a. Premature infants less than 60 weeks' postconceptual age and infants with a history of bronchopulmonary dysplasia, apnea, or need for ventilatory support are at increased risk for apnea and cardiovascular instability following general anesthesia. Spinal anesthesia where appropriate (e.g., inguinal hernia repair) may decrease the likelihood of these postoperative anesthetic complications. However, these infants still require a minimum of 24 hours of cardiorespiratory monitoring postoperatively regardless of the anesthetic technique selected.
      b. Children at significant risk for malignant hyperthermia.
      c. Children with chronic airways disease such as asthma or cystic fibrosis.
      d. Cooperative older children and adolescents with full stomachs undergoing emergency surgery.
   2. **Anatomy.** See Chap. 16.
   3. **Technique**
      a. The procedure may be performed in the lateral decubitus or sitting position. For premature infants and neonates, to limit rostral spread of drug, the patient is positioned in the sitting position. The head is supported upright to prevent upper airway obstruction. A 22-gauge, 1.5-inch spinal needle is generally used for infants. In children older than 2 years, a 25- or 26-gauge needle is preferred.
      b. An IV should be started prior to the block and the patient monitored throughout the procedure. In addition, attention to maintaining normothermia is essential, especially for premature infants and neonates. The infant should remain supine at all times after the spinal is in place, avoiding Trendelenburg or reverse Trendelenburg positioning.
   4. **Drugs and dosage**
      a. Hyperbaric solutions of tetracaine, bupivacaine, and lidocaine are most frequently used.
      b. Increased dosage requirement and shorter duration of action are seen in infants.
      c. **Recommended dosages** (for a T4 level)
         (1) **Tetracaine** 1%, 0.5–1.0 mg/kg in the infant and 0.25–0.5 mg/kg in the child.
         (2) **Lidocaine** 5%, 2 mg/kg in the infant and 1 mg/kg in the child.
         (3) **Bupivacaine** 0.75%, 0.3 mg/kg in both infants and children.
      d. **Duration** of surgical anesthesia averages 90 minutes with tetracaine, less with lidocaine and bupi-

vacaine. Blocks may be prolonged with the addition of epinephrine, 10 μg/kg (up to 0.2 mg), or phenylephrine, 75 μg/kg (up to 2 mg).

5. Complications and contraindications

   a. Blockade recedes from its initial level significantly more rapidly in children than in adults. If blockade is inadequate, supplemental anesthesia must be used cautiously, especially in premature infants and neonates.

   b. Hypotension is very rare in children less than 7–10 years old, perhaps because resting sympathetic vascular tone is lower than in adults. A "high spinal" anesthetic may be heralded only by mottled skin or apnea with bradycardia.

   c. Contraindications are for an adult to receive spinal anesthesia, with particular attention to congenital CNS anatomic defects and a history of grade III–IV intraventricular hemorrhage.

C. Caudal and epidural anesthesia

   1. Indications. These techniques are useful in combination with light general anesthesia for minor and major procedures of the thorax, abdomen, pelvis, and lower extremities, particularly when significant postoperative pain is anticipated (e.g., orthopedic surgery).

   2. Anatomy is as outlined in Chap. 16. Note that the dural sac ends at S3 in the neonate, and therefore, in infants, caution will be needed to avoid dural puncture during placement of the caudal needle.

   3. Technique is as outlined in Chap. 16.

   a. Most caudal and lumbar (not thoracic) epidural anesthetics are placed after induction of general anesthesia.

   b. Caudal anesthesia may be administered as a **single injection** of local anesthetic through a 1.5-inch short-bevel needle in the caudal space. This technique is ideally suited to short procedures with significant postoperative pain such as inguinal hernia repair and circumcision. Alternatively, for longer procedures or prolonged postoperative analgesia, a catheter may be threaded from the sacral epidural space cephalad to an appropriate level. Intermittent boluses or a continuous infusion of local anesthetic with or without narcotic through the catheter may be used. In infants, 22-gauge caudal catheters are placed through 20-gauge, 40- to 50-mm Tuohy needles; older children require 17- or 18-gauge, 90- to 100-mm Tuohy needles and 20-gauge catheters.

   c. Caudal catheters are readily threaded to lumbar or thoracic levels in children less than 7 years of age, in whom the epidural space is not yet extensively vascularized (T6–9 region for thoracic surgery [e.g., pectus excavatum repair], T10–12 for abdominal surgery [e.g., Nissen fundoplication or bowel resections], and L3–4 for pelvic procedures). While easy to place, the caudal catheter has the potential to become more readily contaminated than a more cephalad catheter.

d. **Epidural catheters** may also be placed via the lumbar and thoracic routes. The distance from skin to epidural space is short (1–2 cm) in children, and care must be taken to avoid dural puncture. Loss of resistance is usually accomplished with saline. In older children, 18-gauge Tuohy needles and 20-gauge catheters are used. The use of thoracic epidural catheters is generally restricted to adolescents who can be awake with sedation during the procedure.

4. **Drugs and dosage**

a. In **single-dose caudal anesthesia**, long duration of sensory blockade with minimal motor blockade is desirable. Bupivacaine 0.125–0.25% with epinephrine is bolused according to the formula 0.06 ml of local anesthetic/kg/segment, where number of segments is counted from S5 to the desired level of analgesia. Increasing the concentration of bupivacaine above 0.25% does not appear to improve analgesia. Dosages of bupivacaine up to 3.5 mg/kg result in plasma levels in infants and children below the toxic range for adults.

b. **Caudal or epidural catheter anesthesia**

(1) **Intermittent bolus dosing.** Initially 1% lidocaine, 0.5 ml/kg, followed by 0.5% lidocaine, 0.5 ml/kg every hour as needed, or initially 0.5% bupivacaine, 0.5 ml/kg, followed by 0.25% bupivacaine, 0.25 ml/kg every 1.5–2.0 hours as needed, is recommended.

(2) **Continuous infusion.** An initial loading dose of 0.04 ml/kg/segment of 0.1% bupivacaine with or without fentanyl, 3 μg/ml in infants and children younger than 7 years and 0.02 ml/kg/segment for children older than 7 years, is recommended. An infusion of 0.1% bupivacaine with or without fentanyl, 3 μg/ml at 0.1 ml/kg/hr, is started immediately following the bolus. The infusion rate may be brought up to 0.3 ml/kg/hr as needed, with the total hourly dose of fentanyl not to exceed 1 μg/kg/hr. Infants younger than 1 year generally do not receive fentanyl in the epidural infusion.

c. **Postoperative analgesia** may be provided by infusion through the caudal or epidural catheter. Generally, an infusion of 0.1% bupivacaine with fentanyl, 3 μg/ml at 0.1–0.3 ml/kg/hr, will provide good analgesia without motor blockade. However, some patients benefit from omission of local anesthetic from the infusion, and fentanyl, 0.5–1.0 μg/kg/hr can be used in these patients. Infants younger than 1 year old, as noted in **b**, usually do not receive epidural narcotics in our institution because of concern over postoperative respiratory depression. Bupivacaine 0.1%, 0.1–0.3 ml/kg/hr, is used for infants younger than 1 year.

> **5. Contraindications** are as for spinal anesthesia (see sec. **B.5**).
> **6. Complications** of epidural and caudal anesthesia are discussed in Chap. 16.

D. Brachial plexus blocks (for upper extremity surgery), **penile blocks** (for circumcision), and **ilioinguinal blocks** (for inguinal hernia repair) are also particularly useful regional techniques in the pediatric population. They are described more fully in Chap. 17 and in Gregory's *Pediatric Anesthesia* (see Suggested Reading).

SUGGESTED READING

Cloherty, J., and Stark, A. *Manual of Neonatal Care*. Boston: Little, Brown, 1991.

Dorsch, J., and Dorsch, S. The Breathing System II: The Mapleson Systems. *Understanding Anesthesia Equipment*. Baltimore: Williams & Wilkins, 1984. Pp. 182–196.

Gregory, G. *Pediatric Anesthesia*. New York: Churchill Livingstone, 1989.

Ryan, J., et al. *A Practice of Anesthesia for Infants and Children*. Philadelphia: Saunders, 1986.

29

Anesthesia for Obstetrics and Gynecology

John S. Wadlington

I. **Maternal physiology in pregnancy.** The pregnant woman is physiologically different from the nonpregnant woman in many ways.
   A. **Respiratory system**
      1. Capillary engorgement of the mucosa takes place throughout the respiratory tract. This swelling decreases the size of the glottic opening such that a 6.0- to 6.5-mm endotracheal tube is recommended for intubation to decrease the possibility of airway trauma.
      2. Lung volumes and capacities are not greatly changed in the pregnant patient, but functional residual capacity is decreased 15–20% at term. Also, up to 50% of pregnant women will develop airway closure during normal tidal ventilation, making them more susceptible to atelectasis. These two factors, along with increased oxygen consumption during pregnancy, make the pregnant patient more vulnerable to hypoxia.
   B. **Cardiovascular system**
      1. The blood volume increases markedly throughout the course of pregnancy. Since the plasma volume increases more than the red cell volume increase, a relative dilutional anemia occurs.
      2. Stroke volume increases an average of 30% and heart rate an average of 15%, resulting in a 40% increase in cardiac output. During labor, contractions of the engorged uterus will provide a 300- to 500-ml autotransfusion into the maternal circulation, leading to a further increase in cardiac output. Cardiac output becomes highest immediately postpartum and can reach 80–100% above the prelabor value. Blood pressure is not increased in normal pregnancy, indicating a decrease in peripheral vascular resistance.
      3. Near term, the large gravid uterus may obstruct the aorta and inferior vena cava of the patient when lying supine. This may result in decreased venous return, decreased cardiac output, and decreased uteroplacental blood flow. Left uterine displacement will prevent aortocaval compression when supine.
      4. The pregnant patient becomes hypercoagulable throughout gestation. Factors VII, VIII, X, and fibrinogen become markedly elevated after the first trimester. This hypercoagulable state leads to decreased blood loss at delivery. Normal blood loss is about 500 ml for vaginal delivery and 1000 ml for cesarean section.
   C. **Central nervous system**
      1. The minimum alveolar concentration for inhalation anesthetics is decreased up to 40% during pregnancy. The etiology for this is unclear but may be related to

457

hormonal and endogenous opiate changes during pregnancy.

2. Due to increased intraabdominal pressure, epidural veins become distended, making a bloody tap during placement of an epidural catheter more common.

3. The pregnant patient requires less local anesthetic to produce the same degree of epidural anesthesia than a nonpregnant patient. Reasons for this include the distended epidural veins, which decrease the effective size of the epidural space as well as prevent loss of drug through the intervertebral foramina. Low cerebrospinal fluid protein will increase the unbound fraction of the local anesthetic, resulting in more free active drug. There may also be hormonally induced changes in sensitivity to local anesthetics from increased progesterone levels. Pregnant patients likewise need 30–50% less local anesthetic for subarachnoid anesthesia.

D. **Gastrointestinal system.** The gravid uterus causes a shift in the position of the stomach, resulting in gastric reflux and heartburn in 45–70% of pregnant patients. Gastric emptying is delayed, and the pregnant patient should be considered at risk for aspiration. If general anesthesia is planned, metoclopramide and a nonparticulate antacid should be given routinely and rapid sequence induction used. Exactly when during pregnancy a woman becomes "at risk" for regurgitation is controversial. Plasma gastrin levels are elevated throughout pregnancy, and reduced sphincter tone has been documented as early as 15 weeks into gestation. In general, any patient in her third trimester or with symptoms of esophagitis during pregnancy should have rapid sequence induction.

E. **Renal system.** Renal plasma flow and glomerular filtration may increase up to 50%, leading to increased creatinine clearance and a decrease in normal blood urea nitrogen and creatinine levels.

II. **Labor and delivery**

A. **Labor** can be divided into three stages.

1. The **first stage** begins with the onset of regular contractions and ends with full cervical dilation.

2. The **second stage** extends from full cervical dilation to delivery of the infant.

3. The **third stage** begins with delivery of the infant and ends with delivery of the placenta.

B. **Pain** during the first part of labor is primarily due to uterine contractions and cervical dilation. Nerve fibers that transmit pain during the first part of labor enter the spinal cord from T10 to L1. In late first-stage and early second-stage labor, pain is due to perineal stretching and travels through the S2–S4 segments via the pudendal nerve.

C. **Physiologic changes** during labor tend to accentuate many of the changes already present during pregnancy. Oxygen uptake, which may increase 20% in a normal pregnancy, may increase an additional 60% during painful uterine contractions.

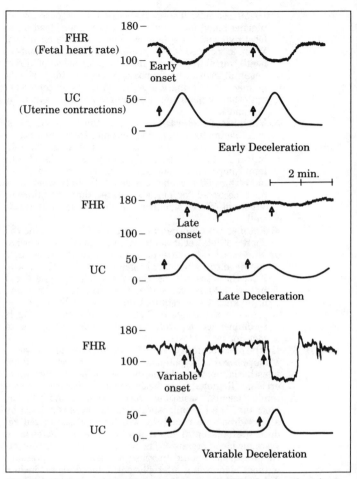

Fig. 29-1. Patterns of periodic fetal heart rate (FHR) decelerations in relation to uterine contractions (UC). See text for details.

    D. Fetal monitoring can provide a fairly accurate assessment of fetal well-being. Normal fetal heart rate ranges from 120–160 beats/min. Monitoring the response of the fetal heart rate to uterine contraction can alert physicians to possible fetal asphyxia or distress (Fig. 29-1).

        1. Early decelerations occur concomitantly with uterine contraction and provide a mirror image of the contraction on the monitor printout. They are thought to be caused by an increase in vagal tone, perhaps from compression of the fetal head, and do not require intervention.

        2. Late decelerations have their beginning and resolution delayed after the onset of uterine contraction by

10–30 seconds. These are caused by a decrease in uterine blood flow during the contraction, leading to fetal hypoxia. Late decelerations are cause for alarm. When associated with loss of normal baseline "beat-to-beat" variability, they may be indicative of direct neonatal myocardial hypoxia. Vigorous efforts should be made to eliminate late decelerations by correcting maternal hypotension and administering oxygen by face mask.

3. **Variable decelerations** are, as the name suggests, variable in duration and appearance from one contraction to the next and are usually associated with umbilical cord compression. They may be associated with fetal compromise when severe (heart rate below 70 for more than 60 seconds) but generally only when they have occurred for periods greater than 30 minutes. Vigorous efforts should be made to correct these as well.

4. **Fetal scalp blood sampling** is used to determine the degree of fetal acidosis from asphyxia when abnormal fetal heart rate patterns cannot be corrected or their significance is unclear. In general, if the pH is above 7.25, the fetus will be vigorous at birth, while a **pH below 7.20** suggests that the fetus is acidotic and asphyxiated and requires immediate delivery. If the pH is in the range of 7.20–7.25, close monitoring is recommended as well as repeat scalp sampling to monitor for acidosis.

III. **Medications commonly used for labor and delivery**

A. **Vasopressors.** Hypotension can result from regional anesthesia, aortocaval compression, or peripartum hemorrhage. Regional anesthesia causes a decrease in systemic vascular resistance resulting from sympathetic blockade. The uteroplacental circulation is regulated by alpha-adrenergic receptors, which when stimulated reduce uteroplacental blood flow despite an increase in systemic blood pressure. The ideal vasopressor for obstetric anesthesia should increase maternal blood pressure without decreasing uteroplacental blood flow. Such a drug should have predominant beta-adrenergic effects and limited alpha effects.

1. **Ephedrine** stimulates both alpha and beta receptors and thus provides cardiac stimulation with a subsequent increase in peripheral and uterine blood flow. **Ephedrine is the drug of choice for treatment of maternal hypotension.**

2. Pure alpha-adrenergic agents like **phenylephrine** and **methoxamine** and mixed alpha agonists such as **epinephrine** and **norepinephrine** are vasoconstrictors that will increase maternal blood pressure at the expense of uteroplacental blood flow. However, phenylephrine in small doses to treat maternal hypotension has been shown to produce no effect on uteroplacental flow. It is used only when ephedrine is ineffective or contraindicated.

B. Oxytocics
  1. Indications. Oxytocics are agents that stimulate uterine contractions. Their primary uses are
    a. To induce or augment labor.
    b. To control postpartum bleeding and uterine atony.
    c. To induce therapeutic abortion.
  2. The most frequently used drugs include the synthetic posterior pituitary hormone, oxytocin (Pitocin), the ergot alkaloids, ergonovine (Ergotrate), and methylergonovine (Methergine).
    a. Oxytocin acts on the uterine smooth muscle to stimulate both the frequency and force of contractions. It also has effects on the cardiovascular system, including a decrease in systolic and especially diastolic blood pressure, tachycardia, and arrhythmias. In high doses, an antidiuretic effect can be seen, leading to water intoxication, cerebral edema, and convulsions in the presence of overzealous IV hydration.
    b. Ergot alkaloids in small doses increase the force and frequency of uterine contractions, followed by normal uterine relaxation. At higher doses, contractions become more intense and prolonged, resting tonus is increased, and tetanic contractions occur. For these reasons, the use of ergot alkaloids is restricted for use in the third stage of labor to control postpartum bleeding. These drugs also have effects on the cardiovascular system, including vasoconstriction and hypertension, especially in the presence of vasopressors. IM administration is recommended, as IV injection has been associated with severe hypertension, convulsions, stroke, retinal detachment, and pulmonary edema.
    c. Prostaglandin $F_{2\alpha}$ has become the third line of therapy following oxytocin and ergot alkaloids for uterine atony. It is given intramyometrially and causes tetanic uterine contraction. Transient hypertension and severe bronchoconstriction have been reported following its use.
C. Tocolytics
  1. These drugs are used to delay or stop premature labor. In general, tocolytics are used for fetuses with gestational ages between 20 and 34–36 weeks. Cervical dilation of less than 4 cm and cervical effacement of less than 80% are associated with a greater likelihood of terminating premature labor.
  2. Indications
    a. To delay or prevent premature labor.
    b. To slow or arrest labor while initiating other therapeutic measures (e.g., steroid therapy to mature fetal lungs).
  3. Contraindications
    a. Chorioamnionitis.
    b. Fetal distress.
    c. Preeclampsia or eclampsia.

4. Specific drugs
  a. Terbutaline and ritodrine, are "selective" beta-2 agonists used to inhibit preterm labor and produce myometrial inhibition. This beta-2 stimulation will also produce bronchodilation and vasodilation and may result in undesirable tachycardia. Metabolic effects include hyperglycemia, hypokalemia, and hyperinsulinemia. It can also produce metabolic (lactic) acidosis. Pulmonary edema may also develop but usually only after 24 hours of therapy. Before beginning treatment with a beta-2 agonist, a baseline electrocardiogram (ECG) should be obtained and preexisting hyperglycemia should be corrected.
  b. Magnesium sulfate is more commonly used for the treatment of preeclampsia (see sec. **VII.C.4**) and is also an effective tocolytic agent. The mechanism of action remains uncertain. Patients receiving magnesium sulfate are more sensitive to both the depolarizing and nondepolarizing muscle relaxants.
  c. Other drugs known for their tocolytic properties are ethanol, prostaglandin synthetase inhibitors, and calcium channel blocking agents. These drugs are inferior to the drugs previously mentioned.

IV. Placental transfer of drugs
  A. Placental transport of anesthetics occurs primarily by passive diffusion as described by Fick's law of diffusion. Briefly, drugs with a high diffusion constant more readily cross the placental membranes. **Factors that promote rapid diffusion** include the following:
    1. Low molecular weight (< 600 daltons).
    2. High lipid solubility.
    3. Low degree of ionization (the more drug in the "free" nonionized form at physiologic pH, the more diffusible).
    4. Low protein binding.
  B. Most of the **agents used to produce sedation, analgesia, or anesthesia** are of low molecular weight, high lipid solubility, relatively nonionized, and minimally protein bound, accounting for their early passage across the placenta.
  C. Muscle relaxants are water soluble and ionized, have high molecular weights, and therefore tend not to cross the placenta.
  D. Damage to the placenta, as seen in hypertension, diabetes, and toxemia, may lead to loss of placental capillary integrity, resulting in nonselective transfer of materials across the placenta.

V. Anesthesia for labor and vaginal delivery (see sec. **XIII** for standards for conduction anesthesia in obstetrics).
  A. Natural childbirth. Many women opt to have no medication at all during labor and delivery. If these patients have any medical problems, however, it would be prudent to know them in advance should the need for an emergency anesthetic arise.
  B. Supplemental medication. Systemic medications are used to relieve pain and anxiety during labor and delivery. There is no ideal medication, as they all cross the

placenta and may depress the fetus. Most commonly used drugs are narcotics such as meperidine (Demerol) and oxymorphone (Numorphan) and agonist-antagonist agents like butorphanol and nalbuphine. Anxiolytics such as diazepam (2.5–10.0 mg) may be used in low doses if needed. Larger doses have been associated with newborn hypotonia and impaired thermal regulation.

C. **Epidural** blockade can provide analgesia through labor and delivery, as well as anesthesia for cesarean section. Epidural analgesia is usually initiated when active labor has been achieved (cervix dilated 5–6 cm in a primipara, 3–4 cm in a multipara). Placement of the epidural earlier than this may slow the progress of labor such that oxytocics may be necessary.

1. **Advantages**
   a. There is a decreased need for systemic pain medications that may produce neonatal depression.
   b. Reducing pain will decrease endogenous catecholamine secretion.
   c. The mother is awake and able to participate in labor and delivery.
   d. It can be used for cesarean section if necessary.
   e. Compared with general anesthesia, there is a lower risk of pulmonary aspiration.

2. **Disadvantages**
   a. Hypotension is the most common problem and can lead to uteroplacental insufficiency.
   b. Progress of labor may be delayed.
   c. Toxic reaction to local anesthetic agents is possible.
   d. Postdural puncture headache is possible.

3. **Contraindications**
   a. Patient refusal.
   b. Coagulation disorder (e.g., in abruption or preeclampsia).
   c. Infection at site.
   d. Hypovolemic shock.

4. **Technique**
   a. A large-bore IV should be placed, and at least 500–1000 ml of crystalloid (preferably warmed) should be infused prior to placement. This will help prevent hypotension as the epidural takes effect.
   b. A 30-ml dose of a nonparticulate antacid should be administered prior to beginning epidural placement.
   c. Baseline vital signs and fetal heart rate should be recorded.
   d. Patients may be in the lateral decubitus or sitting position for lumbar catheter placement (see Chap. 16).

5. **Anesthetics**
   a. A **test dose** of 3 ml of 1.5% lidocaine with epinephrine 1:200,000 should always be given to rule out subarachnoid or intravascular injection.
   b. For analgesia during labor, a **dilute, long-acting local anesthetic** such as bupivacaine 0.25% or 0.125% is commonly used. The dilute solution

should provide adequate analgesia without causing motor blockade or impeding the progress of labor. Incremental doses of 3–5 ml of the selected anesthetic are given every 3–5 minutes until the patient is comfortable (usually T10 for labor and delivery). Blood pressure should be monitored every few minutes to ensure that hypotension has not occurred. Hypotension may be treated with ephedrine, 5–10 mg IV, and repeated as necessary. Theoretically, any local anesthetic can be used (lidocaine 1–2%, chloroprocaine 2–3%, or bupivacaine 0.25–0.5%), although the more concentrated local anesthetics will tend to produce a dense blockade and should be reserved for cesarean sections. Epidural bupivacaine 0.75% is no longer approved for use in obstetric anesthesia because of its association with cardiac arrest in these patients.

c. During the course of labor, the epidural can either be augmented every few hours as needed for patient comfort, or a continuous infusion of a dilute local anesthetic can be used (0.125% bupivacaine).

d. A small amount of **narcotic** such as fentanyl (2–3 µg/ml) added to the infusion may improve the degree of analgesia for the patient.

6. **Complications**

a. **Neurologic complications.** The most common neurologic complication is postdural puncture headache. A dural puncture with an epidural needle is likely to produce headache because of the large needle size (17-gauge) (70% incidence of headache in parturients with "wet-tap"). Bed rest, hydration, and analgesics are the initial treatments of choice. Caffeine preparations have proved to be of some help, although nursing mothers may prefer to avoid this. If after 24–48 hours conservative measures fail, the headache is best treated with an epidural blood patch.

b. **Intravascular injection** is most often heralded by agitation, visual disturbances, tinnitus, and convulsions and may lead to loss of consciousness. If any of these symptoms are noted, the injection should be stopped and immediate attention given to the airway. Seizures may be terminated with 50–150 mg of thiopental IV, and the patient should be given 100% oxygen by mask. In this situation, it is often necessary to intubate the patient and hyperventilate to ensure fetal oxygenation and to offset metabolic acidosis. If cardiovascular collapse occurs, immediate cardiopulmonary resuscitation (CPR) and cesarean delivery are undertaken. Maintenance of left uterine displacement is absolutely vital during this time.

c. **Total spinal anesthesia.** Inadvertent subdural injection of local anesthetic intended for the epidural space may produce total spinal anesthesia. Nausea, hypotension, and unconsciousness may be followed by respiratory and cardiac arrest if appropriate intervention is not made. Should this occur, the patient should be placed supine (with left uterine displacement), ventilated by mask with 100% oxygen using cricoid pressure, and then intubated. Hypotension should be treated with fluids and ephedrine.

D. Spinal "saddle block" in labor and vaginal delivery produces a motor blockade that will interfere with delivery. It can be useful as a last-minute anesthetic if a forceps delivery is required or postpartum for repair of traumatic lacerations of the vagina or rectum.

VI. Anesthesia for cesarean section. The most frequent indications for cesarean section are prior cesarean section, failure to progress, fetal distress, cephalopelvic disproportion, and prior uterine surgery. Anesthetic choice will depend on the urgency of the procedure and the condition of mother and fetus.

A. Regional anesthesia

1. Spinal anesthesia is a simple, rapid, and reliable technique to provide anesthesia for cesarean delivery if no contraindications exist. The patient is hydrated and given metoclopramide and a nonparticulate antacid. The patient may be sitting or in a lateral decubitus position. Lidocaine 5% with 7.5% dextrose, tetracaine 1% with 10% dextrose, or bupivacaine 0.75% in 8.25% dextrose are local anesthetic options. A T4 level is sought, although the patient may still experience visceral discomfort with exteriorization of the uterus. Addition of small amounts of narcotics like fentanyl (10 µg) in combination with the local anesthetic may decrease the incidence of discomfort during the surgery. Subarachnoid morphine 0.1–0.5 mg may be mixed with the local anesthetic for postoperative analgesia.

2. Epidural anesthesia is ideal in patients who are having elective cesarean sections. The dose of anesthetic can be titrated and repeated as necessary. An epidural can be used effectively for an emergency cesarean section in a patient who already has an existing catheter inserted for labor analgesia. A dose of 3% 2-chloroprocaine or 2% lidocaine may be used. Epidural narcotics may be used for postoperative pain control.

B. General anesthesia is the technique of choice for emergency cesarean sections when regional anesthesia is refused or contraindicated, when substantial hemorrhage is anticipated, or when uterine relaxation is required.

1. Advantages

a. Rapid induction allows surgery to be started immediately.

b. Optimal control of airway and ventilation is ensured.

c. Decreased incidence of hypotension in the hypovolemic patient is seen.

2. Disadvantages

       a. The inability to intubate the trachea remains a major cause of maternal morbidity and mortality.

       b. The risk of aspiration is increased.

       c. General anesthetics may cause fetal depression.

   3. Technique

       a. A 10-mg dose of metoclopramide and 30 ml of a nonparticulate antacid are given prior to induction. A large-bore (16-gauge) IV catheter and standard monitoring are used. The patient is positioned supine with left uterine displacement.

       b. The patient breathes 100% oxygen for 3 minutes if time allows or takes 5–6 deep breaths if time is of the essence. The surgeons should prepare and drape the abdomen at this time.

       c. A rapid sequence intubation with cricoid pressure is performed with 4–5 mg/kg of thiopental IV (less if hypotensive from bleeding) and 1.5 mg/kg of succinylcholine IV.

       d. Until delivery, a 50% mixture of nitrous oxide and oxygen is used with either enflurane or isoflurane 0.75–1.0% and a succinylcholine infusion or short-acting nondepolarizing muscle relaxant. Hyperventilation should be avoided because of its adverse effects on uterine blood flow.

       e. As soon as the umbilical cord is clamped, the potent inhalation agent is discontinued, as it can cause uterine atony. The patient may then be given a small amount of narcotic and switched to a balanced (nitrous oxide–narcotic–relaxant) technique.

       f. Oxytocin (Pitocin) (10–20 units) is added to the IV infusion and administered after delivery of the placenta to stimulate uterine contraction.

       g. Extubation is performed when the patient is fully awake.

VII. Preeclampsia and eclampsia

   A. **Preeclampsia** is the syndrome of **hypertension, proteinuria,** and **generalized edema** and has an incidence of about 7% of all pregnancies. When seizures occur, the condition is known as **eclampsia,** which has an incidence of about 0.3%. These disorders do not manifest themselves before the twentieth week of pregnancy and usually abate within 48 hours of delivery. The hypertension in these disorders is defined as a systolic blood pressure greater than 140 mm Hg (or an increase > 30 mm Hg above baseline blood pressure) or a diastolic blood pressure greater than 90 (or an increase > 15 mm Hg above baseline). The condition is most often seen in young nulliparous women but is also associated with hydatidiform mole, multiple pregnancy, diabetes, and Rh incompatibility.

   B. **Pathophysiology of preeclampsia** is thought to be related to immunologic rejection of fetal tissues, resulting in placental vasculitis and ischemia. Decreased placental perfusion results in increased circulating levels of renin, angiotensin, aldosterone, and catecholamines, which lead to generalized vasoconstriction and endothelial damage.

This causes a shift of intravascular fluid into the extravascular space with resultant edema, hypoxemia, and hemoconcentration. Frank disseminated intravascular coagulation (DIC) is rare, but coagulation abnormalities such as thrombocytopenia, increased fibrin split products, and a slightly prolonged partial thromboplastin time may occur. Renal blood flow, glomerular filtration rate, and urine output are reduced. Hyperreflexia occurs, and central nervous system irritability often increases.

C. **Management.** Definitive treatment involves prompt delivery of the fetus. Symptoms usually abate within 48 hours of delivery. Until then, normalization of blood pressure, intravascular volume, coagulation abnormalities, and prevention or termination of seizures are high priorities.

1. **Hypertension**
   a. **Hydralazine** is probably the most commonly used vasodilator because it increases both uteroplacental and renal blood flow.
   b. **Sodium nitroprusside** may be useful for preventing the acute increases in blood pressure that may accompany laryngoscopy or during hypertensive crisis.

2. **Fluid management.** Intravascular depletion should be corrected with crystalloid and may be guided by central venous pressure (CVP) and pulmonary artery lines.

3. **Coagulation abnormalities.** The patient's clotting status should be assessed, especially in severe preeclampsia, and platelets, fresh-frozen plasma, and red cells should be administered as necessary.

4. **Seizures.** Magnesium sulfate is a mild central nervous system depressant and vasodilator. By relaxing the myometrium, it also causes an increase in uteroplacental blood flow. After an initial IV loading dose of 2–4 gm over 15 minutes, a continuous infusion of 1–3 gm/hr is used to maintain therapeutic blood levels of 4–8 mEq/L. Deep tendon reflexes diminish at 10 mEq/L, and respiratory paralysis and heart block may ensue above 12–15 mEq/L. Magnesium causes increased sensitivity to both depolarizing and nondepolarizing muscle relaxants. Magnesium may cross the placenta, resulting in newborn muscle weakness or apnea. Intravenous calcium may counteract this weakness in both mother and newborn, but calcium may also antagonize the anticonvulsant effect of magnesium in the mother.

D. **Anesthesia**
1. **Epidural anesthesia** is recommended for cesarean delivery in the preeclamptic patient who is volume repleted and has a normal clotting profile. Epidural catheters placed early in labor may help to reduce circulating levels of maternal epinephrine and norepinephrine, thus improving uteroplacental perfusion.
2. **Spinal anesthesia** may be associated with sudden severe hypotension from sympathetic blockade in the

presence of severe hypovolemia. Since this may lead to decreased uteroplacental perfusion and fetal asphyxia, it is generally not recommended.

3. **General anesthesia** is employed for emergency cesarean deliveries if the patient has a coagulopathy or other contraindication to regional anesthesia. These patients are particularly prone to soft-tissue edema of the glottic area, making rapid sequence induction particularly difficult. The hemodynamic response to intubation may be blunted by administration of labetalol, 10 mg IV. Systemic and pulmonary hypertension increase the incidence of stroke and pulmonary edema. The sensitizing effects of magnesium on muscle relaxants must be considered.

VIII. **Peripartum hemorrhage** is the major cause of maternal mortality.

A. **Antepartum hemorrhage** is most commonly due to placenta previa or placental abruption.

1. **Placenta previa** occurs when the placenta is implanted at or very near the cervical opening. This can result in bleeding that is usually painless and can vary from minimal spotting to massive hemorrhage. Placenta previa in a patient with a previous cesarean section has a higher incidence of abnormal placental attachment (placenta accreta). The incidence of gravid hysterectomy is higher in this population. If the patient is not actively bleeding and is euvolemic, subarachnoid or epidural anesthesia may be performed. Pelvic examination in patients with placenta previa may also precipitate hemorrhage and should only be done in the operating room with all preparations made for emergency cesarean section. This is called the **"double setup"** and generally consists of the following:

a. Administration of 10 mg of metoclopramide and 30 ml of a nonparticulate antacid.

b. Placement of a large-bore (14- or 16-gauge) IV with a pump set.

c. Blood (2–4 units) in the room.

d. Abdomen prepared and draped by the surgeons.

e. All preparations for general anesthesia with ketamine available.

f. Assistance available.

2. **Placental abruption** is the premature separation of the normally implanted placenta prior to birth. The bleeding is usually painful and may be either external (obvious bleeding from the vagina) or concealed (blood is trapped behind the placenta and remains inside the uterus). Abruption is the most common cause of DIC in pregnancy. Anesthetic management is essentially the same as for placenta previa except that coagulation studies are checked prior to initiating regional anesthesia. Regional anesthesia should only be used in cases of mild abruption when there is no fetal distress, hypovolemia, or coagulopathy. Consumption of coagulation factors and activation of the fibrinolytic system

occur frequently and should be treated with blood products as needed.

B. Intrapartum hemorrhage

1. **Uterine rupture** can occur at any point during labor and delivery.

   a. **Etiologies**

      (1) Separation of prior uterine scar.

      (2) History of previous difficult deliveries.

      (3) Rapid, spontaneous, tumultuous labor.

      (4) Prolonged labor in association with excessive oxytocin stimulation.

      (5) Traumatic rupture such as during a difficult forceps application.

   b. **Anesthetic management** is the same as that for any actively bleeding, acutely hypovolemic patient. It is controversial whether a patient who has had a prior cesarean section should be allowed to deliver vaginally (VBAC—vaginal birth after cesarean section). The concern is possible uterine rupture at the site of a prior incision. In general, patients with a singleton fetus, in vertex presentation, with no other maternal risk factors, are the best candidates for VBAC. Also, dehiscence of a low transverse scar has been shown to be less catastrophic than rupture of a classic vertical incision scar, both to the mother and fetus. It is safe to use regional techniques in these patients because there often is no pain with uterine rupture, and more reliable signs of rupture are a change in uterine tone, contraction pattern, and fetal heart rate.

2. **Vasa previa** is a condition where the umbilical cord of the fetus passes in front of the presenting part. Therefore, the vessels of the umbilical cord are vulnerable to trauma during vaginal examination or during artificial rupture of membranes. Of note is that bleeding in this circumstance is from the fetal circulation only. This obviously puts the fetus at great risk and is a reason for immediate delivery.

C. Postpartum hemorrhage

1. **Retained placenta** occurs in up to 1% of all vaginal deliveries, and it usually requires manual exploration of the uterus. If the patient still has an epidural or spinal block, this will facilitate removal of the placenta. If not, placement of a regional block in a patient who has been bleeding and is probably hypovolemic is contraindicated and may lead to severe hypotension. General anesthesia with a rapid sequence induction and a potent inhalation agent may be necessary. As soon as the uterus is relaxed enough to allow extraction, the potent agent should be turned off to prevent uterine atony and further bleeding. Nitroglycerin up to 500 µg/min IV has been used to relax the uterus and allow removal of the placenta.

2. **Uterine atony** occurs in up to 2–5% of patients. Infusion of crystalloid, colloid, and blood products as

needed should begin when the diagnosis is made. Pharmacologic therapy involves IV oxytocin to cause uterine contracture. If this fails, the ergot preparation methergine, 0.2 mg IM, should be administered. If this fails to result in uterine contraction, then prostaglandin $F_{2\alpha}$ should be injected directly into the uterus by the obstetrician. If these measures fail, then emergency hysterectomy or internal iliac artery ligation may be necessary.

IX. **Amniotic fluid embolism**
   A. **Pathophysiology.** Amniotic fluid embolism occurs in 1/20,000–30,000 deliveries, and most cases are fatal. As many as 10% of the maternal deaths from all causes result from amniotic fluid embolism. The pathogenesis of this disorder involves a tear through the amnion or chorion (opening uterine or endocervical veins) and pressure sufficient to force the fluid into the venous circulation.
   B. **Clinical features.** Typical signs and symptoms include respiratory distress, shock, hemorrhage (from DIC), and coma. Pulmonary edema, cyanosis, altered mental status, and seizures may be presenting symptoms. Coagulopathies and/or renal and respiratory failure may impede delivery.
   C. **Predisposing factors** include a tumultuous or oxytocin-stimulated/augmented labor, meconium in the amniotic fluid, intrauterine fetal demise, abruptio placentae, advanced maternal age, multiparity, and vaginal manipulation or cesarean section.
   D. **Laboratory studies.** The diagnosis may be confirmed by the presence of fetal squamous calls, lanugo hair, vernix, or mucin in the buffy coat of heparinized maternal blood sampled from a pulmonary artery catheter. A rising pulmonary capillary wedge pressure is ominous. Further diagnostic workup consists of serial arterial blood gases, coagulation studies, chest x-ray, and ECG.
   E. **Treatment** consists of CPR and immediate delivery of the fetus. Endotracheal intubation and respiratory support using high FIO_2, positive end-expiratory pressure, diuresis, and blood-product transfusions are used to correct the pulmonary edema and hematologic derangements.

X. **The pregnant patient with cardiac disease.** The incidence of cardiac disease in pregnancy is about 0.4–4.1%. Cardiac lesions most commonly become manifest during times of maximal stress such as the third trimester, during labor and delivery, and in the immediate postpartum period (see sec. I.B).
   A. **Congenital heart disease.** Patients with some forms of congenital heart disease such as patent ductus arteriosus, atrial septal defect, and ventricular septal defect develop pulmonary hypertension. This may progress to the point where the left-to-right shunt is reversed (Eisenmenger's syndrome). Patients with this syndrome tolerate pregnancy poorly because the decreased peripheral vascular resistance aggravates the right-to-left shunt even more.

Anesthesia for patients with this or other forms of cyanotic heart disease, such as tetralogy of Fallot, should minimize decreases in peripheral vascular resistance. Intrathecal opioids are a good choice. If general anesthesia is required, a high-dose narcotic technique is employed.

B. **Valvular disease.** The most important predictor of perioperative complications is the patient's **functional status.** Epidural anesthesia seems to provide some advantage to patients with valvular lesions by attenuating the normally huge increases in cardiac output that occur during labor and delivery. This decreases the strain on the heart. Also, by relieving the pain, there is less tachycardia. Patients with severe aortic stenosis are unable to tolerate the hypotension induced by regional anesthetics, and intrathecal or epidural opioids may be used to provide some degree of analgesia for these patients.

XI. **Anesthesia for nonobstetric surgery during pregnancy**

A. Approximately 1.5% of women undergo nonobstetric surgery during their pregnancy. Maternal morbidity or mortality is unchanged from that of nonpregnant women, but fetal mortality ranges from 5–35%. The **objectives** for this type of surgery are
   1. Maintenance of uteroplacental blood flow.
   2. Maintenance of pregnancy.
   3. Avoidance of teratogenic substances.

B. No anesthetic agent has been proved to be teratogenic in humans.

C. **Nitrous oxide** has been the most extensively investigated drug in terms of its effects on DNA synthesis. Vitamin B_{12}, a cofactor for the enzyme methionine synthetase, is inactivated by nitrous oxide, halting the production of thymidine, which is necessary for DNA synthesis. The time period of exposure in these studies has been prolonged (several days) so it seems unlikely that a single, short exposure would cause any fetal abnormalities.

D. **Recommendations**
   1. Postpone elective surgery until 6 weeks postpartum (when the physiologic changes of pregnancy have returned to normal).
   2. Postpone semi-urgent surgery until the second or third trimester.
   3. Use regional techniques when possible, especially spinal anesthesia, which minimizes fetal exposure to local anesthetic.
   4. Avoid polypharmacy. Limit the anesthetic to as few agents as possible.
   5. Consider pretreating patients who are to receive nitrous oxide with folic acid.
   6. After the sixteenth week of gestation, continuous fetal monitoring may be employed perioperatively. Communication with the obstetrician is important for interpretation of fetal heart rate tracings.
   7. A uterine tocodynamometer should be used to detect preterm labor, especially in the postoperative period.

XII. Anesthesia for gynecologic surgery

A. Laparoscopy

1. Laparoscopy requires pneumoperitoneum, occasional extreme Trendelenburg positioning, and use of electro-coagulation during sterilization procedures.

2. Insufflation of the peritoneal cavity with carbon dioxide causes an elevation of $PaCO_2$ unless ventilation is controlled. Hypercarbia results from decreased pulmonary compliance, decreased functional residual capacity, and absorption of the carbon dioxide used for pneumoperitoneum. Excess carbon dioxide may be eliminated with controlled ventilation 1.5 times the basal requirements. Increased intraabdominal pressure secondary to gas insufflation at pressures of 20–25 cm H_2O produces increases in CVP and cardiac output, secondary to central redistribution of blood volume. Pressures greater than 30–40 cm H_2O produce a decrease in CVP and cardiac output by decreasing right heart filling.

3. **Techniques.** While virtually all anesthetic techniques have been used for laparoscopy, the preferred method in most instances is a balanced nitrous oxide–oxygen–narcotic–muscle relaxant) anesthetic. The additional use of an inhalation agent in low concentrations such as 0.5–1.0% isoflurane or enflurane may also be employed. Local anesthesia consisting of a periumbilical field block with 10–15 ml of 0.5% bupivacaine and light sedation (fentanyl, 50 µg IV) may also be used in appropriate patients. Spinal or epidural techniques are generally not well tolerated because of the increased ventilatory load associated with pneumoperitoneum, unless insufflation is less than 2 liters.

B. Abdominal procedures.
Most of these procedures are performed through a low abdominal incision, and a regional or general anesthetic is appropriate. The patient may experience discomfort from peritoneal tugging. In extensive pelvic and abdominal procedures with large blood loss and fluid shifts, general anesthesia is usually chosen.

C. Vaginal procedures.
Both regional and general anesthetics may be used for these procedures, although regional techniques are more common. When placing the regional anesthetic, having the patient sitting will help ensure adequate sacral anesthesia. Some procedures require extreme Trendelenburg with lithotomy position. This may compromise patient ventilation, necessitating general anesthesia. Major transvaginal procedures may be associated with large occult blood losses, and close monitoring of fluids and blood loss must be maintained.

D. In vitro fertilization (IVF)

1. **Indications.** IVF and embryo transfer have become increasingly popular for the treatment of infertility. The indications for these procedures have been broadened to include infertility due to tubal disease, "male factor" infertility, endometriosis, and idiopathic infer-

tility. Pregnancy rates of 16–20% with IVF emphasize the need for safe and efficient anesthesia.

2. There are two basic **techniques** for oocyte retrieval:

   a. **Laparoscope-guided oocyte aspiration** is the most common technique. A total of two or three abdominal trocar or needle punctures are performed for stabilization of the ovaries and aspiration of the follicles. Many infertility patients have pelvic adhesions from previous abdominal surgery or pelvic pathology or endometriosis. The risk of bowel, bladder, or other organ injury during laparoscopy is increased in these patients. Although general anesthesia is usually utilized, regional techniques may be employed.

   b. **Ultrasonically guided follicle aspiration** is a rapidly growing alternative approach to laparoscopy for oocyte retrieval. The procedure involves percutaneous puncture and aspiration of the follicles using real-time ultrasound through a transabdominal, transvaginal, or transurethral approach. These procedures are often performed under local anesthesia consisting of a suprapubic wheal of 10–15 ml of 0.5% bupivacaine. Benzodiazepine combined with small doses of fentanyl, meperidine, or morphine usually provides satisfactory analgesia and sedation. Spinal anesthesia can also be used for this procedure for maximum patient comfort.

XIII. **Standards for conduction anesthesia in obstetrics** apply to the use of major conduction anesthesia administered to the parturient during labor and delivery. These standards may be exceeded based on the judgment of the responsible anesthesiologist. They are intended to encourage high-quality patient care but cannot guarantee any specific patient outcome. They are subject to revision from time to time as warranted by the evolution of technology and practice.

   A. **Standard I.** Major conduction anesthesia (lumbar or caudal epidural, subarachnoid or bilateral lumbar sympathetic block) shall be initiated and maintained only in locations in which appropriate resuscitation equipment and drugs are immediately available to manage procedurally related problems (e.g., hypotension, respiratory depression, convulsions, and myocardial depression).

   Resuscitation equipment shall include sources of oxygen and suction, equipment to maintain an airway and perform endotracheal intubation, and a means to provide positive-pressure ventilation. Drugs and equipment for cardiopulmonary resuscitation shall be immediately available.

   B. **Standard II.** Major conduction blocks in obstetrics shall be initiated and maintained by or under the direction of a physician with appropriate privileges.

   Physicians must be approved through the institutional credentialing process to administer or supervise the administration of obstetric anesthesia and must be qualified to manage procedurally related complications.

C. **Standard III.** Major conduction anesthesia should not be administered until the patient has been examined and the fetal status and progress of labor evaluated by a qualified physician who is readily available to supervise the labor and to deal with any obstetric complications that may arise.

D. **Standard IV.** An intravenous infusion shall be established before initiation and maintained throughout the duration of major conduction block.

E. **Standard V.** A qualified individual shall monitor continually* the parturient's oxygenation, ventilation, and circulation.

   Anesthetic techniques, drugs, and maternal vital signs shall be documented in the medical record.

F. **Standard VI.** Qualified personnel, other than the anesthesiologist attending the mother, should be immediately available to assume responsibility for resuscitation of the depressed newborn.

   The primary responsibility of the anesthesiologist is to provide care to the mother. If the anesthesiologist is also requested to provide brief assistance in the care of the newborn, the benefit to the child must be compared to the risk of temporarily leaving the mother.

G. **Standard VII.** All patients recovering from major conduction anesthesia shall receive appropriate postanesthesia care.

   1. A postanesthesia care unit (PACU) shall be available to receive patients. The design, equipment, and staffing shall meet requirements of the facility's accrediting and licensing bodies.

   2. When the PACU is not available, equivalent postanesthesia care shall be provided in a suitable location.

H. **Standard VIII.** A physician with appropriate privileges shall remain in the facility to manage anesthetic complications until the patient is accepted by the PACU or equivalent area.

SUGGESTED READING

Barash, P. G. Obstetric Anesthesia. In P. G. Barash, B. F. Cullen, and R. K. Stoelting (eds.), *Clinical Anesthesia*. Philadelphia: Lippincott, 1989.

Briggs, C., Freeman, R., and Yaffe, S. *Drugs in Pregnancy and Lactation* (2nd ed.). Baltimore: Williams & Wilkins, 1986.

The Canadian Preterm Labor Investigators Group. Treatment of preterm labor with the beta-adrenergic agonist ritodrine. *N. Engl. J. Med.* 327:308, 1992.

Clark, S. L., et al. Placenta previa/accreta and prior cesarean section. *Obstet. Gynecol.* 66(1):89, 1985.

Cohen, S. E. Physiological Alterations of Pregnancy: Anesthetic Implications. In *1990 ASA Annual Refresher Course Lectures*. American Society of Anesthesiologists, 1990. No. 171.

---

* Note that *continual* is defined as "repeated regularly and frequently in steady rapid succession," whereas *continuous* means "prolonged without any interruption at any time."

Cunningham, F. G., MacDonald, P. C., and Gant, N. F. *Williams' Obstetrics*. Norwalk, CT: Appleton & Lange, 1989.

DeCherney, A. H., and Levy, G. Oocyte recovery methods in in-vitro fertilization. *Clin. Obstet. Gynecol.* 29(1):171, 1986.

Killam, A. Amniotic fluid embolism. *Clin. Obstet. Gynecol.* 28(1):32, 1985.

Ostheimer, G. W. *Manual of Obstetric Anesthesia*. New York: Churchill Livingstone, 1984.

Rotmensch, H. H., Elkayam, E., and Frishman, W. Antiarrhythmic drug therapy during pregnancy. *Ann. Intern. Med.* 98:487, 1983.

Snider, S. M., and Levinson, G. *Anesthesia for Obstetrics*. Baltimore: Williams & Wilkins, 1987.

30

Ambulatory Anesthesia

Steven Small and Bobbie Jean Sweitzer

I. Patient selection

A. The volume of patients receiving ambulatory anesthesia and surgical care now exceeds the number of inpatient procedures. The determination of patient suitability and type of procedure for outpatient surgery is based on the expertise of the anesthesiologists, surgeons, and supporting staff, as well as proximity to an inpatient facility, although third-party payers have greatly influenced these decisions. Outpatient surgery is not restricted to American Society of Anesthesiologists (ASA) class I and II patients, and ASA class III patients frequently undergo surgery as long as their medical conditions are stable. The patient must be able to cooperate with all instructions and have a suitable escort. Selection of appropriate patients will limit the number of unplanned hospitalizations. Admissions and complications correlate with type of procedure, duration of surgery, and patient age, rather than ASA classification.

B. **Patients inappropriate for outpatient surgery**

1. **Pediatric**

   a. Formerly premature infants of less than 46 weeks' postconceptual age, even if healthy, have an increased risk of postanesthetic apnea. Regardless of type of anesthesia (e.g., general or regional), these infants should be admitted for 12 hours of postoperative apnea monitoring.

   b. Infants with respiratory disease such as severe bronchopulmonary dysplasia, apnea, or bronchospasm.

   c. Infants with cardiovascular disease such as congestive heart failure or hemodynamically significant congenital heart anomalies (e.g., tetralogy of Fallot).

2. **Adult**

   a. ASA III and IV patients who require extended postoperative treatment and monitoring.

   b. Morbidly obese patients with significant respiratory disease.

   c. Patients with a need for complex postoperative pain management.

   d. Patients with significant fever, wheezing, nasal congestion, and cough.

II. Patient preparation

A. **Preoperative screening.** All preoperative screening for outpatient surgery is done by the surgeon following guidelines developed by a multidisciplinary group. Patients are instructed as to the time of expected arrival, appropriate clothing, diet restrictions, duration of surgery, need for escort home, and necessary laboratory tests. Most patients have a hematocrit and urinalysis performed. Patients over the age of 40 or those with cardiovascular or pulmonary problems must have an electrocardiogram and chest x-ray. In special circumstances, additional tests such as coagulation studies, serum electrolytes, or therapeutic drug levels may be necessary.

B. Prehospital instructions

   1. Diet guidelines. In the pediatric population, current NPO recommendations are that children younger than 6 months of age may receive *clear* liquids (not breast milk or formula) up to 2 hours prior to surgery, whereas children older than 6 months of age may receive clear fluids up to 3 hours prior to surgery. (See Chap. 28 for a complete discussion.) Adults are kept NPO after midnight.

   2. Medications. Patients should be instructed to continue their cardiovascular, asthma, pain, anxiety, anticonvulsant, and antihypertensive medications until the time of surgery. Warfarin (Coumadin) should be stopped several days prior to surgery to allow the prothrombin time to return to normal, and most anesthesiologists advocate holding diuretics (other than thiazides used as antihypertensives) on the morning of surgery. Regular insulin should be held the morning of surgery and half the usual NPH dose administered (which should be delayed until the patient reaches the hospital if he or she must travel a significant distance or is coming alone).

   3. Preanesthetic visit. For the convenience of outpatients and families, an evaluation by an anesthesiologist is usually done just prior to the planned procedure. When the surgeon recognizes a potentially serious problem, a consultation with an anesthesiologist should be arranged in advance. A standard history and physical examination are performed, and any significant new problems are explored (e.g., symptoms of an upper respiratory infection or unexplained chest pain). NPO status is confirmed and compliance with preoperative medications determined. The anesthetic plan is discussed, and informed consent is obtained.

III. Anesthetic management

A. Premedication

   1. Anxiolytics. Reassurance and good rapport with the patient may be all that are required. If necessary, midazolam in small doses may be used.

   2. Aspiration prophylaxis. There is some concern as to whether the anxious patient is at risk for aspiration due to higher gastric volume and low pH (see Chap. 1). Treatment of the patient may include

   a. H_2-receptor antagonist (cimetidine).

   b. Metoclopramide.

   c. Nonparticulate antacids.

   3. Narcotics. Fentanyl, 50–100 µg, may be used preoperatively.

B. IV access. A small IV catheter (20-gauge) is started, frequently in an antecubital vein to diminish the pain associated with injection of propofol.

C. Standard monitoring is used (see Chap. 10).

D. General anesthesia

1. **Induction.** Propofol is most commonly used for induction in adults because of its short half-life and reduced incidence of emesis. Lidocaine, 20 mg, is added to each 200 mg of propofol to decrease the pain associated with injection. Small doses of alfentanil or fentanyl may be added. Barbiturates or etomidate may also be used. Halothane is often used for pediatric inductions.

2. **Airway management.** The choice of employing a face mask, a laryngeal mask, or tracheal intubation is discussed in Chaps. 13 and 14. Succinylcholine is used to facilitate intubation for short procedures. Pretreatment with small doses of a nondepolarizing muscle relaxant may minimize the myalgias that follow succinylcholine administration. For longer procedures, an intubating dose of a short-acting nondepolarizing agent is used. Once the trachea is intubated, an orogastric tube is passed to empty the stomach.

3. **Maintenance.** Volatile anesthetics (e.g., halothane, isoflurane, enflurane, desflurane, sevoflurane), with or without nitrous oxide, are commonly used. Propofol and alfentanil infusions are also used in conjunction with nitrous oxide. Supplemental regional anesthetic blocks can reduce general anesthetic requirements and provide early postoperative analgesia.

E. Regional anesthesia

1. **The ideal outpatient technique** involves the use of short-acting drugs with a rapid onset to facilitate quick recovery and discharge. Patient selection is important, as the benefits of regional anesthesia will be negated if heavy sedation is required. A separate room for performing blocks will increase turnover.

2. **Specific blocks**

   a. **Spinal anesthesia**

      (1) Spinal blockade is a fast, predictable, and reliable technique providing adequate conditions for lower abdominal, groin, pelvic, perineal, and lower extremity surgery. The duration can be adjusted by appropriate selection of local anesthetic and occasional use of a spinal catheter (see Chap. 16 for a discussion of spinal anesthesia).

      (2) Procaine and lidocaine are most commonly used in ambulatory surgery (see Chap. 15).

      (3) **Complications**

         (a) **Postdural puncture headache** (PDPH) occurs in 5–10% of outpatients. Patients under 40 years of age and females are at greater risk. Patients need to be informed of the risk of headache and the steps taken to reduce the risk, which might include use of a small gauge needle (e.g., 24ga sprottle) (see Chap. 16). If a PDPH does develop, bed rest, analgesics, and fluid are the best therapy for the first day. If the headache is severe or persists longer than 24 hours, an epidural blood patch should be performed.

(b) **Urinary retention.** Recovery of bladder tone may be delayed 1–2 hours compared with recovery of motor and sensory function. Ureteral catheterization may be required, and persistent inability to void may be an indication for admission.

b. **Epidural anesthesia** is used in the outpatient to decrease the risk of PDPH. Single-dose administration of epidural anesthesia can be provided by a 20- to 22-gauge needle with a low risk of PDPH. When used with a catheter, it provides anesthesia for procedures of uncertain duration. The technique is described in Chap. 16. Lidocaine and 2-chloroprocaine are frequently used (see Chap. 15).

c. **Peripheral nerve blocks**

(1) **IV regional.** The advantages include simplicity, rapidity of onset, and high reliability. Excellent anesthesia results without interference with early ambulation and discharge. Only lidocaine 0.5% can be used. Disadvantages include short duration, lack of postoperative analgesia, and risk of local anesthetic toxicity if the tourniquets fail.

(2) **Brachial plexus blockade** can be performed by the axillary, supraclavicular, or interscalene approach as described in Chap. 17. Lidocaine is the usual anesthetic chosen. Advantages include excellent postoperative analgesia. Disadvantages include the extra time required to perform a block, temporary loss of sensory and motor function of the extremity, and the need to protect an insensate extremity until recovery from blockade.

F. **Monitored anesthesia care** (MAC). During certain procedures, an anesthesiologist may be asked to monitor a patient and provide supplemental medications, sedatives, and/or narcotics. Standard monitoring must be used, and equipment for the administration of general anesthesia must be available.

IV. **Postoperative considerations.** All patients are admitted to a postanesthesia care unit (PACU), and the same considerations as discussed in Chap. 34 apply. Specific considerations in the outpatient include

A. **Pain.** If the patient has pain on admission to the PACU, intravenous supplementation with fentanyl or morphine is given. When awake, the patient is usually given PO acetaminophen (Tylenol, 975 mg), oxycodone (Percocet, 1–2 tablets), or ibuprofen (Motrin, 600 mg).

B. **Nausea and vomiting**

1. **Predisposing factors** include the following:

a. History of emesis after previous anesthetics or motion sickness.

b. Use of narcotics.

c. Use of nitrous oxide.

d. Gastric distention.

e. Severe pain.

      f. The surgical procedure (laparoscopy, orchidopexy, strabismus correction).

      g. Other factors such as postural hypotension or hypoxia.

  2. Treatment

      a. Oxygen.

      b. Droperidol, 0.625 mg IV.

      c. Metoclopramide, 10 mg IV (0.15 mg/kg for pediatric patients).

      d. Compazine 5–10 mg po/pr.

  3. Severe nausea and vomiting may require admission.

C. Discharge criteria

  1. The operative site should be without evidence of abnormal swelling, bleeding, or compromised circulation.

  2. Vital signs should be stable.

  3. The patient should be able to take PO fluids without nausea or vomiting.

  4. The patient should be able to ambulate.

  5. Analgesia should be controlled with PO medications.

  6. The patient must be able to urinate after urologic procedures or axial blockade.

D. Discharge instructions. When the discharge criteria are met, patients may be discharged, provided they have an escort and understand the specific written instructions, which should include the following:

  1. Dietary instructions: clear liquids initially with gradual resumption of normal diet.

  2. Prescriptions with clear instructions including appropriate pain medications.

  3. Patients with residual analgesia from extremity blockade should be given crutches or slings and cautioned to protect the extremity until full function is regained.

  4. Precautions about performing activity requiring concentration (e.g., driving).

  5. Phone number to report postoperative anesthetic concerns or complications.

  6. Surgeon's instructions regarding phone number, follow-up appointment, and anticipated complications.

V. Unanticipated admission. Unanticipated admission rates after outpatient anesthesia range from 0.1–5.0%. Nausea (about 30%), vomiting (about 20%), and pain occur more commonly than adverse drug reaction or other complications related to anesthesia and surgery. Each outpatient facility must have access to an inpatient unit.

SUGGESTED READING

Bailey, P. L., et al. Transdermal scopolamine reduces nausea and vomiting after outpatient laparoscopy. *Anesthesiology* 72:977, 1990.

Clark, G. A., and Power, K. J. Spinal anesthesia for day case surgery. *Ann. R. Coll. Surg. Engl.* 70:144, 1988.

Gold, B. S., et al. Unanticipated admission to the hospital following ambulatory surgery. *J.A.M.A.* 262(21):3008, 1989.

Jorgensen, N. H., and Coyle, J. P. Intravenous droperidol decreases nausea and vomiting after alfentanil anesthesia without increasing recovery time. *J. Clin. Anesth.* 2:312, 1990.

Wetchler, B. V. *Anesthesia for Ambulatory Surgery.* Philadelphia: Lippincott, 1990.

White, P. F. Outpatient Anesthesia: An Overview. In P. F. White (ed.), *Outpatient Anesthesia.* New York: Churchill Livingstone, 1990.

31

Anesthesia Outside of the Operating Room

J. Fredrik Hesselvik

I. **General considerations.** The anesthesiologist may be called on to provide sedation or general anesthesia in locations remote from the familiar surroundings and backup facilities of the operating room. The same principles and requirements for anesthesia equipment and monitoring standards outlined in Chaps. 9 and 10 should be met.

A. **Equipment**

1. Outlets for electrical power, oxygen, nitrous oxide, suction, and scavenging must be available and function properly. Extension tubing and electrical cords should be provided. A central supply of oxygen is a minimum requirement, although some locations may not have a central supply of nitrous oxide. The presence of full reserve tanks for oxygen and nitrous oxide must be checked.

2. A complete anesthesia cart should be available, similar to the one used in the operating room. It should include emergency drugs and equipment.

3. Resuscitation equipment (e.g., defibrillator and medications) must be available.

B. **Work space area** and **patient access** are often limited. A previous site visit to determine these restrictions is helpful.

1. Adequate **monitoring** during the procedure may need to be modified if the anesthesiologist cannot stay in the room (e.g., during irradiation). Alternative methods of monitoring (e.g., through a window or by a television camera) must then be used. Monitoring needs during transport to the postanesthesia care unit (PACU) must be anticipated.

2. It is important to establish **communication** channels, particularly for an emergency.

3. Areas outside the operating room where anesthesia will be performed should be designated as "**approved anesthesia locations.**" Whenever possible, a dedicated person assigned to that area is preferable over a "rotating crew."

II. **Specific situations**

A. **Anesthesia for computed tomography (CT) scan.** During a CT scan, the patient is required to be immobile for 20–40 minutes. A scan is usually performed without general anesthesia, but children and uncooperative adults (e.g., retarded or head-injured patients) may need sedation.

1. In **adults,** small IV doses of a benzodiazepine (**midazolam**) or a short-acting hypnotic (**thiopental, methohexital, propofol**) can be used for sedation.

2. **Infants and children**

a. In some children **less than 3 months of age,** scans

can be done with no additional sedation. Standard **monitoring** should be used, and capnography with a side-stream sampling tube taped to the patient's nostril or mouth may provide evidence of ventilation, although the end-tidal carbon dioxide (ETCO2) measurement will not be accurate.

b. Chloral hydrate can be used for sedation (30–50 mg/kg PO or per rectum given 30–60 minutes before the procedure). This is associated with a 15% "failure" rate (defined as movement during the scan).

c. **Rectal methohexital** (25–30 mg/kg), has an onset time of 5–10 minutes and a duration of 30–60 minutes. It is important to realize that compared with chloral hydrate sedation, rectal barbiturates can induce a state of general anesthesia and therefore require full monitoring by an anesthesiologist (see Chap. 28).

d. Most children will require **inhalational anesthesia.** A patent airway may be maintained by use of a laryngeal mask airway or tracheal intubation.

e. Patients recover in the **PACU.**

B. **Anesthesia for magnetic resonance imaging (MRI).** Anesthetizing a patient in the MRI suite presents several challenging problems related to the physical environment.

1. The "tunnel" in which the patient is placed is long and narrow (2 m by 0.5 m) and does not allow **access** to the patient during the procedure.

2. There is a constant **magnetic field** present, which will exert a strong pull on any equipment containing ferromagnetic materials (e.g., steel gas tanks and batteries) and will also interfere with mechanical components (solenoids) in automated noninvasive blood pressure monitors and ventilators. Any person working around an MRI scanner should be extremely careful not to have ferromagnetic materials on them, as they can become dangerous missiles. Magnetically-encoded credit cards are erased by the magnetic field.

3. During scans, **radiofrequency signals** are present that disturb electronic monitoring devices and produce a loud rhythmic noise, making it difficult to hear breath and heart sounds.

4. The **duration** of the MRI procedure is approximately 1 hour, and absolute immobility is required during the actual scans, which take 5–8 minutes each. General anesthesia via endotracheal tube or laryngeal mask airway will be necessary for most infants and children.

a. **Anesthesia**

(1) For reasons of safety and convenience, **general anesthesia** is induced in an area remote from the magnetic field. For children, an inhalation induction with halothane–oxygen–nitrous oxide is employed. After loss of consciousness, an IV is placed and the airway secured by placement of a laryngeal mask airway or endotracheal tube. Anesthe-

sia is maintained with 0.4–0.5% halothane and 60% nitrous oxide with spontaneous ventilation.

(2) When stable, the patient is moved into the magnet area and connected to a specially modified anesthesia machine, which contains nonferrous metal.

b. **Monitoring**

(1) An automated **blood pressure** cuff and a sidestream sampling **carbon dioxide analyzer** can be used with long extension tubing.

(2) The standard **electrocardiogram** (ECG) will be disturbed during scans and may cause a skin burn by induced currents in the cables. A specialized, gated ECG monitor is available. To minimize the risk of burns and interference, the cables should be kept as straight as possible.

(3) Standard, unmodified **pulse oximeters** cannot be used during the scan, as they interfere with imaging and are themselves susceptible to interference by the scanner. For accurate monitoring, it is necessary to remove the oximeter from the MRI room and shield the cable and probe completely. A special pulse oximeter (Nonin, Biochem) functions within the MRI environment, and the sensor should be placed as far from the center of the magnetic field as possible.

(4) A **television camera** can be used to visualize the patient within the scanner, as the anesthesiologist stays outside of the room during the scan.

C. **Anesthesia for neuroradiology.** Neuroradiologic procedures include diagnostic intracranial arteriography, embolization of intracranial arteriovenous malformations or aneurysms, embolization of extracranial arteriovenous malformations, and diagnostic or radiofrequency ablation for trigeminal neuralgia.

1. **Intracranial vascular procedures**

a. Anesthetic **goals** include maintaining patient consciousness to facilitate neurologic evaluation, providing sedation to allow patients to be immobile during dye injection, and maintaining stable hemodynamics.

b. **Sedation** is required to minimize the discomfort associated with arterial puncture and dye injection. Narcotic (e.g., fentanyl, 50–200 µg, or butorphanol, 0.5–2.0 mg), in combination with midazolam (0.5–2.0 mg) or propofol (10–40 mg), will produce adequate analgesia.

c. Hyperosmolar contrast dye and IV fluid administration lead to a brisk diuresis requiring **Foley catheterization.**

d. An **arterial line** is frequently placed or transduced from the femoral artery catheter sheath. Both phenylephrine and nitroglycerin must be available.

e. **Hypertension** must be avoided, as this may increase the risk of hemorrhage or aneurysm rupture.

    f. Embolization procedures are long and place the patient at risk for untoward embolic events. With sudden neurologic deterioration, **emergency airway management and intubation** may be required.

    g. Children and patients with neurologic defects may require a **general anesthetic.** A nitrous oxide–narcotic–relaxant technique with intubation and controlled ventilation is preferred. Potent inhalation agents cause cerebral vasodilation and should be avoided. Likewise, hypoventilation is deleterious, and the $ETCO_2$ should be maintained in the range of 28–35 mm Hg. Stable hemodynamics during a smooth emergence are desirable (see Chap. 24).

2. Embolization for control of extracranial vascular lesions presents potential problems of hemorrhage, hemodynamic instability, and aspiration. Typed and cross-matched blood should be available, large-bore IV access must be obtained, and endotracheal intubation may be required for airway control.

3. Trigeminal neuralgia. Neurolytic block of the trigeminal nerve and its branches has been used effectively in the management of chronic pain. In general, a local anesthetic block is performed to reproduce the anesthesia that will accompany permanent thermogangliolysis.

    a. Diagnostic local anesthetic block of the trigeminal ganglion. Standard monitoring is used, and a brief period of loss of consciousness is induced to allow needle placement in the trigeminal ganglion by way of the foramen ovale. Either methohexital 1% (0.5–1.0 mg/kg) or propofol (1–2 mg/kg) is used. Once the needle is placed using fluoroscopy, a test dose of local anesthetic is injected, and the patient's neurologic examination is evaluated. This requires an awake patient who is fully cooperative.

    b. Neurolytic lesion of the trigeminal ganglion. Once the degree of anesthesia induced by the temporary trigeminal block is deemed to be satisfactory, permanent neurolytic block may be performed. Neurolytic techniques include alcohol or glycerol injection, surgical rhizotomy, and thermogangliolysis. An arterial line is placed, as hypertension is common during gangliolysis. The anesthetic technique is identical to that used for diagnostic local anesthetic block of the trigeminal ganglion, and the resulting hypertension is controlled with esmolol, labetalol, and/or nitroprusside. Airway support may be difficult in these patients when the block needles are in place.

D. Anesthesia for cyclotron therapy. Proton beam radiation therapy is used in the treatment of arteriovenous malformations, pituitary tumors, and retinoblastomas. The irradiation is painless, but targeting and exact positioning may often take several hours, during which the patient's head must remain in a fixed position. To achieve this, the head is usually placed in a frame locked to the positioning device.

1. In **adults,** placement of small pins or screws in the skull can be performed by infiltrating with 2% lidocaine with epinephrine. If "ear bars" are used, a satisfactory ear block can be performed by injection of 3 ml of 2% lidocaine with epinephrine SQ in the outer ear canal. Sedation is usually not recommended, as patient cooperation is required.

2. For **children**, a general anesthetic is usually administered, and the airway is maintained with a laryngeal mask airway or endotracheal tube. The procedure is typically performed daily for about 4 weeks; a propofol induction (3 mg/kg) and maintenance infusion (approximately 75 μg/kg/min) through an indwelling Broviac or Hickman catheter is a suitable technique. Whenever possible, spontaneous ventilation should be allowed. Though the anesthesiologist must leave the room during the brief period of radiation, standard monitoring is employed and supplemented with a television camera.

E. **Anesthesia for radiation therapy.** Children receiving radiation therapy often require general anesthesia.

1. A typical treatment course is 3–4 times a week for a 4-week period. It is desirable to choose an anesthetic that allows rapid recovery with minimal risk of nausea and vomiting.

2. The first radiation procedure may be quite time-consuming (1 to several hours), since molds must be taken and measurements performed. Subsequent treatments are usually much shorter (< 30 minutes).

3. Many patients will have indwelling venous access (such as a Broviac catheter) in place for chemotherapy. IV induction and maintenance with a propofol infusion (see sec. **D.2**) is a suitable technique. A combination of midazolam, glycopyrrolate, and ketamine IM may be required in children with difficult venous access.

F. **Electroconvulsive therapy (ECT)** is used in the treatment of major depression for patients who have not responded to medications, are debilitated by serious side effects, or are acutely suicidal. Patients who suffer from delusions, hallucinations, or profound psychomotor retardation are less responsive to medication, and thus early ECT is preferred for them as well. Of those receiving ECT, 75–85% have a favorable response. Usually a series of 6–10 treatments is required 2–3 times a week for a clinical response. During ECT, the electrical stimulus produces a grand mal seizure consisting of a tonic phase lasting 10–15 seconds, followed by a 30- to 50-second clonic phase.

1. **Physiologic effects of ECT**

a. An increase in cerebral blood flow and cerebral metabolic rate, which leads to an increase in intracranial pressure (ICP).

b. An initial vagal discharge manifested as bradycardia and mild hypotension.

    c. This is followed by sympathetic nervous system activation consisting of hypertension and tachycardia, which persists for 5–10 minutes. ECG changes are common and may include PR prolongation, increased QT interval, T-wave inversions, and atrial or ventricular arrhythmias.

    d. Increased intraocular and intragastric pressure may also occur.

2. Anesthetic goals

    a. Providing amnesia and a rapid return to consciousness.

    b. Prevention of damage from tonic-clonic contracture (e.g., long bone fracture).

    c. Control of the hemodynamic response.

3. Absolute contraindications to ECT include the patient with intracranial hypertension (elevated ICP).

4. Relative contraindications to ECT include an intracranial mass lesion (with normal ICP), intracranial aneurysm, recent myocardial infarction, angina, congestive heart failure, untreated glaucoma, major bone fractures, thrombophlebitis, pregnancy, and retinal detachment.

5. Anesthetic management

    a. Premedication is generally not indicated, as sedatives may prolong emergence. Anticholinergics do not decrease the initial bradycardia seen with ECT and, in fact, may interact with central anticholinergic effects of tricyclic antidepressants, leading to post-ECT confusion and delirium.

    b. An IV is started, standard monitors are applied, and the patient is preoxgenated with 100% oxygen.

    c. Anesthesia is generally provided with methohexital (0.5–1.0 mg/kg) and succinylcholine (0.25–0.5 mg/kg), and the patient is hyperventilated. This increases seizure duration by 20%.

    d. A mouth gag is placed, and a unilateral or bilateral electrical stimulus is applied.

    e. The nature and duration of the induced seizure should be monitored with either an electroencephalogram (EEG) or the "isolated arm" technique. With the latter, the blood supply to one arm is interrupted by an inflated blood pressure cuff prior to injecting the muscle relaxant. This facilitates monitoring the resulting seizure.

    f. The patient is ventilated with oxygen by face mask until spontaneous ventilation has resumed. Agitation and hypertension may require treatment after ECT.

    g. Various agents are used to attenuate the cardiovascular response to ECT, among them labetalol, 10–20 mg IV, and esmolol, 40–80 mg IV. Other medications that may be useful include atropine, nitroglycerin, nitroprusside, and propranolol.

    h. Other anesthetics may be used; however, thiopental prolongs emergence, diazepam raises seizure threshold, and propofol reduces seizure duration.

      i. The patient's **underlying medical condition** may require special intervention prior to ECT.

        (1) Patients with **hiatus hernia** and **reflux** may require aspiration prophylaxis and rapid sequence intubation.

        (2) Patients with **severe cardiac dysfunction** may require invasive monitoring.

        (3) Patients with **intracranial lesions** should be monitored with an arterial line, have tight hemodynamic control, and be hyperventilated prior to ECT.

        (4) **Pregnant** patients require intubation and should have fetal monitoring and left uterine displacement.

      j. Rarely an induced seizure will not spontaneously terminate. Ventilation with 100% oxygen must be continued, and the seizure should be terminated within 3 minutes with thiopental (1–2 mg/kg).

G. Psychiatric drug interactions. The patient for ECT may be treated with mood-altering drugs that have potent effects and side effects and important interactions with anesthetic drugs.

  1. Tricyclic antidepressants (TCA). Drugs in this class include amitriptyline (Elavil), fluoxetine (Prozac), imipramine (Tofranil), nortriptyline (Pamelor), and doxepin (Sinequan). These agents are used along with monoamine oxidase inhibitors and ECT therapy for the treatment of depression. They are also used for the treatment of chronic pain.

    a. The **mechanism of action** of TCAs is to prevent the reuptake of norepinephrine and serotonin, thus potentiating their effects. However, these agents may chronically deplete catecholamine stores.

    b. **Adverse effects** are common and include sedation, dry mouth, urinary retention, and tachycardia.

    c. Anesthetic considerations

      (1) Treatment with TCAs should not be discontinued prior to elective surgical procedures.

      (2) The ECG must be monitored for changes, which include a prolonged PR interval, widened QRS complex, and T-wave changes.

      (3) Hemodynamic control is best provided by direct-acting agents such as phenylephrine for a vasopressor or nitroprusside for a vasodilator.

      (4) Pancuronium should be avoided in these patients, as severe tachydysrhythmias may occur.

      (5) Clonic movements and EEG evidence of seizure activity may occur with low inspired concentrations of enflurane in patients taking TCAs.

      (6) Neuroleptic malignant syndrome occurs in 0.5–1.0% of patients treated with antipsychotic medications (see Chap. 18).

  2. Monoamine oxidase (MAO) inhibitors. Drugs in this class include isocarboxazid (Marplan) and phenelzine (Nardil). These drugs inhibit the enzyme monoamine oxidase and increase intracellular concentrations of amine neurotransmitters such as dopamine, epinephrine, norepinephrine, and serotonin. These agents are used in the treatment of depression, obsessive-compulsive disorders, and chronic pain.

  a. **Adverse effects** include hepatotoxicity, hemodynamic instability, and interactions with narcotics. Inhibition of MAO activity can result in increased availability of norepinephrine to postsynaptic receptors; thus tyramine-containing foods may cause hypertensive crises, and orthostatic hypotension may occur due to the accumulation of octopamine (a false neurotransmitter).

  b. Uncommon **adverse interactions** may occur between opioids and MAO inhibitors and may be manifested by hypertension, hypotension, tachycardia, diaphoresis, seizures, hyperthermia, respiratory depression, and coma. Meperidine has been most often incriminated, and the mechanism is unclear but may include reduced opioid metabolism, formation of toxic metabolites, and opioid-induced mass sympathetic nervous system discharge.

  c. **Anesthetic considerations**

    (1) MAO inhibitors are no longer discontinued prior to elective surgery.

    (2) Induction with barbiturates or benzodiazepines is acceptable, but central nervous system and respiratory depressant effects may be accentuated in patients with hepatic dysfunction from such agents.

    (3) Nitrous oxide and volatile anesthetics are safe for use.

    (4) If vasoactive agents are required, direct-acting agents are chosen (see sec. **1.c**).

    (5) Meperidine should be avoided in patients taking MAO inhibitors.

    (6) Both fentanyl and morphine can be used.

3. **Lithium carbonate** is used in bipolar affective disease to prevent manic episodes. It mimics sodium in excitable cells and accumulates in cells, where it inhibits hormonal activation of adenylate cyclase and results in decreased response of receptors to neurotransmitters.

  a. **Therapeutic plasma levels** are 0.5–1.5 mEq/L.

  b. **Toxicity** occurs at concentrations in excess of 1.5 mEq/L. Toxicity is manifested by sedation, muscle weakness, widening of the QRS complex, atrioventricular block, hypotension, and seizures.

  c. **Anesthetic considerations**

    (1) Treatment with lithium should not be discontinued prior to surgery.

    (2) The sedative effects of lithium will decrease anesthetic requirements for volatile and IV agents.

    (3) The duration of action of succinylcholine and nondepolarizing relaxants may be prolonged by lithium. Train-of-four monitoring is suggested.

4. **Phenothiazine/butyrophenone.** Drugs in this class

include chlorpromazine (Thorazine), thioridazine (Mellaril), fluphenazine (Prolixin), and haloperidol (Haldol).

a. Their **mechanism of action** involves dopamine antagonism, and they have a high therapeutic index.

b. They have a range of **clinical effects** including sedation, alpha-adrenergic blockade, antiemetic effects, anticholinergic effects, hypothermia, endocrine changes, extrapyramidal symptoms, and neuroleptic malignant syndrome. Extrapyramidal symptoms are common, and occasionally irreversible tardive dyskinesia may occur in 5–10% of patients treated for several months.

c. **Anesthetic considerations**

(1) Extrapyramidal symptoms may impair anesthetic care and airway management, as tardive dyskinesia often results in involuntary choreoathetoid movements and acute dystonia may lead to tremor, rigidity, and contraction of the facial and neck muscles. IV diphenhydramine will reverse the latter effects.

(2) The sedative effect of these agents may lower anesthetic requirements.

(3) At high doses, these medications may cause alpha-adrenergic blockade, causing a reduction in systemic vascular resistance and blood pressure. Potential intraoperative hypotension may be exaggerated.

(4) The respiratory depressant effect of opioids is enhanced by these agents.

(5) Phenothiazines can cause hypothermia through an effect on the hypothalamus, and this may contribute to exaggerated heat loss in the operating room.

SUGGESTED READING

Caroff, S. N., et al. Malignant hyperthermia susceptibility in neuroleptic malignant syndrome. *Anesthesiology* 67:20, 1987.

Firestone, S. Radiological Procedures. In J. F. Ryan et al. (eds.), *A Practice of Anesthesia for Infants and Children.* Philadelphia: Saunders, 1986. Pp. 221–227.

Gaines, G. Y., III, and Rees, D. I. Electroconvulsive therapy and anesthetic considerations. *Anesth. Analg.* 65:1345, 1986.

Messick, J. M., MacKenzie, R. A., and Nugent, M. Anesthesia at Remote Locations. In R. D. Miller (ed.), *Anesthesia.* New York: Churchill Livingstone, 1990. Pp. 2061–2088.

Michaels, I., et al. Anesthesia for cardiac surgery in patients receiving monoamine oxidase inhibitors. *Anesth. Analg.* 63:1041, 1984.

Patteson, S. K., and Chesney, J. T. Anesthetic management for magnetic resonance imaging: Problems and solutions. *Anesth. Analg.* 74:121, 1992.

Sedgwick, J. V., Lewis, I. H., and Linter, S. P. K. Anesthesia and mental illness. *Int. J. Psychiatry Med.* 20:209, 1990.

Stack, C. G., Rogers, P., and Linter, S. P. K. Monoamine oxidase inhibitors and anesthesia. *Br. J. Anesth.* 60:222, 1988.

Stoelting, R. K. *Pharmacology and Physiology in Anesthetic Practice* (2nd ed.). Philadelphia: Lippincott, 1991. Pp. 365–383.

Stoelting, R. K., Sierdorf, S. F., and McCammon, R. L. *Anesthesia and Co-Existing Disease* (2nd ed.). New York: Churchill Livingstone, 1988. Pp. 717–727.

32

Anesthesia for Trauma and Burns

William H. Campbell

Trauma

I. **Initial evaluation of the trauma patient**
  A. **Airway**
    1. Since hypoxemia poses the greatest immediate threat to the trauma patient, the focus of the anesthesiologist should be on the airway. All multiple trauma patients should be assumed to have **a cervical spine injury** and **a full stomach.**
    2. All patients should have initial **stabilization of the cervical spine** before any airway manipulation. Manual immobilization can be instituted, keeping the head in a neutral position. Sand bags can be placed on either side of the head and joined by tape across the forehead. Stabilization can also be accomplished with a rigid (Philadelphia) collar, but soft collars are ineffective for immobilizing the neck.
    3. All secretions, blood, or vomitus from the oropharynx and any existing foreign bodies (dentures, teeth) should be removed. If the airway is patent and ventilation is adequate, supplemental oxygen and close monitoring of the patient should be provided while other resuscitative measures are begun. The anesthesiologist should always be prepared to secure the airway immediately.
    4. **Patients requiring intubation**
      a. **The awake patient.** Depending on the nature of the injuries, the ability of the patient to cooperate, and the general stability of the patient, several options are available (see Chap. 13):
        (1) Awake nasal or orotracheal intubation with or without the use of a fiberoptic scope.
        (2) Blind nasal intubation.
        (3) Rapid sequence intubation.
      b. **The combative patient.** A rapid sequence induction is often the most expedient approach, provided there are no anatomic problems precluding neuromuscular blockade. Hypoxemia must always be excluded in an agitated patient. Blind nasal intubation may be attempted, but sedating these patients to control their agitation may lead to serious airway compromise.
      c. **The unconscious patient.** Generally an orotracheal intubation is the safest and most expeditious approach.
    5. If the patient arrives with an **esophageal obturator airway** or **esophageal gastric tube airway,** endotracheal intubation should be performed before removing these devices, as vomiting frequently occurs with removal.

B. **The intubated patient.** The position of an endotracheal tube should be verified by auscultating for breath sounds bilaterally and by use of a portable end-tidal CO_2 detector. The endotracheal tube should be secured and adequate ventilation and oxygenation ensured.

C. **Circulation** is initially assessed by palpating for pulses and then obtaining a blood pressure.

1. **Intravenous access.** IV lines already in place should be checked to ensure that they are functioning well. At least two large (16-gauge minimum) catheters are required, and these lines should be placed above the level of the diaphragm in patients with injuries of the abdomen (and the potential for major venous disruption) to preclude the translocation of fluid into extravascular sites. IV access below the level of the diaphragm is only helpful if obstruction or disruption of the superior vena cava is a consideration.

2. If peripheral venous cannulation fails, **percutaneous subclavian or femoral vein cannulation** is faster than a surgical cutdown and has a similar complication rate. Although the internal and external jugular veins are options, access to these structures is frequently hindered due to immobilization of the head and neck for a suspected cervical spine injury. Introducer sheaths (7.0–8.5 Fr) are often placed percutaneously into a large central vein to obtain greater fluid flow rates.

3. If these approaches prove unsuccessful, **surgical cutdowns** should be performed. The saphenous vein at the ankle or the thigh and the antecubital venous system (i.e., the basilic or cephalic veins) are acceptable options. Intraosseous infusion is also an option but is better suited for the pediatric patient (see Chap. 28).

4. **Military antishock trousers (MAST)** or **pneumatic antishock garments (PASG)** have been advocated in the past as a temporizing maneuver to improve cardiac and venous filling. However, this effect is of questionable value, and their use is associated with a number of complications (e.g., compartment syndrome and ischemia of the lower extremities). They are probably most useful in stabilizing fractures of the lower extremities and pelvis.

5. **Volume resuscitation** begins immediately with the establishment of venous access.

a. Most trauma patients are hypovolemic and will respond to the administration of crystalloid. Blood replacement can usually be deferred until blood typing and cross-matching have been completed.

b. Those patients who do not respond to rapid infusion of crystalloid are candidates for transfusion of type-specific, non-cross-matched blood as soon as it is available (this should usually be within 15 minutes of their arrival).

c. Rarely a patient is moribund despite rapid infusion of crystalloid, and low-titer, type O-negative, non-cross-matched blood may be lifesaving.

    d. Controversy still exists regarding the use of colloid (i.e., albumin and hetastarch) in resuscitation. Albumin is not generally used as a first-line therapy for the management of hypovolemia. Colloids such as the dextrans are not used in the management of hemorrhagic shock because of problems related to coagulopathy.

  6. Volume resuscitation may require concomitant **vasopressor** support to provide an adequate perfusion pressure.

D. History

  1. Patients, family members, and prehospital care personnel should be questioned about the events surrounding an **accident.**

  2. An abbreviated **past medical history** should be obtained, including allergies, medications, and past surgical history.

  3. Mechanisms of injury determine the pattern of injury, allowing the clinician to focus the treatment priorities for each patient.

    a. Blunt trauma, usually from motor vehicle accidents or falls, results in widespread energy transfer to the body and thus multiple injuries in various anatomic locations.

    b. Penetrating trauma, usually from knives and bullets, results in injuries that are generally confined to the penetration track (high-velocity gunshot wounds may also cause tissue disruption in areas adjacent to the penetration track).

E. Physical examination

  1. Frequent monitoring of vital signs provides an ongoing assessment of neurologic, cardiovascular, and pulmonary stability.

  2. Obvious **sites of hemorrhage,** as well as less obvious sites (e.g., chest, abdomen, pelvis, thighs), must be assessed for evidence of blood loss.

  3. Neurologic deficits and **vascular compromise** must be investigated without delay.

F. Diagnostic studies

  1. Laboratory studies include type and cross-matching, complete blood count, platelet count, prothrombin time, activated partial thromboplastin time, electrolytes, glucose, blood urea nitrogen, creatinine, urinalysis, and, if indicated, toxicologic screening.

  2. Radiographic studies should include a lateral cervical spine film, a chest x-ray, and an anteroposterior (AP) view of the pelvis on all patients with blunt trauma. A chest x-ray is obtained as a minimum in patients with penetrating injuries of the trunk.

    a. Lateral radiographs of the cervical spine must include the C7–T1 interface and be of sufficient quality to delineate the structures of interest clearly (i.e., soft tissues and bones).

    b. If the patient's clinical condition will allow time for additional studies, **open-mouth odontoid** and **AP views** of the neck should be obtained (standard trauma cervical spine series). The open-mouth odontoid view is necessary for evaluation of the C1–C2 articulation.

c. If the clinical evaluation demonstrates a patient with significant neck pain and tenderness but no evidence of fracture or dislocation on the plain radiographs, **computed tomography** (CT) and **magnetic resonance imaging** (MRI) may be helpful in delineating an occult injury.

3. **A 12-lead electrocardiogram (ECG)** should be obtained on all major trauma patients.

4. Special studies such as intravenous pyelography, angiography, and CT scans are ordered as needed.

G. **Monitoring** is dictated by the severity of the patient's injuries and preexisting medical problems.

1. An **arterial line** is useful in patients who are hemodynamically unstable, or are intubated and will require frequent arterial blood gas sampling.

2. A **central venous pressure line** should be considered to assess fluid administration, administer vasoactive drugs, or establish additional IV access.

3. A **pulmonary artery line** may be helpful in patients with known left ventricular dysfunction, severe coronary artery disease, valvular heart disease, or multiple organ system involvement. Placement is planned according to the time available and the clinical status of the patient.

II. Specific injuries

A. **Intracranial and spinal cord trauma.** See Chap. 24.

B. **Facial trauma.** Brisk oral or nasal bleeding, broken teeth, or vomitus may occlude the airway, complicating airway management. Emergency cricothyroidotomy or tracheostomy may be lifesaving in such cases.

1. **Maxillary fractures** are grouped by the **Le Fort classification** (Fig. 32-1).

a. **Type I (transverse or horizontal).** The body of the maxilla is separated from the base of the skull above the level of the palate and below the level of the zygomatic process.

b. **Type II (pyramidal).** Vertical fractures through the facial aspects of the maxilla extend upward to the nasal and ethmoid bones.

c. **Type III (craniofacial dysjunction).** Fractures extend through the frontozygomatic suture lines bilaterally, across the orbits, and through the base of the nose and the ethmoid region.

d. **Intracranial hemorrhage, cerebral contusions,** and **cervical spine trauma** are common coexisting injuries.

e. **Le Fort and related fractures** are frequently associated with skull fractures and **cerebrospinal fluid rhinorrhea.** Thus, in Le Fort II and especially Le Fort III fractures, nasal intubation and placement of nasogastric tubes are contraindicated.

2. **Mandibular fractures**

a. Malocclusion, limitation of mandibular movement,

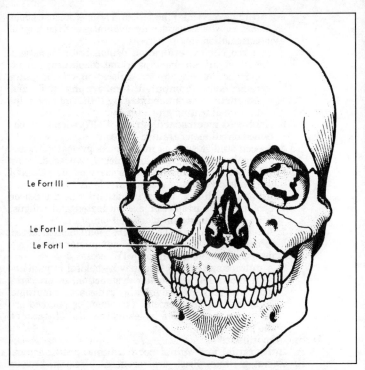

Fig. 32-1. The Le Fort classification. (Reprinted with permission from P. Rosen et al. [eds.], *Emergency Medicine: Concepts and Clinical Practice* [2nd ed.]. St. Louis: Mosby, 1988. P. 407.)

    loose or missing teeth, sublingual hematoma, or swelling at the fracture site will complicate airway management.

    b. Posterior displacement of the tongue producing airway obstruction is frequently seen in association with bilateral condylar or parasymphyseal fractures of the mandible. Simple forward traction on the tongue often provides relief.

    c. Awake nasal intubation is recommended if the nose has not been severely traumatized.

3. Ocular trauma usually requires general anesthesia for repair. Special consideration must be given to open-eye injuries, as discussed in Chap. 25.

4. Anesthetic management. Most displaced facial fractures require general anesthesia for repair. Many soft-tissue injuries can be treated using local anesthesia, although children usually require general anesthesia. Airway compromise is the principal concern, and induction may require awake nasal intubation, fiberoptic laryngoscopy, or tracheostomy under local anesthesia.

C. Neck trauma may be manifested by cervical spine injury, airway injuries presenting as obstruction, subcutaneous emphysema, hemoptysis, dysphonia, or hypoxemia, esophageal tears, and major vascular injuries.

1. **"Clothesline" injuries** occur from direct trauma to the upper airway and may not be accompanied by an open neck wound. Additional injuries include complete laryngotracheal transection and laryngeal fractures.

2. With **penetrating trauma**, initial management includes direct compression of involved vessels to control hemorrhage and prevent air embolism. Direct intubation of open airway defects can be lifesaving.

3. Associated **thoracic injuries**, such as pneumothorax and hemorrhage from injury to the great vessels, may occur with lower neck injuries.

D. Chest trauma

1. Chest trauma can involve injuries to the trachea or larynx, heart, great vessels, thoracic duct, esophagus, lung, or diaphragm.

2. **Rib fractures** are a common feature of major thoracic trauma and mandate ruling out a pneumothorax by chest x-ray. First-rib fractures should alert the clinician to the potential for associated internal injuries. Multiple rib factures most commonly involve ribs 7–10 and are often associated with lacerations of the spleen or liver.

3. A **"flail chest"** refers to the paradoxical inspiratory retraction and expiratory expansion of an unstable chest wall segment that result from sequential segmental rib fractures. The hypoxemia and respiratory failure that accompany flail chest and other major chest injuries are predominantly a reflection of underlying pulmonary contusion.

4. **Subcutaneous emphysema** may indicate the presence of a pneumothorax; however, laryngeal or tracheal trauma may also result in subcutaneous emphysema. Pneumothorax and hemothorax may lead to respiratory and cardiovascular collapse. If these conditions are present or highly suspected, chest tubes should be placed under local anesthesia prior to induction of general anesthesia. Central line insertion (particularly by the subclavian route) should be avoided on the side opposite an injury because of the consequences of bilateral pneumothorax. However, the ipsilateral side should be avoided if a concomitant major venous injury is suspected.

5. **Anesthetic management**

   a. Patients with significant chest injuries almost always require general anesthesia.

   b. Intubation and mechanical ventilation may have to be prolonged into the postoperative period.

   c. If there is any suspicion of a pneumothorax and a chest tube has not been placed, nitrous oxide should be avoided. Airway pressures must also be closely monitored during positive-pressure ventilation.

   d. A hemorrhaging lung must be isolated before blood floods the uninjured side. Double-lumen endotracheal tube placement under these circumstances may be lifesaving (see Chap. 21).

e. Regional anesthesia (i.e., intercostal nerve blockade or thoracic epidural anesthesia) is frequently useful for multiple rib fractures where pain can cause chest wall splinting, regional hypoventilation, and progressive hypoxemia.

E. Heart and great-vessel trauma

1. A fractured sternum, recurrent hemothorax, pericardial tamponade, and ECG changes (persistent sinus tachycardia and other dysrhythmias, nonspecific ST-segment and T-wave changes, and overt ischemia) are all signs of **cardiac trauma.**

2. A widened mediastinal profile and lack of clarity of the aortic knob on chest x-ray mandate **emergency angiography** to rule out traumatic aortic rupture.

3. **Myocardial contusion** is the most common injury resulting from nonpenetrating cardiac trauma and thus should be considered in all multiple trauma patients. Two-dimensional echocardiography combined with serial ECG and creatine kinase–MB determinations provides the highest yield in diagnosing myocardial contusion.

4. The **subclavian arteries** are subject to injury with hyperextension of the neck and shoulder.

5. With major injuries of the heart and great vessels, **cannulation of large peripheral veins for transfusion** is absolutely essential. However, femoral vessels should be spared if possible, since they may be the access site for emergency angiography or cardiopulmonary bypass. IV catheters should not be placed in the lower extremities if there is a high suspicion of injury to the inferior vena cava.

6. **Anesthetic management**

a. These patients are often **severely hypovolemic** and may have compromised cardiac function as well. Cardiopulmonary bypass may be required.

b. **Ketamine** is often the best choice for induction, but use of this drug must be weighed against its risk in patients with concomitant head injury.

F. Abdominal trauma

1. **Penetrating abdominal wounds** (with the exception of gunshot wounds) are initially evaluated by local wound exploration in stable patients to determine whether the peritoneal cavity has been violated. If the exploration is equivocal, diagnostic peritoneal lavage or abdominal CT scan is performed.

2. All patients with **gunshot wounds of the abdomen** are surgically explored.

3. With **impalement injuries** (e.g., stab wounds or falls onto sharp objects), the penetrating object, if still present in the wound, will usually be removed in the operating room after anesthesia has been induced and the patient stabilized. Removal in an uncontrolled environment may result in exsanguinating hemorrhage and death.

4. **Blunt trauma** may result in intraabdominal or retro-peritoneal bleeding.
   a. The **spleen** is the most frequently injured abdominal organ in blunt trauma. Symptoms include abdominal or referred shoulder pain (Kehr's sign), abdominal rigidity, and a falling hematocrit or hypotension.
   b. The **liver** frequently fractures with blunt abdominal trauma, often leading to massive blood loss.

G. **Genitourinary trauma**
   1. All multiple trauma patients should have a **Foley catheter** placed. However, if pelvic or perineal injury has occurred as evidenced by blood at the meatus, a perineal hematoma, or a high-riding prostate, retrograde urethrography should be performed before urethral catheterization.
   2. All patients with penetrating abdominal or back injuries and those with significant hematuria following blunt trauma should have a **kidney-ureter-bladder (KUB)** examination and undergo **intravenous pyelography.**
   3. Eighty-five percent of renal injuries can be managed nonoperatively, but patients with refractory hypotension should go directly to the operating room for exploration.
      a. **Ureteral laceration** is managed by surgical exploration after locating the disruption by retrograde urography.
      b. Seventy percent of patients with blunt injury of the **bladder** have an associated pelvic fracture. Contusions may be treated nonoperatively, but rupture usually requires exploration.
      c. Injury to the **urethra** is indicated by the inability of the patient to void or by the clinical signs of injury (see sec. 1). Diagnosis is by urethrography, and treatment consists of suprapubic cystostomy for urinary diversion and control of hemorrhage. Most disruptions can undergo delayed repair.

H. **Peripheral vascular trauma**
   1. **Peripheral pulses** should be checked routinely in all extremities during the evaluation of trauma patients. Early arteriography is advisable when any doubt exists.
   2. **Anesthetic management** should focus on the recognition of hypovolemia secondary to uncontrolled hemorrhage. Once volume resuscitation has been effected, regional anesthesia (spinal and epidural anesthesia) may be useful in selected cases.

I. **Orthopedic trauma**
   1. All **fractures or dislocations** that compromise nerve or vascular function must be reduced immediately, as they constitute surgical emergencies (e.g., radial nerve injury with humeral shaft fractures and aseptic necrosis of the femoral head with hip dislocation).
   2. **Upper extremity**
      a. Severe depression or hyperabduction of the shoulder

girdle can stretch or tear the brachial plexus. Horner's syndrome may be evident if the cervical sympathetic chain is damaged.

b. When the shoulder is struck hard from the side, the medial end of the clavicle may be dislocated upward or retrosternally. Pressure on the trachea in a retrosternal dislocation may cause life-threatening airway compromise.

c. Dislocation of the glenohumeral joint can cause axillary nerve injury.

d. Fractures of the humeral shaft, especially the middle or distal part, are frequently associated with radial nerve injury.

e. Neurovascular compromise of the forearm can occur with fracture or dislocation of the elbow.

f. Median nerve compression is a possibility with fractures at the wrist.

g. Fractures of the elbow or direct trauma to the forearm may cause edema of the anterior compartment of the forearm. The anterior compartment is a closed space, and pressure on the blood vessels will result in ischemic necrosis. Early fasciotomy is indicated.

3. Pelvis

a. Patients who have sustained pelvic injuries can be divided into one of three major categories:

(1) **Exsanguinating hemorrhage** from external bleeding in open fractures or from retroperitoneal hematoma in closed fractures (0.5–1.0%). These patients almost always present with either severe hypotension or cardiac arrest and rarely respond to resuscitative measures.

(2) **Hemodynamically stable** with a relatively uncomplicated course (75%). Urgent or elective surgery for repair of bony and ligamentous pelvic disruptions may be required.

(3) An intermediate group in **critical condition** with varying degrees of overall injury, hemorrhage, and hemodynamic instability (25%).

b. Initial management for these injuries, in addition to addressing the ABCs, includes the application of MAST trousers pending pelvic angiography (with or without therapeutic embolization to control hemorrhage) and external pelvic fixation.

c. Fat embolism can occur with pelvic and major long-bone fractures (see Chap. 18).

d. Crush injuries are associated with **hyperkalemia** and **myoglobinemia** if large amounts of muscle tissue are devitalized. Early administration of loop diuretics and alkalinization of the urine may prevent acute renal failure due to rhabdomyolysis and myoglobinuria.

4. Lower extremity

a. Fractures of the **tibia** and **fibula** are the most common major skeletal injuries and can be associated with neurovascular trauma.

b. Whenever a fracture of the **femur** or **pelvis** is present, blood loss may be much greater than evident from superficial inspection.

c. Hip fractures are common in the elderly, whose clinical picture is often dominated by other complicating medical illnesses. Traction is used initially for pain relief, but most fractures require open reduction and internal fixation to ensure adequate healing and function and to avoid the complications of prolonged immobilization.

d. Regional and combined techniques are usually excellent choices for patients with isolated hip fractures. Options include

(1) Spinal anesthesia, using hypobaric (with affected side up) or hyperbaric (with affected side down) techniques.

(2) Epidural anesthesia, alone or in combination with general anesthesia.

(3) Peripheral nerve block (i.e., femoral and sciatic nerves).

(4) General anesthesia, usually necessary in the multiple trauma patient.

5. Extremity reimplantation

a. Indications. In general, these procedures are performed only on the upper extremities and only in patients who are otherwise stable. An amputated arm, hand, or digit will not be reimplanted if it has sustained severe crush injury or has been torn from attachments to major nerves and blood vessels. Reimplantations may be extremely lengthy procedures, occasionally in excess of 24 hours.

b. Anesthetic management

(1) General anesthesia is usually chosen, due to the long duration of these procedures. However, a combined technique will reduce anesthetic requirements and provide for postoperative analgesia (especially with catheter placements, rather than single-dose brachial plexus blocks). The potential risk of arterial injury during axillary brachial plexus blockade should be kept in mind, as the resulting hematoma may compromise efforts at reimplantation.

(2) During general anesthetics, the head must be repositioned at frequent intervals (e.g., every 1–2 hours) to avoid pressure-induced scalp ulceration and hair loss. Water blankets or well-padded sponge blocks should be used to minimize pressure on susceptible peripheral nerves (e.g., ulnar, sciatic, sural). The endotracheal tube cuff pressure should be periodically assessed, as nitrous oxide will diffuse into the cuff over time.

III. The pediatric trauma patient

A. General considerations

1. A clear understanding of the salient anatomic and physiologic differences between adults, children, and infants as well as a working knowledge of the specific

anesthetic considerations for this patient population is required of all anesthesiologists (see Chaps. 27 and 28).

2. **Blunt trauma** predominates in children, usually from falls or motor vehicle accidents. Multiple injuries are the rule rather than the exception, but diagnosis is often more difficult because of the child's inability to provide an accurate history.

B. **Anesthetic considerations**
   1. **Surgical cricothyroidotomy** is rarely performed in the infant or small child due to the technical difficulties encountered in performing the procedure.
   2. Although the pediatric trauma patient frequently presents with significant **blood loss,** the alteration in vital signs may be minimal.
   3. **Intraosseous infusion** is an acceptable procedure for critically ill and injured pediatric patients in whom venous access cannot be established (see Chap. 28).
   4. The small child who is **hypothermic** may be refractory to therapy for shock. While the child is exposed during initial evaluation and management, overhead heaters or thermal blankets will be needed to maintain body temperature.

IV. **The pregnant trauma patient**
   A. **General considerations**
      1. Pregnancy must always be suspected in any trauma patient of childbearing age (see Chap. 29 for management of the pregnant patient). The pregnant uterus is prone to injury because of its size.
      2. Because the fetus is highly dependent on its mother for its oxygen requirements, an **uninterrupted supply of oxygenated blood** must be provided to the fetus at all times.
         a. **Compression of the vena cava by the uterus** reduces venous return to the heart, thereby decreasing cardiac output and exacerbating shock. Unless a spinal injury is suspected, the pregnant patient should be transported and evaluated on her left side.
         b. If **MAST** are used, the abdominal compartment must not be inflated.
      3. Although diagnostic irradiation poses a risk to the fetus, necessary **radiographic studies** should be obtained.
   B. **Treatment**
      1. If the mother's condition is stable, the status of the fetus or the extent of uterine injury will determine further management.
      2. A fetus that shows no signs of distresss should be monitored with external ultrasound. Since premature labor is always a possibility in these patients, an external tocotransducer must be used to detect the onset of contractions. Should premature labor ensue, therapy may be initiated with beta agonists.
      3. When a viable fetus shows signs of distress despite resuscitative measures, a cesarean delivery must be performed expeditiously. A nonviable fetus should be

managed conservatively in utero by optimizing maternal oxygenation and circulation.

4. Primary repair of all maternal wounds must be attempted in a critically injured mother carrying a viable gestation, even at the expense of fetal distress.

Burns

I. Pathophysiology

A. **Deep thermal injury** destroys skin, the body's barrier to the external environment. Skin plays a vital role in thermal regulation, fluid and electrolyte homeostasis, and protection against bacterial infection. Thus, significant heat loss, massive fluid shifts and protein losses, and infections (local as well as systemic) are seen in patients with severe thermal injuries. There is also a diffuse alteration in the permeability of cell membranes to sodium, resulting in generalized cellular swelling. Microvascular injury results from local damage by heat and from the release of vasoactive substances from the burned tissue. Therefore, edema occurs in both burned and unburned tissues.

B. In **electrical burns,** it is thermal energy that actually destroys tissue, particularly those tissues with high resistances such as skin and bone. It is difficult to predict the precise location and extent of tissue damage.

C. In **chemical burns**, the degree of injury depends on the particular chemical, its concentration, duration of contact, and the penetrability and resistance of the tissues involved. Some substances producing chemical burns, such as phosphorus, are absorbed systemically, producing significant and often life-threatening injury.

D. **Infections and drug reactions** may also cause dermal injury.

1. **Staphylococcal scalded skin syndrome** is a disease in children caused by an exotoxin from an infecting strain of coagulase-positive *Staphylococcus aureus*.

2. **Toxic epidermal necrolysis** is a disease of adults in which the skin sloughs in large sheets. Although it is similar in appearance to staphylococcal scalded skin syndrome, it is a different disorder that may accompany drug reactions.

II. Preoperative evaluation

A. **Burns are a form of trauma**, thus the ABCs should be initially assessed (see Trauma, sec. I).

B. Size of the **burn** should be estimated as a percent of the total body surface area (%TBSA).

1. The **rule of nines** guides estimations (Fig. 32-2).

   a. **Adults**

   (1) The head and both of the upper extremities represent 9% TBSA each.

   (2) The anterior trunk, posterior trunk, and both of the lower extremities represent 18% each.

   (3) The perineum represents 1%.

   b. **Infants and children.** Because of the different

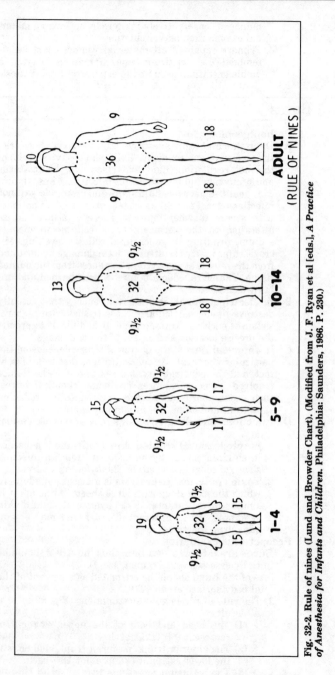

Fig. 32-2. Rule of nines (Lund and Browder Chart). (Modified from J. F. Ryan et al [eds.], *A Practice of Anesthesia for Infants and Children*. Philadelphia: Saunders, 1986. P. 230.)

proportions of body surface area relative to patient age, reference must be made to the proper burn chart when calculating %TBSA to avoid significant errors (Fig. 32-2).

2. **Another practical method** to estimate %TBSA is that the area of the patient's hand will cover about 1% TBSA.

C. The **depth of the burn** determines therapy (i.e., conservative management versus excision and grafting). Burn depth is difficult to determine visually; however, there are some useful guidelines.

1. The area under a **partial-thickness burn** should have normal or increased sensitivity to pain and temperature and should blanch with pressure.

2. A **full-thickness burn** will be anesthetic and will not blanch.

III. Perioperative management

A. Cardiovascular system

1. **Fluid loss**

   a. During the first 24–48 hours, massive evaporative losses and sequestration of fluid in the extracellular compartment (third-spacing) are to be expected. Aggressive fluid repletion will be necessary to prevent hypotension, hypoperfusion, and shock.

   b. The composition of lost or sequestered fluid is very similar to that of plasma (i.e., the fluid has a high protein content).

   c. **Fluid replacement** consists of crystalloid, usually Ringer's lactate, with or without the addition of colloid.

   d. **Standard protocols** for fluid replacement use body weight in kilograms and %TBSA burned.

   (1) **Parkland formula** (most commonly used at the MGH): 4.0 ml of Ringer's lactate/kg/%TBSA burn/24 hr.

   (2) **Brooke formula:**

   1.5 ml of crystalloid/kg/%TBSA burn/24 hr.
   plus
   0.5 ml of colloid/kg/%TBSA burn/24 hr.
   plus
   2000 ml of 5% dextrose in water/24 hr.

   e. Generally, half the calculated fluid deficit is administered during the first 8 hours postburn and the remainder over the next 16 hours. The patient's daily maintenance fluid requirements are given concurrently.

   f. Acceptable colloids include albumin and hetastarch (hydroxyethyl-substituted amylopectin).

   g. The end points of fluid therapy are hemodynamic stability and maintenance of an adequate urine output. In extensive burns, it is imperative that fluid management be followed with appropriate invasive monitoring and laboratory studies.

2. **A fall in cardiac output and arterial blood pressure** may occur in the immediate postburn period

despite adequate volume resuscitation. The etiology of this phenomenon remains unclear but may be related to circulating factors that depress myocardial contractility.

3. **Capillary integrity** is reestablished by 36–72 hours after the initial injury, allowing resorption of fluid from the interstitial space and decreasing the need for fluid infusion. At this juncture, a "diuretic phase" may begin.

4. A **hypermetabolic state** develops 3–5 days following the burn injury. This may result in a two- to threefold increase in cardiac output, which persists for weeks to months. However, gram-negative sepsis may cause continued depression of cardiac output in some patients.

5. **Chronic postburn hypertension** may be seen in young children (usually boys) who have sustained extensive burns. The syndrome usually develops within 2 weeks of injury and may result from elevated endogenous catecholamine levels.

6. **Circumferential burns of the abdomen** may produce increased intraabdominal pressure, which can reduce cardiac output by decreasing venous return.

B. **Respiratory system**

1. **Circumferential full-thickness burns of the thorax** can cause hypoventilation and decrease functional residual capacity, leading to hypoxia. Emergency escharotomies are frequently required.

2. **Thermal injury of the face and upper airway** is a common occurrence, but burns involving the lower respiratory tract are infrequent. However, during a fire in a closed space or when heated noxious vapors are inhaled, inhalation injury may occur. This should be suspected in the presence of burns of the head or neck; singed nasal hairs; swelling of the mucosa of the nose, mouth, lips or throat; a brassy cough; or carbonaceous sputum. Both upper airway and pulmonary parenchyma may be severely affected, leading to adult respiratory distress syndrome.

3. Before airway edema occurs, **endotracheal intubation** should be performed **expeditiously.** Continued swelling and distortion of the soft tissues will progress at a rapid rate rendering intubation difficult, if not impossible.

4. The **inhalation of toxic fumes** may result in physical damage to the tracheobronchial tree and cause systemic effects such as cyanide toxicity and carbon monoxide poisoning.

   a. **Combustion of polyurethane-containing products** (e.g., insulation and wall paneling) releases hydrogen cyanide, a cellular poison that leads to tissue hypoxia and death.

   b. **Carbon monoxide poisoning** occurs when carbon monoxide combines with hemoglobin, displacing oxygen (carbon monoxide is bound more than 200 times as firmly as oxygen) and shifting the oxyhemoglobin curve to the left. Tissue hypoxia ensues.

(1) Carbon monoxide toxicity may be difficult to diagnose because carboxyhemoglobin is visually the same as oxyhemoglobin, and PaO_2 measurements are in the normal range (unless there is underlying pulmonary parenchymal injury). Therefore, one must maintain a high index of suspicion when evaluating burn patients and obtain carboxyhemoglobin levels when indicated.

(2) The half-life of carboxyhemoglobin is directly related to the inspired oxygen concentration (FIO_2); it is 5–6 hours when breathing room air, but 30–60 minutes while breathing 100% oxygen. Hyperbaric oxygen at 3 atmospheres further reduces carboxyhemoglobin half-life to 20–30 minutes. Thus, treatment consists of supplemental oxygen (hyperbaric oxygen in severe cases) and supportive care until the carbon monoxide is eliminated.

(3) The ambient atmosphere during a fire is low in oxygen and high in carbon monoxide, so all burned patients, especially those burned within a closed space, may have sustained some degree of tissue **hypoxia** with their thermal injury. Therefore, oxygen administration should begin at the scene.

5. The **inhalation of particulate matter** (i.e., smoke and soot) results in mechanical obstruction of the airways.

C. Central nervous system. A high incidence of encephalopathy occurs in burned patients.

D. Renal blood flow may be decreased from

1. Prerenal factors (see Chap. 4).

2. Intrinsic renal factors specific to burn trauma, these include tubular obstruction secondary to rhabdomyolysis and hemoglobinuria from hemolysis. The former is most common in electrical injury, while the latter is seen following severe cutaneous burns (see Chap. 4 for appropriate therapy).

E. Gastrointestinal system

1. Gastrointestinal function is diminished immediately following burn injury secondary to the development of gastric and intestinal ileus. Because of the danger of pulmonary aspiration of gastric contents, the stomach should be adequately vented with a nasogastric tube, particularly in patients unable to protect their airway.

2. Serum enzyme changes indicative of liver damage are sometimes evident in the early postburn period.

3. Curling's ulcers (mucosal erosion) will occur at variable times after major burns, leading to life-threatening gastric hemorrhage or perforation. These seem to be more common in children than in adults. Therapy consists of antacids and H_2 antagonists.

4. Other gastrointestinal complications of burns include esophagitis, tracheoesophageal fistula (from prolonged intubation and the presence of a nasogastric tube), acalculous cholecystitis, and mesenteric artery thrombosis.

F. **Endocrine system.** The stress of a burn injury causes marked changes in catecholamine, corticosteroid, and glucagon levels. Increases in these catabolic hormones result in loss of muscle and accelerated nitrogen breakdown.

G. **Musculoskeletal system.** Circumferential burns of the extremities can lead to vascular compromise from compartment syndrome. **Escharotomy** is required to prevent ischemic necrosis of distal structures, particularly the digits.

H. **Hematologic system**
   1. **Microangiopathic hemolytic anemia** can occur.
   2. **Thrombocytopenia,** secondary to increased platelet aggregation and trapping of platelets in the lungs, is seen early in the postburn period and is followed by an increase in the platelet count 10–14 days following the injury. This elevation will persist for several months.
   3. **Sepsis** can lead to disseminated intravascular coagulation as well as bone marrow suppression.

I. **Bacterial infection**
   1. **Infection of burned areas** delays healing and prevents successful skin grafting. Bacterial invasion of underlying tissues may result in septicemia.
   2. **The most common organisms involved** are staphylococci, beta-hemolytic streptococci, and the gram-negative rods such as *Pseudomonas* and *Klebsiella.*
   3. **Local treatment** consists of topical antimicrobials:
      a. **Silver nitrate** (0.5%). Methemoglobinemia is a rare complication.
      b. **Mafenide cream** (10%) may cause metabolic acidosis if absorbed, as it is a carbonic anhydrase inhibitor.
      c. **Silver sulfadiazine** (1%). Leukopenia is the main disadvantage but reverses with discontinuation.
      d. **Povidone-iodine** elevates serum iodide levels and is contraindicated in any patient with renal dysfunction.
   4. **Sepsis** may also be inhibited by using temporary biologic dressings, which may be allografts (cadaver skin, amnion) or xenografts (porcine). "Artificial skin," which is manufactured from collagen and cultured epidermis, grown in vitro from a patient's own cells, is still being investigated.
   5. The use of **systemic antibiotics** is limited to treatment of documented systemic infection (as opposed to colonization) and as prophylaxis prior to surgical procedures.

IV. **Anesthetic considerations**
   A. **General considerations**
      1. **Early excision and grafting of burned areas** is now a widely accepted procedure. Thus, patients are brought to the operating room in the acute phase of injury, when they may still be unstable. Special em-

phasis should be placed on correcting acid-base and electrolyte disturbances as well as coagulopathies. Adequate colloid and blood products should be ordered in advance.

2. During the **chronic phase of burns,** when reconstructive procedures are performed, altered pharmacokinetics, drug tolerance, and extremely difficult airways are the main considerations.

B. **Monitoring and intravenous access**

1. Often **IV access** will still be in place from the initial resuscitation. Large-bore IVs are mandatory to allow for massive fluid replacement.

2. In massive burns, there may be no unburned skin on which to place **ECG pads.** However, after induction, electrodes can be stitched onto the skin, or alternatively, needle electrodes may be used.

3. **Arterial lines** are indispensable for continuous blood pressure monitoring and to facilitate frequent blood sampling. Almost any artery can be used; the site will depend on the availability of unburned areas. If all appropriate sites are burned, the line may have to be placed through the burn wound after the area has been prepared in a sterile fashion.

4. **Central venous pressure lines** are useful, both for monitoring central volume and as central access for drug infusions.

5. A **pulmonary artery catheter** may be required for optimal management of patients with cardiac disease.

C. **Airway.** Obtaining an adequate mask fit may be difficult because of edema in the early phases of burn injury or because of scars and contractures later on. These same processess can render burn patients difficult to intubate.

D. **Muscle relaxants**

1. **Succinylcholine** is absolutely **contraindicated 24 hours to 2 years following major burns,** as it can produce profound hyperkalemia and cardiac arrest.

2. **Nondepolarizing relaxants** are used when muscle relaxation is required. Burn patients show a "resistance" to these drugs (diminished response to conventional doses), in some cases requiring three- to fivefold higher doses than are sufficient in nonburned patients.

E. **Anesthetics**

1. There is no single preferred agent or combination of agents.

   a. **Ketamine** may have advantages in patients with extensive burns with uncertain volume status.

   b. For dressing changes, **nitrous oxide–oxygen** can be used as an analgesic, with small amounts of ketamine for supplementation.

2. These patients may have **greatly increased narcotic requirements** due to tolerance and increases in the apparent volume of distribution for drugs. It is important to provide adequate analgesia.

F. **Temperature regulation.** The most comfortable body temperature for a burn patient is about 100°F (38°C). In the burn intensive care unit, such acute patients are cared for in warmed, humidified rooms. Every effort should be made to maintain normothermia during transport and surgery. The operating room, IV fluids, and blood products should be warmed and inspired gases heated and humidified. Pediatric patients should be placed under a radiant heat source and on a warming blanket whenever possible.

G. **Immunosuppression.** The immune system is suppressed for weeks to months following burn injury, and unfortunately, the wound itself serves as an excellent medium for bacterial growth. Thus, every attempt should be made to practice aseptic technique when handling patients or inserting intravascular lines.

H. **Postanesthetic care.** It is important to maintain normothermia while transporting patients back to the intensive care unit, since shivering may contribute to graft loss. Supplemental oxygen should be given until patients are fully recovered from anesthesia because of their high metabolic rate (i.e., high oxygen consumption) and frequent intrapulmonary shunting.

SUGGESTED READING

Baud, F. J., et al. Elevated blood cyanide concentrations in victims of smoke inhalation. *N. Engl. J. Med.* 325:1761, 1991.

Capan, L. M., Miller, S. M., and Turndorf, H. *Trauma Anesthesia and Intensive Care.* Philadelphia: Lippincott, 1991.

Grande, C. M. Trauma anesthesia and critical care. *Crit. Care Clin.* 6:1990.

Nicholls, B. J., and Cullen, B. F. Anesthesia for trauma. *J. Clin. Anesth.* 1:115, 1988.

Philips, T. F., Soulier, G., and Wilson, R. F. Outcome of massive transfusion exceeding two blood volumes in trauma and emergency surgery. *J. Trauma* 27:903, 1987.

Trunkey, D. Initial treatment of patients with extensive trauma. *N. Engl. J. Med.* 324:1259, 1991.

Vanstrum, G. S. (ed.). *Anesthesia in Emergency Medicine.* Boston: Little, Brown, 1989.

33

Transfusion Therapy

Douglas Hansell

I. **Indications for transfusion therapy.** Blood component transfusion is usually performed because of decreased production, increased utilization/destruction or loss, or dysfunction of a specific blood component (red cells, platelets, or coagulation factors).

A. **Anemia**

1. **Hemotocrit.** The main reason for transfusing red cells is to maintain oxygen carrying capacity to the tissues. Healthy individuals or individuals with a chronic anemia can usually tolerate a hematocrit (Hct) of 20–25%, assuming normal intravascular volume. In patients with coronary or peripheral arterial disease, it is clinical practice to maintain higher hematocrits (28–30%), although the efficacy of this has not been proved.

2. If a patient is anemic preoperatively, the **etiology** should be clarified. It may be secondary to decreased production (marrow suppression), increased loss (hemorrhage), or destruction (hemolysis).

3. **Estimating blood volumes**

a. Intraoperative blood transfusion is dependent on **red cell loss.** This can be roughly estimated by measuring blood in suction canisters, weighing sponges, and checking blood loss on the drapes.

b. **Estimated allowable blood loss** (EABL) can be calculated as follows:

$$EABL = (Hct_{starting} - Hct_{allowable})$$
$$\times BV/Hct_{starting}$$

Blood volume (BV) in an adult is approximately 7% of lean body mass or approximately 70 ml of blood/kg of body weight.

c. Estimating the **volume of blood to transfuse** can be calculated as follows:

$$Volume\ to\ transfuse = (Hct_{desired} - Hct_{present})$$
$$\times BV/Hct_{transfused\ blood}$$

B. **Thrombocytopenia.** Spontaneous bleeding is unusual with platelet counts above 20,000, but for surgical hemostasis, counts above 50,000 are preferable. Thrombocytopenia is due to either decreased bone marrow production (chemotherapy, tumor infiltration, alcoholism) or increased utilization or destruction (hypersplenism, idiopathic thrombocytopenia purpura, drug effects [heparin, H_2 blockers]). It is also seen with massive blood transfusion (see sec. **IX.A.1**).

C. **Coagulopathy.** Bleeding associated with documented factor deficiencies or prolonged clotting studies (prothrombin time, partial thromboplastin time) mandates replacement therapy to maintain normal coagulation function. See secs. **II** and **IX** for a discussion of coagulopathy.

II. Coagulation studies. The most important clue to a clinically significant bleeding disorder in an otherwise healthy patient remains the history. Prior surgical bleeding, gingival bleeding, easy bruising, epistaxis, or menorrhagia in women should raise concern. There are many tests available to measure the coagulation system. However, in interpreting the various laboratory tests, the clinician must remember that the coagulation system is a complex interplay of platelets and coagulation factors. There is no single test that measures the integrity of the entire coagulation system.

A. Partial thromboplastin time (PTT) is performed by adding particulate matter to a blood sample to activate the intrinsic coagulation system. Normal values for the PTT are between 25 and 37 seconds and depend on normal levels of clotting factors in the intrinsic coagulation system. The test is sensitive to decreased amounts of coagulation factors and is elevated in a patient on heparin therapy. The PTT will also be abnormal if there is a circulating anticoagulant present (i.e., lupus anticoagulant, antibodies to factor VIII). The clinician should remember that an abnormal PTT does not necessarily correlate with clinical bleeding. Aggressive correction of an abnormal PTT in surgical patients is not always indicated, unless the patient is actively bleeding.

B. Prothrombin time (PT) is a measure of the extrinsic coagulation system and is measured by adding tissue factor to a blood sample. While both PT and PTT are affected by levels of factors V and X, prothrombin, and fibrinogen, the PT is specifically sensitive to deficiencies of factor VII. The PT is normal in deficiencies of factors VIII, IX, XI, XII, prekallikrein, and high-molecular-weight kininogen.

C. Bleeding time reflects the interaction of platelets with the vessel endothelium leading to formation of an initial clot. An abnormal bleeding time usually reflects dysfunctional or diminished platelets. Abnormal or decreased von Willebrand's factor (platelet adhesion) or fibrinogen (diminished fibrin strands) can also result in an elevated bleeding time. The standard Ivy bleeding time is most commonly used. This test is performed by producing a standardized incision (5 mm long × 2 mm deep) on the forearm with a blood pressure cuff inflated. The bleeding time reflects the time to initial clot formation. The test is somewhat technician dependent, and reproducible results are more likely when a standardized template or automated device is used to make the incision. Normal bleeding time in our hospital is under 9 minutes.

D. Activated clotting time (ACT) is a modified whole blood clotting time in which diatomaceous earth is added to a blood sample to activate the intrinsic clotting system. The ACT is the time until clot formation. A normal ACT is between 90 and 130 seconds. The ACT, a relatively easy and expedient test to perform, is useful in monitoring heparin therapy in the operating room.

E. **Thrombin time** is performed by adding thrombin to anticoagulated plasma. The thrombin time is a sensitive measure of the conversion of fibrinogen to fibrin. Patients with abnormal or low fibrinogen levels may have only minimally elevated PT or PTT, whereas they will have a prolonged thrombin time. The thrombin time is also prolonged in the face of heparin therapy.

F. **Euglobin lysis time** is a measure of fibrinolytic activity. If a patient has increased fibrinolytic activity, the euglobin lysis time will be shorter than the normal 2 hours.

G. **Fibrin split products.** When fibrinolysis occurs, plasmin degrades both fibrin and fibrinogen. Fibrin split products reflects the amount of degradation products in the circulation. The half-life of these fragments is approximately 9 hours, and they are removed by the liver, kidney, and endothelial cells. These fibrin fragments also interfere with normal coagulation by impairing platelet function and the normal formation of fibrin clot.

III. **Blood typing and cross-matching**

A. Donor and recipient blood is typed in the red cell surface ABO and Rh systems and screened for antibodies to other cell antigens. Cross-matching involves directly mixing the patient's plasma with the donor's red cells to establish that hemolysis does not occur from any undetected antibodies. An individual's red cells have either A, B, AB, or no surface antigens. If the patient's red cells are lacking either surface antigen A or B, then antibodies will be produced against it. A person who is type B will have anti-A antibodies in the serum, and a type O individual (having neither A nor B surface antigens) will have circulating anti-A and anti-B antibodies. Consequently, a person who is type AB will not have antibodies to either A or B and can receive red blood cells from any blood type. **Type O blood** has neither A nor B surface antigens and is the **universal red cell donor.**

B. **Rh surface antigens** are either present (Rh-positive) or absent (Rh-negative). Individuals who are Rh-negative will develop antibodies to the Rh factor when exposed to Rh-positive blood. This is not a problem with the initial exposure, but with subsequent exposures hemolysis will occur due to the circulating antibodies. This can be a particular problem during pregnancy. The anti-Rh antibodies are IgG and freely cross the placenta. In Rh-negative mothers who have developed Rh antibodies, these antibodies are transmitted to the fetus. Obviously, if the fetus is Rh-positive, massive hemolysis will occur, causing fetal death. RhoGAM, an Rh blocking antibody, prevents the Rh-negative patient from developing anti-Rh antibodies. RhoGAM should be given to individuals who receive Rh-positive blood and to Rh-negative mothers delivering Rh-positive babies (some fetal maternal blood mixing occurs at delivery). The recommended dosage is 1 dose (approximately 300 μg/vial) for every 15 ml of Rh-positive blood transfused.

C. If an emergency blood transfusion is needed, **type-specific (ABO) red cells** can usually be obtained within minutes if the patient's blood type is known. If type-specific blood is unavailable, type O Rh-negative red cells should be transfused. Type-specific blood should be substituted as soon as possible to minimize the amount of type O plasma (containing anti-A and anti-B antibodies) transfused.

IV. **Blood component therapy** (Table 33-1)

  A. **General considerations**

    1. One unit of **packed red blood cells** (hematocrit about 70%, volume about 250 ml) will usually raise the hematocrit of a euvolemic adult by 2–3% once equilibration has taken place.

    2. One unit of **platelets** increases the platelet count 5000–10,000. If thrombocytopenia is due to increased turnover (due to development of antiplatelet antibodies) or if platelets are dysfunctional, platelet transfusions will be less efficacious. Single-donor or HLA-matched platelets may be required.

  B. **Technical considerations**

    1. **Compatible infusions.** Blood products should not be infused with 5% dextrose solutions, as they cause hemolysis, or with lactated Ringer's, which contains calcium, which may induce clot formation. Sodium chloride 0.9%, albumin (5%), and fresh-frozen plasma are all compatible with red blood cells.

    2. **Blood filters** (80 micron) should be used for all blood components to remove debris and microaggregates. Leukocyte filters may be used to remove white blood cells in patients with a history of febrile reactions and to prevent alloimmunization to foreign leukocyte antigens. Platelets should be transfused through a 170 micron blood filter.

  C. **Future therapy.** Fluosol-DA 20% is a synthetic fluorocarbon that has been tested in humans. However, since its oxygen carrying capacity is limited, it cannot function as a complete blood substitute. Free hemoglobin solutions are also being investigated as a potential alternative or supplement to blood transfusions.

V. **Plasma substitutes.** Various colloid products are available commercially. Their main limitations are their cost and the dilution of red cells and coagulation factors that occurs with their administration.

  A. **Albumin** is available in either an isotonic 5% solution or a hypertonic 20% and 25% solution. Albumin is plasma that has been pasteurized, eliminating the infectious transfusion risk. It has an intravascular half-life of 10–15 days.

  B. **Dextran.** Dextran 70 (Macrodex) and dextran 40 (Rheomacrodex) are high-molecular-weight polysaccharides. Dextran 70, having a higher molecular weight, is not filtered by the kidney. The dextrans have relatively short half-lives (2–8 hours) and are either excreted or metabolized. Dextrans decrease platelet adhesiveness and depress factor VIII activity. Blood coagulation changes are commonly seen with dextran dosages greater than 1.5 gm/kg. Anaphylactoid reactions have been seen in ap-

Table 33-1. Blood components available

Component	Composition	Volume	Indications
Whole blood	RBCs; WBCs; platelets; plasma	500 ml	Increases both RBC and plasma volume (platelets and WBCs nonfunctional after 72 hours; deficient in factors VII, V)
RBCs	RBCs; WBCs; platelets; reduced plasma	250 ml	Increase RBCs in symptomatic anemia
Leukocyte-poor RBCs (prepared by filtration or centrifugation)	RBCs; $< 5 \times 10^8$ WBCs; few platelets; minimal plasma	200 ml	Increase RBCs; prevent febrile reactions due to leukocyte antibodies
Saline-washed packed RBCs	RBCs; $< 5 \times 10^8$ WBCs; no platelets; no plasma	180 ml	Increase RBCs; reduce risk of allergic reaction to plasma proteins
Platelet concentrate	$> 5 \times 10^{10}$ platelets; RBCs; WBCs; plasma	50 ml	Bleeding from thrombocytopenia or thrombocytopathy
Fresh-frozen plasma	Plasma with all coagulation factors; no platelets	220 ml	Treatment of some coagulation disorders
Cryoprecipitate	Fibrinogen; factors VIII, XIII; von Willebrand's factor	15 ml	Deficiency of factor VIII, XIII, fibrinogen; von Willebrand's disease
Lyophilized VIII	Factor VIII with trace plasma proteins	25 ml	Factor VIII deficiency (hemophilia A)
Lyophilized II, VII, IX, X	Factors II, VII, IX, X	25 ml	Hereditary deficiency
Lyophilized IX	Factor IX with trace plasma proteins	25 ml	Factor IX deficiency (hemophilia B)

RBCs = red blood cells; WBCs = white blood cells.

proximately 1% of patients. These reactions can be avoided by injecting a blocking dextran (20 ml of Promit), which binds the patient's dextran binding antibodies.

C. **Hydroxyethyl starch (Hespan)** is manufactured from amylopectin. After infusion, hydroxyethyl starch is stored in the endothelial cells of the liver for a prolonged time. The starch can cause an increase in serum amylase for several days, which may confuse the diagnosis of pancreatitis. While a decrease in factor VIII levels and decreased platelet function can be seen, hydroxyethyl starch dosages up to 1 gm/kg have been used without adverse bleeding problems. Anaphylactoid reactions are rare.

VI. Pharmacologic therapy

A. **Erythropoietin** increases red cell mass by stimulating proliferation and development of the erythroid precursor cells. Initially it was used to correct anemia in patients with chronic renal failure; however, it is beginning to be used to increase preoperative hematocrits. Erythropoietin may also be used to increase red cell mass prior to preoperative autologous donation. Patients taking erythropoietin should be supplemented with iron and folate. Side effects of hypertension and seizures have been reported in renal failure patients. Initial recommended dosages in renal patients range from 50–100 IU/kg IV or SQ 3 times a week. An appreciable increase in red cell production is seen within 4–6 weeks of starting therapy.

B. **Aminocaproic acid (Amicar)** inhibits fibrinolysis by interfering with plasminogen activators. Fibrinolysis is the naturally-occurring process by which fibrin clot is broken down. Plasmin, converted from the proenzyme plasminogen, digests fibrin. By interfering with the activation of plasmin, aminocaproic acid decreases the breakdown of fibrin clot. Consequently, aminocaproic acid is only helpful when fibrinolysis is believed to play a role in bleeding (e.g., after cardiopulmonary bypass and transurethral resection of the prostate [TURP]). It may also play a role in reversing the effects of tissue plasminogen activator (tPA) or streptokinase. Aminocaproic acid should not be administered if the possibility of disseminated intravascular coagulation (DIC) exists. IV dosing recommendations are a 5-gm loading dose over 1 hour followed by an infusion of 1 gm/hr.

C. **Desmopressin (DDAVP)** is an antidiuretic hormone that is known to be helpful in patients with hemophilia A (factor VIII deficiency) and in patients with classic von Willebrand's disease. Desmopressin increases endothelial cell release of von Willebrand's factor, factor VIII, and plasminogen activator. Desmopressin has also been helpful in patients with platelet defects associated with uremia. The dosage of desmopressin is 0.3 μg/kg. Tachyphylaxis may occur if dosing is greater than every 48 hours. The IV dose should be given slowly, as hypotension may result. Water intoxication and hyponatremia are possible complications in awake patients taking PO fluids.

D. **Aprotinin** has been shown to be effective in diminishing blood loss after cardiopulmonary bypass. Aprotinin inhibits fibrinolysis by inhibiting plasmin and may also protect platelet membrane receptors responsible for platelet adhesion. Aprotinin is administered by continuous IV infusion (short serum half-life), starting prior to cardiopulmonary bypass and continued through the completion of surgery. Adverse reactions include allergic reactions and contact activation of the extrinsic coagulation pathway. Renal toxicity has been seen in patients receiving large doses. Its efficacy outside of cardiac surgery has not been proved, but it would appear to be theoretically useful in cases with excessive fibrinolysis (bleeding after TURP or liver transplantation).

VII. **Conservation/salvage techniques**

A. **Autologous donation** usually begins 4–5 weeks prior to surgery and can greatly reduce the chance or amount of homologous blood transfusion. The length of the predonation period is limited by the length of time that blood can be stored, currently 35 days. If the red cells are frozen, predonation time can be lengthened almost indefinitely. Current blood bank guidelines require a predonation hemoglobin of at least 11 gm/dl, donations no more frequently than every 3 days, and no donations in the 72 hours prior to surgery. Most patients tolerate autologous donation without complication. In heart disease patients, some centers infuse crystalloid at the time of donation to maintain euvolemia. Patients with severe aortic stenosis or unstable angina are not candidates for autologous donation. Since the vast majority of fatal transfusion reactions are due to clerical errors, autologous blood should **not** be transfused unless indicated.

B. **Isovolemic hemodilution.** Preoperative or intraoperative hemodilution entails phlebotomizing a patient of one or more units of fresh whole blood while replacing the lost volume with either colloid or crystalloid. By using isovolemic hemodilution prior to intraoperative blood loss, fresh autologous blood is available for later reinfusion. Also by hemodiluting a patient to a hematocrit of 30% or less, any blood loss intraoperatively will constitute more plasma loss and less red cell loss. The phlebotomized blood is returned to the patient after surgical blood loss is complete. Obviously if surgical blood loss is extreme, the fresh autologous blood should be transfused before any homologous blood. It should also be remembered that the autologous blood has a hematocrit similar to the patient's preoperative hematocrit, as opposed to packed red blood cells, which have a hematocrit of approximately 70–80%. While hemodilution alone may not eliminate the need for homologous transfusion, when used in combination with preoperative autologous donation, it can certainly decrease the need for homologous units. Hemodilution can also be very helpful in situations where platelet function is altered intraoperatively (i.e., cardiopulmonary bypass), since the phlebotomized blood has normal platelets and clotting factors when reinfused.

C. **Cell saver/scavenger.** Intraoperative autotransfusion utilizes blood collected from the surgical field by a double-lumen suction device. Heparinized normal saline is infused through one lumen so that the blood is anticoagulated as it is suctioned from the surgical field. The aspirated and heparinized blood is filtered and collected in the reservoir. The blood is then centrifuged to remove plasma and any debris. The red cells are suspended in normal saline and then recentrifuged. The washed red cells are then ready for reinfusion. The hematocrit of these processed units is approximately 50%. The processing time takes approximately 3 minutes. These units are washed packed red blood cells deficient in plasma, clotting factors, and platelets.

VIII. Complications of blood transfusion therapy
A. Transfusion reactions
1. **Acute hemolytic transfusion reactions.** Hemolytic transfusion reactions are estimated to occur in 1/30,000 transfusions, and most are due to clerical errors. Symptoms of anxiety, agitation, chest pain, flank pain, headache, dyspnea, chills, or fever may indicate an acute hemolytic transfusion reaction. In patients under general anesthesia, signs may include fever, hypotension, unexplained bleeding (DIC), or hemoglobinuria. If a transfusion reaction is suspected, the following steps should be followed:
   a. Stop transfusion.
   b. Send unused donor blood and a fresh patient sample to the blood bank to be recross-matched.
   c. Send blood samples for free hemoglobin, haptoglobin, Coombs' test, and DIC screening. Pink plasma in a spun sample indicates at least 20 mg/dl of free hemoglobin.
   d. Treat hypotension with fluids and vasopressors as indicated.
   e. Consider corticosteroids.
   f. Preserve renal function by increasing renal blood flow and maintaining brisk urine output (IV fluid, furosemide, mannitol).
   g. Be alert for DIC.
2. **Nonhemolytic transfusion reactions.** Allergic or febrile transfusion reactions occur and are usually due to antibodies against donor white cells or plasma proteins. These patients may complain of anxiety, pruritus, or mild dyspnea. Under general anesthesia these patients may develop fever, flushing, hives, tachycardia, and mild hypotension. The transfusion should be stopped and a hemolytic transfusion reaction ruled out. If the reaction is only urticaria or hives, the transfusion should be slowed, and antihistamines (diphenhydramine, 25–50 mg IV) and glucocorticoids (hydrocortisone, 50–100 mg IV) may be given. In patients with known febrile or allergic transfusion reactions, leukocyte-poor red cells (leukocytes removed by filtration or centrifugation) may be given and the patient pretreated with antipyretics (acetaminophen, 650 mg) and an antihistamine. Anaphylactic reactions occur rarely (1/800) and may be more common in

patients with an IgA deficiency. These reactions are usually due to plasma protein reactions. Patients with a history of transfusion anaphylaxis should only be transfused with washed red cells (plasma-free).

B. Metabolic complications of blood transfusions

1. **Potassium (K^+).** Changes in K^+ concentration are common with rapid blood transfusion, but seldom of clinical importance. With storage, red cells leak K^+ into the extracellular storage fluid. However, with transfusion and replenishment of cellular energy stores, this is rapidly corrected.

2. **Calcium.** Citrate, which binds calcium, is used as an anticoagulant in stored blood products. Consequently, rapid transfusion may cause a decreased ionized calcium level but is usually not a problem clinically, as the infused citrate is rapidly metabolized by the liver. However, hypocalcemia may become a problem in patients with impaired liver function, during the anhepatic phase of liver transplantation, in hypothermic patients, or in patients with decreased hepatic blood flow. Ionized calcium levels should be followed, as total serum calcium measures the citrate-bound calcium and may not accurately reflect free serum calcium.

3. **Acid-base status.** Banked blood is acidic due to accumulated red cell metabolites. However, the actual acid load to the patient is minimal. Acidosis in the face of severe blood loss is more likely due to hypoperfusion and will improve with volume resuscitation. Alkalosis is not uncommon following massive blood transfusion. Citrate metabolism contributes to alkalosis, since metabolism of one citrate molecule generates three bicarbonate molecules. Metabolization of lactate also generates significant bicarbonate.

C. Infectious complications of blood transfusions

1. **Hepatitis**

a. **Hepatitis B.** The risk of hepatitis B infection from a blood transfusion has decreased since testing donated blood for hepatitis B antigen became routine in 1971. The current risk is estimated to be between 1/200 and 1/300 per unit transfused. While the majority of infections are usually asymptomatic, long-term morbidity may be significant.

b. **Hepatitis C.** The incidence of non-A, non-B hepatitis is estimated to be 5%. However, with the advent of routine testing for hepatitis C antigen, the incidence of non-A, non-B hepatitis may approach that of hepatitis B.

c. **Pooled products** have an increased risk proportional to the number of donors.

2. **Human immunodeficiency virus (HIV).** With the recent advent of antibody testing, the risk of transfusion-associated HIV has been estimated to be about 1/150,000 per unit transfused in the United States. Often several years elapse before sequelae of infection are apparent.

3. **Cytomegalovirus (CMV).** The incidence of trans-

fusion-associated CMV infection in previously noninfected patients is quite high. The prevalence of CMV antibodies in the general population is approximately 70% by adulthood, so it can be assumed that most of the blood transfused is CMV contaminated. Usually the infection is asymptomatic, but immunosuppressed patients and neonates may have severe reactions. CMV-negative blood may be available for these patients, but it must be specifically requested.

4. **Epstein-Barr virus (EBV).** Approximately 90% of blood donors are EBV antibody–positive, but clinically significant post-transfusion disease in immunocompetent patients is rare. The reasons for this are not entirely clear. The role of EBV in lymphoproliferative disease has not been fully defined.

5. **Lymphotrophic viruses.** Retroviruses, in addition to being the etiologic agent for acquired immunodeficiency syndrome (AIDS), have been implicated as the causal agents in some leukemias and lymphomas. Human T-cell lymphotrophic virus-I (HTLV-I) is known to cause a T-cell leukemia/lymphoma, and there is clinical evidence that this virus is transmitted by transfusion. HTLV-II has also been associated with hairy-cell leukemia, and HTLV-III is synonymous with HIV (see sec. 2).

6. **Bacterial infections.** Exclusion of donors with evidence of infectious disease and the storage of blood at 4°C reduce the risk of transmitted bacterial infection. In addition, fresh blood is bactericidal due to white cells, complement, and immunoglobulin. Occasional contamination by organisms that can grow at 4°C (e.g., *Pseudomonas*) has been known to occur but is rare. However, bacterial contamination of warm blood is a concern, and for this reason blood must be kept refrigerated prior to transfusion. This is a particular problem with platelets that are stored at room temperature. The impact on the individual patient depends on the size of the bacterial inoculum and the immunocompetence of the recipient.

7. **Parasitic infections** are rare in the United States and Europe but are commonly a concern elsewhere. Transfusion-associated malaria is common in endemic countries, as are filariasis and trypanosomiasis (Chagas' disease). Toxoplasmosis has been transmitted by blood transfusion, but in immunocompetent adults the infection is usually asymptomatic. To reduce the risk of parasitic infections, individuals who have recently traveled to endemic areas are asked not to donate blood.

D. **Immunologic complications of blood transfusions.** Blood transfusions are known to affect the immune system. Transfusion-induced immunosuppression through impaired cell-mediated immunity and increased prostaglandin E production may occur, but the clinical impact is unknown.

IX. **Perioperative coagulopathy**

A. **Coagulopathy of massive transfusion** is rarely seen prior to the transfusion of greater than 1.0–1.5 complete blood volumes, assuming the patient had a normal coagulation profile, normal platelet count, and normal platelet function to start.

1. **Thrombocytopenia.** Diffuse oozing and failure to form clot after a massive blood transfusion are almost always due to thrombocytopenia. The decreased platelet count is due to the transfusion of platelet-poor blood products. Clinical bleeding is unlikely with platelet counts above 50,000. If a blood loss of one blood volume is expected, platelets should be available **in the operating room** but not transfused unless there is clinical evidence of bleeding. In adults, 5–10 units of platelets may be required, and in children, 0.3 units/kg.

2. **Clotting factors.** The normal human body has tremendous reserves of clotting factors. In addition, the patient receives small amounts of the stable clotting factors in the plasma with each unit of red cells. Bleeding from factor deficiency in the face of massive transfusion is usually due to diminished levels of fibrinogen (factor I) and labile factors (V, VIII, IX). Bleeding from hypofibrinogenemia is unusual unless the fibrinogen level is below 75 mg/dl. In some patients, factor VIII levels actually increase with massive transfusion and are believed to be due to endothelial cell release. Labile clotting factors are administered in the form of fresh-frozen plasma. Six units of platelets contain the equivalent of 1 unit of fresh-frozen plasma. If the patient is known to be factor deficient (e.g., from warfarin therapy, liver disease), then the threshold for transfusion of fresh-frozen plasma should be lower.

B. **Disseminated intravascular coagulation (DIC)** refers to the diffuse systemic activation of the clotting system.

1. **Etiologies.** DIC is usually caused by infections, shock, or tissue injury, is a complication of pregnancy (amniotic fluid embolism, premature placental separation, septic abortion), or is a complication of extracorporeal circulation. Endothelial cell damage with exposure of collagen may be the cause of DIC seen in shock and infections. DIC may also be seen in hemolytic reactions, head injury (brain tissue is highly thromboplastic), burns, fat embolism, and malignancies.

2. **Clinical features.** When the clotting system is diffusely activated and fibrin forms, the body compensates by attempting to lyse fibrin clots. Plasmin is activated, and diffuse fibrinolysis ensues. The resulting clinical picture is usually one of bleeding (due to consumption of the coagulation factors and platelets), as opposed to diffuse thrombosis. DIC will result in increased fibrin degradation products, and advanced DIC will also result in thrombocytopenia and hypofibrinogenemia.

3. **Treatment** of DIC involves treating the precipitating cause and support with appropriate blood products.

The use of heparin to decrease fibrin formation in DIC remains controversial. After correction of the underlying problem, transfusion of fresh-frozen plasma and platelets may be indicated to correct diffuse bleeding.

C. Chronic liver disease. With the exception of factor VIII and von Willebrand's factor, which are manufactured by the endothelium, most of the coagulation factors are made by the liver. Consequently, in patients with severe liver disease, the production of coagulation factors may be impaired. Factor replacement can be accomplished with fresh-frozen plasma (10–15 ml/kg of body weight). Patients with liver disease may also have decreased clearance of activated clotting factors. With increased circulating activated clotting factors, patients may have an ongoing consumptive coagulopathy, similar to DIC. Since the liver is also instrumental in removing the by-products of fibrinolysis, in patients with severe liver disease circulating fibrin split products may be elevated, also contributing to coagulopathy.

D. Vitamin K deficiency. Vitamin K is required by the liver for production of factors II, VII, IX, and X and proteins C and S. Since vitamin K cannot be synthesized by humans, interference with vitamin K absorption will cause a coagulopathy (see Chap. 5). Clinically this is manifested as a prolonged PT. These patients can be treated with vitamin K (10–15 mg SQ or IV each day for 3 days). If faster correction is required, fresh-frozen plasma (10–15 ml/kg) can be used.

E. Pharmacologic intervention

1. **Heparin** acts by accelerating the effect of antithrombin III. Heparin's half-life is short. If patients are anticoagulated with heparin, stopping the heparin for approximately 2–4 hours will usually reverse the effect. If faster reversal is required, protamine, a natural antagonist, may be used. Protamine (1 mg for every 100 units of heparin remaining in the patient) should be given slowly, as adverse reactions (hypotension, hypersensitivity reactions) are common.

2. **Warfarin** (Coumadin) is a vitamin K antagonist inhibiting hepatic production of factors II, VII, IX, and X, and proteins C and S. The half-life of warfarin is approximately 35 hours, requiring days for reversal. If quick reversal of warfarin is required, active factors can be given in the form of fresh-frozen plasma (10–15 ml/kg). Vitamin K (10–15 mg IV or SQ) can also be given for warfarin reversal, but its effect is unpredictable and slow.

3. **Nonsteroidal anti-inflammatory drugs (NSAIDs)** inhibit platelet aggregation by interfering with the cyclooxygenase pathway. **Aspirin** permanently inhibits the pathway for the lifespan of the platelet. Since the half-life of platelets in circulation is approximately 4 days, once aspirin is taken approximately 10 days are required before platelet function returns to normal. The other NSAIDs reversibly inhibit the cyclooxygen-

ase pathway. Once the drugs have been cleared from the body, platelet function returns to normal. Consequently, platelet function is dependent on the individual half-life of the particular drug.

4. **Tissue plasminogen activator (tPA).** Recombinant tPA (Activase) has been available for the past few years. tPA is a naturally occurring enzyme that converts plasminogen into its active form, plasmin, which breaks down fibrin clot. It is used to treat cardiac ischemia and evolving infarct and may serve a role in the treatment of strokes, pulmonary emboli, and peripheral vascular occlusions. tPA has a very short half-life. Clinically, it is given as a loading dose followed by an infusion. Approximately 80% of tPA is cleared by the liver within 10 minutes of stopping the infusion; however, fibrinogen levels will remain depressed for up to 24–36 hours. If emergency surgery is required after tPA therapy, it should be delayed at least 20–30 minutes after cessation of tPA infusion to allow drug clearance. The hypofibrinogenemic state can be corrected with fresh-frozen plasma or cryoprecipitate.

5. **Streptokinase,** a protein isolated from beta-hemolytic streptococci, is an indirect activator of plasminogen. The indications for streptokinase are similar to those for tPA. Ongoing fibrinolysis stops within a few hours of stopping the streptokinase infusion; however, fibrinogen levels may remain low for up to 24–36 hours.

X. **Special considerations**
  A. **Classic hemophilia or hemophilia A** is due to an abnormality of factor VIII. Classic hemophilia constitutes 90% of patients with congenital coagulation abnormalities and has an incidence of 1/10,000. It is a sex-linked recessive trait, affecting males almost exclusively.

1. **Clinical features.** The diagnosis should be suspected in a patient with an elevated PTT, normal PT, and normal bleeding time. Clinical bleeding is related to the level of factor VIII activity (normal activity is 100%):
   a. < 1% activity — spontaneous bleeding.
   b. 1–5% activity — bleeding after minor trauma.
   c. > 5% activity — infrequent bleeding.
   Since these patients have normal platelet function, they are able to form the initial clot, and they will have normal bleeding times. However, since they are unable to stabilize the blood clot, bleeding will recur.

2. **Treatment** consists of lyophilized factor VIII, cryoprecipitate, or desmopressin. A dosage of 1 unit/kg of factor VIII will raise the activity of factor VIII by approximately 2%. Activity levels of 20–40% are recommended prior to surgery. The half-life of factor VIII is 8–12 hours. Since up to 20% of patients will eventually develop resistance due to antibodies against factor VIII, factor VIII activity levels should be measured pretransfusion and post-transfusion. Patients with resistance must then be treated with high-dose factor

VIII, activated factor IX, or plasmapheresis. Since most hemophiliacs require frequent support with clotting factors, a high percentage have been exposed to HIV. Over 80% of these patients are believed to be HIV antibody–positive as well as seropositive for hepatitis. Recombinant factor VIII holds great hope for decreasing the infectious risks for hemophiliacs.

B. Hemophilia B, or Christmas disease, is due to a factor IX abnormality. It also is sex-linked, occurring almost exclusively in males, and has an incidence of 1/100,000. Clinically, these patients present similarly to patients with classic hemophilia. These patients will have an abnormal PTT and a normal PT and bleeding time. Therapy consists of factor IX concentrates or fresh-frozen plasma. For surgical hemostasis, activity levels of 50–80% are necessary (0.5–0.8 units/ml). A dosage of 1 unit/kg of factor IX will raise the activity of factor IX by 1%. The half-life of factor IX is approximately 24 hours.

C. von Willebrand's disease is actually a combination of diseases associated with abnormalities of von Willebrand's factor. von Willebrand's factor is a glycoprotein manufactured by megakaryocytes and endothelial cells and has three known functions: It serves as an anchor for platelet adhesion to collagen, it interlinks platelets (aggregation) in clot formation, and it protects and stabilizes VIII. von Willebrand's disease is most commonly inherited in an autosomal dominant pattern with variable penetrance.

    1. Clinical features. Clinically, these patients most commonly have episodes of mucocutaneous bleeding, excessive epistaxis being the most common presentation. The bleeding tendency of these patients is quite variable.

    2. Laboratory studies. The most common laboratory finding is a prolonged bleeding time, although the PTT may also be prolonged.

    3. Treatment for these individuals include desmopressin (see sec. **VI.C**) and/or cryoprecipitate. Desmopressin (0.3 µg/kg) is known to increase endothelial cell release of von Willebrand's factor. Plasma products may also be required for an actively bleeding patient. Cryoprecipitate (1 unit/10 kg/day) is preferred; however, fresh-frozen plasma may also be used if cryoprecipitate is unavailable. In patients with acquired von Willebrand's disease, high-dose IV gamma globulin (1 gm/kg for 2 days) has been successfully used.

D. Sickle cell anemia. Sickle cell (SC) disease has a prevalence of approximately 1% in the black population in the United States. Sickle cell disease is caused by the substitution of valine for glutamic acid on the beta chain of hemoglobin. Homozygotes for this substitution have clinical sickle cell disease (as well as double heterozygotes SC or beta-thalassemia).

    1. Clinical features. In these patients, the abnormal hemoglobin will polymerize and cause a sickling deformity of the red cell under certain conditions (hypoxia, hypothermia, acidosis, and dehydration). The red cells also have a shortened survival time of 12 days (normal being 120 days), leading to an anemia and extramedullary hematopoiesis.

2. The **anesthetic management** of these patients remains controversial. It has been common practice to give patients red cell transfusions to raise hematocrits and decrease the relative proportion of hemoglobin S red blood cells. Guidelines in the past have suggested transfusing to an end point of having 70% hemoglobin A and less than 30% hemoglobin S cells confirmed by hemoglobin electrophoresis prior to major surgery. Due to the risk of transfusion-associated infections, this practice has recently been questioned. Currently, a multicenter trial is underway examining whether preoperative transfusion for major surgery is indicated. Attention to certain anesthetic issues can lessen the risk of intraoperative sickling. Since hypoxia is a known precipitant of sickling, these patients should be well oxygenated at all times, with close monitoring of oxygen saturation. Acidosis should be avoided and the threshold for blood gas monitoring low. Patients should be well hydrated to maintain intravascular volume and ensure adequate tissue perfusion (preventing systemic acidosis). Hypothermia should also be avoided, since it is also known to precipitate sickle cell crises, probably due to increased blood viscosity and stasis. Interestingly, successful cardiopulmonary bypass has been reported in patients with sickle cell disease. Preoperative partial exchange transfusion to lower hemoglobin S to under 30% is a common but not universal practice. The dilutional effect of going on bypass with crystalline prime or blood prime appears protective. Neonates are usually protected from sickle crisis for the first few months of life due to persistent fetal hemoglobin (hemoglobin F). Patients with sickle cell trait are usually asymptomatic and do not require preoperative transfusion.

E. **Jehovah's Witness patients** create a practical and ethical challenge for anesthesiologists. Their religious faith prohibits them from accepting transfusions of blood or blood products (fresh-frozen plasma, platelets, cryoprecipitate, or albumin). Blood conservation measures are crucial in these patients (see sec. **VII**). Most Jehovah's Witnesses will allow transfusion of intraoperatively phlebotomized blood (see sec. **VII.B**) as long as the blood remains in continuity with the body (i.e., the blood tubing must always remain connected to the patient). Jehovah's Witnesses have successfully undergone major surgeries, including cardiopulmonary bypass, with attentive planning. Erythropoietin may show promise in these patients by allowing an increased red cell mass and allowing increased intraoperative phlebotomy and autodonation. However, it should be noted that currently one vial of erythropoietin contains 2.5 mg of human albumin. It is incumbent on the anesthesiologist to discuss fully the implications of the patient's decision not to accept blood.

Whatever the decision, it is important to document the decision regarding blood product transfusion in the chart and also to have the patient sign the statement showing agreement.

SUGGESTED READING

Colman, R. W., et al. *Hemostasis and Thrombosis: Basic Principles and Clinical Practice.* Philadelphia: Lippincott, 1987.

CONSENSUS conference. Fresh-frozen plasma: Indications and risks. *J.A.M.A.* 253:551, 1985.

CONSENSUS conference. Platelet transfusion therapy. *J.A.M.A.* 257:1777, 1987.

CONSENSUS conference. Perioperative red blood cell transfusion. *J.A.M.A.* 260:2700, 1988.

Cooper, J. R. Perioperative considerations in Jehovah's Witnesses. *Int. Anesthesiol. Clin.* 28:210–215, 1990.

D'Ambra, M. N., and Risk, S. C. Aprotinin, erythropoietin, and blood substitutes. *Int. Anesthesiol. Clin.* 28:237, 1990.

Esseltine, D. W., Baxter, M. R., and Bevan J. C. Sickle cell states and the anaesthetist. *Can. J. Anaesth.* 35:385, 1988.

Flaharty, K. K., Grimm, A. M., and Vlasses, P. H. Epoetin: Human recombinant erythropoietin. *Clin. Pharm.* 8:769, 1989.

Fruchtman, S., and Aledort, L. M. Disseminated intravascular coagulation. *J. Am. Coll. Cardiol.* 8(6):159B–167B, 1986.

Goodnough, L. T., et al. Increased preoperative collection of autologous blood with recombinant human erythropoietin therapy. *N. Engl. J. Med.* 321:1163, 1989.

Hogman, C. F. Immunologic transfusion reactions. *Acta Anaesthesiol. Scand. [Suppl.]* 89:4, 1988.

Messmer, K. F. The use of plasma substitutes with special attention to their side effects. *World J. Surg.* 11:69, 1987.

Murray, D., et al. Coagulation changes during packed red cell replacement of major blood loss. *Anesthesiology* 69:839, 1988.

Ratnoff, O. D., and Forbes, C. D. *Disorders of Hemostasis.* Philadelphia: Saunders, 1991. Pp. 1–604.

Sane, D. C., et al. Bleeding during thrombotic therapy for acute myocardial infarction: Mechanisms and management. *Ann. Intern. Med.* 111:1010, 1989.

Solem, J. O., and Vagianos, C. Perioperative blood salvage. *Acta Anaesthesiol. Scand. [Suppl.]* 89:71, 1988.

34

The Postanesthesia Care Unit

Luca Bigatello

I. **General considerations.** The postanesthesia care unit (PACU) provides close monitoring and care to all patients emerging from general anesthesia, regional anesthesia, or monitored anesthesia care (MAC), as stipulated by the American Society of Anesthesiologists' (ASA) Standards for Postanesthesia Care (see Appendix). Selected patients remain in the PACU overnight, such as those following carotid endarterectomy or extensive procedures with large transfusion requirements. Recovery from anesthesia is usually uneventful, but complications may be sudden and life-threatening. A recent prospective study of more than 12,000 patients reported a 7% incidence of significant complications in the PACU. The most common events were hypotension, dysrhythmias, hypertension, and respiratory complications. A dedicated nursing staff and a designated anesthesiologist should be available at all times. Equipment and drugs for routine care (oxygen, suction, monitoring of vital signs) and advanced support (ventilators, transducers, infusion pumps, and equipment for cardiopulmonary resuscitation) must be available. Portable radiographs and quick access to laboratory values are essential.

II. **Admission to the PACU**

A. On arrival in the PACU, supplemental oxygen is routinely administered to all patients, and vital signs are recorded.

B. If the patient is unstable, the operating room anesthesiologist must remain with the patient until the PACU team feels ready to assume responsibility for the patient's care.

C. The operating room anesthesiologist should provide the admitting nurse with a succinct but complete **report.** If the intraoperative course was complicated in any way or if preexisting clinical conditions warrant it, the physician in charge of the PACU should also receive the report.

1. Patient identification and age, surgical procedure and diagnosis, a brief summary of prior medical history, routine medications, allergies, and preoperative vital signs, as well as any specific features such as blindness, deafness, personality disorder, or language barrier that may impact on care.

2. A description of the location and size of IV catheters.

3. **Medications** administered, including premedication, routine medications continued intraoperatively, antibiotics, anesthetic drugs used for induction and maintenance, narcotics, muscle relaxants, and reversal agents, as well as intraoperative use of vasoactive drugs, antihypertensives, and antiarrhythmics.

4. **Anesthetic course,** with particular emphasis on problems such as a difficult intubation, hemodynamic instability, electrocardiographic (ECG) changes, laryngospasm, bronchospasm, and airway secretions.

5. **Exact nature of the surgical procedure.** A member of the surgical team should inform the PACU nurse regarding surgical issues that may be relevant in the immediate postoperative period (e.g., location and care of drains and restrictions on positioning).

6. **Fluid balance.** The amount and type of fluid administered, estimated blood loss, and urine output are reported. Laboratory values obtained intraoperatively should be reported, as well as pertinent information regarding the adequacy of hemostasis.

III. **Monitoring.** Close observation by a vigilant PACU nurse is important. The nurse-patient ratio for routine cases is 3 : 1. This is increased to 1 : 1 for patients at high risk (e.g., children under 3 years of age, patients with significant preexisting medical problems, or those who have suffered intraoperative complications). Vital signs are monitored and charted at regular intervals according to the acuity of the patient.

A. **Electrocardiogram (ECG).** Continuous recording of one or more leads of the ECG is widely used in the PACU.

B. **Pulse oximetry** is used for all patients, as it allows continuous, noninvasive measurement of arterial oxygen saturation.

C. **Hemodynamic monitoring** (see Chap. 10)

1. **Arterial blood pressure** is measured at regular intervals during recovery from anesthesia.

2. **Central venous pressures** are transduced when present.

3. **Pulmonary artery catheters.** Patients with pulmonary artery catheters are not admitted to the PACU but rather to the surgical intensive care unit.

IV. **Airway difficulties**

A. **Upper airway obstruction** may occur during recovery from general anesthesia or sedation. The most common cause is obstruction due to the tongue's falling backward and occluding the airway. Cardinal signs are lack of air movement, intercostal and suprasternal retractions, and abdominal wall motion unaccompanied by chest wall elevation. Principles of airway management are outlined in detail in Chap. 13.

1. Incomplete recovery from **general anesthesia** (including muscle relaxants) and excessive **sedation** is associated with hypoventilation and decreased strength and coordination of airway reflexes. The airway should be supported with a nasal or oral airway and, if necessary, reintubated to ensure adequate gas exchange.

2. **Laryngospasm** may occur during emergence from general anesthesia or as a consequence of mechanical irritation of the glottis by secretions, blood, or foreign bodies. The pathophysiology and treatment of laryngospasm are discussed in Chap. 18.

3. **Edema of the airway** as manifested by inspiratory **stridor** may occur from surgical manipulation during procedures such as bronchoscopy, esophagoscopy, and excision of laryngeal and tracheal masses. It may also

be a consequence of traumatic intubation, a hyperinflated cuff (particularly in children), an allergic reaction, or intraoperative positioning in the Trendelenburg position for a prolonged period. Treatment of upper airway obstruction secondary to edema includes the following:

a. Head elevation.

b. Administration of warmed, humidified oxygen by face mask.

c. Nebulization of racemic epinephrine: 2.25% solution, 0.5–1. ml in 2–3 ml of normal saline, which may be repeated in 20 minutes and every 2–4 hours as needed.

d. Corticosteroids can be delivered by metered dose inhaler (beclomethasone, 2–4 puffs) or intravenously (dexamethasone, 4–8 mg IV q6h for 24 hours). The efficacy of steroid therapy in this setting has not been clearly demonstrated.

e. Fluid restriction and diuresis may be indicated when large fluid volumes have been administered in the operating room.

f. Reintubation with a smaller sized endotracheal tube may be required.

4. **Wound hematoma.** Thyroid and parathyroid surgery, neck dissections, and carotid endarterectomies may cause airway obstruction secondary to hematoma formation. Airway obstruction is caused by acute, massive edema of the soft tissues of the neck due to obstruction of venous and lymphatic drainage. Wound hematomas must be treated rapidly. The surgeon must be notified and an operating room prepared. The anesthesiologist must support the airway with bag-mask ventilation with 100% oxygen, followed by intubation of the trachea under direct vision before the patient becomes severely distressed. A smaller sized endotracheal tube may be required for reintubation. Distortion of the airway evolves rapidly, and laryngoscopic visualization is generally more difficult than what clinical symptoms may suggest. If endotracheal intubation cannot be accomplished in a patient in respiratory distress and the surgeon is not available, the wound must be opened at the bedside to relieve pressure. This *may* temporarily improve the patient's condition and make airway management easier, although edema is unaffected. In most circumstances, surgical evacuation is a rapid and simple procedure.

5. **Vocal cord paralysis.** Unilateral or bilateral vocal cord paralysis may occur after surgical manipulation near the recurrent laryngeal nerves (e.g., thyroid and parathyroid surgery, thoracotomy, or tracheal procedures). The risk of bilateral vocal cord paralysis is highest after total thyroidectomy for cancer, where neoplastic infiltration beyond the thyroid capsule may make identification of the recurrent laryngeal nerves impossible. Paralysis of the vocal cords may be transient or permanent. If the nerves have simply been

bruised, function will eventually resume, while transection results in permanent paralysis.

B. **Hypoventilation** may be secondary to a decrease in respiratory rate, tidal volume, or both. Decreased alveolar ventilation will cause hypercarbia, hypoxemia, acidosis, carbon dioxide narcosis, and ultimately apnea. Several factors may lead to hypoventilation in the immediate postoperative period.

1. **Decreased ventilatory drive**
   a. Decreased ventilatory drive may occur as a result of **central nervous system (CNS) injury** following head trauma or neurosurgery.
   b. More commonly, **residual anesthesia** reversibly depresses ventilatory drive (see Chap. 11). Both residual volatile anesthesia and opioids are potent respiratory depressants; the overnarcotized patient shows a typical clinical picture characterized by analgesia, a slow respiratory rate, and a tendency to become apneic when unstimulated.
      (1) **Narcotic-induced respiratory depression** may be reversed by administering the pure opiate antagonist naloxone (Narcan). Naloxone will reverse the analgesia, respiratory depression, and other receptor-mediated effects. Incremental doses of 40–80 μg IV are titrated to effect (e.g., an increase in ventilation or wakefulness). Reversal of CNS depression occurs within 1–2 minutes and lasts for 30–60 minutes.
      (2) **Oversedation secondary to benzodiazepines.** Flumazenil (Mazicon) is a benzodiazepine receptor antagonist.
         (a) The dosage for reversal of conscious sedation is 0.2 mg IV, titrated to a total dose of 1 mg over a 5-minute interval.
         (b) For known or suspected benzodiazepine overdose, 0.2 mg is given IV and titrated up to a maximum dose of 5 mg.
         (c) The onset of reversal occurs within 1–2 minutes with peak effect at 6–10 minutes. The half-life is 54 minutes. For resedation, repeated doses may be given at 20-minute intervals. Patients with respiratory depression secondary to benzodiazepine overdose may require intubation and mechanical ventilation.

2. **Inadequate reversal of neuromuscular blockade.** Muscle weakness, secondary to residual neuromuscular blockade may be noted clinically by the presence of spasmodic twitching, generalized weakness, and fatigue. Muscle function can be assessed with clinical criteria or a twitch monitor. Criteria for reversal of neuromuscular blockade are discussed in Chap. 12. Special situations must be considered in the differential diagnosis: myasthenia gravis, pseudocholinesterase deficiency, succinylcholine-induced phase II block, myasthenic syndromes (Eaton-Lambert syn-

drome), administration of aminoglycoside antibiotics, and anticholinesterase overdose. Symptoms of cholinergic crisis include muscle weakness, bradycardia, wheezing, abundant salivation, and abdominal cramping.

3. **Upper airway obstruction** (see sec. A) may cause hypercapnia and hypoxemia.

4. **Excessive pain** following thoracotomy or upper abdominal surgery may cause splinting and a reduction in tidal volume, resulting in hypoventilation and the development of atelectasis. This is preventable by providing adequate analgesia (e.g., patient-controlled analgesia, epidural) and chest physical therapy.

5. **Preexisting lung disease**

   a. Patients with restrictive disease states (obesity, severe scoliosis, massive ascites, or pregnancy) may be more prone to develop hypoventilation.

   b. Patients with chronic obstructive pulmonary disease (COPD) must perform increased work of breathing to maintain gas exchange under normal circumstances. These patients may retain carbon dioxide in the postoperative period secondary to bronchospasm, airway secretions, and surgical trauma.

   c. Chest physical therapy to stimulate deep breathing and coughing, bronchodilator therapy, and analgesia are particularly important in this group of patients.

6. **Bronchospasm** in the postoperative period is common in patients with COPD, asthma, or a recent respiratory tract infection. The onset of bronchospasm is generally precipitated by mechanical airway irritation or the presence of secretions. Wheezing may also be seen in pulmonary edema, endobronchial intubation, aspiration pneumonitis, and pneumothorax. Physical examination, arterial blood gases, and chest radiographs will confirm the diagnosis. Treatment of bronchospasm is discussed in Chap. 18.

7. **Pneumothorax** may complicate surgical procedures such as thoracotomy, mediastinoscopy, bronchoscopy, high retroperitoneal dissections (nephrectomy and adrenalectomy), and following back surgery for scoliosis. Insertion of central venous lines and performance of regional nerve blocks of the upper extremities are also possible etiologies. A high index of suspicion is necessary, as a large or tension pneumothorax may cause severe respiratory distress. Treatment is discussed in Chap. 18.

C. **Hypoxemia.** Arterial oxygen desaturation is a relatively common event during recovery from anesthesia. Physical signs associated with hypoxia include cyanosis, altered mental status (agitation), dyspnea, tachycardia, dysrhythmias, and hypertension. Hypoxemia should always be ruled out before beginning treatment of these symptoms. Common causes of hypoxemia during recovery from anesthesia include the following:

1. **Atelectasis** results in a decrease in lung volumes induced by mucus plugging, hypoventilation, or general anesthesia. Deep breathing, coughing, and chest physiotherapy are effective in reexpanding areas of alveolar collapse. Larger areas of atelectasis should be suspected in the presence of refractory hypoxemia and a chest x-ray that reveals segmental or lobar **lung collapse**. In patients who do not respond to aggressive chest physiotherapy, fiberoptic bronchoscopy should be performed to remove secretions.

2. **Upper airway obstruction** (see sec. **A**).

3. **Hypoventilation** (see sec. **B**).

4. **Diffusion hypoxia** due to the washout of nitrous oxide during emergence from general anesthesia. This is short-lived and easily prevented by the administration of high inspired concentrations of oxygen by face mask.

5. **Bronchospasm** (see sec. **6**).

6. **Aspiration** of gastric contents should always be considered in the differential diagnosis of postoperative hypoxia. Possible risk factors for aspiration include a difficult airway, anesthesia administered by face mask, a full stomach, history of gastroesophageal reflux, obesity, and retching and vomiting on emergence. The chest radiograph may reveal a discrete infiltrate but often is not diagnostic for several hours after the event. In most patients, it is reasonable to wait for the results of Gram's stain and sputum cultures prior to beginning antibiotic therapy. Supplemental oxygen should be provided.

7. **Pulmonary edema** may be secondary to left ventricular failure or increased pulmonary capillary permeability. Cardiogenic pulmonary edema may be revealed by dyspnea, orthopnea, jugular venous distention, an S_3 gallop, and wheezing. Factors that can precipitate acute cardiogenic pulmonary edema include fluid overload, myocardial ischemia and infarction, and rapid atrial fibrillation. "Permeability" pulmonary edema in the immediate postoperative course may be secondary to head injury (neurogenic pulmonary edema), aspiration, transfusion reaction, anaphylaxis, sepsis, or upper airway obstruction (negative-pressure pulmonary edema). Evaluation should include auscultation of the chest, analysis of arterial blood gases, examination of a 12-lead ECG, and obtaining a chest radiograph. Invasive monitoring with a central line or a pulmonary artery catheter may be necessary. Therapy of pulmonary edema may include the administration of supplemental oxygen, diuretics, vasodilators, inotropic agents, endotracheal intubation, and mechanical ventilation with positive end-expiratory pressure.

8. **Pneumothorax** (see sec. **B.7**).

9. **Pulmonary embolism** must be considered in the differential diagnosis of acute dyspnea and hypoxemia, although it seldom occurs in the immediate postoperative period. The pulmonary artery angiogram is the most specific diagnostic procedure. Diagnosis and man-

agement of pulmonary embolism are outlined in Chap. 18.

D. **The intubated patient.** Patients may be admitted to the PACU intubated. Common reasons include

1. **Delayed emergence** from general anesthesia. This can be due to either volatile or intravenous agents. Reversal of narcotic overdose may be facilitated by administration of a narcotic antagonist; however, it may be prudent simply to allow the respiratory depression to resolve while mechanically supporting ventilation.

2. **Inadequate reversal of neuromuscular blockade.** If maximal pharmacologic reversal of nondepolarizing blockade has already been administered (neostigmine, 0.06–0.07 mg/kg, or edrophonium, 1 mg/kg), further reversal should not be attempted, and the patient should be ventilated until full recovery.

3. **Potential for airway obstruction.** Surgical procedures that may mandate postoperative intubation for airway protection include major head and neck reconstruction, drainage of pharyngeal abscesses, mandibular wiring or banding, and surgery for trauma of the face and neck. These patients should not be extubated until fully awake.

4. **Full stomach.** The presence of recently ingested food in the stomach mandates extra attention to full recovery of pharyngeal reflexes prior to extubation.

5. **Hemodynamic instability.** It is important to postpone extubation until patients are hemodynamically stable. A sedated and ventilated patient is more safely managed in these circumstances.

6. **Poor gas exchange.** Inadequate oxygenation and carbon dioxide elimination often resolve in the PACU as the effects of anesthesia, surgery, and positioning fade. If they do not, transfer to an intensive care unit is appropriate.

7. **Hypothermia** may be associated with altered mental status, muscle weakness, and the potential for severe shivering during rewarming. In the presence of severe hypothermia (< 94°F), one should delay extubation until patients are rewarmed.

8. **Adequate ventilation and gas exchange** must be ensured. Spontaneous ventilation through a "T-piece" may be sufficient in some patients, while others may require full support with mechanical ventilation. A portable chest radiograph should be obtained in all patients requiring prolonged postoperative intubation to rule out pulmonary pathology and to ensure proper positioning of the endotracheal tube. The anesthesiologist in the PACU should establish a plan regarding weaning and assess the need for a prolonged stay or transfer to an intensive care unit.

9. **Guidelines for extubation**

a. **Adequate breathing pattern.** Patients should be able to sustain spontaneous unlabored ventilation with a slow respiratory rate (< 20–25 breaths/min).

         b. Adequate lung volumes. A vital capacity of 1 liter and a tidal volume greater than 300 ml are generally associated with successful extubation in adults.

         c. Full recovery of muscle strength as assessed by clinical examination. An inspiratory force greater than -25 cm H_2O is usually adequate.

         d. Adequate oxygenation with minimal supplemental oxygen (FiO_2 0.30–0.40).

         e. Before proceeding with extubation, the PACU anesthesiologist should be aware of potential **airway problems** in the event that reintubation is necessary.

         f. Oxygen 100% is administered, and the endotracheal tube, mouth, and pharynx are suctioned. The cuff is deflated, and the tube is removed following a positive-pressure breath. Oxygen 100% is supplied by face mask, SaO_2 is monitored (if available), and the patient is assessed for signs of airway obstruction or respiratory insufficiency.

V. Hemodynamic problems

    A. Hypotension is a common postoperative problem. Accuracy of the value must be determined and artifact excluded prior to beginning therapy. The patient's medical history and intraoperative record are quickly reviewed with particular attention focused on instability and the adequacy of volume replacement. Hypotension may result from

        1. Inadequate venous return

            a. Hypovolemia. Signs and symptoms of hypovolemia include thirst, dry mucous membranes, tachycardia, and oliguria. Continued bleeding should be excluded by physical examination and hematocrit. A fluid bolus (250–500 ml of crystalloid) should be given. If the patient is anemic, volume replacement with red blood cells is appropriate. Persistent hypotension following adequate volume replacement will necessitate the placement of a Foley catheter and invasive monitoring (e.g., central venous pressure or pulmonary artery line).

            b. Mechanical limitation to venous return may be secondary to increased intrathoracic or extracardiac pressure. This may occur with mechanical ventilation, tension pneumothorax, or pericardial tamponade. Chest radiographs, echocardiography, and invasive monitoring may aid in diagnosis and therapy (see Chap. 18).

        2. Decreased vascular tone. Vasodilatation may cause hypotension despite adequate intravascular volume. This can be seen with spinal and epidural anesthesia, anaphylactoid and anaphylactic reactions, sepsis, and adrenal insufficiency. Vasodilatation may be seen following administration of antihypertensive, antiarrhythmic, and anticonvulsant medication, as well as during rewarming from hypothermia. Therapy consists of volume replacement, restoration of vascular tone (e.g., usually with phenylephrine), and treatment of specific etiologies (e.g., allergic reaction, adrenal insufficiency). Invasive monitoring may be required.

3. **Myocardial dysfunction.** Potential etiologies include myocardial ischemia, infarction, congestive heart failure, sepsis, hypothyroidism, arrhythmias, and negative inotropic drugs (e.g., beta blockers, calcium channel blockers, and antiarrhythmics). A 12-lead ECG must be obtained to evaluate ischemia and rhythm disturbances. Invasive monitoring may be indicated, and treatment is discussed in Chap. 18.

B. **Hypertension** following emergence from general anesthesia can be caused by pain, agitation, hypoxemia, hypercarbia, increased intracranial pressure (ICP), and bladder distention. Chronic hypertension is often associated with elevated blood pressure in the immediate postoperative period, particularly if antihypertensive medications are held preoperatively.

1. **Management** starts with identifying its etiology and correcting the underlying cause. Under some circumstances, pharmacologic treatment of hypertension may be unnecessary or even dangerous (e.g., hypertension secondary to ICP). Moderate hypertension (30% elevation over preoperative values) is generally not harmful. Tight control of blood pressure may be indicated in particular circumstances, such as following intracranial surgery or for those patients with ischemic heart disease or a known aortic or cerebral aneurysm.

2. **Adequate oxygenation and ventilation** should be ensured and pain relief provided.

3. **Short-acting medications** are preferred, since postoperative hypertension may be short-lived. Hypertension can be effectively treated with drugs such as
   a. **Labetalol,** 5–10 mg IV.
   b. **Propranolol,** 0.5-mg increments IV.
   c. **Nifedipine,** 5–10 mg SL.
   d. **Hydralazine,** 5–20 mg IV.
   e. **Nitroglycerin,** begun at 20 μg/min IV.
   f. **Sodium nitroprusside** titrated to effect.
   g. **Trimethaphan** titrated starting with a dose of 1 mg/min.

C. **Dysrhythmias** in the immediate postoperative period may be secondary to increased sympathetic stimulation, myocardial ischemia, hypoxia, increased ICP, electrolyte imbalance, or drug toxicity. Benign arrhythmias such as premature atrial contractions and unifocal premature ventricular contractions generally do not require specific treatment and subside within a short period of time. In the presence of more serious rhythm disturbances, supplemental oxygen should be delivered and proper treatment begun while the etiology is investigated. Specific pharmacologic therapy of arrhythmias is outlined in Chap. 18.

1. **Supraventricular arrhythmias.**
   a. **Sinus tachycardia** is common and may be second-

ary to pain, agitation, hypovolemia, or fever. It does not require treatment unless associated with hypotension or myocardial ischemia.

b. **Sinus bradycardia** may result from the administration of narcotic analgesics, beta blockers, or vagal stimulation. Severe hypertension, increased ICP, and profound hypoxemia are potential causes that must be excluded.

c. Rapid supraventricular rhythms include **paroxysmal tachycardia, nodal tachycardia, atrial fibrillation,** and **flutter.** These may cause myocardial ischemia if untreated.

d. **Treatment**

   (1) **Beta antagonists** (propranolol, 0.5–5.0 mg IV, or esmolol, 10–60 mg IV).

   (2) **Verapamil** (2.5–5. mg IV).

   (3) **Adenosine** (6–12 mg IV).

   (4) **Digoxin** (0.25-mg IV increments titrated to a maximum of 1.0–1.5 mg).

   (5) **Synchronized cardioversion** if accompanied by severe hypotension.

2. **Ventricular arrhythmias.** If premature ventricular contractions are multifocal, occur in runs, or are associated with R-on-T phenomenon, they may indicate inadequate myocardial perfusion and must be treated.

a. A 12-lead **ECG** should be obtained.

b. **Lidocaine,** 1.5 mg/kg IV bolus, is given followed by an infusion at 1–4 mg/min.

c. **Ischemia** or **hypokalemia** is treated.

d. **Ventricular tachycardia** and **ventricular fibrillation** are obvious emergencies.

D. **Myocardial ischemia and infarction.** ECG changes compatible with ischemia are a relatively frequent postoperative occurrence. When abnormalities suggestive of ischemia are observed, a 12-lead ECG must be obtained and compared with a previous one if available. New-onset ST-segment changes (> 1-mm ST elevation or depression) should be considered indicative of ischemia until proved otherwise.

1. **T-wave changes.** Changes in the configuration of the T-wave (inversion, flattening, pseudo-normalization) not associated with abnormalities of the ST segment may be seen with lead placement, electrolyte changes, hypothermia, or manipulation of the pericardium. Nonspecific T-wave changes must be considered within the clinical context and should not automatically mandate a "rule-out myocardial infarction" routine. If the clinical scenario suggests ischemia, the patient must be aggressively treated.

2. **ST-segment changes.** ST-segment elevation or depression is a highly specific sign of myocardial ischemia.

a. **Treatment** should begin with correction of factors that may precipitate ischemia: hypoxia, tachycardia, hypotension, or hypertension. Supplemental oxygen should be administered, adequate analgesia achieved, rate-related ischemia should be controlled with beta antagonists (IV **esmolol, propranolol,** or **labetalol**), and IV **nitroglycerin** should be administered.

b. The ECG must be monitored, and a **cardiology consultation** should be obtained.

c. **Persistent ischemia** despite aggressive therapy (unstable angina) may require invasive monitoring, placement of an intraaortic balloon pump, cardiac catheterization, percutaneous angioplasty, or emergency revascularization.

VI. Oliguria

A. **Etiologies. Oliguria** is defined as a urine output of less than 0.5 ml/kg/hr, which in the postoperative period is generally secondary to hypovolemia, hypotension, or low cardiac output. Postrenal causes include catheter obstruction, intraoperative ureter transection, bladder perforation, and renal vein compression from high intraabdominal pressure.

B. **Diuretics should not be routinely administered,** as they may worsen hypovolemia and confound diagnostic studies. Once intravascular volume and blood pressure have been optimized, urine electrolytes should be checked, and diuresis may be stimulated with loop diuretics (furosemide, 5–20 mg IV), low-dose dopamine (1–3 μg/kg/min), or mannitol (12.5–25.0 gm IV).

VII. Neurologic problems

A. **Delayed awakening**

1. **Hypoxemia, hypercarbia, and hypotension** should always be excluded.

2. In the absence of severe hypotension or hypoxia, delayed awakening is usually secondary to **residual anesthesia** (see sec. **IV.B.1.b.**).

3. The possibility of **neurologic damage** should be considered when obtundation occurs (particularly in the presence of known cerebrovascular disease) following either severe intraoperative hemodynamic instability, head trauma, or intracranial surgery. If a focal deficit or altered mental status is present in a neurosurgical patient, the surgeon should be immediately notified. Subdural hematoma, intracerebral hemorrhage, or edema may produce these changes and may be amenable to treatment.

4. **Metabolic causes** include hyperglycemia, hypoglycemia, sepsis, and electrolyte or acid-base derangements.

5. **Emergence delirium** is characterized by excitement, occasionally alternating with lethargy, disorientation, and inappropriate behavior. Supplemental oxygen must be administered and a neurologic examination performed to rule out focal deficits. Hypoxemia, acidosis, hyponatremia, hypoglycemia, fever, sepsis, severe pain, and alcohol withdrawal should all be considered. Drugs administered during and after anesthesia should be reviewed: Ketamine may produce hallucinations, benzodiazepines and narcotics may cause paradoxical agitation and confusion in the elderly, scopola-

mine and atropine may produce delirium, and phenothiazines, butyrophenones, and metoclopramide may cause dysphoric reactions. **Physostigmine** (0.5–2.0 mg IV prn) may be administered specifically to reverse anticholinergic agitation or nonspecifically to improve delirium in some patients. Small doses of narcotics or benzodiazepines will provide sedation and smooth emergence in others.

B. **Focal neurologic deficits** may occur following neurosurgical procedures or carotid artery surgery or may be the result of an intraoperative stroke or direct peripheral nerve damage secondary to surgery or improper positioning. Prompt communication with the surgeon and support of the airway and circulation are critical.

VIII. **Pain.** Since pain is a predictable response to the trauma of surgery, adequate analgesia should begin in the operating room and be supplemented as needed in the PACU. Many factors affect the incidence and severity of postoperative pain. Thoracic, upper abdominal, and orthopedic surgery are associated with a high degree of pain. Marked preoperative anxiety and fear tend to be associated with increased postoperative pain.

A. **Opiates** remain the mainstay of postoperative analgesia. IV opiates result in adequate pain relief more rapidly than do IM doses.

   1. **Morphine,** in incremental doses of 2–4 mg, may be repeated every 10–30 minutes until adequate analgesia is achieved. In children above 1 year of age, 15–20 μg/kg/IV or IM can be safely administered at 30- to 60-minute intervals.

   2. **Meperidine** in doses of 25–50 mg is similarly effective but must be avoided in patients taking monoamine oxidase (MAO) inhibitors.

   3. Mixed narcotic agonist-antagonists include **nalbuphine** (0.1 mg/kg IV) and **butorphanol** (1- to 2-mg increments). Although less predictable than the pure agonists in their analgesic action, these compounds do not depress ventilatory drive to the same extent.

B. **Nonsteroidal anti-inflammatory drugs** (e.g., ketorolac), **adjuvant therapy** with hydroxyzine (Vistaril), spasmolytics, and sedative and neuroleptic drugs may decrease the need for narcotic analgesia.

C. **Regional anesthesia** can be effectively carried out in the PACU. Epidural and intercostal blocks and blocks of the upper or lower extremities can provide excellent analgesia.

D. Specialized modalities for postoperative pain control (**patient-controlled analgesia, continuous epidural analgesia**) are frequently instituted in the PACU.

IX. **Nausea and vomiting** are common sequelae of general anesthesia (see Chap. 11). The incidence is increased in young adults, in certain surgical procedures (eye and ear surgery, laparoscopy), and with specific drugs (i.e., narcotics). Therapy is directed toward correcting specific causes (e.g., hypotension) and may include the use of antiemetics.

A. All **phenothiazines** and **butyrophenones** have antiemetic properties. Droperidol (0.625–1.25 mg), promethazine (Phenergan, 12.5–25.00 mg), and prochlorperazine
(Compazine, 10 mg) are among the most effective. All of
these compounds are dopaminergic antagonists and have
the potential to elicit dystonic reactions, particularly in
patients with Parkinson's disease.

B. **Metoclopramide** (Reglan, 10 mg IV) may inhibit the
central stimulus for emesis and increase gastric motility.

C. **Omeprazole** (Prilosec, 20 mg PO) inhibits $H^+ - K^+$
adenosinetriphosphatase and thus inhibits gastric acid
secretion.

X. **Hypothermia**

A. Decreased body temperature on arrival to the PACU is
common, due to the many causes of heat loss during
surgery. Significant hypothermia is accompanied by vasoconstriction, which may cause peripheral hypoperfusion
and metabolic acidosis. Hypothermia may impair platelet
function, affect cardiac repolarization, and cause T-wave
abnormalities on the ECG.

B. During rewarming, **shivering** is a common occurrence.
Oxygen consumption and carbon dioxide production may
increase two- to threefold, which is undesirable in patients with coronary artery disease or severe COPD.
Supplemental oxygen should be provided, and shivering
may be attenuated by the administration of small doses of
meperidine (25 mg IV) or **hydroxyzine** (50–100 mg IV
or IM). Hypothermia should be treated with warming
blankets, fluid warmers, or warming lights. Hypotension
can occur during rewarming and is treated with volume
expansion or a vasopressor.

C. Hypothermia is particularly dangerous in **newborns** and
infants, resulting in acidosis and hypotension.

XI. **Hyperthermia.** Increased body temperature in the immediate postoperative period is uncommon. Preexisting infection
may cause hyperthermia, particularly after drainage or manipulation of infected tissues. Other possible etiologies include the following:

A. **Malignant hyperthermia.** Hyperthermia is a late sign
of malignant hyperthermia and is generally preceded by
hypercapnia, muscular rigidity, and tachyarrhythmias.
Malignant hyperthermia should always be considered in
the differential diagnosis of an unexpected rise in body
temperature in the perioperative period. Diagnosis and
treatment of malignant hyperthermia are outlined in
Chap. 18. Dantrolene is the treatment of choice.

B. **Pulmonary** complications may be an early cause of fever.
Atelectasis classically causes fever on the first postoperative day, not in the PACU. Aspiration of gastric contents
during anesthesia may cause fever early in recovery.

C. **Thyroid storm** is rare but may be life-threatening if not
recognized promptly.

D. **Neuroleptic malignant syndrome** is a rare cause of
hyperthermia. This syndrome is difficult to distinguish
from malignant hyperthermia and may occur at any time

during therapy with neuroleptic drugs and also for a variable period of time after discontinuation of these agents. Treatment is discussed in Chap. 31.

E. Administration of **meperidine** to patients receiving MAO inhibitors may cause hyperpyrexia and death. The pathogenesis of this reaction is unknown. Mild reactions have apparently been reported with other narcotics (see Chap. 31).

F. **Symptomatic treatment** should be individualized to each patient. It seems wise to limit treatment of fever to those situations where significant hyperthermia is perceived as potentially dangerous, such as in young children or patients with compromised respiratory or cardiac reserve. External cooling with ice packs or cooling blankets and **acetaminophen** (Tylenol suppositories, 650–1300 mg or 10 mg/kg in children) are indicated.

XII. **Recovery from regional anesthesia**

A. **Regional blocks** (e.g., brachial and lumbosacral plexus, ankle block) do not require monitoring in the PACU, as long as there is no evidence of acute complications (e.g., intravascular or intrathecal injection, pneumothorax). Postoperative monitoring is indicated if heavy sedation was administered or if the surgical procedure requires it (e.g., carotid surgery performed with a cervical plexus block).

B. **Spinal and epidural anesthesia.** Recovery from peridural blockage progresses from most cephalad to caudal dermatomes. While sensory blockade tends to wane first, complete recovery of motor function may follow the return of painful sensation. If recovery seems unduly delayed, a neurologic examination should be performed and a neurologic consultation obtained to investigate the possibility of spinal cord compression from epidural hematoma. Criteria for discharge after spinal and epidural anesthesia vary among institutions but should include evidence that sensory and motor blockade is receding and that sympathetic blockade has resolved. Patients should be hemodynamically stable and not require vasopressors.

XIII. **Criteria for discharge.** All patients are observed for a minimum of 30 minutes at the Massachusetts General Hospital. Selected surgical procedures require a longer observation period (i.e., post-thyroidectomy patients remain for 4 hours). Patients must be easily arousable and oriented to their preoperative status. They should be hemodynamically stable and able to maintain adequate ventilation and protect their airway. Pain should be under acceptable control, and nausea should be absent or minimal. Normal body temperature should have been reached, and adequate intravenous access should be secured for inpatients. Discharge must be authorized by the PACU anesthesiologist following discussion with the PACU nurse. Decisions should be made regarding the nature of analgesia on the floor such as need for continuous ECG monitoring, oxygen therapy, and chest physiotherapy. A discharge note should be written in the chart by the PACU anesthesiologist. If the discharge criteria are not met, the patient remains in the PACU. A limited number of patients are monitored overnight in the PACU. Transfer is then made either to the floor or to an intensive care unit as appropriate.

SUGGESTING READING

Breslow, M. J., et al. Changes in T-wave morphology following anesthesia and surgery: A common recovery-room phenomenon. *Anesthesiology* 64:398, 1986.

Cooper, J. B. et al. Effects of information feedback and pulse oximetry on the incidence of anesthesia complications. *Anesthesiology* 67:686, 1987.

Coté, C. J., et al. A single-blind study on pulse oximetry in children. *Anesthesiology* 68:184, 1988.

Greene, N. M. Uptake and elimination of local anesthetics during spinal anesthesia. *Anesth. Analg.* 62:1013, 1983.

Guze, B. H., and Baxter, R. L. Neuroleptic malignant syndrome. *N. Engl. J. Med.* 313:163, 1985.

Pedersen, T., Eliasen, D., and Henriksen, H. A prospective study of risk factors and cardiopulmonary complications associated with anesthesia and surgery: Risk indicators of cardiopulmonary morbidity. *Acta Anesthesiol. Scand.* 34:144, 1990.

Teplick, R. S., Welch, J. P., and Ford, P. J. Monitoring Devices for Vascular Surgery: Basic Principles, Limitations, and Proper Functioning. In M. Roizen (ed.), *Anesthesia for Vascular Surgery*. New York: Churchill Livingstone, 1990.

Appendix. American Society of Anesthesiologists' Standards for Postanesthesia Care

These Standards apply to postanesthesia care in all locations. These Standards may be exceeded based on the judgment of the responsible anesthesiologist. They are intended to encourage high quality patient care, but cannot guarantee any specific patient outcome. They are subject to revision from time to time as warranted by the evolution of technology and practice.

STANDARD I

ALL PATIENTS WHO HAVE RECEIVED GENERAL ANESTHESIA, REGIONAL ANESTHESIA, OR MONITORED ANESTHESIA CARE SHALL RECEIVE APPROPRIATE POSTANESTHESIA MANAGEMENT.

1. A Postanesthesia Care Unit (PACU) or an area which provides equivalent postanesthesia care shall be available to receive patients after surgery and anesthesia. All patients who receive anesthesia shall be admitted to the PACU except by specific order of the anesthesiologist responsible for the patient's care.
2. The medical aspects of care in the PACU shall be governed by

(From the American Society of Anesthesiologists Standards for Postanesthesia Care. American Society of Anesthesiologists, Park Ridge, IL.)

policies and procedures which have been reviewed and approved by the Department of Anesthesiology.
3. The design, equipment, and staffing of the PACU shall meet requirements of the facility's accrediting and licensing bodies.
4. The nursing standards of practice shall be consistent with those approved in 1986 by the American Society of Post Anesthesia Nurses (ASPAN).

STANDARD II

A PATIENT TRANSPORTED TO THE PACU SHALL BE ACCOMPANIED BY A MEMBER OF THE ANESTHESIA CARE TEAM WHO IS KNOWLEDGEABLE ABOUT THE PATIENT'S CONDITION. THE PATIENT SHALL BE CONTINUALLY EVALUATED AND TREATED DURING TRANSPORT WITH MONITORING AND SUPPORT APPROPRIATE TO THE PATIENT'S CONDITION.

STANDARD III

UPON ARRIVAL IN THE PACU, THE PATIENT SHALL BE REEVALUATED AND A VERBAL REPORT PROVIDED TO THE RESPONSIBLE PACU NURSE BY THE MEMBER OF THE ANESTHESIA CARE TEAM WHO ACCOMPANIES THE PATIENT.

1. The patient's status on arrival in the PACU shall be documented.
2. Information concerning the preoperative condition and the surgical/anesthetic course shall be transmitted to the PACU nurse.
3. The member of the Anesthesia Care Team shall remain in the PACU until the PACU nurse accepts responsibility for the nursing care of the patient.

STANDARD IV

THE PATIENT'S CONDITION SHALL BE EVALUATED CONTINUALLY IN THE PACU.

1. The patient shall be observed and monitored by methods appropriate to the patient's medical condition. Particular attention should be given to monitoring oxygenation, ventilation, and circulation. While qualitative clinical signs may be adequate, quantitative methods are encouraged.
2. An accurate written report of the PACU period shall be maintained. Use of an appropriate PACU scoring system is encouraged for each patient on admission, at appropriate intervals prior to discharge, and at the time of discharge.
3. General medical supervision and coordination of patient care in the PACU should be the responsibility of an anesthesiologist.
4. There shall be a policy to assure the availability in the facility of a physician capable of managing complications and providing cardiopulmonary resuscitation for patients in the PACU.

STANDARD V

A PHYSICIAN IS RESPONSIBLE FOR THE DISCHARGE OF THE PATIENT FROM THE POSTANESTHESIA CARE UNIT.

1. When discharge criteria are used, they must be approved by the Department of Anesthesiology and the medical staff. They may vary depending upon whether the patient is discharged to a hospital room, to the ICU, to a short stay unit, or home.
2. In the absence of the physician responsible for the discharge, the PACU nurse shall determine that the patient meets the discharge criteria. The name of the physician accepting responsibility for discharge shall be noted on the record.

35

Perioperative Respiratory Insufficiency

Barbara A. Ryan

I. **Overview.** Respiratory insufficiency is a condition in which gas exchange by the lungs is inadequate to meet metabolic demands. Respiration refers to gas exchange at the cellular level, while ventilation refers to the movement of gas by the lungs. Respiratory insufficiency may develop at any point during the perioperative period and it may also occur in patients with medical disorders. Anesthesiologists are often consulted to assist with management of the airway, pulmonary problems, or ventilatory support.

II. **Etiology of respiratory failure**
   A. **Ventilatory failure**
      1. **Chemoreceptors and control of ventilation.**
         a. **Central** control of ventilation is by chemoreceptors located on the surface of the medulla. Alterations in cerebrospinal fluid (CSF) pH are the major stimuli for these receptors. The main determinant of CSF pH is the $PaCO_2$ due to the permeability of carbon dioxide across the blood-brain barrier. Very small changes in $PaCO_2$ (2–3 mm Hg) rapidly alter minute ventilation.
         b. **Peripheral** chemoreceptors are located in the carotid and aortic bodies and are also sensitive to small changes in $PaCO_2$. Patients with chronic obstructive pulmonary disease (COPD) may have carbon dioxide retention and diminished sensitivity of these receptors to abnormalities in $PaCO_2$. These patients rely on hypoxia as a stimulus to the peripheral chemoreceptors, so that increasing the inspired FiO_2 may result in further hypoventilation.
         c. Many drugs cause depression of chemoreceptor sensitivity including narcotics, barbiturates, inhalation anesthetics, and benzodiazepines.
         d. Intracranial pathology that interrupts the vascular supply to the medulla (trauma, neoplasm, or major cerebrovascular accidents) will result in altered ventilation.
      2. **Neuromuscular dysfunction**
         a. **Upper motor neuron** lesions can disrupt phrenic nerve function (C3–C5), resulting in diaphragmatic paralysis and apnea. Lesions arising at the mid to lower cervical spine region can impair intercostal and expiratory muscle function. These lesions include neoplasms, demyelinating disorders, syringomyelia, and trauma.
         b. **Lower motor neurons** supplying the respiratory muscles may be interrupted by trauma or regional anesthesia or affected by diseases including polyneuritis (Guillain-Barré syndrome), amyotrophic lateral sclerosis, and the various neuropathies.

      c. **Neuromuscular junction disorders** include myasthenia gravis, Eaton-Lambert syndrome, botulism toxin, organophosphate compounds, and residual neuromuscular blockade.

  3. **Increased airway resistance** is the most common cause of ventilatory failure (see Chap. 3).

  4. **Respiratory muscle dysfunction.** Muscle weakness may result from a number of causes including disuse atrophy, neuromuscular disease, hypoperfusion, hypoxia, hypercapnia, old age, and malnutrition. Diaphragmatic dysfunction is common in the postoperative period following thoracic or upper abdominal procedures and can last for weeks.

  5. **Chest wall abnormalities.** Loss of compliance of the chest wall may significantly impair ventilation (see Chap. 3).

  6. **Decreased lung compliance.** Parenchymal or pleural processes may impair lung expansion (i.e., pleural effusions, hemothorax, pneumothorax, pneumonia, pulmonary fibrosis, and empyema).

  7. **Increased dead space.** Dead space refers to lung areas that are ventilated but not perfused. Normal anatomic dead space is about 150 ml or 2 ml/kg. Increased dead space will produce hypercapnia unless minute ventilation also increases. Etiologies include severe parenchymal diseases (diffuse pneumonia, respiratory distress syndrome) and pulmonary emboli.

B. Altered oxygenation

  1. **Hypoventilation** (see sec. **A**). This form of hypoxia is always accompanied by hypercapnia and may be corrected by supplemental oxygen.

  2. **Ventilation-perfusion ($\dot{V}/\dot{Q}$) mismatch.** Average minute ventilation is approximately 5 L/min. This is matched by cardiac output, giving a typical $\dot{V}/\dot{Q}$ ratio of 1.0. Ventilated but not perfused alveoli increase dead space, producing a greater effect on the $PaCO_2$. At the other extreme, $\dot{V}/\dot{Q}$ approaches zero when the alveoli are perfused but not ventilated, representing true **shunt** with a dramatic drop in PaO_2. Intrapulmonary shunting may also occur through arteriovenous fistulas. Extrapulmonary right-to-left shunting may occur through patent atrial or ventricular septal defects or a patent ductus arteriosus. $\dot{V}/\dot{Q}$ mismatch is the major cause of hypoxemia. Etiologies include retained pulmonary secretions, bronchoconstriction, COPD, pneumonia, pulmonary edema, and other interstitial lung diseases. Hypoxemia secondary to shunting, however, is quite refractory to oxygen therapy.

  3. **Diffusion impairment.** Under normal conditions, capillary blood rapidly equilibrates with PAO_2, rendering diffusion impairment an uncommon cause of hypoxemia. The diffusion path from alveolar gas to red blood cells may be increased in diseases such as asbestosis, sarcoidosis, collagen vascular diseases, diffuse interstitial fibrosis (Hamman-Rich syndrome), and alveolar cell carcinoma. Hypoxemia secondary to diffusion im-

pairment is readily correctable with supplemental oxygen.

C. Decreased oxygen supply

1. **Reduced cardiac output** or **decreased oxygen-carrying capacity** (severe anemia) may contribute to respiratory failure by decreasing oxygen supply.

2. **Pulmonary hypertension,** primary or secondary, may impair $\dot{V}/\dot{Q}$ matching. Sustained increases in pulmonary artery pressure result in medial hypertrophy and intimal thickening. Etiologies include vasoconstriction, obstruction (pulmonary embolism), and obliteration (emphysema, arteritis). Hypoxia has a constrictor effect on the pulmonary vasculature. This effect, called hypoxic pulmonary vasoconstriction, is an important regulatory mechanism that controls blood flow to ventilated lung. It may also be an important mechanism for the development of severe pulmonary hypertension and right heart failure in chronic and acute respiratory failure.

3. **Decreased oxygen delivery.** Shifts to the left in the oxygen-hemoglobin dissociation curve facilitate oxygen uptake, but enhanced hemoglobin binding attenuates unloading of oxygen to tissues. Factors associated with a leftward shift include hypothermia, alkalemia, hypocapnia, decreased 2,3-diphosphoglycerate concentration, and some hemoglobin variants.

D. Increased oxygen demand

1. **Increased oxygen consumption.** Basal oxygen consumption averages 200–250 ml/min. Increases in metabolic rate may raise oxygen consumption 20-fold. Common etiologies include fever, increased muscle activity (shivering, seizures), and sepsis.

2. **Increased carbon dioxide production.** The respiratory quotient (RQ) is the ratio of carbon dioxide production to oxygen consumption. This ratio is normally 0.8 in the adult and varies with diet. Pure carbohydrate metabolism yields an RQ of 1.0, and fat metabolism yields the lowest RQ of 0.7. An RQ greater than 1.0 can result from anaerobic metabolism or fat synthesis from excessive carbohydrate ingestion.

III. Diagnosis of respiratory failure

A. Clinical findings. Signs of impending respiratory failure include a respiratory rate less than 6/min or greater than 30/min, shallow respirations, use of accessory respiratory muscles, discoordinate motions of the chest and abdomen, severe bronchospasm, or cyanosis.

B. Arterial blood gas analysis

1. **Normal arterial PO$_2$ (PaO$_2$)** averages 80–100 mm Hg and declines with age due to shunting of blood through areas of lung with closed airways. A PaO$_2$ less than 60 mm Hg signifies impending respiratory failure.

2. **Normal PaCO$_2$** averages 34–45 mm Hg. A PaCO$_2$ greater than 50 mm Hg indicates respiratory failure. PaCO$_2$ rises about 4–5 mm Hg/min of apnea.

3. **Normal pH** averages 7.36–7.44 and is dependent on

HCO_3^- and $PaCO_2$ according to the Henderson-Hasselbalch equation:

$$pH = 6.1 + \log (HCO_3^- /0.03\ PaCO_2)$$

where $6.1 = pK_a$ of H_2CO_3
$0.03 =$ solubility coefficient of carbon dioxide

Acute changes in minute ventilation produce corresponding changes in both pH and PCO_2; for each 10 mm Hg change in PCO_2, the pH will change by 0.08 in the opposite direction. Chronic carbon dioxide retention produces less significant pH changes due to compensatory metabolic changes.

IV. **Treatment**
  A. **Supplemental oxygen.** Hypoxemia is the primary clinical indication for oxygen therapy. Supplemental oxygen can be administered via low- and high-flow systems.
   1. **Low-flow systems** produce highly variable FiO_2 ranges that are inversely proportional to peak inspiratory flow rate, tidal volume, and minute ventilation.
      a. **Nasal cannulas** are well tolerated up to flow rates of 4 L/min. Flows above 4 L/min for prolonged periods may dry the nasal mucosa, resulting in irritation and bleeding. The nasal passages must be patent, although nose breathing is not required due to the effective anatomic reservoir of the upper airway.
      b. **Simple masks** provide an FiO_2 higher than nasal cannulas by increasing oxygen flow rates and adding reservoir space.
      c. **Masks with reservoir bags attached** ("nonrebreathing masks") may increase FiO_2 further, although lack of a tight seal limits the achievable FiO_2 to 0.60–0.80.
   2. **High-flow systems** must provide gas flows to meet the average peak inspiratory flow rate (approximately 40 L/min).
      a. **Venturi masks** deliver a relatively constant FiO_2 ranging from 0.24–0.5 by entraining a set ratio of room air along with oxygen. The inspired FiO_2 is independent of both minute ventilation inspiratory flow rates up to a maximum of 40 L/min. As the FiO_2 increases to 0.4 or greater, higher oxygen flow rates are required secondary to the higher oxygen-air entrainment ratio, and the patient's needs are more likely to exceed the flow capability of the system. In this situation, the actual inspired FiO_2 will be lower than indicated.
      b. **Humidified systems** have the advantage of delivering particulate water to the airways, although the maximum FiO_2 obtainable depends on inspiratory flow rate and mask fit. Usually 0.6 is the maximum, but up to 0.8 is possible when two aerosol generators are placed in parallel. This system can be applied by simple face mask, face tent, or trach mask.

    c. High-flow humidification systems can deliver > 100 L/min and therefore can provide up to 1.0 FiO_2.

    d. Mask or nasal continuous positive airway pressure (CPAP) provides high flow and humidification up to an FiO_2 of 1.0. It also maintains positive airway pressure at end exhalation, resulting in increased functional residual capacity (FRC). CPAP requires a snug, airtight mask seal, which may be poorly tolerated by some patients and may produce gastric distention with an increased risk of aspiration. Gastric distention may be relieved by continuous nasogastric suctioning while mask CPAP is used.

B. Mobilization and removal of secretions. Excessive pulmonary secretions, changes in viscosity, and inability to clear secretions effectively are common problems and may impair both ventilation (by increasing lower airway resistance) and gas exchange (impaired $\dot{V}/\dot{Q}$).

    1. Humidification of gases. The upper airway is quite efficient at warming and humidifying inspired gases to 37°C and 100% humidity (which contains 44 ml H_2O/L). True humidifiers will evaporate water to individual molecules or water vapor, unlike nebulizers, which produce particulate water in the form of various sized droplets. Larger droplets will simply deposit in the upper airways. Alveolar deposition occurs at particle sizes of 2–5 μm. The goal of humidification and aerosol nebulization (water, saline) is to improve mobilization of retained secretions by increasing water content and decreasing viscosity.

    2. Intravascular hydration. Maintaining adequate intravascular volume may be of benefit in preventing dry, inspissated secretions.

    3. Chest physical therapy. Properly performed percussion and vibration of the chest with postural drainage and coughing are effective means of clearing secretions and preventing mucus plugging. Incentive spirometry (maximum deep inspiration with end-inspiratory hold) is effective in mobilizing secretions and treating atelectasis.

    4. Mucolytics. Acetylcysteine (Mucomyst, 2–5 ml of 5–20% solution q6–8h by nebulizer) decreases mucus viscosity by reducing the disulfide bonds of the mucus glycoproteins. It may produce bronchorrhea and precipitate bronchospasm in susceptible patients. It is occasionally useful in select patients with thick, inspissated secretions and should be administered with a bronchodilator to prevent bronchospasm.

    5. Suctioning. Pain, sedation, underlying severe illness, or debilitation can severely limit a patient's ability to cough and clear secretions adequately. Blind nasotracheal suctioning effectively clears tracheal secretions and stimulates coughing but may be associated with hypoxemia, tachycardia, vagal stimulation, laryngospasm, bronchoconstriction, and tissue trauma.

    6. Bronchoscopy can be employed to remove secretions

and thick mucus plugs from the tracheobronchial airways.

7. **Minitracheostomies** provide a direct route for removal of secretions in the patient requiring frequent suctioning. The technique for insertion involves placement of a 4.0-mm uncuffed tube through the cricothyroid membrane into the trachea. This can also be used for administration of medications and oxygen and for temporary ventilation in airway emergencies. The small lumen is inadequate for spontaneous ventilation, and only limited positive-pressure ventilation is possible. Secretions must be thin enough to be suctioned through a No. 8 catheter, the only size that can fit through the minitracheostomy. Complications from insertion include intratracheal bleeding, hematoma, subcutaneous emphysema, pneumothorax, esophageal perforation, and hoarseness.

C. **Pharmacologic therapy**

1. **Increased airway resistance.** Pharmacologic agents used in treating this common cause of altered ventilation and gas exchange are discussed in Chap. 18.

2. **Stridor.** Pharmacologic treatment is discussed in Chaps. 18 and 34.

3. **Central nervous system (CNS) depressants.** Numerous drugs produce depression of central chemoreceptors, resulting in hypoventilation and apnea. These drugs and reversal agents are discussed in Chap. 34.

4. **Skeletal muscle relaxants.** Incomplete reversal of these drugs may lead to ventilatory failure and inadequate airway protection. Monitoring and reversal of muscle relaxants are discussed in Chap. 12.

D. **Pain control.** Therapeutic modalities are discussed in Chaps. 16 and 37.

E. **Intubation.** See Chap. 13 for indications and technique.

F. **Mechanical ventilation** becomes necessary when spontaneous ventilation is insufficient for adequate gas exchange. New microprocessor-controlled mechanical ventilators provide nearly unlimited variability in gas delivery patterns and are more capable of meeting the needs of a wide variety of critically ill patients.

1. **Traditional modes of ventilation** (volume-cycled positive-pressure ventilation).

a. **Control mode ventilation (CMV)** delivers a preset tidal volume (V_T) at a preset frequency independent of patient effort. No provisions for gas delivery on patient demand are included. This mode has few ICU indications and is suitable only for use in the operating rooms or with apneic patients.

b. **Assist-control ventilation** combines CMV with the ability to provide patient-triggered positive-pressure breaths at the same preset V_T. The patient therefore determines the frequency of ventilation with the safety feature of a backup preset rate in the event of apnea. Increased patient triggering can produce variable degrees of respiratory alkalosis.

c. **Assist ventilation** provides a preset V_T only upon patient triggering. This mode is seldom used.

d. **Intermittent mandatory ventilation (IMV)** provides a preset V_T at a preset frequency with regularly spaced intervals while allowing spontaneous patient-generated breaths, without positive-pressure assist, in between. Synchronized IMV (SIMV) is similar to IMV except preset tidal volume breaths are coordinated with spontaneous breaths, thus avoiding "stacking" of a mechanical breath during spontaneous inspiration or expiration. Spontaneous ventilation requires opening of a demand valve in some ventilators. The effort required is machine variable and usually minimal, although it may be significant in patients with marginal reserve. Other ventilators have continuous fresh gas flow at high flow rates, avoiding the need to open a demand valve.

2. **Newer ventilator modes**

a. **Inspiratory pressure support ventilation (IPS)** applies a preset positive pressure while the frequency, inspiratory flow rate, and inspiratory time are determined by the patient. When triggered by the patient, the system rapidly pressurizes to the preset level and remains there until inspiratory flow rate decreases to about 25% (machine variable) of the peak flow rate. At this time, gas flow stops and exhalation begins. IPS may be used as a primary means of ventilatory support in the patient with spontaneous respiratory efforts. The pressure level is adjusted to a point that provides adequate tidal volume and comfortable breathing at a rate $\leq$ 20 breaths/min. IPS, as a sole mode of ventilation, should be used cautiously in patients with unstable respiratory drive or changing airway resistance (due to bronchospasm, secretions, pain, or anxiety) because the IPS requires patient triggering, and the V_T can vary widely with changing airway resistance. Conversely, the stable preset pressure level may be preferable for the patient in whom wide pressure swings (possible on a volume ventilator during changes in airway resistance) could be detrimental, such as the patient with a bronchopleural fistula, airway trauma, or recent airway surgery. IPS may be combined with IMV or SIMV to decrease the work of spontaneous breathing or overcome the resistance of endotracheal tubes. Tapering IPS levels, either combined with CPAP trials or alone, is a useful weaning method, particularly for the difficult-to-wean patient.

b. **Pressure-controlled inverse-ratio ventilation (PC-IRV)** is a pressure-controlled, volume-variable mode with a lengthened inspiratory-expiratory (I/E) ratio. In this mode, rapid system pressurization and prolonged positive pressure during inspiration may progressively recruit collapsed alveoli and fill alveolar units with slower time constants. Peak airway pressures tend to be lower, but mean airway pressures will increase with increasing inspiratory time. Shortening the expiratory time may produce intrinsic positive end-expiratory pressure (autoPEEP), which will decrease alveolar collapse but may not be tolerated hemodynamically. This mode is generally used in patients with severe respiratory distress syndrome and refractory hypoxemia requiring high FIO_2 and positive end-expiratory pressure (PEEP). Although oxygenation may improve in many cases, several recent studies of small groups of patients show conflicting rates of improvement and survival.

c. **High-frequency ventilation (HFV)**
   (1) There are three **types** of HFV.
      (a) **High-frequency positive pressure ventilation (HFPPV)** delivers compressed gas at a frequency of 60–120 breaths/min, with V_T of 3–5 ml/kg and an I/E < 0.3.
      (b) **High-frequency jet ventilation (HFJV)** delivers jets of compressed gas at high pressure (15–20 psi) through a small-bore cannula at frequencies of 100–600, V_T of 2–5 ml/kg, and an I/E of approximately 1 : 2–1 : 8.
      (c) In **high-frequency oscillations (HFO)**, gas is forced into the lungs at inspiration and actively sucked out on expiration at frequencies of 60–3600/min and V_T of 1–3 ml/kg.
   (2) **The mechanism of gas transport and exchange** in HFV is uncertain but likely involves two fundamental processes: convection and molecular diffusion.
   (3) **Indications.** Despite theoretic advantages (less barotrauma, improved oxygenation), HFV has been shown to be superior to conventional modes in few settings. HFJV has been used successfully for unilateral ventilation in thoracotomies and lung resections, during laryngoscopy and bronchoscopy, and in the treatment of patients with bronchopleural fistulas. In the difficult intubation or airway emergency, HFJV via a 14 gauge cannula or via minitracheostomy through the cricothyroid membrane may be lifesaving.

d. **Airway pressure release ventilation (APRV)** is a form of CPAP ventilation with transient releases in airway pressure to lower ambient pressures during exhalation. Clinical experience with this newer mode is limited, though it appears to be more effective in improving alveolar ventilation rather than oxygenation and may therefore be useful in the treatment of airflow obstruction.

3. **Noninvasive mechanical ventilation (Bi-PAP)** is a method that combines CPAP with intermittent positive-pressure ventilation delivered through an air-

tight face or nasal mask. Indications include nocturnal hypoventilation, acute or chronic respiratory failure in which long-term ventilatory support and difficult weaning may be anticipated, and end-stage respiratory failure in the patient awaiting lung transplantation in whom tracheal intubation would limit the chance for transplantation.

4. **Ventilator settings** (for conventional IMV modes).

   a. **Tidal volume (V_T)** is set at 10–15 ml/kg, which has been shown to decrease atelectasis, improve compliance, and eliminate the need for "sigh" breaths (intermittent larger V_T breaths). Higher V_T will increase alveolar pressure with possible increased dead space, decreased cardiac output, and barotrauma.

   b. **Respiratory rate** is usually set at 8–10 and subsequently adjusted to the desired $PaCO_2$. In choosing between respiratory rate and V_T to adjust for hypoventilation, a greater increase in minute ventilation is obtained by increasing the V_T compared with an equivalent increase in respiratory rate due to the relatively constant dead space (150 ml in the normal adult) per breath.

   c. **FIO_2** is often initially set at 1.0 in ICU patients to ensure adequate oxygen saturation and also to estimate the degree of alveolar-to-arterial oxygen gradient (A-a DO_2). It should then be reduced to a level required to maintain oxygen saturation in the range of 95–100%.

   d. **Positive end-expiratory pressure (PEEP)** is a super atmospheric pressure maintained at end exhalation. CPAP is essentially PEEP applied to a spontaneously ventilating patient and is present throughout the respiratory cycle.

      (1) The **overall effect** of PEEP (CPAP) is an increased FRC and improved oxygenation.

      (2) The **mechanism** includes distention of patient alveoli, prevention of alveolar collapse with exhalation, recruitment of closed alveoli, and redistribution of lung water from dependent regions (though total lung water does not decrease and probably increases).

      (3) **Application of low levels of PEEP** (3–5 cm) is commonly used as a compensatory mechanism to restore "physiologic PEEP" normally provided by epiglottic closure and upper airway resistance. Low levels of CPAP during weaning may improve FRC and oxygenation when compared to spontaneous ventilation without CPAP.

      (4) **Detrimental effects** of PEEP include decreased cardiac output (due to decreased venous return as a result of increased intrathoracic pressure), potential risk of barotrauma, increased intracranial pressure, and alteration in renal function causing increased ADH levels and fluid retention.

(5) The **major indication** for PEEP is to maintain adequate arterial oxygen saturation at an FIO_2 below toxic levels (< 0.5–0.6) using the minimal amount of PEEP necessary to reduce barotrauma or untoward hemodynamic effects.

e. **Inspiratory-to-expiratory time (I/E)** is generally set at 1 : 2 and then adjusted as necessary to allow for complete exhalation. Longer expiratory times may be needed in patients with obstructive diseases such as emphysema or asthma to prevent air trapping and the development of autoPEEP.

f. **Flow pattern or wave form configuration options** include square, sinusoidal, constant, decelerating, and accelerating waves. Often the ventilator mode determines the flow pattern; for instance, PC-IRV utilizes decelerating inspiratory flow, IMV patterns can be adjusted from sinusoidal to square wave, and pressure support ventilation flow patterns are variable depending on set pattern and patient breathing pattern. Otherwise, patterns are adjusted to promote optimal distribution of ventilation and to avoid regional hyperinflation with increased risk of barotrauma. **Expiratory flow retardation** is theoretically of use in obstructive airway disease. By applying a flow-restricting device on the exhalation limb of the circuit, smaller airways that tend to collapse may be stented open, simulating in effect the pursed lip breathing of the COPD patient. Unlike PEEP, airway pressure returns to zero, but mean airway pressure increases.

G. **Hemodynamic support**

1. Therapeutic measures directed toward restoring the circulation and improving oxygen delivery include inotropic and vasoactive drugs and volume and blood product replacement.

2. Treatment is more complicated in the patient with **severe respiratory failure and increased pulmonary vascular resistance.** There are no parenterally available selective pulmonary artery vasodilators, and the side effect of systemic vasodilatation is often not tolerated in these patients. Systemic vasoconstrictors also constrict the pulmonary vessels, worsening the pulmonary artery hypertension in these patients. Nitric oxide is currently under investigation as a selective pulmonary artery vasodilator when administered by the inhaled route, which delivers the molecule to ventilated alveoli only, theoretically improving $\dot{V}/\dot{Q}$ matching and oxygen saturation. Systemic vasodilatation does not seem to occur due to the rapid uptake and inactivation of nitric oxide by hemoglobin. Nitric oxide may also produce local bronchodilatation.

H. **Musculoskeletal paralysis** can decrease oxygen consumption by inhibiting excess muscle activity. In addition, this can improve ventilation by preventing noncompliance with the ventilator when sedation alone is inadequate. Indications for paralysis include severe respiratory failure with hypoxemia, respiratory acidosis, and high peak inspiratory pressures. Nondepolarizing muscle relaxants (curare, vecuronium) are given by continuous IV infusion and must be accompanied by sedation and analgesia.

I.   Deliberate hypothermia is employed for severely hypoxic patients on high levels of FIO_2 and PEEP when no further method to improve oxygenation is available by decreasing oxygen consumption and carbon dioxide production. Hypothermia is accomplished by a cooling blanket or ice packs and should be accompanied by sedation and skeletal muscle paralysis to avoid shivering. Temperatures below 32° C should be avoided due to an increase in incidence of arrhythmias.

J.   Extracorporeal membrane oxygenation (ECMO) is the venovenous or venoarterial exchange of oxygen into and carbon dioxide out of extracorporeal blood. Use of ECMO in adults with respiratory failure has not improved mortality compared with conventional therapy (for pediatrics see Chap. 28). Since ECMO does not prevent the progression of parenchymal injury in the adult, its usefulness is limited to providing support for ventilation.

V. Complications of therapy

A.   Oxygen toxicity. High concentrations of oxygen in lung zones with low $\dot{V}/\dot{Q}$ may result in alveolar collapse secondary to absorption atelectasis. High concentrations of oxygen over long periods are detrimental to lung tissue causing interstitial fibrosis, and adverse effects of inspiring 100% oxygen occur within a matter of hours. FIO_2 greater than 0.5 for more than 2 days may produce toxic parenchymal changes.

B.   Barotrauma. Positive-pressure ventilation is associated with an increased incidence of barotrauma. Mechanisms may include high peak inspiratory pressure, high mean airway pressure, high inflation volumes, or simply the underlying lung pathology. Alveolar overdistention seems to be most commonly associated with barotrauma. The mechanism of injury is local rupture of an alveolar wall with air extravasation through the bronchovascular sheath into the pulmonary interstitium, the mediastinum, pericardium, peritoneum, pleural space, or subcutaneous tissue. Pneumothorax can rapidly progress to tension pneumothorax with cardiovascular collapse in the mechanically ventilated patient.

C.   Bronchopleural fistula. A persistent bronchopleural leak can be produced or aggravated by positive-pressure ventilation and can result in persistent lung collapse and hypoventilation with large air loss and respiratory acidosis. A bronchopleural fistula is usually treated conservatively by minimizing tidal volume or inspiratory pressure, PEEP, inspiratory time, flow rates, and level of chest tube suction. In severe respiratory acidosis, other modes of ventilation may be required such as independent lung ventilation or HFJV.

D.   Hemodynamic dysfunction. Positive-pressure ventilation and PEEP adversely affect cardiovascular performance by increasing airway and intrathoracic pressure. The adverse cardiovascular effects of PEEP in particular may be substantial.

1. **Right ventricular filling** is limited by increased intrathoracic pressure that reduces venous return. When alveolar pressure exceeds pulmonary vascular pressure, pulmonary blood flow is limited by alveolar pressure rather than left atrial pressure, producing an increase in pulmonary vascular resistance. As a consequence, RV afterload increases and RV ejection fraction decreases.

2. **Left ventricular (LV) filling** is limited by reduced RV output and decreased LV diastolic compliance. Increased RV size also affects LV performance by stiffening the interventricular septum and shifting it to the left. LV afterload may decrease during positive-pressure ventilation. Increased pleural pressure with resulting decreased transmural LV pressure may explain the improvement in stroke volume often seen in the patient with LV dysfunction who is exposed to mechanical ventilation.

3. **Cardiovascular effects of weaning.** Decreased intrathoracic pressure during weaning redistributes intravascular volume from peripheral to central compartments. LV transmural pressure also increases when intrathoracic pressure is decreased. As a result, central venous pressure, left ventricular end-diastolic pressure, and pulmonary capillary wedge pressure may increase. These changes can impair weaning success, particularly in the patient with borderline pulmonary function, coronary artery disease, or LV dysfunction.

E. **Infection.** Nosocomial pneumonia is common in patients requiring mechanical ventilation. Bacterial colonization of the gastrointestinal and upper respiratory tract (usually with gram-negative bacilli) is a frequent occurrence in the intensive care unit patient and is directly proportional to the severity of illness. Nebulizers and ventilatory circuits can also become colonized.

VI. **Weaning from mechanical ventilation.** The rate of withdrawal of ventilation generally varies with the duration of ventilation. Rapid weans can follow transient periods of ventilation such as recovering from anesthesia, drug overdose, or an acute asthma exacerbation. Longer weaning periods are required with more extensive dysfunction such as with CNS injury, trauma, or COPD.

A. **Measurements of weaning potential**

1. **Respiratory pattern and rate.** One of the most useful indicators is the respiratory pattern and rate. Tachypnea is the earliest sign of unsuccessful weaning and is the most consistent negative predictor.

2. **Subjective symptoms** (dyspnea, fatigue) are also of great value and very often predict failure of weaning before objective findings are apparent.

3. **Ventilatory parameters** are simple bedside measure-

ments of muscle strength that are useful to predict muscle endurance when trends are followed. Measurements that suggest ability to wean include

a. Tidal volume > 5 ml/kg.
b. Vital capacity > 10 ml/kg.
c. Negative inspiratory force > − 25 cm H_2O.
d. Minute ventilation > 10 L/min.

4. Oxygenation. Patients requiring high FiO_2 or high PEEP/CPAP to maintain a PaO_2 greater than 65 mm Hg or an SaO_2 greater than 90% are not ready to wean.

5. Hemodynamic and metabolic stability. Overall clinical stability is an obvious though occasionally overlooked requirement for weaning. Continued need for pressor support or unresolved critical illness such as sepsis precludes weaning attempts.

6. Nutrition. Inadequate nutrition produces muscle weakness and atrophy, which will hamper or prohibit weaning. Excessive caloric intake, particularly carbohydrates, increases carbon dioxide production, placing increased demands on ventilation.

B. Weaning techniques. Readiness for weaning is more important than the particular method used. Clinical judgment along with trial and error best determines which method to attempt. Key to all methods is observation for early signs and symptoms of failure to avoid overfatigue, distress, or hemodynamic compromise.

1. IMV weaning allows partial support as mandatory ventilator breaths are reduced and the patient gradually assumes the entire work of spontaneous breathing. T-piece or CPAP trials are then attempted or extubation is done from low IMV levels, particularly in the patient who cannot tolerate breathing through smaller endotracheal tubes without some support.

2. CPAP or T-piece weans are performed by discontinuing mechanical ventilation and placing the patient on a Briggs T piece. The patient thus assumes all of the work of breathing during such a wean, and the frequency and duration of such trials are increased until mechanical ventilation is no longer required.

3. Pressure support weaning consists of gradual reduction of inspiratory pressure from one that may completely unload the respiratory muscles to a level where all work is assumed by the patient. Signs of failure are a decreasing tidal volume and an increasing respiratory rate.

VII. Chest tube function (Fig. 35-1). The management of chest tubes requires an understanding of the mechanics of the various drainage systems. The **Pleur-Evac** is the most common system for drainage of the pleural space. The Pleur-Evac is a derivative of the traditional "three bottle system," where the proximal bottle traps the drainage, the middle bottle is the "water seal" that prevents air or fluid from being drawn into the thorax, and the distal bottle regulates the level of suction that is applied to the pleural cavity. Application of constant vacuum to the suction-control chamber produces a steady stream of bubbles and subatmospheric

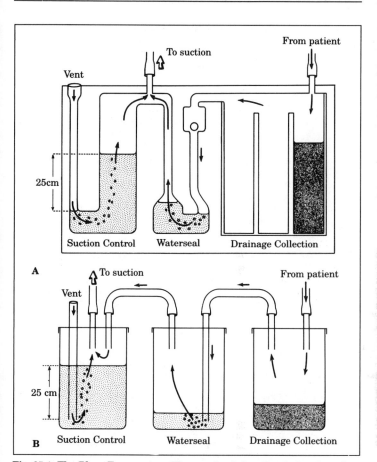

Fig. 35-1. The Pleur-Evac system. The proximal chamber is for pleural drainage, the middle (the "water seal") prevents air or fluid from being drawn into the thorax, and the distal regulates the level of suction.

pressures in all three chambers. The negative pressure is independent of strength of the wall suction and depends only on the height of the water column in the suction-control chamber. Chest tubes are connected to either of the following: water seal, if minimal air or fluid drainage is expected (e.g., following pneumonectomy); or to suction, if significant drainage is expected (e.g., following cardiac surgery or thoracic lobectomy).

A. **Examination of a Pleur-Evac system**
   1. The **water level** in the water seal chamber should vary with respiration if the chest tube is patent and properly placed.
   2. The presence of bubbling in the water seal chamber with inspiration indicates a **bronchopleural leak.**

The current systems have a means of grossly quantifying the size of the leak. Massive leaks or continuous inspiratory and expiratory leaks are suggestive of large airway or parenchymal tears (intraparenchymal chest tube placement), and these patients can decompensate when suction is applied to the tube due to large loss of minute volume.

VIII. Respiratory function calculations

A. Compliance = change in volume/change in pressure. Normal values are approximately 100 ml/cm H_2O in the normal lung and approximately 70 ml/cm H_2O in the mechanically ventilated lung. Dynamic characteristics (V_T/peak pressure) measure both compliance and resistance components (including upper airway and tubing resistance). Static compliance of the lungs and chest wall = V_T/plateau pressure. Plateau pressure is obtained by occluding the expiratory limb at end inspiration and measuring pressure proximally at flow = zero. This eliminates the resistance of ventilator tubing, the endotracheal tube, and the upper airway from the calculation. Both assume constant relaxed respiratory muscles. Static compliance below 30 ml/cm H_2O indicates a severe abnormality. Spontaneous ventilation cannot be maintained due to the tremendous work required for lung inflation.

B. The **alveolar gas equation** calculates the alveolar-arterial oxygen gradient ($A - a\, DO_2$).

$$A - a\, DO_2 = P_AO_2 - PaO_2$$

$$P_AO_2 = (P_B - PH_2O)(FIO_2) - PaCO_2[FIO_2 + (1 - FIO_2)/RQ]$$

where P_AO_2 = alveolar oxygen tension
P_B = barometric pressure
PH_2O (saturated vapor pressure of H_2O) = 47 mm Hg at 1 atmosphere and 37°C.
RQ = respiratory quotient (usually about 0.8)
The equation may be simplified for clinical use to:
$P_AO_2 = (P_B - PH_2O)(FIO_2) - PaCO_2/RQ$

C. Oxygen content of blood (CaO_2) = oxygen bound to hemoglobin + oxygen dissolved in blood.

$$CaO_2 = (1.36\ ml\ O_2/gm\ Hgb)\ (gm\ Hgb/dl\ blood)\ (SaO_2) + (PaO_2)\ (0.003\ ml\ O_2/mm\ Hg/dl\ blood)$$

D. The **Fick equation** is used to calculate cardiac output or oxygen consumption when one of the two variables is known.

$$CO = \dot{V}O_2/ (CaO_2 - C\bar{v}O_2)$$

where CO = cardiac output (dl/min)
$\dot{V}O_2$ = oxygen consumption (ml/min)
CaO_2 and $C\bar{v}O_2$ are the O_2 contents of arterial and mixed venous blood (ml/dl) respectively

The Fick principle assumes that the amount of oxygen in the inspired gas is constant and equal to the amount added to the blood that flows through the lungs. Interpretation of calculated results must be done with skepticism given these assumptions. The amount of extrapulmonary shunt and the FIO_2 in the lung can change and errors in measuring mixed venous oxygen occur. O_2 consumption is normally 3–4 ml/min/kg. Oxygen consumption can also be calculated by measuring oxygen differences in inspiratory and expiratory gases.

E. The **shunt equation** calculates the ventilation-perfusion inequality or physiologic shunt:

$$\dot{Q}sp/\dot{Q}t = (CcO_2 - CaO_2)/(CcO_2 - C\bar{v}O_2)$$

where $\dot{Q}sp/\dot{Q}t$ = physiologic shunt/total lung blood flow
CcO_2 = O_2 content of pulmonary capillary blood
CaO_2 = arterial O_2 content
$C\bar{v}O_2$ = mixed venous O_2 content

This equation assumes $CcO_2 = CaO_2$ (alveolar oxygen content), which implies a constant FIO_2 throughout the lung. It is therefore usually determined at 100% or 21% FIO_2. Overestimation of shunt occurs when poorly ventilated alveoli (with lower than estimated FIO_2) are present. The magnitude of shunting is also directly related to cardiac output, and therefore changes of cardiac output must be taken into consideration. The arteriovenous oxygen difference is often estimated (from the oxygen-hemoglobin dissociation curve) rather than measured. This can lead to large inaccuracies in estimating shunt.

F. **Carbon dioxide production ($\dot{V}CO_2$)** is measured by collecting expired gas in an impermeable "Douglas" bag over a known period of time during steady-state ventilation.

$$\dot{V}CO_2 \text{ (cc/min)} = (FECO_2)(\dot{V}E) \text{ at STP}$$

where $FECO_2$ = concentration of expired CO_2
$\dot{V}E$ = measured expired minute ventilation
STP refers to gases at standard temperature and pressure.

G. **Oxygen consumption,** in addition to being estimated by the Fick equation, can be calculated by measuring the difference between inspired and expired oxygen, similar to measurement of $\dot{V}CO_2$ described in **F.** The same method employing the Douglas bag is used.

H. V_D/V_T represents the **physiologic dead space as a fraction of the tidal volume** and is a useful measure of lung dysfunction. Values greater than 0.6 are often incompatible with weaning from mechanical ventilation.

$$V_D/V_T = (PaCO_2 - P\bar{E}CO_2) / PaCO_2$$

where $P\bar{E}CO_2$ = average CO_2 in expired gas collected over time (several minutes)

SUGGESTED READING

Hurford, W. E. Effect of positive pressure ventilation on cardiovascular function. *Curr. Opinion Anesthesiol.* 2:789, 1989.

Kacmarek, R. M., and Stoller, J. K. *Current Respiratory Care.* Toronto, Philadelphia: Decker, 1988.

Kirby, R. R., Banner, M. J. and Downs, J. B. *Clinical Application of Ventilatory Support.* New York: Churchill Livingstone, 1990.

Martin, J., and Tobin, M. D. Mechanical Ventilation. In J. Martin, and M. D. Tobin, *Critical Care Clinics,* Vol. 6, No. 3. Philadelphia: Saunders, 1990.

Nunn, J. F. *Applied Respiratory Physiology.* Boston: Butterworth, 1987.

III

Patient Care
in Other Settings

36

Adult, Pediatric, and Newborn Resuscitation

Larry B. Scott

I. **Overview.** Cardiopulmonary resuscitation (CPR) in the operating room falls within the realm of responsibilities of the anesthesiologist. Although a team approach to resuscitation is mandatory, anesthesiologists, with their knowledge of physiology and pharmacology, are uniquely suited to lead the effort. In light of this responsibility, anesthesiologists should be familiar with the basic resuscitation protocols and the ongoing developments and controversies in the field of CPR. Time is of the essence in resuscitation efforts. Even appropriately applied basic life support (BLS) does not reliably produce adequate cerebral and myocardial perfusion to prevent permanent damage. Early initiation of advanced cardiac life support (ACLS) is therefore crucial for a good outcome. It has been determined that initiation of BLS within 4 minutes and ACLS within 8 minutes can lead to a greater than 40% survival rate. This 40% survival rate is the highest that has been reported for any major study of outcome after cardiac arrest. Most studies have been performed in cities with a population of less than 500,000 and have reported a survival rate of less than 18%. The survival rate of cardiac arrests occurring out of the hospital in large cities (population greater than 500,000) is 1–2%. The survival rate of in-hospital cardiac arrests is up to 14%.

II. **Cardiac arrest**

A. The **diagnosis** of cardiac arrest must be made with certainty prior to any resuscitative efforts, since the performance of BLS and ACLS is not without morbidity. The absence of a palpable pulse in a major vessel (carotid or femoral) in an unconscious patient is diagnostic of a cardiac arrest. The following may be suggestive as well:

1. Asystole, ventricular fibrillation, or ventricular tachycardia on an electrocardiogram.
2. Inaudible heart sounds.
3. Absent blood pressure.
4. Cyanosis, lack of bleeding in the surgical field, or "dark blood."
5. Failure of pulse oximeter.
6. Sudden decrease in end-tidal carbon dioxide.

B. **Etiologies.** Cardiac arrest is a final common pathway for many pathophysiologic disturbances. Treatment of these abnormalities may aid in the resuscitation effort or prevent a recurrence. The following may lead to a cardiac arrest:

1. Hypoxemia.
2. Acid-base disturbances.
3. Derangements of potassium, calcium, and magnesium.
4. Hypovolemia.
5. Hypotension.
6. Electrocution.

7. Adverse drug effects.
8. Surgical manipulation and trauma.
9. Underlying arrhythmias.
10. Mechanical derangements (e.g., pericardial tamponade, tension pneumothorax).

C. **Pathophysiology.** With the onset of a cardiac arrest, effective blood flow ceases, resulting in tissue hypoxia, anaerobic metabolism, and accumulation of cellular waste. Vital organ function is compromised, and permanent damage ensues unless reversed within minutes. Acidosis, resulting from anaerobic metabolism, results in systemic vasodilation, pulmonary vasoconstriction, and a decreased responsiveness to the actions of catecholamines.

III. **Adult resuscitation**

A. **Basic life support.** When a person becomes or is found unconscious, a cardiac arrest should be suspected. Simultaneously, the first person on the scene should summon help and assess the patient. Once it has been determined that the patient cannot be aroused, the "ABCs" of resuscitation should be followed, with assessment at each stage before treatment is rendered.

1. **Airway and breathing.** The airway should be assessed by placing an ear over the patient's mouth to listen and feel for air movement, at the same time looking at the chest to detect respiratory efforts. If the airway appears to be obstructed, use the "head tilt/chin lift" or "jaw thrust" maneuver to open the airway, and reassess. If effective ventilation is still absent, begin rescue breathing. Two slow breaths should be delivered initially, to be followed by 12 breaths/min. Slow breaths at low airway pressures are used to prevent gastric distention. The effectiveness of the rescue breathing should be assessed by observing chest movement and feeling and hearing air return at the mouth.

2. **Circulation.** The circulation is then assessed by feeling for a pulse in the carotid artery for 5–10 seconds. If a pulse cannot be palpated, then artificial circulation should be provided by external chest compression. The patient should be on a firm surface with the head on the same level as the thorax. The rescuer should place the heel of one hand on the patient's sternum, two finger-breadths above the xiphoid process. The other hand may either sit on top of the first, interlocking the fingers, or it may grasp the wrist of the first hand. The rescuer's shoulders should be directly over the patient, and the elbows should be locked for effective compressions. The sternum should be depressed 1.5–2.0 inches in a normal-sized adult, and the compression should account for 50% of each compression-relaxation cycle. Compressions should be delivered at a rate of 80–100/min.

3. **One rescuer versus two rescuers.** Single rescuers should perform chest compressions at a rate of 80–100/min, with a compression-ventilation ratio of 15 : 2. With two rescuers, the compression-ventilation ratio should be 5 : 1.

        4. Reassessment. The rescuer should check for the return of spontaneous cardiopulmonary activity after the first four cycles and then after every couple of minutes.

B. Advanced cardiac life support should supplement, but not replace, BLS efforts. ACLS is the definitive treatment of cardiac arrest with endotracheal intubation, electrical defibrillation, and pharmacologic intervention. BLS is still necessary, however, to maintain vital organ perfusion and to make the delivery of drugs to the central circulation possible.

        1. Intubation. The airway should be controlled as soon as possible to ensure the delivery of oxygen during the resuscitation effort. An attempt should be made to establish a good mask airway prior to intubation attempts. Once oxygenation has been achieved with a bag-mask setup, intubation should be done by the most experienced person available with minimal disruption of other resuscitative measures. Once in place, the endotracheal tube may be used to deliver essential medications if IV access has not already been established. Epinephrine, lidocaine, and atropine may be administered by the endotracheal route. Dilution of these drugs in up to 10 ml of sterile saline will ensure a more complete delivery of the medications. There is some evidence that the peak drug concentrations are lower with endotracheal as opposed to IV administration; higher doses, therefore, may be warranted if the endotracheal route is used.

        2. Defibrillation. Cardiac arrest may result from a variety of arrhythmias (e.g., ventricular fibrillation, ventricular tachycardia, asystole, and heart block). As the time of arrest progresses, the rhythm tends to deteriorate to those that are more difficult to convert. Therefore, early attempts at defibrillation are crucial to a successful outcome from CPR. A solitary precordial thump is recommended for patients with a witnessed cardiac arrest if a defibrillator is not available. As soon as the equipment is available, attempts at electrical conversion of the rhythm should be instituted. Three shocks should be delivered in rapid succession to take advantage of the decrease in transthoracic impedance that occurs with each shock. The energy level for the initial series of shocks should be 200, 300, and 360 joules, respectively. If unsuccessful, the subsequent shocks should all be at 360 joules and should be repeated after every pharmacologic manipulation. If ventricular fibrillation recurs following a successful defibrillation, then the energy level that was previously successful should be used. It is the responsibility of the person operating the defibrillator to ensure the safety of the resuscitation team and thus to make certain that no one is in contact with the patient at the time of defibrillation. Lower energies and synchronization of the shock with the patient's rhythm are used for supraventricular arrhythmias and hemodynamically stable ventricular tachycardia.

3. **Pacing.** The etiology of the cardiac arrest may be a high-grade heart block. In this situation, profound bradycardia ensues, and attempts at defibrillation are not warranted. If atropine and/or isoproterenol is not successful in increasing the heart rate, a means of temporary pacemaking should be utilized. The fastest way to achieve temporary pacing is with an external pacemaker. If these are not available, however, attempts should be made to pass a transvenous pacing wire into the central circulation while CPR continues.

4. **Intravenous access.** An adequate means to deliver medications and fluid is imperative for successful resuscitation. The most desirable route of drug administration is into the central circulation, since that is the site of action. Internal or external jugular, subclavian, femoral, or long peripheral lines may be used. The internal jugular and femoral veins are desirable because of the relative ease of insertion, fewer complications, and less interruption of the resuscitative efforts during insertion. The antecubital veins are the next most desirable and are fairly effective if the extremity is elevated and a large volume is used to flush the medications toward the central circulation.

5. **Medications**
   a. **Oxygen.** Because of the profound tissue hypoxemia present, 100% oxygen should be provided to all cardiac arrest victims by positive-pressure ventilation. In the case of a hemodynamically stable patient with arrhythmias, oxygen should be provided through a face mask.
   b. **Fluid** replacement with crystalloid or colloid solutions is indicated in patients with known intravascular volume depletion. In the usual cardiac arrest scenario, however, fluid should be used only to keep IV lines open and flush medications toward the central circulation.
   c. **Epinephrine.** No method of CPR tested to date, with the possible exception of open-chest CPR, can reliably provide vital organ blood flow sufficient to prevent ischemic injury. It has been determined that the addition of adrenergic agents to CPR greatly improves outcome. Epinephrine is currently the mainstay of pharmacologic therapy in cardiac arrest. The beneficial effect of epinephrine in this setting is thought to be a result of its alpha-adrenergic effects. It has even been postulated that its beta-adrenergic effects are actually harmful in CPR. Epinephrine causes profound vasoconstriction in the noncerebral and noncoronary vascular beds, thus shunting blood toward these vital organs. This vasoconstriction may actually decrease cardiac output while at the same time increasing cerebral and myocardial blood flows. Fears about possible adverse effects of the beta effects of epinephrine have led to a search for a better alpha agonist in the cardiac arrest setting. Methoxamine, phenyleph-

rine, and norepinephrine have all been compared to epinephrine for this purpose. At the time of this writing, although the initial data on norepinephrine look promising, epinephrine remains the adrenergic agent of choice. The optimal dosage of epinephrine in the cardiac arrest setting is also a subject of much debate. The current recommended dosage of epinephrine in the cardiac arrest setting is 0.5–1.0 mg IV, to be repeated every 5 minutes.

d. Lidocaine is the drug of choice for ventricular ectopy, including refractory ventricular fibrillation. Indications for use include ventricular fibrillation, ventricular tachycardia, and premature ventricular complexes that are frequent (greater than 6/min), closely coupled, occurring in runs of two or more, or multifocal in configuration. The initial dose of lidocaine in the cardiac arrest setting is 1 mg/kg IV. Lidocaine may be repeated as a 0.5 mg/kg bolus every 8 minutes to a total dose of 3 mg/kg. A continuous infusion of lidocaine at a rate of 2–4 mg/min should be instituted after successful resuscitation. The dosage of lidocaine should be reduced in patients with reduced cardiac output, hepatic dysfunction, or advanced age.

e. Bretylium is indicated for the treatment of ventricular arrhythmias and fibrillation resistant to other therapies. Caution must be exercised in its use, however, since it may result in hypotension several minutes after administration through postganglionic adrenergic blockade. Bretylium is given as an initial 5 mg/kg bolus, followed by doses of 10 mg/kg every 15 minutes (if necessary), to a total dose of 30 mg/kg. If successful, bretylium should be administered as an infusion of 1–2 mg/min for arrhythmia prophylaxis.

f. Procainamide should be used to suppress ventricular arrhythmias when lidocaine is contraindicated or has failed. Procainamide may be given in 50-mg boluses every 5 minutes or as a continuous infusion of 20 mg/min up to a total dose of 1 gm. This initial loading phase of procainamide administration should be terminated when the arrhythmia is suppressed, hypotension occurs, or the QRS complex is widened by 50% of its original size. When the arrhythmia is suppressed, a maintenance infusion of 1–4 mg/min should be initiated. The procainamide dosage should be reduced in the presence of renal failure.

g. Atropine is useful in the treatment of hemodynamically significant bradycardia or atrioventricular (AV) block occurring at the nodal level. Atropine increases the rate of sinus node discharge and enhances AV node conduction by its vagolytic activity. For bradycardia or AV block, atropine should be administered as a 0.5-mg bolus and repeated (if necessary) every 5 minutes to a total dose of 2 mg.

In the case of asystole, atropine should be given as a 1-mg bolus and repeated in 5 minutes if needed.

h. Isoproterenol is a pure beta-sympathomimetic agonist that is useful in the treatment of hemodynamically significant bradycardia that has not responded to atropine. Isoproterenol should be used as a temporary measure while a pacemaker is being inserted. The infusion rate of 2–10 μg/min should be titrated to the desired heart rate.

i. Verapamil is a calcium channel blocker with powerful depressant effects on the AV node. It is therefore very useful for the treatment of hemodynamically stable paroxysmal supraventricular tachycardia (PSVT) that uses AV node conduction and that has not responded to vagal maneuvers. The initial dose should be 2.5–5.0 mg IV, and subsequent doses of 5–10 mg IV should be administered every 15–30 minutes if the PSVT continues. Unfortunately, verapamil also has vasodilating and negative inotropic properties that can result in hypotension, exacerbation of congestive heart failure, bradycardia, and enhancement of accessory conduction in patients with Wolff-Parkinson-White syndrome. The hypotension associated with verapamil may be reversed by the administration of calcium chloride, 0.5–1.0 gm IV.

j. Propranolol, like all beta-blocking agents, acts by competing with agonists at beta-adrenergic receptors. Propranolol may be used in the treatment of hemodynamically stable PSVT and is occasionally useful in the treatment of ventricular arrhythmias. The initial dose of propranolol should be 0.25–0.5 mg IV, and subsequent doses can be increased to 1 mg or higher and given every 5 minutes until the rhythm is controlled. Propranolol, as opposed to verapamil, is not a direct-acting negative inotropic agent. Propranolol decreases inotropy only in situations where the patient is dependent on sympathetic input to maintain inotropy. Propranolol does not cause vasodilation and therefore is not as likely to cause hypotension as verapamil. Propranolol may, however, cause bronchospasm in susceptible patients.

k. Calcium. Multiple studies have failed to demonstrate a beneficial effect of calcium administration in CPR. In fact, there is evidence to demonstrate that high levels of calcium may be detrimental in the cardiac arrest setting. Therefore, calcium should only be used in the treatment of cardiac arrest when documented hyperkalemia, hypermagnesemia, or ionized hypocalcemia exists or in the setting of calcium channel blocker toxicity. Calcium chloride, 2–4 mg/kg IV, should be used in these situations and repeated as necessary.

l. Sodium bicarbonate should be used in the treatment of cardiac arrests only in the setting of preexisting acidosis or hypokalemia and then only when the standard ACLS protocol has been followed and failed. The initial dose of bicarbonate should be 1 mEq/kg IV, and subsequent doses of 0.5 mEq/kg may be given every 10 minutes (as indicated by arterial blood gas results). It has been determined that bicarbonate administration is actually detrimental in the cardiac arrest setting, and its indiscriminate use should be discouraged.

6. **Specific American Heart Association (AHA) ACLS protocols (flow charts)**
   a. Ventricular fibrillation (Fig. 36-1).
   b. Ventricular tachycardia (Fig. 36-2).
   c. Asystole (Fig. 36-3).
   d. Electromechanical dissociation (Fig. 36-4).
   e. Paroxysmal supraventricular tachycardia (Fig. 36-5).
   f. Bradycardia (Fig. 36-6).
   g. Ventricular ectopy (Fig. 36-7).

7. **Open-chest CPR** has been shown in multiple studies to produce higher organ blood flows, higher resuscitation and survival rates, and better neurologic outcome than closed-chest CPR. Open-chest CPR requires specialized training and equipment and should be performed only by persons specifically trained in its delivery. Open-chest CPR is indicated for cardiac arrest associated with
   a. Penetrating chest trauma.
   b. Anatomic deformity of the chest that prevents adequate closed-chest compression (including severe chronic obstructive pulmonary disease and crushed chest injury).
   c. Hypothermia.
   d. Ruptured aortic aneurysm.
   e. Cardiac tamponade.
   f. Situations when the chest is already open.
   g. Failure of adequately applied closed-chest CPR.

8. **When to terminate CPR.** Although studies have revealed that the probability of the patient's surviving until discharge from the hospital approaches zero as the resuscitation time exceeds 30 minutes, there are no absolute guidelines for when to terminate resuscitative efforts. It is left up to the discretion of the physician in charge to determine when the failure of the cardiovascular system to respond to adequately applied BLS and ACLS indicates that the patient is no longer viable. There should be meticulous documentation of the resuscitative effort by the physician in charge, including the reasons for terminating the effort.

9. **"Do not resuscitate"** orders place the anesthesiologist in a particularly sensitive situation when the patient suffers a cardiac arrest in the operating room or postanesthesia care unit. In this scenario, the patient should be resuscitated because of the possibility that the arrest was precipitated by a therapeutic maneuver rather than the patient's underlying dis-

Witnessed arrest
↓
Check pulse — if no pulse
↓
Precordial thump
↓
Check pulse — if no pulse

Unwitnessed arrest
↓
Check pulse — if no pulse

↓
CPR until a defibrillator is available
↓
Check monitor for rhythm — if VF or VT
↓
Defibrillate, 200 joules
↓
Defibrillate, 200–300 joules
↓
Defibrillate with up to 360 joules
↓
CPR if no pulse
↓
Establish IV access
↓
Epinephrine, 1:10,000, 0.5–1.0 mg IV push
↓
Intubate if possible
↓
Defibrillate with up to 360 joules
↓
Lidocaine, 1 mg/kg IV push
↓
Defibrillate with up to 360 joules
↓
Bretylium, 5 mg/kg IV push
↓
(Consider bicarbonate)
↓
Defibrillate with up to 360 joules
↓
Bretylium, 10 mg/kg IV push
↓
Defibrillate with up to 360 joules
↓
Repeat lidocaine or bretylium
↓
Defibrillate with up to 360 joules

Fig. 36-1. AHA ACLS protocol for ventricular fibrillation.

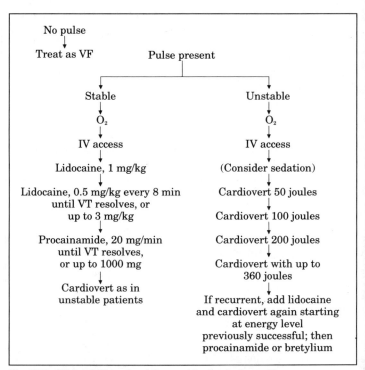

No pulse
↓
Treat as VF

Pulse present

Stable   Unstable

O₂   O₂
↓   ↓
IV access   IV access
↓   ↓
Lidocaine, 1 mg/kg   (Consider sedation)
↓   ↓
Lidocaine, 0.5 mg/kg every 8 min   Cardiovert 50 joules
until VT resolves, or   ↓
up to 3 mg/kg   Cardiovert 100 joules
↓   ↓
Procainamide, 20 mg/min   Cardiovert 200 joules
until VT resolves,   ↓
or up to 1000 mg   Cardiovert with up to
↓   360 joules
Cardiovert as in   ↓
unstable patients   If recurrent, add lidocaine
                                    and cardiovert again starting
                                    at energy level
                                    previously successful; then
                                    procainamide or bretylium

Fig. 36-2. AHA ACLS protocol for ventricular tachycardia.

If rhythm is unclear and possibly ventricular
fibrillation, defibrillate as for VF. If asystole is present
↓
Continue CPR
↓
Establish IV access
↓
Epinephrine, 1:10,000, 0.5–1.0 mg IV push
↓
Intubate when possible
↓
Atropine, 1.0 mg IV push (repeated in 5 min)
↓
(Consider bicarbonate)
↓
Consider pacing

Fig. 36-3. AHA ACLS protocol for asystole.

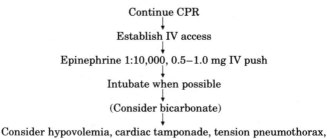

Continue CPR
↓
Establish IV access
↓
Epinephrine 1:10,000, 0.5–1.0 mg IV push
↓
Intubate when possible
↓
(Consider bicarbonate)
↓
Consider hypovolemia, cardiac tamponade, tension pneumothorax, hypoxemia, acidosis, pulmonary embolism

Fig. 36-4. AHA ACLS protocol for electromechanical dissociation.

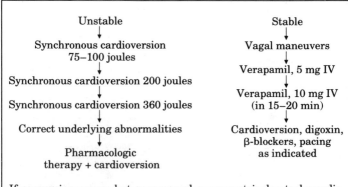

Unstable	Stable
↓	↓
Synchronous cardioversion 75–100 joules	Vagal maneuvers
↓	↓
Synchronous cardioversion 200 joules	Verapamil, 5 mg IV
↓	↓
Synchronous cardioversion 360 joules	Verapamil, 10 mg IV (in 15–20 min)
↓	↓
Correct underlying abnormalities	Cardioversion, digoxin, β-blockers, pacing as indicated
↓	
Pharmacologic therapy + cardioversion	

If conversion occurs but paroxysmal supraventricular tachycardia recurs, repeat electrical cardioversion is *not* indicated. Sedation should be used as time permits.

Fig. 36-5. AHA ACLS protocol for paroxysmal supraventricular tachycardia.

ease. This course of action should be discussed preoperatively with the patient (if competent), the patient's family, the primary physician, and the surgeon.

IV. **Pediatric resuscitation.** The need for CPR in the pediatric age group is a fairly rare occurrence after the neonatal period. Outcome after cardiac arrest occurring out of the hospital in the pediatric population is poor, with a survival until discharge of less than 10%. Pediatric cardiac arrests are usually the result of hypoxia from respiratory failure or airway obstruction. Initial efforts should be directed toward securing the airway and ensuring adequate ventilation.

A. **Basic life support.** The basic considerations for resuscitation of the pediatric patient are the same as for the adult (airway, breathing, and circulation). Modifications of the rate and magnitude of compressions and ventila-

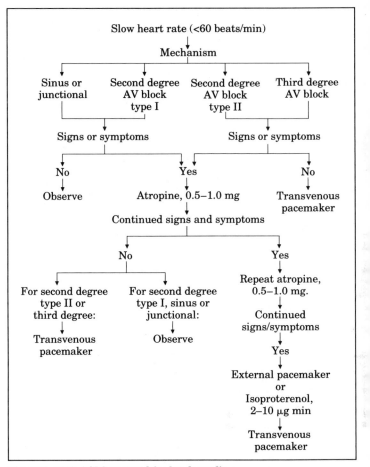

Slow heart rate (<60 beats/min)
↓
Mechanism

Sinus or junctional — Second degree AV block type I — Second degree AV block type II — Third degree AV block

Signs or symptoms   Signs or symptoms

No → Observe

Yes → Atropine, 0.5–1.0 mg
↓
Continued signs and symptoms

No   Yes

For second degree type II or third degree: → Transvenous pacemaker

For second degree type I, sinus or junctional: → Observe

Repeat atropine, 0.5–1.0 mg.
↓
Continued signs/symptoms
↓
Yes
↓
External pacemaker
or
Isoproterenol, 2–10 µg min
↓
Transvenous pacemaker

No → Transvenous pacemaker

Fig. 36-6. AHA ACLS protocol for bradycardia.

tions, as well as of the hand position for compressions, are necessary because of anatomic and physiologic differences (Table 36-1). Detailed below are differences between pediatric and adult resuscitation techniques.

1. **Airway.** Controlling the airway to ensure adequate ventilation is the most important factor for successful pediatric resuscitation. Maneuvers to establish the airway are the same as in the adult, with two important exceptions. First, hyperextension of an infant's neck for the head tilt/chin lift maneuver may actually lead to airway obstruction because of the small diameter and ease of compression of the immature airway. Second, submental compression while performing the chin lift can lead to airway obstruction by pushing the tongue into the pharynx. Ventilations should be given

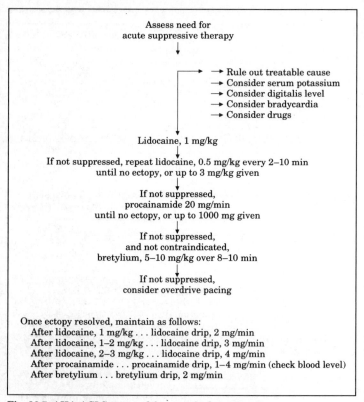

Assess need for
acute suppressive therapy

→ Rule out treatable cause
→ Consider serum potassium
→ Consider digitalis level
→ Consider bradycardia
→ Consider drugs

Lidocaine, 1 mg/kg

If not suppressed, repeat lidocaine, 0.5 mg/kg every 2–10 min
until no ectopy, or up to 3 mg/kg given

If not suppressed,
procainamide 20 mg/min
until no ectopy, or up to 1000 mg given

If not suppressed,
and not contraindicated,
bretylium, 5–10 mg/kg over 8–10 min

If not suppressed,
consider overdrive pacing

Once ectopy resolved, maintain as follows:
    After lidocaine, 1 mg/kg . . . lidocaine drip, 2 mg/min
    After lidocaine, 1–2 mg/kg . . . lidocaine drip, 3 mg/min
    After lidocaine, 2–3 mg/kg . . . lidocaine drip, 4 mg/min
    After procainamide . . . procainamide drip, 1–4 mg/min (check blood level)
    After bretylium . . . bretylium drip, 2 mg/min

Fig. 36-7. AHA ACLS protocol for ventricular ectopy.

slowly with low airway pressures to avoid gastric distention and should be of sufficient volume to cause the chest to rise and fall. Once the presence of an arrest has been established, two initial breaths should be given; subsequent ventilation rates vary with age and are provided in Table 36-1.

2. **Circulation.** The carotid artery in infants (< 1 year) is difficult to palpate because of their relatively short necks. The brachial or femoral artery should therefore be used to establish pulselessness in an infant. The carotid artery should be used in all other patients. Once pulselessness has been established, chest compressions should be initiated. The chest compression rates and depths vary with age and are provided in Table 36-1. The compression phase should take up 50% of the entire compression-relaxation cycle. Chest compressions in infants may be delivered using two fingertips applied to the sternum or by encircling the chest with both hands and using the thumbs on the sternum. The sternum should be depressed 0.5–1.0 inch with each compression. The correct position in infants is

Table 36-1. Pediatric cardiopulmonary resuscitation

Age	Ventilations/min	Compressions/min	Ventilation-Compression Ratio	Depth (inches)
Infant	20–24	100–120	1 : 5	0.5–1.0
Young child (1–4 years)	20	100	1 : 5	1.0–1.5
Older child (> 4 years)	16	80	1 : 5	1.5–2.0

determined by drawing an imaginary line between the nipples. The fingers should be placed one finger-breadth below the intersection of this imaginary line and the sternum. In older children the correct hand position is determined as in adults, and one hand is used to depress the sternum 1.0–1.5 inch.

3. **One rescuer versus two rescuers.** For both one- and two-rescuer scenarios in pediatric patients, a 5 : 1 compression-ventilation ratio should be maintained. A pause should occur at the end of the fifth compression to allow for adequate ventilation.

4. **Reassessment.** The pediatric patient should initially be reassessed after 10 compression-ventilation cycles to check for the return of spontaneous cardiopulmonary activity. Thereafter, resuscitation attempts should be halted every couple of minutes for reassessment.

B. **Advanced cardiac life support.** The majority of pediatric cardiac arrests occur in infants less than 1 year old. Respiratory and idiopathic (sudden infant death syndrome) etiologies predominate in this age group. Interestingly, over 90% of pediatric arrests present as asystole or bradycardia rather than ventricular arrhythmias. When faced with a pediatric arrest, the first consideration should be the rapid initiation of BLS. ACLS should be an extension, not a replacement of BLS. Once again, anatomic and physiologic differences dictate that drug dosages and defibrillator current be calculated based on the patient's weight.

1. **Intubation.** Control of the airway and ensurance of adequate ventilation are paramount in pediatric resuscitation. Endotracheal tube size should be based on the patient's age (tube size [mm ID] = age/4 + 4 for children over 2 years old). Once the endotracheal tube is in place, it can be used to administer atropine, epinephrine, and lidocaine until adequate IV access is established.

2. **Defibrillation.** Defibrillator paddles 4.5 cm in diameter should be used for infants and 8 cm in diameter for older children. The energy level for the initial shock should be 2 joules/kg. If this energy level is unsuccessful, the dose should be increased to 4 joules/kg and repeated twice if necessary. If 4 joules/kg is unsuccess-

ful, an attempt should be made to find a treatable cause such as hypoxemia, acidosis, or hypothermia. After each pharmacologic manipulation, defibrillation should be reattempted with an energy level of 4 joules/kg. If fibrillation should recur after a successful defibrillation, repeat attempts should be at the energy level that was previously successful. For cardioversion, the dose should be started at 0.2 joules/kg and escalated to 1.0 joules/kg as needed.

3. **Pacing.** In the case of symptomatic bradycardia or heart block unresponsive to atropine, an attempt should be made to treat the patient pharmacologically with isoproterenol. The initial dosage is 0.1 µg/kg/min, subsequently titrated to effect. If the rhythm disturbance does not respond to pharmacologic treatment, pacing should be established with external and then transvenous pacing.

4. **Intravenous access.** Central venous access is the preferred route of drug administration in the cardiac arrest setting. It permits a more rapid onset of action and a higher peak concentration of medications. If the standard routes are not successful, the femoral vein can be used to access the central circulation if a catheter of suitable length is employed. If central access is impossible, peripheral IVs can be used if they are flushed with sufficient fluid to ensure central delivery of the drugs. The intraosseous route may also be used in children. A bone marrow or spinal needle is inserted into the tibial plateau to gain access to the bone marrow. If none of the above is available, the endotracheal tube may be used to deliver essential medications if they are diluted in 2–5 ml of normal saline to ensure their delivery to the pulmonary vasculature.

5. **Medications.** The medications described in the adult ACLS section apply here as well. The proper dosage must be calculated based on the child's weight as outlined in Table 36-2. One important exception is epinephrine. There is evidence in the pediatric CPR literature that doses higher than the current AHA recommendations (10 µg/kg) are more effective in achieving a return to spontaneous circulation. It has, therefore, been advocated that doses of 100–200 µg/kg be used following the failure of the initial 10 µg/kg dose (Table 36-2).

6. **Specific ACLS protocols.** The protocols described in the adult ACLS section apply here as well. The appropriate drug dosages and defibrillation energies must be calculated based on the patient's weight, as previously described.

V. **Newborn resuscitation.** It has been estimated that up to 6% of newborns require resuscitation after delivery, and this rises to 80% in newborns weighing less than 1500 gm. Therefore, at least one person who is skilled in neonatal resuscitation should be present at every delivery. Newborn resuscitation can be divided into four phases: stimulation and

Table 36-2. Drugs used in pediatric advanced life support

Drug	Dose	How supplied	Remarks
Atropine sulfate	0.02 mg/kg/dose	0.1 mg/ml	Minimum dose of 0.1 mg (1.0 ml)
Calcium chloride	20 mg/kg/dose	100 mg/ml (10%)	Give slowly
Dopamine hydrochloride	2–20 µg/kg/min	40 mg/ml	α-Adrenergic action dominates at 15–20 µg/kg/min
Dobutamine hydrochloride	5–20 µg/kg/min	250 mg/vial lyophilized	Titrate to desired effect
Epinephrine hydrochloride	0.1 ml/kg (0.01 mg/kg)	1 : 10,000 (0.1 mg/ml)	1 : 1000 must be diluted
Epinephrine infusion	Start at 0.1 µg/kg/min	1 : 1000 (1 mg/ml)	Titrate to desired effect (0.1–1.0 µg/kg/min)
Isoproterenol hydrochloride	Start at 0.1 µg/kg/min	1 mg/5 ml	Titrate to desired effect (0.1–1.0 µg/kg/min)
Lidocaine	1 mg/kg/dose	10 mg/ml (1%) 20 mg/ml (2%)	
Lidocaine infusion	20–50 µg/kg/min	40 mg/ml (4%)	
Norepinephrine infusion	Start at 0.1 µg/kg/min	1 mg/ml	Titrate to desired effect (0.1–1.0 µg/kg/min)
Sodium bicarbonate	1 mEq/kg/dose or 0.3 × kg × base deficit	1 mEq/ml (8.4%)	Infuse slowly and only if ventilation is adequate

suctioning, airway management, chest compressions, and delivery of resuscitation drugs and fluids. Resuscitation of the newborn is labor intensive and as such may require up to three persons. One rescuer should manage the airway, the second rescuer monitors the newborn and provides chest compressions, and the third person establishes IV access and administers the medications and fluids.

A. **Assessment.** Time is of the utmost importance in neonatal resuscitation. Profound hypoxemia may result from delays in initiating care. Hypoxemia will lead to acidosis, which may cause persistence of the fetal circulation and worsening of the hypoxemia.

1. The **APGAR scoring system** is an objective assessment of the physiologic well-being of the child that is

Table 36-3. The APGAR score

Clinical sign	Points assigned		
	0	1	2
Appearance	Cyanotic	Acrocyanotic	Pink
Pulse (determined either by auscultation of the precordium or by palpation of the umbilical artery)	< 60	60–100	> 100
Grimace or reflex irritability to oropharyngeal suctioning	No response	Weak cry	Vigorous cry
Activity or muscle tone	Flaccid	Weak	Good
Respiratory effort	Apnea	Irregular	Regular

done at 1 and 5 minutes after birth (Table 36-3). Newborns with an APGAR score of 0–2 require the immediate initiation of CPR. Those with scores of 3–4 require bag and mask ventilation. Neonates with scores of 5–7 require supplemental oxygen and stimulation.

2. **Clinical assessment** of the newborn's respiratory activity, heart rate, and color may be a better method than waiting the full 1 minute to assess the APGAR score, since the time lag in initiating resuscitative efforts will be eliminated. The respiratory activity should be evaluated by watching the newborn's chest rise and fall and auscultation of breath sounds. The heart rate may be ascertained by auscultation or by palpating the pulse in the base of the umbilicus.

B. **Four phases of newborn resuscitation**
   1. **Stimulation and suctioning**
      a. **Warming.** The neonate should be thoroughly dried and placed in a prewarmed environment after birth to minimize heat loss. Neonates do not tolerate a cold environment, and hypothermia can exacerbate acidosis.
      b. **Suctioning.** The newborn should be placed on its back or its left side in the Trendelenburg position to encourage venous return and drainage of secretions. The head should be turned to the side with the neck placed in a neutral position. The mouth and nose should be suctioned with a bulb syringe to remove blood, mucus, or meconium. Suctioning attempts should be limited to 10 seconds with oxygen supplied between attempts. The heart rate should be monitored during suctioning, since bradycardia may result from vagal stimulation or as a result of hypoxemia.

c. Infants born with thick meconium in the amniotic fluid should have their hypopharynx suctioned after delivery of the head using a DeLee trap. The trachea should then be intubated and suction applied to the endotracheal tube as it is removed. This step should be repeated until the trachea is cleared of meconium. The suction should be applied directly to the endotracheal tube, since meconium is too viscous to be aspirated through a suction catheter. The presence of thin meconium does not warrant endotracheal intubation.

d. Stimulation. Drying and suctioning are adequate stimulation to lead to respiratory activity in most newborns. Additional measures that may be used include gently rubbing the newborn's back and slapping the soles of the feet.

2. Airway management

a. Positive-pressure ventilation with 100% oxygen should be provided in the following situations:

(1) Apnea.

(2) Cyanosis.

(3) Heart rate below 100 beats/min.

b. A bag and mask unit should be attempted initially. The chest should be observed and auscultated to determine the adequacy of ventilation. The initial breath may require airway pressures as high as 30–40 cm H_2O and should be held for 2 seconds to permit adequate lung expansion. All breaths should be at the lowest pressure possible (while ensuring adequate chest expansion) to prevent gastric distention. Gastric distention may lead to further respiratory compromise and should be relieved. Assisted ventilation should be continued until spontaneous respirations are present and the heart rate is greater than 100 beats/min.

c. Endotracheal intubation should be used when

(1) Bag and mask ventilation is ineffective.

(2) Tracheal suctioning is needed (e.g., meconium aspiration).

(3) Prolonged ventilatory assistance is anticipated.

3. Chest compressions. The heart rate should be evaluated after adequate ventilation with 100% oxygen has been performed for 30 seconds. If the heart rate is less than 100 beats/min, assisted ventilation should be continued. If the heart rate is less than 80 beats/min and not rising, or less than 60 beats/min, chest compressions are required as well. The sternum should be depressed 0.5–0.75 inch at a rate of 120 times/min. The compression-ventilation ratio in neonates is 3 : 1. The compression should last for 50% of the entire compression-relaxation cycle. The compressions should be stopped periodically to check the spontaneous heart rate and should be terminated when the intrinsic rate is greater than 80 beats/min. Assisted ventilation should continue until the newborn's respiratory attempts are deemed adequate.

4. **Delivery of resuscitation drugs and fluids.** If the heart rate remains below 80 beats/min despite adequate ventilation with 100% oxygen and chest compressions, then resuscitation drugs should be administered. Although other veins may be used, the umbilical vein provides the best vascular access for a resuscitation. The umbilical vein is the largest and thinnest of the three umbilical vessels. It should be cannulated with a 3.5–5.0 Fr umbilical catheter after the cord has been prepared and trimmed. Sterile umbilical tape should be placed at the base of the cord to prevent bleeding. The catheter should be placed below the skin level and blood should be freely aspiratable. Care must be taken not to permit air into the system, since a neonate who requires resuscitation certainly will have a significant right-to-left shunt. If no vascular access is available, the endotracheal tube may be used to administer epinephrine, atropine, lidocaine, and naloxone. The drugs may be diluted in 1–2 ml of normal saline to ensure their delivery to the pulmonary vasculature.

5. **Drug and fluid dosages**
    a. **Oxygen** (100%) should be used in all resuscitation situations. Concerns about oxygen toxicity are not warranted in life or death situations.
    b. **Epinephrine.** The beta effects of epinephrine are important in neonatal resuscitation to increase the intrinsic heart rate. Epinephrine should be used for asystole or for a heart rate less than 80 despite adequate oxygenation and chest compressions. The dose is 10–30 μg/kg IV or endotracheal and should be repeated every 5 minutes.
    c. **Naloxone** is a specific opiate antagonist and should be used in the resuscitation setting when neonatal depression occurs after maternal administration of narcotics. The initial dose should be 10 μg/kg IV, IM, SQ, or endotracheal. The dose may be repeated every 2–3 minutes. The respiratory efforts of the child must be monitored for an extended period of time after narcotic reversal, since the duration of action of naloxone is shorter than that of narcotics. An acute withdrawal reaction may be precipitated in the child of a narcotic-addicted mother.
    d. The routine use of **sodium bicarbonate** is not recommended, although it may be considered in prolonged arrests to relieve myocardial depression and to optimize the actions of catecholamines, since both are depressed by acidosis. Intraventricular hemorrhage in premature infants has been associated with the osmolar load occurring with bicarbonate administration. A neonatal preparation of sodium bicarbonate (4.2% or 0.5 mEq/ml) should be used to prevent this from occurring. The initial dose should be 1 mEq/kg IV given over 2 minutes. Subsequent doses of 0.5 mEq/kg may be given every 10 minutes and should be guided by blood gases.

e. **Atropine calcium** and **glucose** are not recommended for use in neonatal resuscitation unless specifically indicated.

f. **Fluids**
   (1) **Hypovolemia** should be considered in the setting of
      (a) Peripartum hemorrhage.
      (b) Hypotension.
      (c) Weak pulses.
      (d) Persistent pallor, despite adequate oxygenation and chest compressions.
   (2) Albumin 5%, lactated Ringer's solution, or O-negative whole blood cross-matched with maternal blood may be used for resuscitation. The volume should be 10 ml/kg and repeated as necessary.

SUGGESTED READING

American Heart Association. Standards and guidelines for cardiopulmonary resuscitation (CPR) and emergency cardiac care (ECC). *J.A.M.A.* 255:2095, 1986.

Becker, L. B., et al. Outcome of CPR in a large metropolitan area—where are the survivors? *Ann. Emerg. Med.* 20:355, 1991.

Eisenberg, M. S., Bergner, L., and Hallstrom, A. H. Cardiac resuscitation in the community. *J.A.M.A.* 241:1905, 1979.

Geller, S. A., Elliot, P. L., and Rogers, M. C. Update on cardiopulmonary resuscitation. *Adv. Anesth.* 3:323, 1986.

Gregory, G. A. Resuscitation of the newborn. *Anesthesiology* 43:255, 1975.

Milner, A. D. Resuscitation of the newborn. *Arch. Dis. Child.* 66:66, 1991.

Paradis, N. A., and Koscove, E. M. Epinephrine in cardiac arrest: A critical review. *Ann. Emerg. Med.* 19:128, 1990.

Safar, P. *Cardio-Pulmonary-Cerebral-Resuscitation.* Philadelphia: Saunders, 1981.

Schleien, C. L., et al. Controversial issues in cardiopulmonary resuscitation. *Anesthesiology* 71:133, 1989.

Todres, I. D., and Rogers, M. C. Methods of external cardiac massage in the newborn infant. *J. Pediatr.* 86:781, 1975.

37

Pain

Kenneth Blazier

I. Pain and the anesthesiologist

A. Acute pain. Anesthesiologists play a unique role in the treatment of acute pain. Intraoperative blockade of afferent stimuli, or the central response to such, is the hallmark of successful anesthetic management. Once the patient leaves the postanesthesia care unit (PACU), responsibility for further analgesic management increasingly rests with a group of clinicians in which the anesthesiologist plays a major role. New techniques such as patient-controlled analgesia (PCA) and epidural opioids have expanded this role. In difficult cases, such as when pain is expected to persist (e.g., after a noncurative cancer operation), or when pain patterns do not fit the objective findings, an inpatient "pain consult" is often sought for adjustment of pharmacotherapy, for diagnostic and therapeutic nerve blocks, or for other interventions ranging from (permanent) neurolysis to placement of catheters for prolonged drug delivery.

B. Chronic pain

1. Patients with long-standing symptoms are referred to anesthesiologist consultants for diagnosis as well as therapy. Few other specialists are prepared to perform selective nerve blocks to judge the importance of an individual facet joint, nerve root, or sympathetic chain within a symptom complex. Prognostic importance also attaches to local anesthetic blockade performed to simulate neurolysis, for example, of intercostal nerves in a patient with malignant involvement of the chest wall or of the celiac plexus in a patient with inoperable pancreatic cancer. Therapeutic trials of local anesthetics and corticosteroids instilled into the epidural space or into suspected "trigger points" are also performed.

2. Apart from technical facility with neural blockade, anesthesiologists are consulted to help manage patients whose pain has a more obscure anatomic basis. Chronic neuropathic, myofascial, or idiopathic pain is often managed medically, the regimen for which is a consensus between specialists in anesthesia, psychiatry, and neurology. Familiarity with analgesic, anxiolytic, antiinflammatory, anticonvulsant, and antidepressant drugs has led anesthesiologists to serve as valuable consultants and members of comprehensive pain management teams.

II. Pain pathways

A. Nociceptors (pain receptors). Pain usually arises from one of three areas: skin, deep tissues (including bone), and body organs (viscera).

1. **Cutaneous nociceptors**

   a. Cutaneous nociceptors respond to strong pressure over a wide area of skin (usually > 1 cm^2) by high-threshold **mechanoreceptors** that transmit through rapidly conducting (5–25 m/sec) myelinated A-delta fibers.

b. **Polymodal receptors** respond to thermal and chemical irritation and pressure transmitted through slower unmyelated C-fibers (< 2 m/sec) as well as A-delta fibers (see Chap. 15).

2. **Deep nociceptors** are polymodal.

3. **Visceral nociceptors** are not clearly delineated. A-delta and C-fibers have been associated with the heart, lung, and other organs. Deep tissue and visceral pain may be referred to distant cutaneous sites that share dorsal horn, spinal, or other central nervous system (CNS) pathways (i.e., diaphragmatic irritation may cause shoulder pain, and myocardial ischemia may cause jaw or arm pain).

B. **Afferents.** The primary afferents associated with pain transmission are the myelinated A-delta and the unmyelinated C-fibers whose cell bodies are located in dorsal root ganglia. From whatever source, nearly all pain fibers enter the dorsal horn of the spinal cord through the dorsal root. Stimulation of A-delta fibers yields "first" pain: sharp, prickling, localized, and rapid in onset. C-fibers mediate "second" pain: dull, aching, poorly localized, and prolonged. Visceral afferents reach the spinal cord through sympathetic, parasympathetic, and splanchnic nerves. Dorsal horn processing of afferent input takes place in a cascade system arrayed in six laminae. Most A-delta fibers terminate in Rexed's laminae I, II (substantia gelatinosa), and V, while C-fibers terminate in I and II. Rexed's lamina V also receives pain afferents from visceral and deep tissue sources.

C. **Dorsal horn neurons.** The most popular of the many proposed classifications for dorsal horn neurons is based on skin stimulation. There are three primary types:

1. **Wide dynamic range neurons** respond to mechanical as well as noxious stimuli and are located mainly in Rexed's laminae I, II, and V.

2. **Nociceptive-specific neurons** are activated only by painful stimuli and are found in a number of lamina.

3. **Non-nociceptive-specific neurons** respond primarily to innocuous stimuli but are also capable of responding to intense noxious stimuli and are primarily located in laminae III and IV (nucleus proprius).

D. **Transmitters.** Numerous neurotransmitters have been isolated throughout the nervous system. In one area a transmitter may inhibit neuronal depolarization, while elsewhere it may excite. A partial list of neurotransmitters involved in nociception includes substance P, somatostatin, enkephalin, neurokinins A and B, serotonin, glutamate, aspartate, cholecystokinin, and calcitonin gene-related peptide.

E. **Ascending pathways.** Classically, the spinothalamic and spinoreticular tracts have been associated with pain transmission. Spinothalamic tract neurons originate from Rexed's laminae I and IV–VI in the dorsal horn and decussate within the segment of entry. Most of these fibers ascend in the ventrolateral spinal cord, yet some project through dorsolateral funiculi bilaterally. The pathway terminates in one of several thalamic nuclei: either the ventral posterolateral, the posterior complex, or the submedian nuclei. The spinoreticular tract is less anatomically distinct. These neurons arise from lamina V and ascend in the contralateral ventrolateral quadrant along with spinothalamic fibers. Spinomesencephalic, spinocervical, and spinohypothalamic tracts also participate in nociception.

F. **Descending inhibition.** Wall and Melzack proposed the **gate control theory of pain,** whose basic idea is that a spinal "gate" modulates dorsal horn transmission of pain. Two distinct descending inhibitory systems exist.

1. The first originates in the raphe nuclei, a collection of serotonergic neurons in the middle of the brainstem. These cells project to the dorsal horn by way of the dorsolateral funiculus and directly inhibit dorsal horn cells or activate an inhibitory segmental interneuron that uses enkephalin as a transmitter.

2. The other inhibitory pathway originates in the medulla and uses norepinephrine as its transmitter. Its precise anatomic route is unclear. Stimulation of these cells as well as those of the raphe nuclei causes naloxone-reversible analgesia.

III. **Chemical mediators of pain**

A. **Peripheral algesic substances** activate nociceptors during acute injury or inflammation. Acetylcholine, histamine, serotonin, bradykinin, prostaglandins, adenosine triphosphate, and hydrogen and potassium ions can act alone or synergistically. Many of these and others under investigation (e.g., lymphokines, monokines, interleukins) are white blood cell products.

B. **Neuropeptides** function in primary sensory as well as inhibitory ("modulatory") roles. **Substance P,** an 11-amino acid peptide, is a major sensory transmitter of primary pain afferents; other peptides with possible roles include cholecystokinin, angiotensin II, and vasoactive intestinal peptide. Analgesic peptides include somatostatin, calcitonin gene-related peptide, and **endorphins.** The last includes several families of opioid peptides, each with part of their structure resembling morphine, but with other regions having actions distinct from narcotics (e.g., immune modulation). Endorphins and their receptors are found in the dorsal horn (where they inhibit substance P release), periaqueductal gray, raphe nucleus, and limbic structures. Beta endorphin is derived from the same precursor as adrenocorticotropic hormone, and both are cosecreted during stress.

C. **Monoamines** include dietary amino acids (glycine) or their enzymatically produced derivatives (e.g., catecholamines from tyrosine or serotonin from tryptophan). Catecholamines function as excitatory sympathetic transmitters and also are released systemically as hormones that sensitize nociceptors. Yet norepinephrine and serotonin pathways not only transmit key inhibitory brainstem signals to dorsal horns but also mediate in the analgesia produced by morphine.

IV. **Acute pain.** Whether the result of surgical intervention, trauma, or medical disease, acute pain can disrupt and delay recovery. The anesthesiologist has a wide variety of options to interrupt pain pathways at a number of points.

   A. **Nonsteroidal antiinflammatory drugs (NSAIDs)** (Table 37-1)

      1. **Effect.** NSAIDs decrease pain by inhibiting the enzyme cyclooxygenase, thereby preventing the synthesis of prostaglandins, key mediators of pain associated with inflammation. NSAIDs bind to peripheral proteins that leak into the damaged site and are locally concentrated in the acidic environs of the damaged tissue. An additional spinal site of action has been demonstrated.

      2. **Indications.** NSAIDs are valuable in the treatment of mild to moderate pain when used alone. In addition, they can be combined with other classes of analgesics for severe pain. Individual responses to different NSAIDs are variable. Therefore, a trial of different NSAIDs may be warranted.

      3. NSAIDs share common **side effects** including renal dysfunction, gastric irritation and ulceration, and reversible platelet dysfunction.

      4. **Parenteral NSAID.** The recent introduction of an injectable nonsteroidal (ketorolac) represents an advance in the treatment of acute postoperative pain, particularly with orthopedic and thoracic surgery (see **Ketorolac** in Appendix).

   B. **Opioids** (Table 37-2)

      1. All opioids act on **membrane receptors.** The nomenclature for opioid classification reflects the type and degree of receptor activation. Pure agonists (e.g., morphine sulfate, codeine, oxycodone, and meperidine) activate the **mu receptor.** Mixed agonist-antagonists (e.g., butorphanol, pentazocine, nalbuphine) selectively activate other opioid receptors (i.e., kappa, delta, and sigma) while partially or completely blocking activity at mu receptors. These drugs have been promoted as having a ceiling on respiratory depression. They appear also to plateau in their analgesic capabilities. Partial agonists (e.g., buprenorphine, dezocine) only partially stimulate a receptor, thereby producing a submaximal effect. If partial agonists or mixed agonist-antagonists are administered to opioid-tolerant patients, they may precipitate withdrawal.

      2. **Parenteral opioids** are the primary method of pain control for moderate to severe pain. Dosages are calculated based on weight, age, type of procedure, and the presence of tolerance. Allowing for potency differences, even opioids of a single class may evoke variable responses in a single individual, and so empiric trials of different opioids are often worthwhile. See Table 37-2 for comparative dosage information.

      3. **Side effects** include respiratory depression, sedation,

Table 37-1. Analgesic adjuncts

Generic name	Proprietary name	Typical oral dosage (mg)	Typical parenteral dosage (mg)
NSAIDs			
Aspirin		650 q3–4h	
Ibuprofen	Motrin, Advil	200–800 q6h	
Naproxen	Naprosyn	250–500 q12h	
Indomethacin	Indocin	25–50 q8–12h	Rectal 25–50 q8–12h
Choline magnesium trisalicylate	Trilisate	1000–1500 q12h	
Ketorolac	Toradol	10 mg q4–6h	15–60 IM/IV q6h
Diclenofac	Voltaren	50–75 q8–12h	
Sulindac	Clinoril	150–200 q12h	
Fenoprofen	Nalfon	200 q4–6h	
Piroxicam	Feldene	20 q24h	
Etodolac	Lodine	200–400 q6–8h	
Acetaminophen	Tylenol	325–650 q4–6h	
Antidepressants			
Amitriptyline	Elavil	25–250 hs	
Imipramine	Tofranil	25–150 hs	
Desipramine	Norpramin	25–150 hs	
Phenelzine	Nardil	15 q8–24h	
Doxepin	Sinequan	25–50 q8–24h	
Fluoxetine	Prozac	20 q12–24h	
Anxiolytics, antispasmodics			
Diazepam	Valium	2.5–10.0 q6–8h	5–10 IV q4–6h
Clonazepam	Klonopin	0.5–1.0 q8h	
Alprazolam	Xanax	0.5–1.0 q8h	
Lorazepam	Ativan	1–2 q12h	0.5–1.0 IM/IV q6–8h
Chlordiazepoxide	Librium	5–10 q6–8h	50–100 IM/IV q8h
Cyclobenzaprine	Flexeril	10–20 q8h	
Baclofen	Lioresal	5–20 q8h	
Methocarbamol	Robaxin	1000–1500 q8h	
Hydroxyzine	Vistaril, Atarax	50–100 q6h	50–100 IM q4–6h
Anticonvulsants			
Carbamazepine	Tegretol	100–200 q12h	
Phenytoin	Dilantin	50–100 q8h	
Valproate	Depakene	100–400 q8h	
Antiemetics, major tranquilizers			
Prochlorperazine	Compazine	5–10 q8h	5–10 IM q3–4h

Table 37-1. (continued)

Generic name	Proprietary name	Typical oral dosage (mg)	Typical parenteral dosage (mg)
Metoclopramide	Reglan	10–15 q6–8h	10 IM/IV q4–6h
Promethazine	Phenergan	25–50 q4–6h	12.5–25.0 IM q4–6h
Chlorpromazine	Thorazine	10–25 q6h	25–50 IM q3–4h
Haloperidol	Haldol	0.5 q8h	1–2 IM/IV q6h
Droperidol	Inapsine	5–15 q8h	0.625–1.25 q6h
Other			
Bethanechol chloride	Urecholine	10–50 q6–8h	2.5–5.0 SQ 16–8h
Docusate sodium	Colace	50–200 qd	
Dextroamphetamine	Dexedrine	5–10 q6–8h	

nausea and vomiting, urinary retention, pruritus, and ileus.

C. **Patient-controlled analgesia** (PCA)

1. Patients receiving PCA are given control of a computer-controlled infusion device to administer an analgesic either IV, SQ, or epidurally. This type of analgesia leads to a higher level of patient comfort and satisfaction than do conventional (prn IM) regimens. It can be modified for pediatric use so that the family or nurse controls the child's degree of analgesia. Disadvantages of PCA include cost, need for medical supervision and trouble-shooting, and potential for medication error and overdose.

2. **PCA opioid agonists** (Table 37-3)

   a. **Morphine.** A loading dose of 2–4 mg of morphine sulfate PCA bolus every 5 minutes is given until the patient is comfortable. The PCA morphine bolus dosage is then ordered in a range of 0.5–1.5 mg with a specific lockout interval (e.g., q6min), thus limiting the hourly maximum dose to 10–15 mg. A continuous basal infusion of morphine (e.g., 0.5–1.0 mg/hr for adults and 10–30 µg/kg/hr for children) may be useful at night to permit uninterrupted sleep but may be associated with an increased ileus rate and faster onset of tolerance.

   b. **Hydromorphone** (Dilaudid) may be employed when there is a need to administer high-potency/high-concentration preparations for opiate-tolerant patients or patients who have side effects from morphine.

   c. **Meperidine** may also be used for patients with side effects from morphine and hydromorphone.

3. Additional orders are required for prn opioids and

Table 37-2. Opioids

Generic name	Proprietary name	Potency	Typical parenteral dose (mg)	Typical oral dose (mg)	Oral to parenteral ratio
Agonists					
Morphine		1	10	30–60	3–6
Codeine		1/12	120	180	1.5
Oxycodone	Percocet, Tylox	1/3	—	30	N/A
Hydromorphone	Dilaudid	6	1.5	7.5	5
Methadone	Dolophine	1	10	20	2
Levorphanol	Levo-Dromoran	5	2	4	2
Meperidine	Demerol	1/8–1/10	75–100	300	3–4
Fentanyl	Sublimaze	10	0.1	—	N/A
Heroin		2	5	60	12
Propoxyphene	Darvon	1/5	—	65	N/A
Agonist-antagonists					
Butorphanol	Stadol	5	2	—	—
Nalbupine	Nubain	1	10	—	N/A
Pentazocine	Talwin	1/6	60	180	3
Partial agonists					
Buprenorphine	Buprenex	25	0.4	—	N/A
Dezocine	Dalgan	1	10	—	N/A

N/A = not available.

Table 37-3. Patient-controlled analgesia

	Bolus range (mg)	Lockout range (min)	Hourly limit range (mg)	Basal range (mg/hr)
Morphine	0.5–2.5	6–15	10–20	0–1.0
Meperidine	10–25	6–15	100–200	0–1.0
Hydromor-phone	0.2–1.0	10–20	1–4	Minimal

hypnotics or sedatives. Careful observation for side effects is essential.

   D. **Regional techniques** impede nociceptive afferent and spinal pain transmission (Table 37-4).

      1. **Local infiltration.** The use of 0.25% bupivacaine infiltrated into the incision site provides excellent early pain relief, especially in the pediatric population.

      2. **Nerve blocks** (see Chap. 17) are useful for both intraoperative anesthesia and postoperative analgesia.

      3. **Epidural catheters** represent the most common regional neuraxial technique (see Chap. 16).

         a. **Local anesthetics** may be used to achieve intraoperative surgical anesthesia, whereas dilute concentrations (bupivacaine 0.1%) may be used postoperatively along with an opioid.

         b. **Epidural opioids** bind to specific receptors in the **substantia gelatinosa** region of the dorsal column of the spinal cord. Efficacy is dependent on lipid solubility, concentration, and volume of distribution. Bolus administration may include preservative-free morphine (3–5 mg) or fentanyl (50–100 μg). A continuous infusion of fentanyl (10 μg/ml or 3 μg/ml) may also be used. Epidural opioids may cause systemic side effects (e.g., nausea, vomiting, pruritus, urinary retention) as well as sedation.

         c. **Combinations** of dilute local anesthetic with opioid successfully block nociception with minimal motor blockade. Epidural infusions using bupivacaine (0.1%) and fentanyl (10 μg/ml) are employed for orthopedic, gynecologic, general, and thoracic surgical patients. The infusion rate ranges from 3–10 ml/hr. Occasionally, the fentanyl concentration is decreased to 3 μg/ml.

         d. **Drug selection.** The choice of opioid, local anesthetic, a concurrent NSAID, or a combination of the three depends on the operative site and the desired degree of analgesia.

         e. **Management problems**

            (1) **Inadequate analgesia.** When pain is not well controlled with an epidural infusion, the infusion rate or concentration is increased, and supplemental parenteral narcotic administration may be necessary. Concentrated local anesthetics are not administered outside of a monitored

Table 37-4. Epidural solutions for postoperative analgesia

Bupivacaine	Fentanyl (μg)	Rate (min)	Indications
0.1%	10	3–10	Most operations in adults; "standard"
0.1%	3	3–10	Pediatrics, pulmonary disease, or excessive sedation with standard mixture
0.1%	0	5–10	Pulmonary disease, narcotic sensitivity, sedation with 3 μg/ml of fentanyl mixture
0	10	5–10	Local anesthetic allergy, neuromuscular disease
0.25%	0	3.0–6.5	Orthopedic surgery unresponsive to more dilute solutions, complete sympathetic blockade

Naloxone (Narcan) dose for reversal of severe respiratory depression: 0.4 mg IV prn respiratory rate < 4. Repeat as necessary.
Naloxone (Narcan) infusion: 5 μg/kg/hr. Titrate upward to effect.

setting (e.g., operating room, PACU, intensive care unit). To confirm epidural function, a bolus of 5–10 ml of the epidural solution the patient is receiving is given. If there is no response within 10–20 minutes, the catheter is replaced or the patient is started on alternative systemic analgesia.

(2) **Catheter disconnections.** In a witnessed disconnect, the terminal inch of catheter is wiped with an alcohol swab, cut off, and reattached to a new sterile adapter hub. In an unwitnessed disconnect, the catheter is removed and then replaced, or the patient is placed on systemic medications. Epidural catheter entry sites must be inspected daily for signs of infection. In general, they are removed after 4–7 days of use.

(3) **Treatment of side effects.** Pruritus, urinary retention, and nausea are easily treated with the opioid antagonist naloxone (0.04–0.1 mg IV prn). Profound sedation and respiratory depression may require higher doses (0.1–0.4 mg IV prn). These doses may also partially reverse analgesia. A continuous, titrated naloxone infusion (5–10 μg/kg/hr) is often useful to reverse respiratory depression while permitting analgesia. The risk of delayed respiratory depression after epidural opioids is inversely proportional to the lipid solubility. This risk is greatest for epidural morphine, but it is still a rare event with an incidence of less than 1%. The risk of delayed respiratory depression after epidural narcotics is potentiated by coadministered CNS

depressants such as parenteral opioids, barbiturates, and benzodiazepines. Additional risk factors include increasing age, respiratory disease, and factors that encourage cephalad flow of drug such as increased thoracic and abdominal pressure, spinal level of injection, and dose of opioid.

   (4) Epidural analgesia is **converted to oral analgesics** (e.g., acetaminophen 325 mg with oxycodone, 5 mg) when the patient is eating.

4. **Intrathecal catheters** may be used for both short- and long-term analgesia. Commonly used catheters are either 20-gauge, 28-gauge, or 32-gauge. They are used most frequently for obstetric procedures, orthopedic surgery, general/vascular surgery, and cancer pain. Spinal opioids provide excellent postoperative analgesia, although as for epidural techniques, infection remains the greatest risk. Spinal opioids are chosen based on length of analgesia desired, potency, and potential side effects. This mode of analgesia is usually restricted to patients in a monitored setting (e.g., PACU overnight or intensive care unit) or for those with cancer pain. The following agents have been used:

   a. **Preservative-free morphine** (Duramorph or Astramorph, 0.25–1.0 mg). Characteristics include low lipid solubility, slow onset (30–60 minutes), long duration (12–24 hours), and high potential for side effects.

   b. **Meperidine** (preservative-free, 25–50 mg) has both opioid and local anesthetic properties and is used most commonly as an anesthetic for obstetric, perineal, and lower abdominal procedures. Characteristics include high lipid solubility, fast onset (4 minutes), short duration (90 minutes), and moderate incidence of side effects.

   c. **Fentanyl** (5–25 µg) is commonly administered along with spinal local anesthetic to prolong the duration of a primary anesthetic. It is also used for postoperative analgesia and cancer pain. Characteristics include high lipid solubility, fast onset (minutes), moderate duration (1.5–3.0 hours), and low incidence of side effects.

   d. **Sufentanil** (3–10 µg) is used in a fashion similar to that of fentanyl. Characteristics include high lipid solubility, fast onset (minutes), short duration (1–2 hours), and low incidence of side effects.

5. **Interpleural analgesia** has been used to treat acute pain following thoracotomy, gastrectomy, splenectomy, mastectomy, or cholecystectomy. It has also been used to provide analgesia for patients with herpes zoster and rib fractures and those with chronic pain associated with pancreatitis, the postthoracotomy syndrome, and upper extremity reflex sympathetic dystrophy.

   a. **Technique.** Patients are placed in the lateral decubitus position, and the seventh or eighth rib is identified in the posterior axillary line. A 17-gauge

Tuohy-Weiss needle is advanced to the superior surface of the rib, the stylet is withdrawn, and a glass syringe containing saline is attached. The needle is walked off the superior surface of the rib until a "loss of resistance" is appreciated as the needle enters the pleural space. The syringe is removed, and an epidural catheter is threaded 5–6 cm in a posterior direction into the pleural space. The catheter should be aspirated to exclude accidental puncture of the lung parenchyma or a blood vessel.

   b. Dosage. A 20-ml dose of bupivacaine 0.5% with epinephrine is injected every 6–10 hours.

E. Alpha-2 adrenergic agonists. Clonidine and dexmedetomidine are alpha-2 adrenergic agonists. Clonidine is used as an antihypertensive, as an agent to suppress the signs of opiate withdrawal, and as an analgesic that inhibits CNS sympathetic activity. Clonidine, whether given IV or administered into the epidural or intrathecal space, causes sedation and profound analgesia, but no respiratory depression. Clonidine potentiates the analgesic action of narcotics, providing excellent analgesia with a lower risk of narcotic side effects. Aside from its cardiovascular effects (e.g., hypotension and rebound hypertension after abrupt discontinuation of chronic therapy), clonidine is well tolerated. A series of highly selective, centrally active alpha-2 adrenergic agonists are under development to provide analgesia and anesthesia and decrease the sympathoadrenal response to the stress of anesthesia and surgery.

V. Chronic pain syndromes are both varied and complex in their manifestations. Prior to starting any therapy, a careful review of the history, physical findings, other diagnostic studies, and opinions of other consultants is necessary.

A. Significant **behavioral changes** often are present when pain of any etiology has persisted for more than a few months. Irritability, insomnia, dependency on family members, dependency on drugs, and lack of motivation are common. **Depression** is frequent enough to warrant empiric therapy. Tricyclics and monoamine oxidase inhibitors not only act on analgesic pathways directly but also affect neuromodulators such as endorphins. Side effects include drowsiness, which is helpful when these drugs are administered at bedtime.

B. Low back pain occurs at some point in at least 50% of all adults due to multiple, often coexistent mechanisms. Occult disease (e.g., retroperitoneal tumor) must be excluded, anatomic derangements (e.g., bony fragments) characterized thoroughly, and surgical options (e.g., foraminotomy) considered with orthopedists or neurosurgeons prior to selecting nonsurgical management. Sensorimotor function, including tenderness and pain on flexion or extension of the spine and extremities, should be documented at each stage of treatment. Bowel or bladder dysfunction argues for aggressive surgical intervention, as does a persistent decrease in motor power or sensation.

1. **Epidural steroid injections**
   a. **Indications** for epidural steroid therapy for low back pain include patients with disk herniation and the postlaminectomy syndrome. Each of these conditions may cause nerve root irritation with subsequent edema and swelling. Epidural steroid administration will decrease pain and inflammation in many patients and is especially attractive when coexistent disease places the patient at increased operative and anesthetic risk.
      (1) **Protrusion of the intervertebral disk** may lead to nerve compression or cauda equina syndrome. Pain and paresthesias in the lower extremities may ensue and progress to muscle weakness and paralysis, as well as loss of sexual function, bowel, and bladder control. Acute nerve entrapment leading to sudden progression of neurologic symptoms should be considered a neurosurgical emergency, and immediate consultation must be obtained.
      (2) **Spinal stenosis** is produced by either congenital, traumatic, or degenerative narrowing of the spinal canal. This narrowing is usually accompanied by painless bilateral leg weakness and/or neurogenic claudication relieved with rest.
      (3) **When a patient with low back pain fails more conservative treatment** and there has been no progression of neurologic symptoms (e.g., foot drop or bowel and bladder dysfunction), epidural steroid injection is indicated.
   b. **Technique.** With the patient in the prone position, a 22-gauge $2\frac{1}{2}$- or $3\frac{1}{2}$-inch spinal needle (Quincke point) is advanced under fluoroscopic guidance into the epidural space. A permanent x-ray is taken to verify needle placement. After an appropriate test dose, 75 mg of triamcinolone (3 ml of Aristocort 2.5%) in 10 ml of 0.125% or 0.25% bupivacaine is injected, and the patient is observed for signs of adverse reaction. Local trauma due to needle insertion may produce an exacerbation of back pain for a few days following the injection. Patients are reevaluated in 2 weeks. If the patient is substantially improved and satisfied with this level of improvement, no further therapy is needed. If there is only some improvement or the symptoms have returned, repeat block is indicated. If pain is worse after the first injection, a different modality (e.g., substitution of one brand of glucocorticoid for another or injection at a different site) should be tried. No more than three injections in a 12-week period should be performed.
2. **Paravertebral spinal nerve root block**
   a. **Indications** are to determine the contribution of a particular nerve root to a patient's overall pain syndrome and to reduce pain due to irritation of a previously identified root.

   b. Technique. With the patient prone, a skin mark is
   made above the root foramen (the lateral margin of
   the vertebral body as it joins the transverse process).
   Using fluoroscopy, a 10-cm, 22-gauge needle is inserted 5–8 cm lateral to the midline and advanced
   toward the skin mark at an angle of 45 degrees
   posterior to the plane of the back. When the transverse process is reached, the needle is withdrawn
   and redirected caudally until a paresthesia is elicited. Once the needle tip is confirmed to be near the
   foramen by fluoroscopy, 1–2 ml of either lidocaine
   (1% with epinephrine 1 : 200,000) or bupivacaine
   (0.5% with epinephrine 1 : 200,000) is injected in
   divided doses, and the patient is observed for a
   change in pain intensity. Ideal dermatomal anesthesia may not result from injection of a single root.
   Any extreme pain during injection may indicate an
   intraneural injection and mandates immediate repositioning of the needle. A permament x-ray is
   taken for verification of needle position. Glucocorticoid may be added to the local anesthetic to reduce
   edema and scarring (see sec. **B.1.b**).
  3. Facet joint injections
   a. Indications. Clinically, facet joint pathology is
   suspected when low back pain is referred to the
   buttock or thighs and the patient is able to perform
   forward flexion but is limited in extension and
   rotation of the spine.
   b. Technique. With the patient prone or turned
   slightly lateral with one knee drawn toward the
   chest to open the facet maximally, a $1\frac{1}{2}$-inch, 22-
   gauge spinal needle is advanced into the facet joint
   under fluoroscopic guidance. A characteristic loss of
   resistance is felt when penetration is achieved.
   Verification is accomplished by obtaining lateral
   fluoroscopic views. A dose of 1–2 ml of bupivacaine
   (0.5% with 1 : 200,000 epinephrine) or tetracaine
   (1% with 1 : 200,000 epinephrine) is administered,
   and a permanent x-ray is obtained. Corticosteroid
   may be added for therapeutic effect.
 C. Myofascial pain
  1. Myofascial pain syndrome can be quite debilitating
   and confused with disk or facet joint disease. It is
   important to distinguish discrete trigger points from a
   diffuse myofascial pain syndrome, as the latter may be
   a symptom of systemic disease. Hyperirritable sites in
   muscle and connective tissue, termed trigger points,
   result from trauma, fatigue, or tension and can produce
   reflex muscle spasm, ischemia, and pain. Trigger
   points are tender nodules or rope-like cords.
  2. Anesthetic technique. A 1- to 3-ml dose of local
   anesthetic (either 1% lidocaine or 0.5% bupivacaine)
   with corticosteroid (triamcinolone 0.1% or 0.25%) in a
   mix of 10–25 mg (i.e., 1 ml) of steroid plus 9 ml of
   anesthetic is injected into each trigger point. Injections
   may be repeated 5–7 days apart to deliver up to 75

mg/month for no more than 3 months. Patients should respond quickly to therapy. The need for frequent treatments may indicate misdiagnosis or concomitant psychological dysfunction. Use of NSAIDs, muscle relaxants (benzodiazepines), or cooling and stretching trigger points may also be performed.

D. Occipital neuralgia

   1. Pain involving the occipital nerve frequently follows neck injury and can be treated with selective nerve blocks. Patients usually complain of aching pain in the suboccipital region that may radiate across the scalp or into the neck and have a lancinating retroorbital component.

   2. Anesthetic technique. The greater occipital nerve is blocked as it crosses a line drawn from the greater occipital protuberance to the mastoid process (superior nuchal line). After palpation of the occipital artery, 3–5 ml of either 1% lidocaine, 0.25% bupivacaine, or a 50 : 50 mixture of 0.5% bupivacaine and 1% lidocaine with 10–20 mg of triamcinolone (Aristocort 1%, 1–2 ml) is injected on either side of the arterial pulse. A paresthesia or pressure dysesthesia may or may not be elicited. Generally, a series of three injections is sufficient to provide pain relief for an extended period of time.

E. Reflex sympathetic dystrophy (RSD) typically occurs after a trivial injury and is associated with an alteration of the nervous system, resulting in heightened sympathetic outflow. When this alteration follows direct nerve trauma that leads to persistent neural deficit, the term **causalgia** is used.

   1. The hallmark of this syndrome is an exquisitely painful body part (usually a limb). The pain is characterized as a burning sensation with exquisite sensitivity to stimuli (**hyperesthesia**) and progression of pain with repetitive innocuous stimuli (**hyperpathia**). Single innocuous stimuli (e.g., light touch) may also produce pain (allodynia). Typically starting in a small, discrete area, the pain intensifies over time and spreads proximally from its origin.

   2. Characteristic changes are noted when RSD becomes progressive. The skin, which is typically cold, adopts a smooth, glassy appearance with decreased hair growth and sweating. The end stage is significant for disuse atrophy and marked osteoporosis.

   3. Anesthetic technique. Diagnosis and treatment of RSD and causalgia depend on relief of pain following sympathetic blockade.

   a. Stellate ganglion (cervicothoracic) block

   (1) With the patient in the supine position and using fluoroscopic guidance, a 22-gauge $1\frac{1}{2}$- or $2\frac{1}{2}$-inch needle is advanced posteriorly between the trachea and carotid artery. The target is the prevertebral fascia on the anterolateral surface of C7. A 15-ml dose of 1% lidocaine, 0.25% bupivacaine, or a 50 : 50 solution of 1% lidocaine

and 0.5% bupivacaine is slowly injected. Cervical plexus, phrenic, superficial, or recurrent laryngeal nerve anesthesia is common. **Horner's syndrome** (ptosis, enophthalmos, miosis, and anhidrosis) is typically seen, although this sign alone is not pathognomonic for successful sympathetic blockade of the upper extremity.

(2) **Postblock alterations.** The **galvanic skin response** is a change in voltage potential on an electrocardiogram that has limb leads placed on dorsal and volar surfaces of the hand or foot in response to an abrupt noise or painful stimulus. Abolition of the galvanic skin response and an increase in temperature of 10°F or higher are evidence of sympathetic blockade.

(3) This block can be performed intermittently or continuously through a catheter. A total of 5–10 ml of 0.25% bupivacaine can be injected 3–4 times a day at a rate of 1 ml/min.

b. Alternatively, **sympathetic blockade of the upper extremity** may be achieved with placement of local anesthetic into the interpleural space (see sec. **IV.D.5**). Bupivacaine, 75–100 mg in either 0.25% or 0.5% concentration, is given 4 times a day.

c. **Lumbar sympathetic block.** The L2 vertebra is identified with fluoroscopy and the skin marked in the manner described in sec. **B.2.b** for paravertebral spinal nerve root block. A 10- to 15-cm, 22- or 20-gauge needle is inserted just below the twelfth rib and directed toward the body of L2 with the needle bevel facing laterally. When the transverse process is encountered, the needle is redirected cephalad to contact the vertebral body. The needle tip is advanced slightly beyond the anterior projection of the vertebral body and confirmed with fluoroscopy. A total of 15–30 ml of 1% lidocaine, 0.25% bupivacaine, or a 50 : 50 solution of 1% lidocaine and 0.5% bupivacaine is given in divided doses and the limb monitored for effect. This technique may be performed using a catheter technique to provide intermittent injections (10–20 ml of 0.5% bupivacaine 4 times a day) or a continuous infusion (4–8 ml/hr of 0.125–0.25% bupivacaine). A minimum of 7 days' treatment with aggressive physical therapy is recommended.

d. **Intravenous regional sympathetic block.** Adrenergic antagonist drugs may alter the sensitivity of nociceptors. Potential agents include guanethidine, bretylium, reserpine, labetalol (10–30 mg in 30–50 ml of normal saline) or 0.5% lidocaine in a tourniquet-isolated limb for a minimum of 20 minutes.

F. **Postherpetic neuralgia (PHN)**
1. PHN is an extremely painful complication of acute varicella zoster infection, occurring most commonly in

the elderly and immunocompromised. The patient experiences persistent severe burning pain in the same distribution as the original infection.

2. **Anesthetic techniques.** PHN has been reported to respond to sympathetic blocks as described above, provided these blocks are performed during or shortly after (< 6 weeks) the acute attack. PHN in the thoracic distribution may be treated with intermittent intercostal or interpleural nerve blocks or continuously with epidural local anesthetic infusions. Long-established PHN is difficult to treat and is usually managed in the same way as neuropathic pain (see sec. **G.**).

G. **Neuropathic pain**

1. Neuropathic pain results from an aberration of nerve physiology or anatomy seen with alcoholic and diabetic neuropathies as well as following amputation and partial spinal cord damage.

2. **Anesthetic techniques**

a. **Lancinating pain,** secondary to the spontaneous firing of nociceptors or nerve fibers, is treated with anticonvulsants such as carbamazepine, phenytoin, or clonazepam. Burning dysesthesias are commonly treated with tricyclic antidepressant drugs such as amitriptyline or doxepin. For refractory pain, a combination of amitriptyline and fluphenazine has been tried with success. An added benefit of sedating antidepressants is to give an evening dose to prevent the insomnia commonly seen with neuropathic and other forms of chronic pain.

b. **Intravenous infusion of local anesthetic** may be used to treat neuropathic pain, particularly if associated with mononeuropathies (e.g., in diabetes mellitus). If an IV infusion of 100–300 mg of 1% lidocaine over 20–30 minutes provides long-lasting relief, the patient may benefit from a trial of oral mexiletine hydrochloride, 150–200 mg 3 or 4 times a day. Careful follow-up with periodic blood levels is prudent.

VI. **Cancer pain.** Treatment of cancer pain is multifaceted and may require pharmacologic intervention combined with counseling, nursing care, pastoral and social services, nerve blockade, surgery, radiation therapy, chemotherapy, and hospice care. Cancer pain is often a dynamic process with remissions and exacerbations paralleling the disease course. The etiology of an individual's cancer pain must be aggressively investigated and suitably treated at the time of its presentation and during each exacerbation.

A. **Pharmacologic therapy**

1. **NSAIDs** are a useful first line of therapy in cancer pain, particularly since metastatic lesions to bone often cause prostaglandin-mediated inflammation and pain.

2. **Oral opioids.** Propoxyphene and codeine are initiated first. Addition of more potent opioids such as methadone or time-released morphine (MS Contin) may

follow. Every effort is made to keep the outpatient comfortable for as long as possible on oral medications administered "by the clock." Prn "rescue" doses of short-acting medications such as immediate-release morphine tablets or elixir, oxycodone, or hydromorphone may be required (see Table 37-2). Opioid dosage may be increased until either pain is successfully treated or side effects interfere. Sedation is a common problem and can be treated with the addition of dextroamphetamine (6 mg q6h). An added benefit of this combination is increased analgesia.

3. **Parenteral opioids** are used when oral medications fail. The appropriate parenteral dosage is calculated using oral to parenteral conversion data (see Table 37-2), and the patient is started on an intermittent IV or subcutaneous regimen. Since patients develop significant tolerance to opioids after prolonged therapy, withdrawal must be anticipated and avoided when changing the route of a patient's medication (see sec. **IV.B**). PCA lends itself well to treating severe cancer pain with the help of skilled outpatient nursing services (see Table 37-3).

4. **Alternate routes.** Transdermal delivery of opioids, such as the fentanyl patch, is an alternative to the oral route as the treatment of choice for cancer patients. Transdermal fentanyl is available in doses that deliver 25, 50, 75, and 100 μg/hr. Patches are worn for 48–72 hours and achieve a steady-state blood level within 12–24 hours. The consistency of blood levels and the circumvention of an unreliable oral route without resort to injections may be ideal. Unfortunately, transdermal opioids appear to induce tolerance as quickly as continuous infusions, and nausea remains a frequent side effect. Rectal and sublingual opioid administration are other alternatives.

5. **Long-term neuraxial opioids**
   a. High systemic doses of opioids can be avoided with the introduction of neuraxial opioids through a temporary epidural catheter. Preservative-free morphine (2–4 mg) is started on a twice daily dosing schedule. Dosage is increased by 1 mg/dose and/or the schedule is changed (e.g., to 3 times a day) as needed. Parenteral or oral "rescue" doses (e.g., 10–20 mg of morphine elixir q2h prn) are administered during the epidural trial protocol. Patients should be kept on a minimum of 25% of their regular daily dose of systemic opioid to prevent the abstinence syndrome. Combinations of narcotic and local anesthetic provide excellent analgesia and allow opiate receptors to "reset" and become more sensitive to narcotics.
   b. If a trial of epidural opioids is successful, the catheter may be tunneled or surgically implanted for long-term use over several months. Patients are sent home or to a hospice with a dosing schedule in

place, and they will require close follow-up by a skilled nursing service.

6. **Side effects.** All opioids, especially when given in high dosage, generate side effects, as discussed in sec. **IV.B.3.** Constipation is controlled by initiating bowel stimulants and stool softeners whenever opioid therapy is begun. Urecholine may be required to treat urinary retention.

7. **Neurolytic blocks.** The decision to perform a neurolytic block is based on the nature of the patient's malignancy, anticipated life expectancy, medical status, and response to other therapeutic options. Any neurolytic block must first be simulated using local anesthetic alone to assess a particular nerve's contribution to cancer pain. Neurolytic blocks can then be performed with 50–100% ethanol or 6–10% phenol. Ethanol is more likely to have a permanent effect but has a higher tendency to produce painful neuropathies.

Celiac plexus blockade is performed to relieve visceral pain due to pancreatic and upper abdominal tumors.

a. **Technique.** With the patient prone and under fluoroscopic control, 15-cm, 20-gauge needles are inserted bilaterally just below the twelfth rib and directed medially to contact the body of L1. The left-sided needle is advanced cephalad to the transverse process 1–2 cm anterior to the L1 body or until aortic pulsations are felt. Renograffin dye (50%), 2–5 ml, mixed 1 : 1 with sterile saline is instilled to demonstrate a periaortic outline. The right-sided needle is advanced 1–2 cm. Undiluted renograffin, 2–5 ml, is injected to demonstrate a pericaval outline. An irregular outline on either side mandates repositioning of the needle to avoid a psoas muscle injection. Tracking of dye under the diaphragm or toward spinal roots also mandates repositioning. Either 25 ml of 0.25% bupivacaine with 1 : 200,000 epinephrine or a 50 : 50 mixture of 1% lidocaine with 1 : 200,000 epinephrine and 0.5% bupivacaine with 1 : 200,000 epinephrine is injected in divided doses per needle. If pain is relieved, this may be followed after 24 hours by 25 ml per needle of 50% alcohol in 1% lidocaine or 7% phenol in water.

b. **Complications** include temporary (although sometimes persistent) hypotension and diarrhea; intrathecal, epidural, or intramuscular injection of neurolytic agent may result in sexual dysfunction, lower extremity dysesthesias, or paraplegia secondary to spinal artery syndrome; pneumothorax; bowel perforation; kidney or liver puncture; and retroperitoneal hemorrhage.

8. **Neurosurgical procedures** have been employed to treat refractory benign and malignant pain (i.e., percutaneous neurectomy, dorsal rhizotomy, cordotomy).

A thorough discussion of this subject is beyond the scope of this chapter.

SUGGESTED READING

Abram, S. E., ed. *Cancer Pain*. Boston: Kluwer, 1989.

Bonica, J. J. *The Management of Pain* (2nd ed.). Philadelphia: Lea & Febiger, 1990.

Carr, D. B. Opioids. *Int. Anesthesiol. Clin. North Am.* 25:273, 1986.

Carr, D. B., and Lipkowski, A. W. Mechanisms of opioid analgesic actions. In M. C. Rogers et al. (eds.) *Principles and Practice of Anesthesiology*. St. Louis: Mosby-Yearbook, 1992, Pp. 1105–1130.

Carr, D. B., et al. (eds.). *Acute Pain Management: Operative or Medical Procedures and Trauma. Clinical Practice Guideline*. Rockville, MD: Agency for Health Care Policy and Research, Public Health Service, U.S. Department of Health and Human Services, February 1992. AHCPR No. 92-0032.

Carrette, S., et al. A controlled trial of corticosteroid injections into facet joints for chronic low back pain. *N. Engl. J. Med.* 325:1002, 1991.

Cousins, M. J., and Bridenbough, P. O. *Neural Blockade in Clinical Anesthesia and Management of Pain* (2nd ed.). Philadelphia: Lippincott, 1988.

Covino, B. G. Interpleural regional analgesia: An editorial. *Anesth. Analg.* 67:427, 1988.

Davis, J. L., et al. Peripheral diabetic neuropathy treated with amitriptyline and fluphenazine. *J.A.M.A.* 238:2291, 1977.

Estafanous, F. C. *Opioids in Anesthesia II*. New York: Butterworth, 1990.

Gilman, A. G., et al. *The Pharmacological Basis of Therapeutics*. New York: Pergamon, 1990.

Gybels, J. M., and Sweet, W. H. *Neurosurgical Treatment of Persistent Pain*. Basel: Karger, 1989.

Jacox, A. K., et al. *Cancer Pain Management*. Rockville, MD: Agency for Health Care Policy and Research. Public Health Service. U.S. Department of Health and Human Services, 1993.

Reiestad, F., and Stromskag, K. E. Interpleural catheter in the management of postoperative pain. *Reg. Anesth.* 11:89, 1986.

Snoek, W., Weber, H., and Jorgensen, B. Double blind evaluation of extradural methyl prednisolone for herniated lumbar discs. *Acta Orthopaed. Scand.* 48:635, 1977.

Wall, P. D., and Melzack, R. *Textbook of Pain* (2nd ed.). New York: Churchill Livingstone, 1989.

White, A. H., Derby, R., and Wynne G. Epidural injections for the diagnosis and treatment of low back pain. *Spine* 1:78, 1980.

Appendix

Acetomenophen pr. 40 mg/kg

Commonly Used Drugs

Rebecca Leong

Acetylcysteine (Mucomyst)

Indication	Viscous respiratory secretions
Dosage	Inhaled through nebulizer: 2–5 ml of 5–20% solution q6–8h
Onset	1 min
Duration	4–8 hr
Effect	Disruption of disulfide bonds with reduction of viscosity of pulmonary secretions and increase in mucociliary clearance.
Comments	May cause bronchospasm, bronchial bleeding, nausea, or vomiting
Metabolism	Liver
Elimination	Liver, kidney

Adenosine (Adenocard)

Indications	Paroxysmal supraventricular tachycardia, Wolff-Parkinson-White syndrome
Dosage	6–12 mg IV bolus
Onset	Immediate
Duration	Brief; $t_{1/2} < 10$ sec
Effect	Slow or temporary cessation of AV node conduction as well as conduction through reentry pathways.
Comments	The effects of adenosine are antagonized by methylxanthines such as theophylline. Adenosine is contraindicated in patients with second- or third-degree heart block or sick sinus syndrome. When large doses are given by infusion, hypotension can occur. Not effective in atrial flutter or fibrillation. Asystole for 3–6 sec is not uncommon.

Key to abbreviations:
AV = atrioventricular; CNS = central nervous system; D/W = dextrose in water; ECG = electrocardiogram; IM = intramuscularly; IV = intravenously; LD = loading dose; MD = maintenance dose; NSS = normal saline solution; PO = orally; prn = as needed or indicated; RBCs = red blood cells; SL = sublingually; SQ = subcutaneously; $t_{1/2}$ = redistribution half-life.
* Doses of CNS-depressant drugs are those usually given to healthy 70-kg patients and may vary with the patient's condition or concomitant drug intake. Older or debilitated patients may require smaller doses.

| Metabolism/ Elimination | RBCs and endothelial cells |

Aminocaproic acid (Amicar)

Indications	Fibrinolysis, hemorrhage
Dosage	5 gm/100–250 ml of NSS IV to load followed by 1 gm/hr infusion
Effect	Stabilizes clot formation. Used in cardiac and liver transplantation surgery.
Comments	Contraindicated in disseminated intravascular coagulation.
Metabolism/ Elimination	Renal

Aminophylline (theophylline)

Indications	Bronchospasm, infant apnea

Dosage	LD: 6.0 mg/kg IV at < 25 mg/min
	MD:
	    Young, healthy: 0.7 mg/kg/hr IV × 12 hr, then 0.5 mg/kg/hr IV
	    Elderly: 0.6 mg/kg/hr IV × 12 hr, then 0.3 mg/kg/hr IV
	    Congestive heart failure, liver disease: 0.5 mg/kg/hr IV × 12 hr, then 0.1–0.2 mg/kg/hr IV

Onset	Rapid
Duration	6–12 hr
Effect	Inhibition of phosphodiesterase, resulting in bronchodilation with positive inotropic and chronotropic effects.
Comments	May cause tachyarrhythmias. Follow serum levels closely. Therapeutic level = 10–20 µg/ml.
Metabolism	Liver
Elimination	Kidney

Amiodarone (Cordarone)

Indications	Refractory or recurrent ventricular tachycardia or ventricular fibrillation
Dosage	LD: 800–1600 mg/day PO × 1–3 wk, then 600–800 mg/day PO × 4 wk MD: 100–400 mg/day PO
Onset	2–21 days

Duration	> 24 hr
Effect	Depresses the sinoatrial node and prolongs the PR, QRS, and QT intervals and produces α- and β-adrenergic blockade.
Comments	May cause severe sinus bradycardia, ventricular arrhythmias, AV block, liver and thyroid function test abnormalities, hepatitis, and cirrhosis. Pulmonary fibrosis may follow long-term use. Increases serum levels of digoxin, oral anticoagulants, diltiazem, quinidine, procainamide, and phenytoin.
Metabolism	Liver
Elimination	Intestine

Ampicillin

Indications	Treatment of infection with gram-positive cocci, gram-negative rods; endocarditis prophylaxis (with gentamicin)
Dosage	20 mg/kg (1 gm for most adults) IV q4–8h; mix 1 gm/10 ml of 5% D/W or NSS and administer over 1–5 min.
Onset	Rapid
Duration	Variable
Effect	Interferes with bacterial cell wall formation; bactericidal.
Comments	Not useful for β-lactamase-producing organisms, unless sulbactam (Unasyn) is also given. Not effective against methicillin-resistant *Staphylococcus aureus* or gram-positive rods. May cause a rash in the presence of Epstein-Barr virus infection (mononucleosis). May induce interstitial nephritis.
Metabolism	Negligible
Elimination	Kidney, liver

Amrinone (Inocor)

Indication	Management of acute ventricular failure
Dosage	0.75 mg/kg IV bolus over several minutes, then infuse at 5–10 μg/kg/min. Infusion mixtures (100 mg in 250 ml) must not contain dextrose.
Onset	10 min
Duration	Bolus: 0.5–2.0 hr Infusion: 2.5–12.0 hr
Effect	Increase in cardiac output from both inhibition of phosphodiesterase and direct vasodilation.

Comments	May cause hypotension, thrombocytopenia, ana-phylaxis (contains sulfites).
Metabolism	Liver
Elimination	Kidney

Atenolol (Tenormin)

Indications	Hypertension, β_1-adrenergic receptor blockade
Dosage	PO: 50–100 mg/day IV: 5 mg prn
Onset	PO: 30–60 min IV: 5 min
Duration	PO: > 24 hr IV: 12–24 hr (dose related)
Effect	β_1-Selective adrenergic receptor blockade.
Comments	Relatively cardioselective. High doses block β_2-adrenergic receptors. Relatively contraindicated in congestive heart failure, asthma, and heart block. Caution in patients on calcium channel blockers. Rebound angina may occur with abrupt cessation.
Metabolism	None
Elimination	Kidney, intestine

Atropine

Indications	Bradycardia; antisialagogue

Dosage	For drying secretions: 0.2–0.4 mg IV
	For bradycardia: 0.4–1.0 mg IV
	Pediatric:
	   For preoperative control of secretions: 0.01 mg/kg/dose IV/IM (< 0.4 mg)
	   For bradycardia: 0.02 mg/kg/dose IV (< 0.4 mg)

Onset	IV: Rapid
Duration	Variable
Effect	Competitive blockade of acetylcholine at muscarinic receptors.
Comments	May cause tachyarrhythmias, AV dissociation, premature ventricular contractions, bradycardia (low dose), dry mouth, or urinary retention; crosses blood-brain barrier.
Metabolism	Minimal
Elimination	Kidney (77–94%), liver

Bicarbonate, sodium (NaHCO₃)

Indications	Metabolic acidosis, alkalization of urine, hyperkalemia
Dosage	For metabolic acidosis: IV mEq $NaHCO_3$ = [base deficit × wt (kg) × 0.2–0.3] (subsequent doses titrated against patient's pH) Neonatal solution: 4.2% (~0.5 mEq/ml) Adult solution: 8.4% (~1.0 mEq/ml)
Onset	Rapid
Duration	Variable
Effect	H^+ neutralization.
Comments	May cause metabolic alkalosis, hypercarbia, or hyperosmolality. Administration of hyperosmolar solution to neonates may cause intraventricular hemorrhage. Central hypertonic bolus can cause transiently decreased cardiac output, systemic vascular resistance, and myocardial contractility with hypotension and increased intracranial pressure. Crosses placenta.
Metabolism	Blood
Elimination	Lung (as CO_2), kidney

Bretylium (Bretylol)

Indications	Ventricular fibrillation, ventricular tachycardia
Dosage	For immediately life-threatening ventricular arrhythmias: 5–10 mg/kg IV q15–30 min prn to maximum 30 mg/kg (undiluted) For other ventricular arrhythmias: LD: 5–10 mg/kg IV in 50–100 ml of 5% D/W over 10–20 min repeated once after 1–2 hr prn MD: 5–10 mg/kg IV in 50–100 ml of 5% D/W over 10–20 min q6h or, preferably, as constant infusion, 1–2 mg/min
Onset	Ventricular fibrillation: minutes Ventricular tachycardia: 30–60 min
Duration	6–24 hr
Effect	Initially, release of norepinephrine into circulation, followed by prevention of synaptic release of norepinephrine; suppression of ventricular fibrillation and ventricular arrhythmias; increase in myocardial contractility (direct effect).
Comments	May cause initial hypertension and ectopy, followed by decrease in systemic vascular resistance with hypotension (potentiated by quinidine or procainamide), increased sensitivity to

catecholamines, aggravation of digoxin-induced arrhythmias, or drowsiness.

Metabolism	Minimal
Elimination	Kidney (mostly), liver (very small amount)

Bumetanide (Bumex)

Indications	Edema, hypertension, intracranial hypertension
Dosage	0.5–1.0 mg IV, repeated to a maximum of 10 mg/day
Onset	Immediate, peak diuresis within 15–30 min
Duration	2–4 hr; $t_{1/2}$ = 1.0–1.15 hr
Effect	Loop diuretic with principal effect on the ascending limb of the loop of Henle. Causes increased excretion of Na^+, K^+, Cl^-, and H_2O.
Comments	May cause electrolyte imbalance, dehydration, and deafness. Patients who are allergic to sulfonamides may show hypersensitivity to bumetanide. Effective in renal insufficiency.
Metabolism	Liver, kidney
Elimination	Kidney (45% unchanged), liver

Calcium chloride (CaCl₂)

Indications	Hypocalcemia, hyperkalemia, hypermagnesemia, hypotension
Dosage	For life-threatening hypocalcemia, hypotension: 5–10 mg/kg IV prn (10% $CaCl_2$ = 1.36 mEq Ca^{2+}/ml)
Onset	Rapid
Duration	Variable
Effect	Essential for maintenance of cell membrane integrity, muscular excitation-contraction coupling, glandular stimulation-secretion coupling, and enzyme function.
Comments	May cause bradycardia or arrhythmia (especially with digitalis). Irritating to veins.
Metabolism/ Elimination	Protein bound. Incorporated into muscle, bone, and other tissues.

Calcium gluconate (Kalcinate)

Indications	Hypocalcemia, hyperkalemia, hypermagnesemia, hypotension

Dosage	For life-threatening hypocalcemia, hypotension, hyperkalemia: 15–30 mg/kg IV prn (10% calcium gluconate = 0.45 mEq Ca^{2+}/ml)
Onset	Rapid
Duration	Variable
Effect	See Calcium chloride.
Comments	Ca^{2+} less available than with $CaCl_2$ due to binding to gluconate.
Metabolism/ Elimination	See Calcium chloride.

Captopril (Capoten)

Indications	Hypertension, congestive heart failure
Dosage	LD: 12.5–25.0 mg PO bid MD: 25–150 mg PO bid
Onset	15 min
Duration	4–6 hr (1 hr to peak effect)
Effect	Angiotensin I–converting enzyme inhibition decreases angiotensin II and aldosterone levels. Reduces both preload and afterload in patients with congestive heart failure.
Comments	Can be used in hypertensive emergency. May cause neutropenia, agranulocytosis, hypotension, or bronchospasm. Avoid in pregnant patients. Exaggerated response in renal artery stenosis and with diuretics.
Metabolism	Liver
Elimination	Renal (50% unchanged)

Cefazolin (Ancef, Kefzol)

Indications	Treatment of infection with gram-positive cocci and gram-negative rods
Dosage	10 mg/kg (500–1000 mg for most adults) IV q4–8h; mix in 10 ml of 5% D/W or NSS and administer over 1–5 min.
Onset	Rapid
Duration	Variable
Effect	Interferes with bacterial cell wall formation; bactericidal.
Comments	A first-generation cephalosporin. Not useful for β-lactamase-producing organisms. Approximately 5–10% of patients with penicillin allergy will also react to cephalosporins. Can cause elevated liver function tests, positive Coombs' test. Adjust dosage in presence of renal disease.

Metabolism	Negligible
Elimination	Kidney, liver

Cefotetan (Cefotan)

Indications	Most gram-positive anaerobes, gram-positive cocci
Dosage	1–2 gm IV q12h; mix in 10 ml of 5% D/W or NSS and administer over 1–5 min.
Onset	Rapid
Duration	Variable
Effect	Second-generation cephalosporin; interferes with cell wall synthesis.
Comments	Not effective against *Pseudomonas, Enterobacter, Clostridium difficile,* or methicillin-resistant *Staphylococcus aureus.* Effective against β-lactamase-producing organisms. Can cause disulfiram-like reaction. 5–10% of penicillin-allergic patients will react to cephalosporins. Adjust dosage in presence of renal disease.
Metabolism	Liver, kidney
Elimination	Kidney

Chlordiazepoxide (Librium)*

Indications	Sedation, ethanol withdrawal syndrome
Dosage	5–100 mg IV q4–6h prn (dosage individualized).
Onset	5–30 min
Duration	0.5–4.0 hr
Effect	CNS depression, anticonvulsant effect.
Comments	May cause paradoxical CNS excitation, respiratory depression at high doses. Frequent dosing may result in accumulation of active metabolites.
Metabolism	Liver (to several active metabolites)
Elimination	Kidney, liver

Chlorothiazide (Diuril)

Indications	Edema, hypertension
Dosage	500–2000 mg/day IV in divided doses
Onset	15 min
Duration	2–4 hr (30 min to peak effect)

Effect	Increase in renal excretion of Na^+, Cl^-, K^+, Mg^{2+}, Br^-, I^-, H_2O, with decrease in excretion of Ca^{2+}.
Comments	May cause electrolyte imbalance, dehydration, or glucose intolerance.
Metabolism	Minimal
Elimination	Kidney, liver.

Chlorpromazine (Thorazine)*

Indications	Psychosis, agitation, nausea and vomiting, hiccoughs, sedation, prevention of shivering
Dosage	25–50 mg IV in 25–50 ml of NSS infused slowly (< 2 mg/min) (dosage individualized).
Onset	Rapid
Duration	2–4 hr
Effect	Neuroleptic antipsychotic; CNS depression; suppression of nausea and vomiting.
Comments	May cause hypotension from α-adrenergic blockade. Weak anticholinergic effects may cause extrapyramidal reactions, cholestatic jaundice, alteration of thermoregulation, or neuroleptic malignant syndrome.
Metabolism	Liver
Elimination	Liver, kidney.

Cimetidine (Tagamet)

Indications	Reduction of gastric volume and raising of pH (pulmonary aspiration prophylaxis), hiatus hernia, gastric acid hypersecretion; may be used as prophylaxis for potential anaphylactic reaction
Dosage	300 mg q6h IV/IM/PO (q12h in renal failure)
Onset	PO: 45–90 min
Duration	IV/IM/PO: 4–5 hr
Effect	Antagonism of histamine action on H_2 receptors, with inhibition of gastric acid secretion.
Comments	May cause small increase in creatinine, increase in blood levels of concurrently administered propranolol or benzodiazepines, reduction in activity of some liver microsomal enzymes, potentiation of oral anticoagulants, confusion, or somnolence with repeated dosing.
Metabolism	Liver
Elimination	Kidney (75%)

Ciprofloxacin

Indications	Treatment of gram-positive and gram-negative aerobes, including *Hemophilus influenzae* and *Pseudomonas*
Dosage	PO: 250–750 mg q12h IV: 200–400 mg IV q12h
Onset	30–60 min
Duration	24 hr
Effect	Interferes with bacterial DNA synthesis: bactericidal.
Comments	Serum concentration increased by probenecid. Not effective against *Pseudomonas maltophilia* or anaerobes.
Metabolism	Liver (15%)
Elimination	Kidney, liver

Clindamycin (Cleocin)

Indications	Treatment of infection from gram-positive aerobes and anaerobes
Dosage	600 mg IV q6–8h; administered over 1–5 min
Onset	Rapid
Duration	Variable
Effect	Inhibition of bacterial protein synthesis; bacteriostatic.
Comments	Associated with *clostridium difficile* colitis. Bactericidal against pneumococcus. May prolong neuromuscular blockade.
Metabolism	Liver
Elimination	Kidney, liver

Clonidine (Catapres)

Indication	Hypertension
Dosage	0.1–1.2 mg/day PO in divided doses (2.4 mg/day maximum dose)
Onset	30–60 min
Duration	8 hr (2–4 hr to maximal effect)
Effect	Central α-adrenergic agonist, resulting in decrease in systemic vascular resistance and heart rate.
Comments	Abrupt withdrawal may cause rebound hypertension or arrhythmias. May cause drowsiness, nightmares, restlessness, anxiety, or depres-

sion. IV injection may cause transient peripheral α-adrenergic stimulation.

| Metabolism | Liver |
| Elimination | Kidney (80%), liver (20%) |

Dantrolene (Dantrium)

Indication	Malignant hyperthermia
Dosage	Prophylactic preoperative or intraoperative treatment is generally not recommended.
	If signs of the syndrome develop: 3 mg/kg IV bolus; if syndrome persists after 30 min, repeat dose, up to 10 mg/kg.
Onset	30 min
Duration	8 hr
Effect	Reduction of Ca^{2+} release from sarcoplasmic reticulum.
Comments	Mix 20 mg in 60 ml of sterile water. Dissolves slowly into solution. May cause muscle weakness, gastrointestinal upset, drowsiness, sedation, or abnormal liver function (chronically). Additive effect with neuromuscular blocking agents. Tissue irritant.
Metabolism	Liver
Elimination	Kidney

Desmopressin acetate (DDAVP)

Indications	To improve coagulation in von Willebrand's disease and hemophilia A; used as an antidiuretic hormone
Dosage	0.3 µg/kg IV (dilute in 50 ml of NSS)
Onset	Minutes
Duration	3 hr for von Willebrand's disease, 4–24 hr for hemophilia A; peak effect 15–30 min
Effect	Increases plasma levels of factor VIII activity in patients with hemophilia A and von Willebrand's disease by causing release of von Willebrand's factor from endothelial cells.
Comments	Chlorpropamide, carbamazepine, and clofibrate potentiate the antidiuretic effect. Repeat doses q12–24h will have diminished effect compared to initial dose.
Metabolism	Kidney
Elimination	Unknown

Dexamethasone (Decadron)

Indications	See Hydrocortisone.
Dosage	For most non-life-threatening conditions: 0.50–60 mg/day IV/IM
	For cerebral edema:
	LD: 10 mg IV
	MD: 4 mg IV q6h (tapered over 6 days)
	For life-threatening conditions:
	LD: 1–6 mg/kg IV q2–6h prn
	MD: 20 mg
	Infusion: 3 mg/kg/day
Onset	IV: minutes
Duration	IV: 4–6 hr
Effect	See Hydrocortisone. Has 25 times the glucocorticoid potency of hydrocortisone. Minimal mineralocorticoid effect.
Comments	See Hydrocortisone.
Metabolism	Liver (microsomes)
Elimination	Kidney, liver (15%)

Dextran 40 (Rheomacrodex)

Indications	Inhibition of platelet aggregation; Low-flow states (e.g., vascular surgery); volume repletion in patients refusing blood products
Dosage	LD: 30–50 ml IV over 30 min
	MD: 15–30 ml/hr IV (10% solution)
Onset	Rapid
Duration	4–8 hr
Effect	Immediate, short-lived plasma volume expansion; adsorption to RBC surface, resulting in prevention of RBC aggregation and decrease in blood viscosity; decrease in platelet adhesiveness.
Comments	Administer Promit (Dextran monomer), 20 ml IV, prior to giving dexran 40 to minimize the risk of anaphylaxis. May cause volume overload, anaphylaxis, bleeding tendency, interference with blood cross-matching, or false elevation of blood sugar. Can cause renal failure.
Metabolism	Minimal
Elimination	Kidney (unchanged)

Digoxin (Lanoxin)

Indications	Heart failure, supraventricular tachyarrhythmias
Dosage	LD: 0.5–1.0 mg/day IV in divided doses MD: 0.125–0.5 mg IV qd *Pediatric* (IV/IM in divided doses): 　LD (2–10 yr): 15–35 μg/kg/day 　LD (2 wk–2yr): 30–50 μg/kg/day 　LD (neonates): 15–30 μg/kg/day 　MD: 20–30% of LD qd
Onset	IV: 15–30 min
Duration	IV: 2–6 days
Effect	Increase in myocardial contractility; decrease in conduction in AV node and Purkinje fibers.
Comments	May cause gastrointestinal intolerance, blurred vision, ECG changes, or arrhythmias. Toxicity potentiated by hypokalemia, hypomagnesemia, hypercalcemia. Cautious use in Wolff-Parkinson-White syndrome and with defibrillation. Heart block potentiated by β-blockade and calcium channel blockade.
Metabolism	Minimal
Elimination	Kidney (60–90%); use lower dosage with renal failure.

Diltiazem (Cardizem)

Indications	Angina pectoris, variant angina from coronary artery spasm, atrial fibrillation/flutter, paroxysmal supraventricular tachycardia
Dosage	PO: 30–60 mg q6h, IV: 0.25 mg/kg over 2 min; 2nd bolus 0.35 mg/kg. Infusion: 5–15 ml/hr (5–15 mg/hr); mix 25 ml (125 mg) in 100 ml of 5% D/W.
Onset	PO: 1–3 hr IV: 1–3 min
Duration	PO: Several hours IV: 1–3 hr (2–7 min to peak effect)
Effect	Calcium channel antagonist that slows conduction through sinoatrial and AV nodes, dilates coronary and peripheral arterioles, and reduces myocardial contractility.
Comments	May cause bradycardia and heart block. May interact with β-blockers and digoxin to impair contractility. Causes transiently elevated liver function tests. Avoid use in patients with accessory tracts, AV block, IV β-blockers, or ventricular tachycardia.

Metabolism Liver
Elimination Kidney

Diphenhydramine (Benadryl)*

Indications	Allergic reactions, drug-induced extrapyramidal reactions, sedation
Dosage	10–50 mg IV q6–8h *Pediatric:* 5.0 mg/kg/day IV in 4 divided doses (maximum 300 mg)
Onset	Rapid
Duration	4–6 hr
Effect	Antagonism of histamine action on H_1 receptors; anticholinergic effect; CNS depression.
Comments	May cause hypotension, tachycardia, dizziness, or seizures.
Metabolism	Liver
Elimination	Kidney

Dobutamine (Dobutrex)

Indication	Heart failure
Dosage	Infusion mix: 250 mg in 250 ml of 5% D/W or NSS. Start infusion at 2 µg/kg/min and titrate to effect.
Onset	2 min
Duration	5–10 min
Effect	β_1-, β_2-adrenergic agonist.
Comments	May cause hypertension, arrhythmias, or myocardial ischemia. Can increase ventricular rate in atrial fibrillation.
Metabolism	Liver, nerve endings
Elimination	Kidney, liver

Dopamine (Intropin)

Indications	Hypotension, heart failure, oliguria
Dosage	Infusion mix: 200–800 mg in 250 ml of 5% D/W or NSS For hypotension: infusion at 5–20 µg/kg/min IV titrated against patient response For oliguria: infusion at 1–3 µg/kg/min IV
Onset	5 min
Duration	10 min

Effect	Dopaminergic, α- and β-adrenergic agonist.
Comments	May cause hypertension, arrhythmias, or myocardial ischemia. Primarily dopaminergic effects (increased renal blood flow) at 1–5 μg/kg/min. Primarily α- and β-adrenergic effects at ≥ 10 μg/kg/min.
Metabolism	Kidney, liver
Elimination	Kidney

Droperidol (Inapsine)

Indications	Nausea, vomiting, agitation, sedation, adjunct to neuroleptanesthesia
Dosage	0.625–10.0 mg IV prn (dosage individualized)
Onset	3–10 min
Duration	3–6 hr (30 min to peak effect)
Effect	Apparent psychic indifference to environment, catatonia, antipsychotic effect, antiemetic effect.
Comments	May cause inner anxiety, extrapyramidal reactions, or hypotension (from moderate α-adrenergic and dopaminergic antagonism). Residual effects may persist ≥ 24 hr.
Metabolism	Liver
Elimination	Kidney, liver (10% unchanged)

Enalapril/Enalaprilat (Vasotec)

Indications	Hypertension, congestive heart failure
Dosage	PO: LD: 2.5–5.0 mg qd MD: 10–40 mg qd IV:0.625–5.0 mg q6h
Onset	PO: 1 hr IV: 15 min
Duration	PO: 24 hr (4–6 hr to peak effect) IV: 6 hr (1–4 hr to peak effect)
Effect	Angiotensin-converting enzyme inhibitor; synergistic with diuretics.
Comments	Causes increased serum potassium, increased renal blood flow, volume-responsive hypotension. Subsequent doses are additive in effect. May cause angioedema, blood dyscrasia, lithium toxicity, or worsening of renal impairment.
Metabolism	Liver
Elimination	Kidney (90% unchanged)

Ephedrine

Indication	Hypotension
Dosage	5–50 mg IV q3–4h prn
Onset	Rapid
Duration	1 hr
Effect	α- and β-adrenergic stimulation; induction of norepinephrine release at nerve endings.
Comments	May cause hypertension, arrhythmias, myocardial ischemia, CNS stimulation, decrease in uterine activity or mild bronchodilation. Minimal effect on uterine blood flow.
Metabolism	Liver
Elimination	Kidney (60–75% unchanged)

Epinephrine (adrenaline)

Indications	Heart failure, hypotension, bronchospasm, anaphylaxis, cardiac arrest

Dosage	Infusion mix: 1 mg in 250 ml of 5% D/W or NSS
	For bronchospasm:
	    IV: infusion initially at 0.5 µg/min, then titrated against patient response
	    SQ/IM: 1 : 1000 solution (1.0 mg/ml), 0.1–0.5 ml q10–15 min × 3 prn
	For cardiac arrest: 1–10 ml of 1 : 1000 solution IV (1.0 mg/ml)
	Pediatric (for cardiac arrest):
	    IV: 1 : 10,000 solution, 0.1 ml/kg
	    SQ/IM: 1 : 1000 solution, 0.01 ml/kg/dose q15 min × 3 prn

Onset	IV: Rapid SQ: 3–5 min
Duration	IV: 10 min
Effect	α- and β-adrenergic agonist.
Comments	May cause hypertension, arrhythmias, or myocardial ischemia. With local anesthesia, causes vasoconstriction. Crosses placenta.
Metabolism	Liver, nerve endings
Elimination	Kidney, liver (10%)

Epinephrine, racemic (Vaponefrin)

Indications	Airway edema, bronchospasm
Dosage	Inhaled via nebulizer: 0.5 ml of 2.25% solution in 2.5–3.5 ml of NSS q1–4h prn

Pediatric: Inhaled via nebulizer: 0.5 ml of 2.25% solution in 2.5–3.5 ml of NSS q4h prn

Onset	1–5 min
Duration	2–3 hr
Effect	Mucosal vasoconstriction. See also Epinephrine.
Comments	See Epinephrine.
Metabolism/ Elimination	See Epinephrine.

Ergonovine (Ergotrate)

Indication	Postpartum hemorrhage
Dosage	For postpartum hemorrhage: IV (emergency only): 0.2 mg in 5 ml of NSS over ≥ 1 min IM: 0.2 mg q2–4h prn for ≤ 5 doses; then PO: 0.2–0.4 mg q6–12h × 2 days or prn
Onset	IV: Rapid IM: 2–5 min PO: 5–15 min
Duration	IM/PO: 3 hr
Effect	Constriction of uterine and vascular smooth muscle.
Comments	May cause hypertension from systemic vasoconstriction (especially in eclampsia and hypertension), arrhythmias, coronary spasm, uterine tetany, or gastrointestinal upset. IV route is *only* used in emergencies. Overdosage may cause convulsions or stroke.
Metabolism	Probably liver

Erythromycin

Indications	Treatment of community-acquired pneumonia (e.g., *Legionella, Mycoplasma*), *Chlamydia*, gram-positive cocci, gram-negative rods, spirochetes
Dosage	0.5–1.0 gm IV q6h
Onset	Rapid
Duration	6 hr
Effect	Interferes with microbial RNA translation.
Comments	Bacteriostatic. Gastritis common when given PO.
Metabolism	Liver, kidney
Elimination	Kidney (negligible)

Esmolol (Brevibloc)

Indications	Treatment of tachyarrhythmias, myocardial ischemia
Dosage	Start with 10 mg IV bolus and increase q3min prn to total 100–300 mg; infusion 1–15 mg/min
Onset	Rapid
Duration	3–10 min
Effect	Selective β_1-adrenergic blockade.
Comments	May cause bradycardia, AV conduction delay, hypotension, congestive heart failure; β_2 activity at high doses.
Metabolism	Degraded by RBC esterases
Elimination	Kidney

Ethacrynic acid (Edecrin)

Indications	Edema, hypercalcemia, hypertension
Dosage	0.5–1.0 mg/kg IV (dosage individualized)
Onset	15 min
Duration	2–3 hr
Effect	See Furosemide.
Comments	See Furosemide. Tissue irritant. May potentiate oral anticoagulants. Effective in renal impairment.
Metabolism	Liver
Elimination	Liver (30–40%), kidney (30–65%)

Famotidine (Pepcid)

Indications	Pulmonary aspiration prophylaxis, peptic ulcer disease
Dosage	20 mg IV/PO q12h (dilute in 1–10 ml of 5% D/W or NSS)
Onset	Peak effect within 30 min of administration
Duration	8–12 hr
Effect	Antagonism of histamine action on H_2 receptors.
Comments	May cause confusion.
Metabolism	Kidney
Elimination	Kidney

Flumazenil (Mazicon)

Indication	Reversal of benzodiazepine sedation or overdose
Dosage	For reversal of conscious sedation: 0.2–1.0 mg IV q20min at 0.2 mg/min
	For overdose: 3–5 mg IV at 0.5 mg/min
Onset	1–2 min (6–10 min to peak effect)
Duration	20 min–3 hr
Effect	Competitive inhibition of γ-aminobutyric acid/benzodiazepine receptor in CNS.
Comments	Duration of action dependent on dose and duration of action of administered benzodiazepine and on dose of flumazenil. May induce CNS excitation including seizures, acute withdrawal, nausea, dizziness, agitation.
Metabolism	Liver
Elimination	Liver, kidney

Fluorescein (Fluorescite)

Indication	Assess tissue perfusion
Dosage	10 mg/kg IV rapidly
Onset	Rapid
Duration	Several hours
Effect	Uptake by viable cells only.
Comments	May cause nausea, vomiting, false hemoglobin elevation, or hypersensitivity reactions (with slow infusion).
Metabolism	Minimal
Elimination	Kidney, liver

Furosemide (Lasix)

Indications	Edema, hypertension, intracranial hypertension, renal failure, hypercalcemia
Dosage	2–40 mg IV (initial dose; dosage individualized)
Onset	2–10 min
Duration	2 hr
Effect	Increase in excretion of Na^+, Cl^-, K^+, PO_4^{3-}, Ca^{2+}, and H_2O.
Comments	May cause electrolyte imbalance, dehydration, transient hypotension, deafness, hyperglycemia, or hyperuricemia. Sulfa-allergic patients may exhibit hypersensitivity to furosemide.
Metabolism	Minimal
Elimination	Liver, kidney (mostly)

Gentamicin

Indications	Treatment of infection from gram-negative and gram-positive aerobes (including methicillin-resistant *Staphylococcus aureus*).
Dosage	60–120 mg IV q8–12 h (3–5 mg/kg/day in divided doses q8h); mix in 10–250 ml of 5% D/W or NSS and administer over 15–20 min.
Onset	Rapid
Duration	Variable
Effect	Interferes with bacterial protein synthesis.
Comments	Synergistic with penicillin except in renal failure. Decrease dosage in the presence of renal disease. May cause renal damage, deafness. Precipitates with heparin. May cause or prolong neuromuscular blockade especially following bolus administration, requiring neostigmine or calcium gluconate for reversal. Use with caution in patients with myasthenia gravis, parkinsonism, botulism.
Elimination	Kidney, liver

Glucagon

Indications	Duodenal or choledocal relaxation, hypoglycemia
Dosage	For gastrointestinal relaxation: 0.25–0.5 mg IV q20min prn For hypoglycemia: 0.5–1.00 mg IV q20min For gastrointestinal relaxation: 1 min IV
Onset	For hypoglycemia: 5–10 min (30 min to peak effect)
Duration	For gastrointestinal relaxation: 10–30 min (dose dependent) For hypoglycemia: 1–2 hr
Effect	Gastrointestinal tract relaxation, catecholamine release.
Comments	May cause anaphylaxis, nausea, vomiting, hyperglycemia, or positive inotropic and chronotropic effects. High doses potentiate oral anticoagulants. Use with caution in presence of insulinoma or pheochromocytoma.
Metabolism	Liver, kidney

Glycopyrrolate (Robinul)

Indications	Bradycardia, decreasing gastrointestinal motility, antisialagogue
Dosage	For drying secretions: IV/IM/SQ: 0.1–0.2 mg PO: 1–2 mg For Bradycardia: 0.1–0.2 mg/dose IV *Pediatric:* 0.004–0.008 mg/kg IV/IM up to 0.1 mg
Onset	IV: 1–4 min IM: 30–45 min.
Duration	IV: 2–4 hr IM: 2–7 hr
Effect	See Atropine.
Comments	See Atropine. Doses do *not* cross blood-brain barrier or placenta. Better antisialagogue with less chronotropy than atropine.
Metabolism	Minimal
Elimination	Kidney

Haloperidol (Haldol)*

Indications	Psychosis, agitation
Dosage	1–2 mg IV prn (dosage individualized)
Onset	10–15 min
Duration	≤ 3 days
Effect	Antipsychotic effects due to dopamine receptor antagonism. CNS depression.
Comments	May cause extrapyramidal reactions or very mild α-adrenergic antagonism. Antiemetic effect. May precipitate neuroleptic malignant syndrome.
Metabolism	Liver
Elimination	Liver, kidney

Heparin (Lipo-Hepin, Liquaemin Sodium, Panheprin)

Indication	Anticoagulation
Dosage	For thromboembolism: LD: 5000 units IV. MD: 500–1000 units/hr IV or 5000–10,000 units IV q4–6h. Titrate dosage against partial thromboplastin time or activated clotting time. For cardiopulmonary bypass:

LD: 300 units/kg IV.
MD: 100 units/kg/hr IV. Titrate against activated clotting time or heparin level.

Onset	Immediate
Duration	2–6 hr; $t_{1/2}$ = 1–2 hr (dose dependent)
Effect	Blockade of conversion of prothrombin and activation of other coagulation factors. Decrease in platelet agglutination.
Comments	May cause bleeding, acute reversible thrombocytopenia, allergic reactions, or diuresis (36–48 hr after a large dose). Half-life increased in renal failure and decreased in thromboembolism and liver disease. Does not cross placenta.
Metabolism	Liver
Elimination	Kidney

Hydralazine (Apresoline)

Indication	Hypertension
Dosage	2.5–20.0 mg IV q4h or prn (dosage individualized)
Onset	5–20 min
Duration	2–6 hr; peak effect in 10–80 min
Effect	Relaxation of vascular smooth muscle (arteriole > venule)
Comments	May cause hypotension, reflex tachycardia, systemic lupus erythematosus syndrome, or Coombs'-positive hemolytic anemia. Increases coronary, splanchnic, cerebral, and renal blood flows.
Metabolism	Liver
Elimination	Kidney

Hydrocortisone (SoluCortef)

Indications	Adrenal insufficiency, inflammation and allergy, septic shock, CNS tumors, asthma
Dosage	For non-life-threatening conditions: 50–200 mg IV q2–10h prn For life-threatening conditions: 50 mg/kg IV over several minutes q4–24h not longer than 2–3 days
Onset	60 minutes
Duration	6–8 hr
Effect	Stimulation of gluconeogenesis. Inhibition of peripheral protein synthesis. Membrane stabiliz-

	ing effect. Anti-inflammatory and antiallergic effect. Mineralocorticoid effect.
Comments	May cause adrenocortical insufficiency (Addison's crisis with abrupt withdrawal), delayed wound healing, CNS disturbances, osteoporosis, or electrolyte disturbances.
Metabolism	Liver (reductase)
Elimination	Kidney

Hydroxyzine (Vistaril, Atarax)*

Indications	Anxiety, nausea and vomiting, allergies, sedation
Dosage	IM: 25–100 mg q4–6h PO: 25–200 mg q6–8h *Not* an IV drug
Onset	PO: 15–20 min
Duration	PO: 4–6 hr
Effect	Antagonism of histamine action on H_1 receptors; CNS depression; antiemetic effect.
Comments	May cause dry mouth. Minimal cardiorespiratory depression. IV injection may cause thrombosis. Crosses placenta.
Metabolism	Liver
Elimination	Liver, kidney

Indigo carmine

Indications	Evaluation of urine output. Localization of ureteral orifices during cystoscopy.
Dosage	40 mg IV slowly (5 ml of 0.8% solution)
Onset	10–30 min
Duration	Several hours
Effect	Turns urine blue.
Comments	Hypertension from α-adrenergic stimulation (for about 15–30 min after IV dose).
Metabolism	Minimal
Elimination	Kidney

Indocyanine green (Cardio-Green)

Indication	Cardiac output measurement by indicator dye dilution
Dosage	5 mg IV (diluted in 1 ml of normal saline) rapidly injected into central circulation
Onset	Immediate
Duration	Minutes
Effect	Almost complete binding to plasma protein, with distribution within plasma volume.
Comments	May cause allergic reactions or transient increase in bilirubin. Absorption spectra changed by heparin. Cautious use in patients with iodine allergy (contains 5% sodium iodide).
Metabolism	Minimal
Elimination	Liver

Insulin

Indications	Hyperglycemia, hyperkalemia
Dosage	For hyperglycemia (dosage highly individualized): usually 5–10 units IV/SQ prn (regular insulin) For uncontrolled diabetes: LD: 10–20 units IV (regular insulin) MD: 0.05–0.1 units/kg/hr IV (regular insulin), titrated against plasma glucose level
Onset	SQ: Regular: 30 min Semilente: 30 min NPH: 1–2 hr Lente: 1–4 hr PZI: 4–6 hr Ultralente: 4–6 hr
Duration	SQ: Regular 5–7 hr Semilente: 12–16 hr NPH: 18–24 hr Lente: 18–28 hr PZI: 24–36 hr Ultralente: 30–36 hr
Effect	Facilitation of glucose transport into cells. Shift of $K+$ and Mg^{2+} into cells.
Comments	May cause hypoglycemia, allergic reactions, or synthesis of insulin antibodies. May be absorbed by plastic in IV tubing. When initiating insulin therapy, use Humulin rather than beef or pork insulin to minimize the development of antibodies.

Metabolism	Liver
Elimination	Kidney (<10%)

Isoetharine (Bronkosol, Bronkometer)

Indication	Bronchospasm
Dosage	Inhaled (aerosol or intermittent positive-pressure breathing): 0.25–0.5 ml of 0.5–1.0% solution diluted in 1.5–2.5 ml of NSS given over 15–30 min q4h prn
	Inhaled (metered nebulizer [Bronkometer]): 1–2 puffs (0.34 mg/puff) with 1 min between puffs q4h prn
Onset	5 min
Duration	1–4 hr
Effect	β-Adrenergic stimulation (β_1, β_2), resulting in bronchodilation.
Comments	May cause tachycardia, hypertension, peripheral vascular vasodilation, CNS stimulation, or bronchial irritation. Contains sulfite. Tachyphylaxis and paradoxic bronchospasm can occur with excessive use.
Metabolism	Lung, liver
Elimination	Kidney (10% unchanged)

Isoproterenol (Isuprel)

Indications	Heart failure, heart block, bronchospasm, pulmonary hypertension, β-blocker overdose
Dosage	Infusion mix: 1 mg in 250 ml of 5% D/W or NSS
	IV: Infusion initially at 1 µg/min, then titrated against patient response
	Inhaled (aerosol or intermittent positive-pressure breathing: 0.5 ml of 0.5% solution in 1.5–2.5 ml of NSS over 15–20 min q5h prn
Onset	IV: rapid
	inhaled: 2–5 min
Duration	IV: 1–5 min
	Inhaled: 1–3 hr
Effect	β-Adrenergic agonist
Comments	May cause arrhythmias, myocardial ischemia, hypertension, or CNS excitation. Tachyphylaxis after repeated inhaled doses.
Metabolism	Liver, nerve endings
Elimination	Kidney, liver

Isordil (Isosorbide dinitrate)

Indications	Angina, hypertension, myocardial infarction, congestive heart failure
Dosage	5–20 mg PO q6h
Onset	15–40 min
Duration	4–6 hr; $t_{1/2}$ = 4 hr
Effect	See nitroglycerin
Comments	See nitroglycerin. Tolerance may develop.
Metabolism	Liver
Elimination	Renal

Ketorolac (Toradol)

Indications	Nonopioid, nonsteroidal analgesic for moderate pain. Useful adjunct for severe pain when combined with parenteral or epidural opioids.
Dosage	IM/IV/PO: 30–60 mg, then 15–30 mg q6h PO: 10 mg q4–6h
Onset	10 min
Duration	Variable; $t_{1/2}$ = 4–8 hr
Effect	Inhibits prostaglandin synthesis through an effect on cyclo-oxygenase.
Comments	Potentiates the effect of opioids. Adverse effects are similar to those with other nonsteroidal anti-inflammatory drugs and include peptic ulceration.
Metabolism	Liver
Elimination	Liver, kidney

Labetalol (Normodyne, Trandate)

Indications	Hypertension (including hypertensive crisis); combined α- and β-adrenergic blockade during induced hypotension
Dosage	IV: 5 to 10-mg increments at 5-min intervals, to a total dose of 40–80 mg Infusion: 5 mg/ml mix; start at 0.05 μ/kg/min
Onset	IV: 5 min
Duration	IV: 2–12 hr (5–10 min to peak effect)
Effect	Selective α_1-adrenergic blockade with nonselective β-adrenergic blockade. Ratio of α/β blockade = 1:7.
Comments	May cause bradycardia, AV conduction delays,

bronchospasm in asthmatics, and postural hypotension. Crosses placenta.

| Metabolism | Liver |
| Elimination | Kidney, liver (5%) |

Lidocaine (Xylocaine)

Indications	Ventricular arrhythmias, local/topical anesthesia, adjunct to general anesthesia, cough suppression
Dosage	For arrhythmias: LD: 1 mg/kg IV × 2 (2nd dose 20–30 min after 1st dose) MD: 15–50 μg/kg/min IV (1–4 mg/min)
Onset	10–90 sec
Duration	5–20 min
Effect	Antiarrhythmic effect; sedation; neural blockade.
Comments	May cause dizziness, seizures, disorientation, heart block (with myocardial conduction defect), or hypotension. Crosses placenta. Therapeutic level = 1–5 mg/L. Avoid in patients with Wolff-Parkinson-White syndrome.
Metabolism	Liver
Elimination	Kidney (10% unchanged)

Magnesium sulfate

Indications	Eclampsia, preeclampsia, hypomagnesemia
Dosage	LD: 1–4 gm IV (10 or 20% solution) Infusion: 1–3 ml/min (4 gm/250 ml of 5% D/W or NSS)
Onset	IV: Rapid
Duration	IV: 30 min
Effect	To replete serum magnesium level. For the treatment of seizures associated with eclampsia.
Comments	Potentiates neuromuscular blockade (both depolarizing and nondepolarizing agents). Potentiates CNS effects of anesthetics, hypnotics, and opioids. Toxicity occurs with serum levels ≥ 10 mEq/L. Avoid in patients with heart block; caution in patients with renal failure.
Metabolism	Kidney
Elimination	Kidney

Mannitol (Osmitrol)

Indications	Intracranial hypertension, neurosurgery, prophylaxis/treatment of renal failure, glaucoma, diuresis
Dosage	0.25–1.0 gm/kg IV as 20% solution over 30–60 min (in acute situation, can give bolus of 1.25–25.0 gm over 5–10 min)
Onset	15 min
Duration	2–3 hr
Effect	Increase in serum osmolality resulting in decrease in brain size and amount of intraocular fluid, osmotic diuresis, and transient expansion of intravascular volume.
Comments	Rapid administration may cause vasodilation and hypotension. May worsen or cause pulmonary edema, intracranial hemorrhage, systemic hypertension, or rebound intracranial hypertension. Hyponatremia common.
Metabolism	Minimal
Elimination	Kidney (80% unchanged)

Metaproterenol (Alupent)

Indication	Bronchospasm
Dosage	Inhaled (metered aerosol): 2–3 puffs (0.65 mg/puff) q3–4h prn (maximum 12 puffs/day) Inhaled intermittent positive-pressure breathing: 0.2–0.3 ml of 5% solution in 2.5 ml of NSS q4h
Onset	2–10 min
Duration	Inhaled: 1–4 hr
Effect	β-Adrenergic stimulation (mostly β_2), resulting in bronchodilation.
Comments	May cause arrhythmias, hypertension, CNS stimulation, nausea, vomiting, or inhibition of uterine contractions. Tachyphylaxis can occur.
Metabolism	Liver
Elimination	Liver, kidney

Methyldopa (Aldomet)

Indication	Hypertension
Dosage	250–1000 mg IV/PO q6h prn (maximum 1 gm q6h)
Onset	IV: 1–2 hr
Duration	IV: 10–16 hr

Effect	May be a false neurotransmitter from central α_2 stimulation, resulting in decrease in mean arterial pressure without increase in heart rate or change in cardiac output. Causes decreased tissue catecholamines.
Comments	May cause sedation, psychosis, depression, hypotension, liver damage, or Coombs'-positive hemolytic anemia. Contains sulfite.
Metabolism	Liver
Elimination	Kidney

Methylene blue (methylthionine chloride, Urolene Blue)

Indications	Urinary tract diagnostic aid, pulmonary aspiration test, methemoglobinemia
Dosage	For diagnostic aid: 100 mg (10 ml of 1% solution) For methemoglobinemia: 1–2 mg/kg IV as 1% solution over 10 min, repeated in 1 hr prn
Onset	Immediate
Effect	Low dose promotes conversion of methemoglobin to hemoglobin. High dose promotes conversion of hemoglobin to methemoglobin. Less useful than sodium nitrate and amyl nitrite.
Comments	May cause RBC destruction (prolonged use), hypertension, bladder irritation, nausea, diaphoresis. May inhibit nitrate-induced coronary artery relaxation. Interferes with pulse oximetry for 1–2 min. Useful in patients with glucose 6 phosphate dehydrogenase deficiency.
Metabolism	Tissues
Elimination	Liver, kidney (75% unchanged)

Methylergonovine (Methergine)

Indication	Postpartum hemorrhage
Dosage	IV (emergency only): 0.2 mg in 5 ml of NSS/dose over $\geq$ 1 min IM: 0.2 mg q2–4h prn (< 5 doses) PO (after IM or IV doses): 0.2–0.4 mg q6–12h × 2–7 days
Onset	IV: immediate IM: 2–5 min PO: 5–10 min
Duration	IV/IM: 3 hr
Effect	See Ergonovine.
Comments	See Ergonovine. Hypertensive response less

marked than with ergonovine. IV route is *only* used in emergencies.

Metabolism   Liver, kidney

Methylprednisolone (Solu-Medrol)

Indications	See Hydrocortisone.
Dosage	For non-life-threatening conditions: 10–250 mg IV q4–24h (IV given over 1 min) For life-threatening conditions: 100–250 mg IV q2–6h or 30 mg/kg IV q4–6h for 24–48 hr (given over 15 min) prn
Onset	Minutes
Duration	6 hr
Effect	See Hydrocortisone; has 5 times the glucocorticoid potency of hydrocortisone. Almost no mineralocorticoid activity.
Comments	See Hydrocortisone.
Metabolism	Liver (microsomes)
Elimination	Kidney

Metoclopramide (Reglan)

Indications	Gastroesophageal reflux, diabetic gastroparesis, premedication for patients needing pulmonary aspiration prophylaxis, antiemetic.
Dosage	IV: 10 mg PO: 10 mg
Onset	IV: 1–3 min PO: 30–60 min to peak effect
Duration	IV, PO: 1–2 hr
Effect	Increases gastric and small intestinal motility (which improves emptying) and lower esophageal sphincter tone.
Comments	Rarely may produce extrapyramidal reactions. May exacerbate depression. Dopamine antagonist. Avoid in patients with pheochromocytoma.
Metabolism	Liver
Elimination	Kidney

Metoprolol (Lopressor)

Indications	Hypertension, angina pectoris
Dosage	50–100 mg PO q6–12h
Onset	15 min
Duration	6 hr
Effect	β_1-Adrenergic blockade (β_2-adrenergic antagonism at high doses).
Comments	May cause bradycardia, clinically significant bronchoconstriction (with doses > 100 mg/day), dizziness, fatigue, insomnia. May increase heart block. Crosses placenta and blood-brain barrier.
Metabolism	Liver
Elimination	Kidney

Metronidazole (Flagyl)

Indications	Treatment of infection with anaerobes, some gastrointestinal parasites, *Giardia, Trichomonas*
Dosage	500 mg IV q6h, infused over 10–20 min
Onset	Rapid
Duration	Variable
Effect	Inactivation of bacterial DNA.
Comments	May cause elevation of liver function tests. May cause disulfiram-like reaction, mild leukopenia, convulsions; acute toxic psychosis may occur with coadministration of disulfiram.
Metabolism	Liver (negligible)
Elimination	Kidney, liver

Nadolol (Corgard)

Indications	Angina pectoris, hypertension
Dosage	40–320 mg/day PO
Onset	1–2 hr
Duration	> 24 hr
Effect	Nonselective β-adrenergic blockade.
Comments	May cause severe bronchospasm. (See propranolol.)
Elimination	Kidney (unchanged)

Naloxone (Narcan)

Indications	Reversal of systemic narcotic effects
Dosage	For postoperative narcosis: 0.04- to 0.4-mg doses IV, titrated against patient response q2–3 min *Pediatric:* For postoperative narcosis: 1–10 µg/kg (in increments) IV q2–3 min (up to 0.4 mg), titrated against patient response
Onset	1–2 min
Duration	< 1 hr
Effect	Antagonism of narcotic effects.
Comments	May cause reversal of analgesia, hypertension, arrhythmias, rare pulmonary edema, delirium, or withdrawal syndrome (in narcotic tolerant patients).
Metabolism	Liver
Elimination	Kidney

Nifedipine (Procardia)

Indications	Coronary artery spasm, hypertension, myocardial ischemia
Dosage	PO: 10–40 mg tid SL: 10–20 mg (extracted from capsule)
Onset	PO: 15–20 min SL: 1–5 min
Duration	PO: 6 hr SL: 1–2 hr (30 min to peak effect)
Effect	Blockade of slow calcium channels in heart. Systemic and coronary vasodilation and increase in myocardial perfusion.
Comments	May cause reflex tachycardia, gastrointestinal upset, or mild negative inotropic effects. Little effect on automaticity and atrial conduction. May be useful in asymmetric septal hypertrophy. Drug solution is light sensitive.
Metabolism	Liver
Elimination	Liver, kidney

Nitrite, sodium

Indication	Cyanide poisoning
Dosage	300 mg IV (10 ml of 3% solution) at 2.5–5.0 ml/min. *Pediatric:* 6 mg/kg IV (0.2 ml/kg) (≤ 300 mg) slowly.

	Adult and pediatric administration: Repeat ½ dose 2–48 hr later prn; follow immediately with sodium thiosulfate.
Effect	Formation of methemoglobin, which can then bind with cyanide to form cyanmethemoglobin.
Comments	Give amyl nitrite inhalant, 0.3 ml/min, until sodium nitrite infusion is available. May cause hypotension. May decrease oxygen-carrying capacity of hemoglobin by formation of methemoglobin.

Nitroglycerin (glycerol trinitrate, Nitrostat, Nitrol)

Indications	Myocardial ischemia, hypertension, congestive heart failure, pulmonary hypertension, esophageal spasm, biliary colic
Dosage	Infusion mix: 30–50 mg in 250 ml of 5% D/W or NSS IV: infusion initially at 10 μg/min, then titrated against patient response SL: 0.15–0.6 mg/dose Topical: 2% ointment, 0.5–5.0 inches q4–8h
Onset	IV: 1–2 min SL: 1–3 min PO: 1 hr Topical: 30–60 min
Duration	IV: 10 min SL: 30 min PO: 8–12 hr Topical: 3 hr
Effect	Smooth muscle relaxation, resulting in favorable redistribution of coronary blood flow, coronary and pulmonary vasodilatation, bronchodilatation, and biliary, gastrointestinal, and genitourinary tract relaxation.
Comments	May cause reflex tachycardia, hypotension, headache. Tolerance and dependence with chronic use may be avoided with a 10- to 12-hr nitrate-free period. May be absorbed by plastic in IV tubing. May cause methemoglobinemia at very high doses.
Metabolism	Smooth muscle, liver

Nitroprusside (Nipride)

Indications	Hypertension, induction of deliberate hypotension, congestive heart failure, pulmonary hypertension

Dosage	Infusion mix: 50 mg in 250 ml of 5% D/W or NSS IV: infusion initially at 0.1 µg/kg/min, then titrated against patient response to maximum 10 µg/kg/min (total dose < 1.0–1.5 mg/kg over 2–3 hr)
Onset	Rapid
Duration	10 min
Effect	Smooth muscle relaxation. Arterial $>$ venodilator.
Comments	May cause excessive hypotension, reflex tachycardia. Can accumulate cyanide in the presence of liver dysfunction and can accumulate thiocyanate in the presence of renal dysfunction. Prolonged therapy can be associated with increase in plasma cyanide and thiocyanate. Avoid with Leber's hereditary optic atrophy, tobacco amblyopia, severe liver or renal disease, hypothyroidism, or vitamin B_{12} deficiency. May cause tachyphylaxis. Solution and powder are light sensitive and must be wrapped in aluminum foil or other opaque material.
Metabolism	RBC and tissues
Elimination	Kidney, liver (rhodanase)

Norepinephrine (Levarterenol, Levophed)

Indication	Hypotension
Dosage	Infusion mix: 4 mg in 250 ml of 5% D/W or NSS IV: infusion initially at 1–8 µg/min, then titrated against patient response
Onset	Rapid
Duration	1–2 min
Effect	α- and β-adrenergic agonist (mostly α).
Comments	May cause hypertension, arrhythmias, myocardial ischemia, increased uterine contractility, constricted microcirculation, or CNS stimulation.
Metabolism	Liver, nerve endings
Elimination	Kidney

Octreotide (Sandostatin)

Indication	Somatostatin (anti-serotonin) agent used to treat metastatic carcinoid tumors
Dosage	50 µg IV/SQ prn
Onset	IV: minutes

Duration	IV: up to 12 hr
Effect	A long-acting octapeptide somatostatin analogue. It suppresses secretion of serotonin, gastrin, vasoactive intestinal peptide, insulin, glucagon, and secretin. It is used to treat the symptoms associated with metastatic carcinoid tumors (flushing, bronchospasm, hypotension).
Comments	Clearance of octreotide is reduced in renal failure. May cause transient hypoglycemia, nausea.
Metabolism	Liver
Elimination	Kidney (32% unchanged)

Omeprazole (Losec, Prilosec)

Indications	Gastric acid hypersecretion or gastritis, gastroesophageal reflux
Dosage	20–40 mg PO qd
Onset	1 hr
Duration	24 hr
Effect	Inhibition of H+ secretion
Comments	Increases secretion of gastrin. More rapid healing of gastric ulcer than with H_2 blockers. Effective in ulcers resistant to H_2 blocker therapy. Inhibits some cytochrome P450 enzymes.
Metabolism	Liver
Elimination	Liver, kidney

Oxytocin (Pitocin, Syntocinon)

Indications	Postpartum hemorrhage, induction of labor
Dosage	Infusion mix: 10–40 units in 1000 ml of crystalloid
	For postpartum hemorrhage: IV infusion at rate necessary to control atony (e.g., 0.02–0.04 units/min)
Onset	< 1 min
Duration	< 60 min
Effect	Oxytocic effects, e.g., uterine contraction, milk release. Renal, coronary, and cerebral vasodilation. Reduction of postpartum blood loss.
Comments	May cause uterine tetany and rupture, fetal distress, or anaphylaxis. IV bolus can cause hypotension, tachycardia, arrhythmia.
Metabolism	Liver, kidney, mammary glands
Elimination	Kidney (small amount)

Penicillin G

Indication	Treatment of infection with gram-positive cocci
Dosage	500,000–1,000,000 units IV q4h up to 2,000,000 units q4h for meningitis; mix in 10–250 ml of 5% D/W or NSS and administer over 1–5 min.
Onset	Rapid
Duration	Variable
Effect	Interferes with bacterial cell wall formation; bacteriostatic.
Comments	Not useful for β-lactamase-producing organisms. May induce seizures at high doses. May induce interstitial nephritis. Moderate reduction in dosage required in renal failure. Synergistic with gentamicin except in renal failure. Antisynergistic with tetracycline.
Metabolism	Negligible
Elimination	Kidney, liver

Phenobarbital

Indications	Anticonvulsant, sedative/hypnotic

Dosage	As hypnotic:
	  PO: 100–300 mg
	  IV: 50–150 mg
	As anticonvulsant:
	  PO: 50–100 mg tid
	  IV: 200–300 mg initially, repeated in 6 hr (maximum 1–2 gm/24 hr)
	Pediatric:
	  As hypnotic: 1–3 mg/kg PO
	  As anticonvulsant:
	    IV: 15–50 mg bid–tid
	    Rectal: 2 mg/kg tid

Onset	IV: 5 min
Duration	8–12 hr; maximum CNS depression 15 min after IV dose
Effect	All barbiturates are CNS and respiratory depressants.
Comments	May cause hypotension. Multiple drug interactions through induction of hepatic enzyme systems.
Metabolism	Liver
Elimination	Kidney

Phenoxybenzamine (Dibenzyline)

Indication	Hypertension from catecholamine excess as with pheochromocytoma
Dosage	10–200 mg/day PO (start at 10 mg/day and increase dosage by 10 mg/day every 4 days prn)
Onset	2 hr
Duration	3–4 days
Effect	Noncompetitive α-adrenergic antagonism.
Comments	May cause orthostatic hypotension (which may be refractory to norepinephrine) or tachycardia, stuffy nose.
Metabolism	Liver
Elimination	Liver, kidney

Phentolamine (Regitine)

Indications	Hypertension from catecholamine excess as in pheochromocytoma, extravasation of α-agonist.
Dosage	For catecholamine excess states: IV: 1–5 mg prn for hypertension IV: 2–5 mg, 1–2 hr preoperatively PO: 50 mg q6–8h For extravasation of α-agonist: 5–10 mg in 10 ml of NSS into affected area within 12 hr
Onset	IV: 1–2 min
Duration	IV: 5–10 min
Effect	Competitive α_1- and α_2-adrenergic antagonism, resulting in vasodilatation.
Comments	May cause hypotension, reflex tachycardia, arrhythmias, stimulation of gastrointestinal tract, or hypoglycemia.
Metabolism	Unknown
Elimination	Renal (10%)

Phenylephrine (Neo-Synephrine)

Indication	Hypotension
Dosage	Infusion mix: 10–30 mg in 250 ml of 5% D/W or NSS IV: infusion initially at 10 μg/min, then titrated against patient response IV bolus: 40–100 μg/dose
Onset	Rapid
Duration	15–20 min.

Effect	α-Adrenergic agonist.
Comments	May cause hypertension, reflex bradycardia, constricted microcirculation, uterine contraction, or uterine vasoconstriction.
Metabolism	Liver, intestine

Phenytoin (diphenylhydantoin, Dilantin)

Indications	Seizures, digoxin-induced arrhythmias, refractory ventricular tachycardia, neuralgia
Dosage	For seizures: LD of 10–15 mg/kg IV at < 50 mg/min (up to 1000 mg cautiously, with ECG monitoring)
	For neurosurgical prophylaxis: 100–200 mg IV q4h (IV < 50 mg/min)
	For arrhythmias: 50–100 mg IV at < 50 mg/min q10–15 min until arrhythmia is abolished, side effects occur, or 10–15 mg/kg is given
Onset	3–5 min
Duration	Variable; $t_{1/2}$ = 22 hr
Effect	Anticonvulsant effect. Antiarrhythmic effects similar to those of quinidine or procainamide.
Comments	May cause nystagmus, diplopia, ataxia, drowsiness, gingival hyperplasia, gastrointestinal upset, hyperglycemia, or hepatic microsomal enzyme induction. IV bolus may cause bradycardia, hypotension, respiratory arrest, cardiac arrest, CNS depression. Tissue irritant. Crosses placenta. Significant interpatient variation in dose needed to achieve therapeutic level = 7.5–20.0 µg/ml).
Metabolism	Liver
Elimination	Kidney (< 2% unchanged)

Physostigmine (Antilirium)

Indications	Postoperative delirium, tricyclic antidepressant overdose, reversal of CNS effects of anticholinergic drugs
Dosage	For postoperative delirium: 0.5–2.0 mg IV q15min prn
Onset	3–8 min
Duration	1–2 hr
Effect	Inhibition of cholinesterase, resulting in central and peripheral cholinergic effects.
Comments	May cause bradycardia, tremor, convulsions, hallucinations, psychiatric or CNS depression,

mild ganglionic blockade, or cholinergic crisis. Crosses blood-brain barrier. Antagonized by atropine. Contains sulfite.

Metabolism	Acetylcholinesterase
Elimination	Kidney

Phytonadione (AquaMEPHYTON)

Indication	Deficiency of vitamin K–dependent clotting factors
Dosage	IV: 2.5–25.0 mg at ≤ 1 mg/min. IM/SQ/PO: 2.5–25.0 mg; if 8 hr after IV/IM/SQ dose, prothrombin time is not improved, repeat dose prn.
Onset	IV: 15 min IM: 1–2 hr PO: 6–12 hr
Duration	IV/IM: normal prothrombin time in 12–14 hr
Effect	Promotion of synthesis of clotting factors II, VII, IX, X.
Comments	Excessive dose can make patient refractory to further oral anticoagulation. May fail with hepatocellular disease. IV administration (especially if rapid) occasionally causes hypotension, fever, diaphoresis, bronchospasm, anaphylaxis, or pain at injection site. Crosses placenta.
Metabolism	Liver

Potassium (KCl)

Indication	Severe perioperative hypokalemia
Dosage	20 mEq of KCl may be mixed with NSS in a volumetric burette of 100-ml capacity and administered IV over 30–60 min. A central venous line is preferable for administration.
Onset	Immediate
Duration	Variable
Effect	To correct severe hypokalemia ($K^+ < 2.6$ mEq/L).
Comments	Bolus administration may cause cardiac arrest.

Procainamide (Pronestyl)

Indications	Atrial and ventricular arrhythmias
Dosage	LD: 10–50 mg/min IV until toxicity or desired effect occurs up to 12 mg/kg. Stop if $\geq$ 50% QRS widening or PR lengthening occurs. MD: infusion at 2 mg/kg/hr.
Onset	Immediate
Duration	3 hr (prolonged in renal failure)
Effect	Antiarrhythmic effect.
Comments	May cause increased ventricular response in atrial tachyarrhythmias unless predigitalized, asystole (with AV block), myocardial depression, CNS excitement, blood dyscrasia, systemic lupus erythematosus syndrome, or liver damage. IV administration can cause QRS widening and PR prolongation on the ECG or hypotension from vasodilation. Decrease LD by one-third in congestive heart failure or shock. Hypotensive response may be accentuated with general anesthesia. Therapeutic level = 4–8 mg/L. Contains sulfite.
Metabolism	Liver, plasma (to active metabolite N = acetyl-procainamide)
Elimination	Kidney

Prochlorperazine (Compazine)

Indications	Nausea and vomiting
Dosage	5–10 mg/dose IV ($\leq$ 40 mg/day); 5–10 mg IM q2–4h prn; 25 mg PR q12h prn
Onset	Rapid
Duration	3–4 hr
Effect	Similar to chlorpromazine, with more antiemetic and fewer sedative effects. H_1 blocker.
Comments	May cause hypotension (especially when given IV), extrapyramidal reactions, neuroleptic malignant syndrome, or cholestatic jaundice. Contains sulfites. Caution in liver disease.
Metabolism	Liver
Elimination	Liver, Kidney

Promethazine (Phenergan)

Indications	Allergies, anaphylaxis, nausea and vomiting, sedation
Dosage	12.5–50.0 mg IV q4–6h prn

Onset	3–5 min
Duration	2–4 hr
Effect	Phenothiazine, H_1 antagonist, CNS depression, antiemetic effect.
Comments	May cause mild hypotension or mild anticholinergic effects. May interfere with blood grouping. Relatively free of extrapyramidal effects. Crosses placenta. Contains sulfite. Intraarterial injection can cause gangrene.
Metabolism	Liver
Elimination	Kidney, liver

Propranolol (Inderal)

Indications	Atrial and ventricular arrhythmias, myocardial ischemia, hypertension, hyperthyroidism, hypertrophic cardiomyopathy, migraine headache
Dosage	IV: test dose of 0.25–0.5 mg, then 1–5 mg/dose at $\leq$ 1 mg/min titrated against response PO: 10–40 mg q6–8 h, increased prn *Pediatric:* 0.05–0.1 mg/kg IV over 10 min
Onset	IV: 2 min PO: 30 min
Duration	IV: 1–6 hr PO: 6 hr (90 min to peak effect when given PO)
Effect	Nonspecific β-adrenergic blockade
Comments	May cause bradycardia, AV dissociation, bronchospasm (unusual in low doses), drowsiness (in high doses), hypoglycemia, or, congestive heart failure (unusual in low doses). Crosses placenta and blood-brain barrier. Abrupt withdrawal can precipitate rebound angina.
Metabolism	Liver
Elimination	Kidney, liver

Prostaglandin E₁ (Alprostadil, Prostin VR)

Indications	Pulmonary vasodilator, maintenance of patent ductus arteriosus
Dosage	Starting dose 0.1 μg/kg/min; mix 1–5 mg/250 ml of NSS or 5% D/W
Onset	Immediate
Duration	60 min
Effect	Prostaglandin E_1 will cause vasodilation, inhibition of platelet aggregation, vascular smooth muscle relaxation, uterine and intestinal smooth muscle stimulation.

Comments	May cause hypotension, apnea, flushing, brady-cardia.
Metabolism	Lung
Elimination	Kidney

Protamine

Indication	Reversal of the effects of heparin
Dosage	1 mg/100 units of heparin activity IV at ≤ 5 mg/min
Onset	1 min
Duration	2 hr
Effect	Formation of protamine-heparin complex.
Comments	May cause myocardial depression and peripheral vasodilatation with sudden hypotension or bradycardia. May cause severe pulmonary hypertension, particularly in the setting of cardiopulmonary bypass. Protamine-heparin complex antigenically active. Transient reversal of heparin may be followed by rebound heparinization. Can cause anticoagulation if given in excess relative to amount of circulating heparin (controversial). Monitor response with partial thromboplastin time or activated clotting time.
Metabolism	Blood, liver
Elimination	Kidney

Quinidine gluconate (Quinaglute)

Indications	Atrial and ventricular arrhythmias
Dosage	For acute arrhythmias: 800 mg IV in 50 ml of 5% D/W, giving 300–750 mg at ≤ 16 mg/min (≤ 1 ml/min). Stop IV infusion if 25–50% QRS widening, heart rate < 120, loss of P waves, or arrhythmia is ablated. Avoid IM injection.
Onset	IV: 4–6 min
Duration	PO: 6–8 hr
Effect	Antiarrhythmic effect.
Comments	May cause hypotension (from vasodilation and negative inotropic effects), increased ventricular response in atrial tachyarrhythmias, AV block, QT prolongation, congestive heart failure, mild anticholinergic effects, increase in serum digoxin level, cinchonism, or gastrointestinal upset. May potentiate action of oral anticoagulants. Therapeutic level = 3–6 mg/L.

Metabolism	Liver
Elimination	Kidney (15–40% unchanged)

Ranitidine (Zantac)

Indications	Duodenal and gastric ulcers, reduction of gastric volume and raising of pH, esophageal reflux
Dosage	IV: 50–100 mg q6–8h PO: 150–300 mg q12h
Onset	IV: Rapid PO: 1–3 hr
Duration	IV: 6–8 hr PO: 12 hr (1 hr to peak effect)
Effect	Histamine H_2-receptor antagonist. Inhibits basal, nocturnal, and stimulated gastric acid secretion.
Comments	Doses should be reduced by 50% with renal failure.
Metabolism	Liver
Elimination	Kidney

Ritodrine (Yutopar)

Indication	Premature labor
Dosage	IV (continuous infusion): Mix 150 mg in 5% D/W, infuse 0.10–0.35 mg/min.
Onset	5 min
Duration	2 hr
Effect	β_2-Selective adrenergic receptor agonist that inhibits uterine contractility. Dose-related increases in maternal and fetal heart rate and blood pressure due to β_1 stimulation. Crosses the placenta.
Comments	Pulmonary edema may occur, particularly in patients also given corticosteroids. May cause or increase insulin resistance. Potentiation of cardiovascular effects by magnesium sulfate, potent volatile general anesthetics, parasympatholytics (e.g., atropine). Contains sulfite. Contraindicated in eclampsia, pulmonary hypertension, hyperthyroidism.
Elimination	Kidney (70–90% unchanged)

Scopolamine (hyoscine)*

Indications	Antisialagogue; amnesia, sedation
Dosage	0.3–0.6 mg IV/IM
Onset	IV: 1 min
Duration	Variable
Effect	Anticholinergic effect, CNS depression.
Comments	May cause excitement or delirium, transient tachycardia, hyperthermia, or mild antiemetic effect. Crosses blood-brain barrier and placenta.
Metabolism	Liver
Elimination	Kidney (partly unchanged)

Secretin

Indication	A diagnostic tool in pancreatic disease
Dosage	75 units (10 units/ml) IV dissolved in 7.5 ml of NSS
Onset	Immediate
Duration	2 hr (30 min to peak effect)
Effect	Increases the volume and bicarbonate content of pancreatic juice. Also stimulates gastrin release in patients with gastrinoma (Zollinger-Ellison syndrome).
Comments	Decreased response to secretin occurs in patients after vagotomy, on anticholinergics, or with inflammatory bowel disease.
Metabolism	Liver, blood
Elimination	Kidney

Terbutaline (Brethine, Bricanyl)

Indications	Bronchospasm, premature labor
Dosage	For bronchospasm: 0.25 mg SQ; repeat in 15 min prn (use < 0.5 mg/4 hr); 2.5–5.0 mg q6h PO prn (< 15.0 mg/day) For premature labor: Start at 10 µg/min IV, titrate to a maximum dose of 80 µg/min. *Pediatric:* 3.5–5.0 µg/kg SQ.
Onset	SQ: < 15 min PO: < 30 min
Duration	SQ: 1.5–4.0 hr PO: 4–8 hr
Effect	β-Adrenergic stimulation ($\beta_2 > \beta_1$), resulting in bronchodilation, tocolysis.

Comments	May cause arrhythmias, pulmonary edema, hypertension, hypokalemia, or CNS excitement.
Metabolism	Liver, intestinal wall
Elimination	Kidney

Tetracycline

Indications	Community-acquired pneumonias, *Rickettsia, Chlamydia;* gram-positive and gram-negative aerobes and anaerobes
Dosage	250–500 mg IV: q12h
Onset	Rapid
Duration	12–24 hr; $t_{1/2}$ = 10–18 hr
Effect	Inhibition of protein synthesis; bacteriostatic.
Comments	Many resistant species. Contraindicated in pediatrics, since incorporated into teeth, bone until 3 years of age. Interferes with action of penicillins. Crosses placenta.
Metabolism	Liver, kidney
Elimination	Liver, kidney

Thiosulfate, sodium

Indication	Cyanide poisoning
Dosage	50 ml of a 25% solution infused IV over 10 min; may repeat with 50% of initial dose if signs of cyanide toxicity recur
	Pediatric: 7.5–10.0 gm/m^2 (about 250 mg/kg) (not > 12.5 gm)
Effect	Combines with cyanide to yield thiocyanate.
Comments	Give with amyl nitrite and sodium nitrite.
Elimination	Kidney

Tobramycin

Indications	Treatment of aerobic gram-negative organisms, including *Pseudomonas, Staphylococcus aureus*
Dosage	3–5 mg/kg/day in divided doses q8h; mix in 10–250 ml and administer over 15–20 min.
Onset	Rapid
Duration	Variable (prolonged with renal failure)
Effect	Interferes with bacterial protein synthesis.
Comments	Aminoglycoside, similar to gentamicin.
Elimination	Kidney, liver

Trimethaphan (Arfonad)

Indications	Hypertension, induction of deliberate hypotension
Dosage	Infusion mix: 500 mg in 500 ml of 5% D/W IV: 1–4 mg/min × 5–10 min, then titrated against patient response (usually about 1 mg/min)
Onset	Immediate
Duration	10–15 min (2–10 min to peak effect)
Effect	Ganglionic blockade leading to orthostatic hypotension.
Comments	May cause prolonged hypotension (especially with high doses), bradycardia in elderly, tachycardia in the young. Histamine release, urinary retention, mydriasis, tachyphylaxis. Potentiation of the effects of succinylcholine.
Metabolism	Blood
Elimination	Kidney

Trimethobenzamide (Tigan)

Indications	Nausea and vomiting
Dosage	IM: 200 mg q6–8 prn Rectal: 200 mg q6–8h prn PO: 250 mg q6–8h prn
Onset	IM: 15 min PO: 20–40 min
Duration	IM: 2–3 hr PO: 3–4 hr
Effect	Antiemetic effect.
Comments	May cause hypotension, sedation, extrapyramidal reactions, or mild antihistamine effect.
Metabolism	Liver
Elimination	Kidney, liver

Vancomycin (Vancocin)

Indications	Treatment of infection with gram-positive cocci (including methicillin-resistant *Staphylococcus aureus*) and *Clostridium difficile* colitis.
Dosage	500 mg–1 gm IV over 30–60 min q6–12h
Onset	Rapid
Duration	Variable (prolonged in renal failure); $t_{1/2}$ = 6 hr
Effect	Inhibition of bacterial cell wall formation.

Comments	Effective for β-lactamase-producing gram-positive cocci. Decrease dosage in presence of renal disease. May cause severe histamine release (e.g., "red man syndrome") with rapid administration. Associated with renal damage, deafness. May precipitate with other medications, e.g., chloramphenicol, adrenal corticosteroids, methicillin.
Metabolism	Negligible
Elimination	Kidney, liver

Vasopressin (antidiuretic hormone, Pitressin)

Indications	Diabetes insipidus, gastrointestinal bleeding
Dosage	For diabetes insipidus: 5–10 units IM/SQ q8–12h For gastrointestinal bleeding: 0.1–0.4 units/min IV
Onset	IV: Immediate
Duration	SQ/IM: 2–8 hr (aqueous), 24–42 hr (tannate) IV: 2–8 hr
Effect	Increase in urine osmolality and decrease in urine volume. Smooth muscle contraction, resulting in splanchnic, coronary, muscular, and skin vasoconstriction.
Comments	May cause water intoxication, hypertension, arrhythmias, myocardial ischemia, abdominal cramps (from increased peristalsis), anaphylaxis, gallbladder, urinary bladder, and uterine contraction, pulmonary edema, oliguria, vertigo, or nausea. Patients with coronary artery disease are often treated with concurrent nitroglycerin.
Metabolism	Liver, kidney
Elimination	Kidney

Verapamil (Isoptin, Calan)

Indications	Supraventricular tachycardia, atrial fibrillation or flutter, Wolff-Parkinson-White syndrome, Lown-Ganong-Levine syndrome.
Dosage	2.5–10.0 mg (75–150 μg/kg) IV over ≥ 2-min period. If no response in 30 min, repeat 10 mg (150 μg/kg). *Pediatric:* 0–1 yr: 0.1–0.2 mg/kg IV 1–15 yr: 0.1–0.3 mg/kg IV. Repeat once if no response in 30 min.
Onset	1–10 min

Duration	Hemodynamic effects 10–20 min, AV node effects 2 hr (3–5 min to peak effect)
Effect	Blockade of slow calcium channels in heart. Prolongation of PR and AH intervals with negative inotropy and chronotropy. Systemic and coronary vasodilatation.
Comments	May cause severe bradycardia, AV block (especially with concomitant β-blockade), hypertension, or worsening of congestive heart failure. May increase ventricular response to atrial fibrillation or flutter in patients with accessory tracts.
Metabolism	Liver
Elimination	Liver, kidney

Warfarin (Coumadin, Panwarfin, Athrombin-k)

Indication	Anticoagulation
Dosage	LD: 10–15 mg PO MD: 2–10 mg PO; dosage titrated against prothrombin time
Onset	2–12 hr
Duration	2–5 days (36–72 hr to peak effect)
Effect	Interference with utilization of vitamin K by the liver, thereby inhibiting synthesis of factors II, VII, IX, X.
Comments	May cause bleeding. Crosses placenta. May be potentiated by ethanol, antibiotics, chloral hydrate, cimetidine, dextran, d-thyroxine, diazoxide, ethacrynic acid, glucagon, methyldopa, monoamine oxidase inhibitors, phenytoin, prolonged use of narcotics, quinidine, sulfonamides, congestive heart failure, hyperthermia, liver disease, malabsorption, etc. May be antagonized by barbiturates, chlordiazepoxide, haloperidol, oral contraceptives, hypothyroidism, hyperlipidemia, etc.
Metabolism	Liver
Elimination	Kidney

REFERENCES

American Hospital Formulary Service. *American Hospital Formulary*. Bethesda, MD: American Society of Hospital Pharmacists, 1981.

Behrman, R. E., and Vaughan, V. C., II. *Nelson Textbook of Pediatrics* (14th ed). Philadelphia: Saunders, 1992.

Campbell, J. W., and Frisse, M. (eds). *Manual of Medical Therapeutics* (25th ed.). Boston: Little, Brown, 1983.

DiPalma, J. R. (ed.). *Drill's Pharmacology in Medicine* (4th ed.). New York: McGraw-Hill, 1971.

Gilman, A., et al. (eds.). *The Pharmacological Basis of Therapeutics* (8th ed.). New York: Macmillan, 1990.

Govoni, L. E., and Hayes, J. E. *Drugs and Nursing Implications* (3rd ed.). New York: Appleton-Century-Crofts, 1978.

Graef, J. W., and Cone, T. E., Jr. (eds). *Manual of Pediatric Therapeutics* (3rd ed.). Boston: Little, Brown, 1984.

Jordan, C. D., et al. Normal reference laboratory values. Case records of the Massachusetts General Hospital, *N Engl J Med* 327(10):718, 1992.

Kastrap, E. K. (ed.). *Drug Facts and Comparisons*. St. Louis: Lippincott, 1992.

Osol, A., et al. (eds). *Remington's Pharmaceutical Sciences* (16th ed.). Easton, Pa.: Mack, 1980.

Physicians' Desk Reference (46th ed.). Montvale, N.J.: Medical Economics Company, 1992.

Pribor, H. C., Morrell, G., and Scherr, G. H. *Drug Monitoring and Pharmacokinetic Data*. Park Forest South, Ill.: Pathotex, 1980.

Ritschel, W. A. *Handbook of Basic Pharmacokinetics*. Washington, D.C.: Drug Intelligence Publications, 1976.

Shirkey, H. C. *Pediatric Drug Handbook*. Philadelphia: Saunders, 1977.

United States Pharmacopeial Convention, Inc. *Drug Information for the Health Care Professional. USP Dispensing Information, Vol. IA and IB* (10th ed.). Rockville, MD: United States Pharmacopeial Convention, 1990.

Index

Index

Note: Page numbers followed by f *refer to figures; page numbers followed by* t *refer to tables.*